Radiography: Techniques and Applications

Radiography: Techniques and Applications

Editor: Alberto Ascari

FOSTER ACADEMICS
www.fosteracademics.com

www.fosteracademics.com

FOSTER ACADEMICS

Cataloging-in-Publication Data

Radiography : techniques and applications / edited by Alberto Ascari.
p. cm.
Includes bibliographical references and index.
ISBN 978-1-63242-565-2
1. Radiography, Medical. 2. Radiography, Medical--Digital techniques. 3. Radiography.
I. Ascari, Alberto.
RC78 .R33 2018
616.075 72--dc23

Foster Academics,
118-35 Queens Blvd., Suite 400,
Forest Hills, NY 11375, USA

ISBN 978-1-63242-565-2 (Hardback)

Printed and bound in China.

Contents

Preface

This book has been a concerted effort by a group of academicians, researchers and scientists, who have contributed their research works for the realization of the book. This book has materialized in the wake of emerging advancements and innovations in this field. Therefore, the need of the hour was to compile all the required researches and disseminate the knowledge to a broad spectrum of people comprising of students, researchers and specialists of the field.

Radiology is the technology used for diagnosing various diseases. The radiographs produced during the process are generated by passing X-rays through a patient. Radiology can be divided into medical radiology and industrial radiology. Computed tomography, fluoroscopy, angiography, projectional radiography are some popular forms of medical radiology. While understanding the long-term perspectives of the topics, the book makes an effort in highlighting their impact as a modern tool for the growth of the discipline. It will help the readers in keeping pace with the rapid changes in this field.

At the end of the preface, I would like to thank the authors for their brilliant chapters and the publisher for guiding us all-through the making of the book till its final stage. Also, I would like to thank my family for providing the support and encouragement throughout my academic career and research projects.

Editor

Interactive Ion-Mediated Sap Flow Regulation in Olive and Laurel Stems: Physicochemical Characteristics of Water Transport via the Pit Structure

Jeongeun Ryu[1,2], Sungsook Ahn[1,2], Seung-Gon Kim[1,2¤], TaeJoo Kim[3], Sang Joon Lee[1,2*]

1 Department of Mechanical Engineering, Pohang University of Science and Technology (POSTECH), Pohang, Gyeongbuk, Republic of Korea, 2 Center for Biofluid and Biomimic Research, Pohang University of Science and Technology (POSTECH), Pohang, Gyeongbuk, Republic of Korea, 3 Neutron Science Division, Korea Atomic Energy Research Institute (KAERI), Daejeon, Republic of Korea

Abstract

Sap water is distributed and utilized through xylem conduits, which are vascular networks of inert pipes important for plant survival. Interestingly, plants can actively regulate water transport using ion-mediated responses and adapt to environmental changes. However, ionic effects on active water transport in vascular plants remain unclear. In this report, the interactive ionic effects on sap transport were systematically investigated for the first time by visualizing the uptake process of ionic solutions of different ion compositions (K^+/Ca^{2+}) using synchrotron X-ray and neutron imaging techniques. Ionic solutions with lower K^+/Ca^{2+} ratios induced an increased sap flow rate in stems of *Olea europaea* L. and *Laurus nobilis* L. The different ascent rates of ionic solutions depending on K^+/Ca^{2+} ratios at a fixed total concentration increases our understanding of ion-responsiveness in plants from a physicochemical standpoint. Based on these results, effective structural changes in the pit membrane were observed using varying ionic ratios of K^+/Ca^{2+}. The formation of electrostatically induced hydrodynamic layers and the ion-responsiveness of hydrogel structures based on Hofmeister series increase our understanding of the mechanism of ion-mediated sap flow control in plants.

Editor: Juan Carlos del Alamo, University of California San Diego, United States of America

Funding: This work was supported by PAL through the abroad beam time program of the Synchrotron Radiation Facility Project of the Ministry of Education, Science and Technology (MEST) and performed under the approval of the Photon Factory Program Advisory Committee (Proposal No. 2010G722). This work was also supported by the National Research Foundation of Korea (MRF) grant funded by the Korean government (MSIP) (No. 2008-006991). The funders had no role in study design, data collection and analysis, decision to publish, or preparation of the manuscript.

Competing Interests: The authors have declared that no competing interests exist.

* E-mail: sjlee@postech.ac.kr

¤ Current address: Hydrogen and fuel cell department, Korea Institute of Energy Research (KIER), Daejeon, Republic of Korea

Introduction

Plants transport sap water through specific porous structures and xylem conduits, which are composed of dead cells. Since the geometrical features of xylem conduits are believed to determine hydraulic conductance, xylem water transport is considered a passive process. Nonetheless, plants can pull water above 100 m in height without any mechanical pumps. They have also survived over hundreds or thousands of years by regulating water transport against unfavorable situations such as severe freezing weather and prolonged drought. Interestingly, water transport in plants can be actively modulated through the xylem (a system of inert pipes).

Flow modulation responds to the small molecules and ion concentration in, and pH levels of, the sap water, and the ion-mediated response in vascular plants is considered a major factor in sap flow regulation. The flow rate of tap water is known to be faster than distilled water in plant stems [1]. Ieperen et al. [2] and Zwieniecki et al. [3] explored hydraulic conductance upon perfusion of plant stems using salt solutions of different ionic concentrations. Subsequent studies [4–8] have confirmed the variations in sap flow for a variety of plant species. In particular, enhancement of the ionic effect in embolized stems [9–12] is a plausible mechanism for the maintenance of stable water flow under different environmental conditions, compensating for embolism-induced loss of hydraulic conductance.

Due to interest in active flow regulation, previous studies have investigated the effect of ions on sap flow control in terms of a specific cation, K^+ [2,3,5,8,13]. However, few studies have been conducted on the effect of other ions on sap flow in plants [12,14–16] from a physiological standpoint. Although the ionic effect in plants has been shown in many experiments, its physico-chemical mechanism remains unclear.

Interestingly, ion-mediated sap flow regulation is a unique process that occurs in dead cells [3,17]. This suggests that sap flow regulation differs from the biological process that occurs in a living cell, and can be examined from a physicochemical standpoint. In addition, we noted that sap water in plants contain various ions such as K^+, Ca^{2+}, Mg^{2+}, and Na^+ for optimizing water transport under different environmental conditions [18]. Thus, we considered the interactive effects of ion mixtures on water flow regulation. To characterize ion-responsiveness in vascular plants, we investigated the interactive effects of the type and composition of ions on pit membranes and sap flow by systematically varying the molar ratios of K^+ to Ca^{2+}. These two ions are the major cations in xylem sap water [12,18–20] and are closely associated with water transport in plants. For example, K^+ facilitates water flow by controlling evaporation rates from stomata via guard cell regulation [21] and Ca^{2+} by modulating cell wall structure, stomatal aperture and aquaporin stimulation [22,23].

Synchrotron X-ray and neutron imaging methods allow us to directly monitor ion-responsiveness in the stems of vascular plants in a noninvasive and nondestructive manner. Unlike perfusing solutions, these imaging techniques can be employed to characterize sap flow without exerting an artificial positive pressure, which could induce morphological changes in the plant nanostructure [8,24]. Synchrotron X-ray imaging is advantageous for investigating both the xylem structure of vascular plants and the sap flow in individual xylem levels with sufficient spatial and temporal resolutions [25–27]. On the other hand, the neutron imaging method is usually operated with relatively low flux for an expanded field of view (FOV) to investigate ionic solution uptake over a longer time scale [28]. In addition, the neutron imaging method can detect small changes in light elements such as hydrogen, allowing for *in situ* visualization of water transport in plants [28–33].

In this report, to characterize ion-mediated sap flow regulation in vascular plants from a physicochemical standpoint, the interactive ionic effects of K^+ and Ca^{2+} on sap flow in olive and laurel stems were examined using synchrotron X-ray and neutron imaging methods. Our experimental results on the interactive ionic effects increase our understanding of structural changes in pit membranes and the physicochemical mechanism of active sap flow regulation in xylem conduits.

Materials and Methods

Plant materials and experimental conditions

We selected olive (*Olea europaea* L.) and laurel (*Laurel nobilis* L.) as test samples because they are known to be highly sensitive to ions in sap water [5,8]. Olive and laurel stems were excised at lengths of 15 and 25 cm for X-ray and neutron imaging experiments, respectively, to characterize sap water distribution and regulation in their stems (excluding other factors affected by roots and leaves). Given that the ionic effect increases up to a length of 12 cm and then remains constant for longer stems [11], the length of the excised stems was greater than the critical length to maximize the ionic effects on hydraulic conductance. The bottom ends of the excised stems were dipped in reservoirs containing ionic solutions of different K^+/Ca^{2+} ratios, and the uptake process was monitored using synchrotron X-ray and neutron imaging techniques. During the ascent of ionic solutions, the temperature and humidity of environmental air were maintained at 19 ± 1°C and 95 ± 1% relative humidity (RH). During the experiments, the photosynthetic active radiation was 200 μmol m^{-2} s^{-1}.

Although the physiological ionic ratio of K^+/Ca^{2+} ranges from 3 to 10, depending on environmental conditions [12,18,20], we used ionic solutions with K^+/Ca^{2+} ratios of 0.01, 1, and 100 to characterize the interactive ion-response in sap flow. The total concentration of ions was fixed at 50 mM to explore the effects of ion type and ion composition on hydraulic conductance and to maximize the subsequent ionic effect. Ion-mediated variations of hydraulic conductance are known to be concentration-dependent, but the ionic effect is generally saturated at 20 mM to 50 mM KCl [3,8]. Although a total concentration of 50 mM is greater than the normal xylem sap osmolality in laurel stems, which ranges from 20 to 50 mOsm kg^{-1} and corresponds to 10 to 25 mM KCl [34], this concentration may be biologically harmless. Ionic solutions with varying K^+/Ca^{2+} ratios were produced by mixing 0.5 mM KCl and 49.5 mM $CaCl_2$, 25 mM KCl and 25 mM $CaCl_2$, and 49.5 mM KCl and 0.5 mM $CaCl_2$, respectively.

Synchrotron X-ray micro-imaging and neutron imaging techniques

Synchrotron X-ray micro-imaging experiments were performed at the beamline 14C from the Photon Factory (PF), KEK (High Energy Accelerator Organization), Tsukuba, Japan. Using a white (full-energy spectrum) X-ray beam with an energy of 70 keV, X-ray images with a field of view (FOV) of 1.5×1.5 mm were obtained with a spatial resolution of ~10 μm. X-ray images were recorded consecutively at 3-min intervals. To minimize radiation damages, a mechanical shutter and attenuating plates were employed to expose the sample plants to attenuated X-ray beam only when we captured X-ray images. Iopamidol solution was mixed with the ionic solutions as an X-ray contrast agent to clearly visualize the uptake process of ionic solutions in plant stems.

The neutron imaging experiments were conducted at the neutron radiography facility (NRF) of HANARO (30 MW), Korea Atomic Energy Research Institute (KAERI), Korea. A thermal neutron beam with a mean energy of 14 meV was collimated and detected using a ^{6}LiF/ZnS:Ag scintillator (PSI, Switzerland) and a CCD camera attached with a zoom lens (f 2.0, 135 mm). The thermal neutron flux was 5.07×10^6 neutrons cm^{-2} s^{-1} and the effective beam size was approximately 350×450 mm. The FOV of neutron radiography was 11.3×11.7 cm and each image was expressed at 1340×1300 pixels with a spatial resolution of 50 μm. Neutron images were recorded consecutively for several hours and the total image acquisition time for one image was 41.5 s, which consisted of 40-s exposure and 1.5-s readout. Deuterium oxide (D_2O), which has physiological properties similar to those of H_2O in plants, was employed as a contrast agent in neutron imaging experiments [35–37]. Despite long-term expose to D_2O, we observed no wilting and no morphological changes in the test plants. This implies that D_2O application as a contrast agent does not perceptible damages to the test plants.

Image processing for X-ray and neutron images

The effect of temporal fluctuations in the incident beam intensity on the transmission images was corrected using Octopus software (http://www.xraylab.com). Flat-field correction was adopted to eliminate the CCD dark current noises and the heterogeneity of the beam profile. The corrected image (I') was calculated as follows:

$$I' = \frac{I_{raw}(x,y) - I_{dark}(x,y)}{I_{gain}(x,y) - I_{dark}(x,y)} \times f, \tag{1}$$

where $I_{raw}(x,y)$ is the raw image, $I_{dark}(x,y)$ is the image taken with neither beam nor test sample, $I_{gain}(x,y)$ is the image captured without the sample under the same experimental condition, and f is a scaling factor. The calculations were performed pixel-wise at the lateral and vertical positions x and y, respectively. A median filter was adopted to remove noises embedded in the corrected images.

Although the excised stem segments were fixed, the exact positions of the sample stems could change slightly during long-term observations in neutron imaging experiments. This slight change in sample position was corrected by 2D translation within a fraction of a pixel [38]. After this image-alignment process, the corrected initial image (I'_0) was divided by the subsequent images (I'_n) at time $t=n$, as follows:

$$\tilde{I}'_n(x,y) = \frac{1}{I'_n(x,y)/I'_0(x,y)} \tag{2}$$

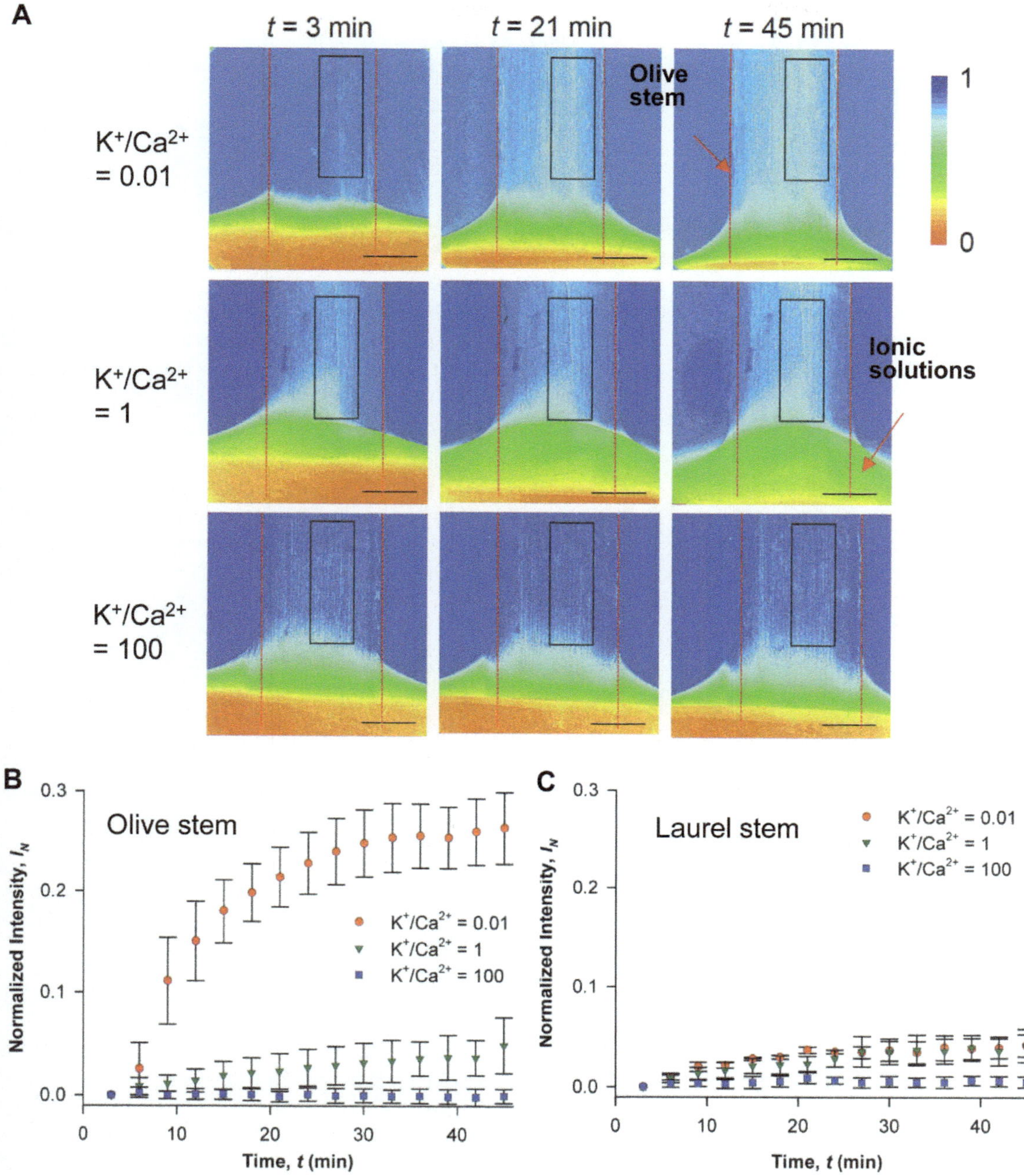

Figure 1. Synchrotron X-ray micro-imaging of the ascent of water containing K^+ and Ca^{2+} in xylem vessels. A) Typical X-ray images showing temporal changes in the spatial distribution of ionic solution uptake mediated by varying K^+/Ca^{2+} ratios from 0.01, 1, to 100 in the excised olive stems. Synchrotron X-ray imaging was employed to observe ionic water uptake directly through the xylem conduits of olive stems with high temporal and spatial resolution. Excised stems with a height of 15 cm took up ionic solutions with different K^+/Ca^{2+} ratios under the same total ion concentration. Intensity-based colored figures in each column show qualitative information regarding water ascent at different ionic ratios: K^+/Ca^{2+} = 0.01 (1st), 1 (2nd), and 100 (3rd), respectively. Light blue color represents the ascent of multi-ionic solutions mixed with iopamidol as a contrast agent. The X-ray image of each column was captured at 3, 21, and 45 min, respectively. Scale bar represents 500 μm. Temporal variations in the normalized X-ray absorption intensities in the region of interest for **B**) olive stems and **C**) laurel stems. Orange circles denote K^+/Ca^{2+} = 0.01; green rotated triangles denote K^+/Ca^{2+} = 1; purple rectangles denote K^+/Ca^{2+} = 100. The normalized intensity values directly represent ionic solution uptake. These figures were derived from three repeated experiments (n = 3) and error bars indicate standard deviations.

This procedure was performed to enhance the sensitivity of detection of light intensity variations during the experiment and to quantitatively compare the uptake behaviors of ionic solutions. The enhanced X-ray and neutron images ($\tilde{I}'_n$) were color-coded into 32 levels and processed with the jet colormap provided by Matlab, respectively.

An 80×30-pixel region of interest (ROI) was selected to quantitatively analyze the X-ray images. The intensity values in the ROI were then averaged and the results in the consecutive images were compared. To show the relative variations in ionic water uptake effectively, normalized intensity (I_N) was determined from the pixel intensities of each image at a time $t=n$ to the corresponding pixel intensities of the first image at $t=0$ (see Eq. (3)).

$$I_N = 1 - \frac{\bar{\bar{I}}'_n}{\bar{\bar{I}}'_0} \quad (3)$$

where $\bar{\bar{I}}'_0$ is the averaged intensity value in the ROI of the initial image and $\bar{\bar{I}}'_n$ represents the averaged intensity value in the ROI of time-consecutive images. I_N quantitatively shows the change in X-ray absorption. In other words, an increase in the average variations of I_N directly corresponded to an increase in ionic solution uptake to replace water already present in a plant.

The relationship between the normalized neutron images and the thickness variation is based on the Beer-Lambert attenuation law [37]. The excised stem segment was assumed to be partitioned into H_2O, D_2O, and dry biomass fractions. The local attenuation coefficient $\mu(x,y,z)$ was assumed to be constant [39]. At time $t=n$, the intensity $\bar{\bar{I}}'_n(x,y)$ of a neutron beam passing the test sample with a thickness δ_n in the z-direction was approximated as:

$$\bar{\bar{I}}'_n(x,y) = \bar{\bar{I}}'_{i,n}(x,y)\, e^{-\left[\mu_{dry}\delta_{dry,n}(x,y)+\mu_{H_2O}\delta_{H_2O,n}(x,y)+\mu_{D_2O}\delta_{D_2O,n}(x,y)\right]}, \quad (4)$$

where $\bar{\bar{I}}'_{i,n}(x,y)$ is the incident beam intensity distribution and $\delta_{H_2O}(x,y)$,$\delta_{D_2O}(x,y)$, and $\delta_{dry}(x,y)$ indicates the hypothetical thickness of H_2O, D_2O, and dry biomass fractions, respectively. Using the initial image ($t=0$) as a reference, the nth image was normalized as $\bar{\bar{I}}'_n(x,y)/\bar{\bar{I}}'_0(x,y)$. In addition, δ_{dry} and $\bar{\bar{I}}'_i$ were assumed to be constant during the experiment. The decrease in H_2O corresponded to an increase in D_2O, which can be expressed as $\delta_{H_2O,n}(x,y) = -\delta_{D_2O,n}(x,y)$. The temporal variation in D_2O thickness ($\Delta\delta_{D_2O}$) in the z-direction up to time $t=n$ at any position (x,y) in the camera plane can be quantified using the following measured beam intensities:

$$\Delta\delta_{D_2O}(x,y) = \delta_{D_2O,n}(x,y) - \delta_{D_2O,0}(x,y) = \frac{1}{\mu_{H_2O}-\mu_{D_2O}} \ln\left[\frac{\bar{\bar{I}}'_n(x,y)}{\bar{\bar{I}}'_0(x,y)}\right]. \quad (5)$$

The thickness $\Delta\delta_{D_2O}$ corresponded to ionic D_2O uptake. The linear attenuation coefficient usually depends on the neutron-beam spectrum. Given that the neutron beam consists of a set of neutrons with different energies, the linear attenuation coefficient is usually increased by integrating over different neutron energies. The measured linear attenuation coefficient of H_2O at NRF[40] was $0.3029 \pm 0.0002\ mm^{-1}$. The linear attenuation coefficient of D_2O was estimated to be $0.0303\ mm^{-1}$.

A threshold value corresponding to a specific neutron absorption intensity was applied to the neutron images captured in this study to evaluate the increased level (h) of ionic solutions. First, intensity values were averaged along the horizontal x direction of the ROI for each stem. The threshold value was then applied consistently to determine the height of the diffusional interface (h) between H_2O and the ionic D_2O among the horizontally averaged intensity values ($\bar{\bar{I}}'_n/\bar{\bar{I}}'_0$). When the value of $\bar{\bar{I}}'_n/\bar{\bar{I}}'_0$ was below the threshold value, the pixel information was thought to represent the contents of D_2O. Changes in h with time were quantitatively compared at different K^+/Ca^{2+} ratios.

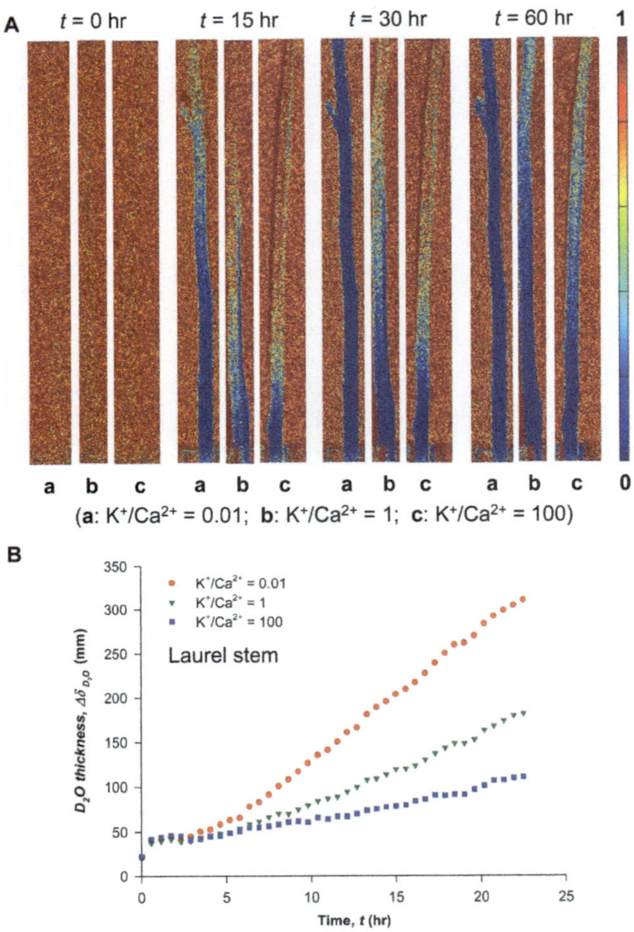

Figure 2. Neutron imaging of ionic solution uptake with different K^+/Ca^{2+} ratios in plant stems. A) Neutron images of ionic solution uptake with K^+/Ca^{2+} ratios of 0.01, 1, and 100 in the excised laurel stems at 0, 15, 30, and 60 h after dipping in the ionic D_2O solution. Ionic D_2O uptake in the excised laurel stems was directly observed using neutron radiography. Each figure provides qualitative information on water ascent at different ionic ratios ($K^+/Ca^{2+}=0.01$ (left), $K^+/Ca^{2+}=1$ (middle), and $K^+/Ca^{2+}=100$ (right)) at 0, 15, 30, and 60 h, respectively. The average diameter of stem segments was approximately 5 mm. Scale bar represents 5 mm. **B)** Temporal variations in ionic D_2O thickness in the laurel stems for 23 h. Orange circles denote $K^+/Ca^{2+}=0.01$; green rotated triangles denote $K^+/Ca^{2+}=1$; purple rectangles denote $K^+/Ca^{2+}=100$.

Results and Discussion

The spatial distribution of the ionic solutions of the same concentration (50 mM) but different K^+/Ca^{2+} ratios in excised olive stems was visualized using synchrotron X-ray imaging (Fig. 1A). The images were selected at time $t=3$, 21, and 45 min. The first, second, and third rows corresponded to K^+/Ca^{2+} ratios of 0.01, 1, and 100, respectively. In particular, the replacement of sap water in the xylem conduits with newly introduced ionic solution could be noninvasively investigated using iopamidol as a nonionic X-ray contrast enhancer. The degree of X-ray absorption change was expressed by color in Fig. 1A with a scale bar on the right ranging from a high increase in X-ray absorption (red) to

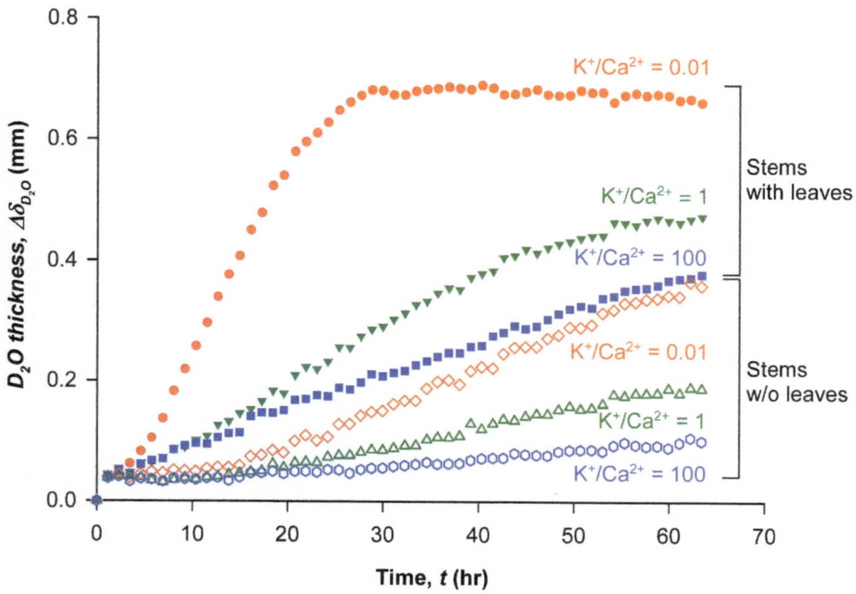

Figure 3. Physicochemical process of ion-mediated sap flow regulation. Effect of K^+/Ca^{2+} ratios on the variations of ionic D_2O thickness in the laurel stems with and without leaves for 64 h. Temporal variations in ionic D_2O contents in the region of interest for the excised laurel stems with leaves (closed symbol) and without leaves (open symbols) were measured using neutron imaging technique for 64 h. Closed orange circles and open orange diamonds denote $K^+/Ca^{2+} = 0.01$; closed green rotated triangles and open green triangles denote $K^+/Ca^{2+} = 1$; and closed purple rectangles and open purple hexagons denote $K^+/Ca^{2+} = 100$.

no change (dark blue). Therefore, the increase in X-ray absorption (and thus the color shift from dark blue) illustrated an increase in ionic solution with iopamidol. Synchrotron X-ray images show local inhomogeneity in the X-ray absorption, as shown in square boxes of Fig. 1A, which represent the ROI in xylem conduits rapidly filling with newly introduced ionic solutions. In the ROI, different xylem conduits pulled-up the ionic solutions at varying speeds.

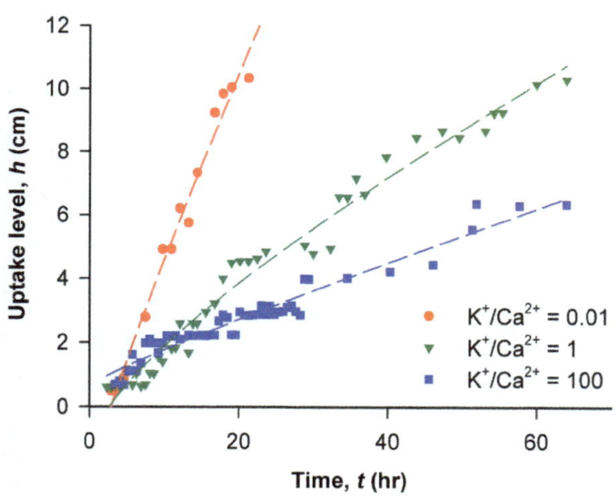

Figure 4. Effect of K^+/Ca^{2+} ratios on the uptake level of ionic solution. Temporal variations in the increase in ionic solutions with three K^+/Ca^{2+} ratios in the excised laurel stems and curve-fitted with 2-D diffusion-convection model. Variations in the increased K^+/Ca^{2+} ratios were quantified using a neutron imaging technique for 64 h. Orange circles denote $K^+/Ca^{2+} = 0.01$; green rotated triangles denote $K^+/Ca^{2+} = 1$; purple rectangles denote $K^+/Ca^{2+} = 100$.

In Figs. 1B and 1C, the overall variation in ionic solution uptake at different K^+/Ca^{2+} ratios was compared using intensity-based analysis of X-ray images. Normalized intensity (I_N) was determined from the pixel intensities of each image at a time $t = t_1$ to the corresponding pixel intensities of the first image at $t = 0$ (Eq. (3)), which quantitatively shows the change in X-ray absorption. An increase in the average variations of I_N directly corresponded to an increase in ionic solution uptake to replace existing water in a plant. The I_N value increased at lower K^+/Ca^{2+} ratios for both systems. The overall change in the normalized intensity (I_N) at $K^+/Ca^{2+} = 0.01$ or 1 was more rapid than at $K^+/Ca^{2+} = 100$ in olive stems in a relatively short time (45 min).

To further investigate the uptake of ionic solutions over longer time scales, neutron imaging techniques were employed with laurel stems. Laurel responded to ions more slowly than olive. Figure 2A shows the time-averaged ionic water uptake by tracing the spatial distribution of D_2O containing varying K^+/Ca^{2+} ratios in excised laurel stems at 0, 15, 30, and 60 h after dipping in ionic D_2O. The degree of neutron transmission was also color scaled as shown in the scale bar on the right of Fig. 2A. In Fig. 2A, blue shift represents better neutron transmission compared with the first image, while red shift represents no transmission change. Therefore, blue color corresponds to ionic D_2O solution uptake and replacing H_2O present in the stems. Assuming the stem samples showed the same initial water potential, the neutron images clearly demonstrated that when the K^+/Ca^{2+} ratio was 0.01, the ionic D_2O uptake was much faster than at higher K^+/Ca^{2+} ratios of 1 or 100 for a longer time scale in the excised laurel stems. The modulation of water uptake according to K^+/Ca^{2+} observed by neutron imaging for an extended time period (65 h) was similar to the results obtained by synchrotron X-ray imaging for short time durations (50 min). These results suggest that the interactive effect of different K^+/Ca^{2+} ratios at a fixed concentration (50 mM) has a considerable influence on the water uptake process, irrespective of plant species or time scale.

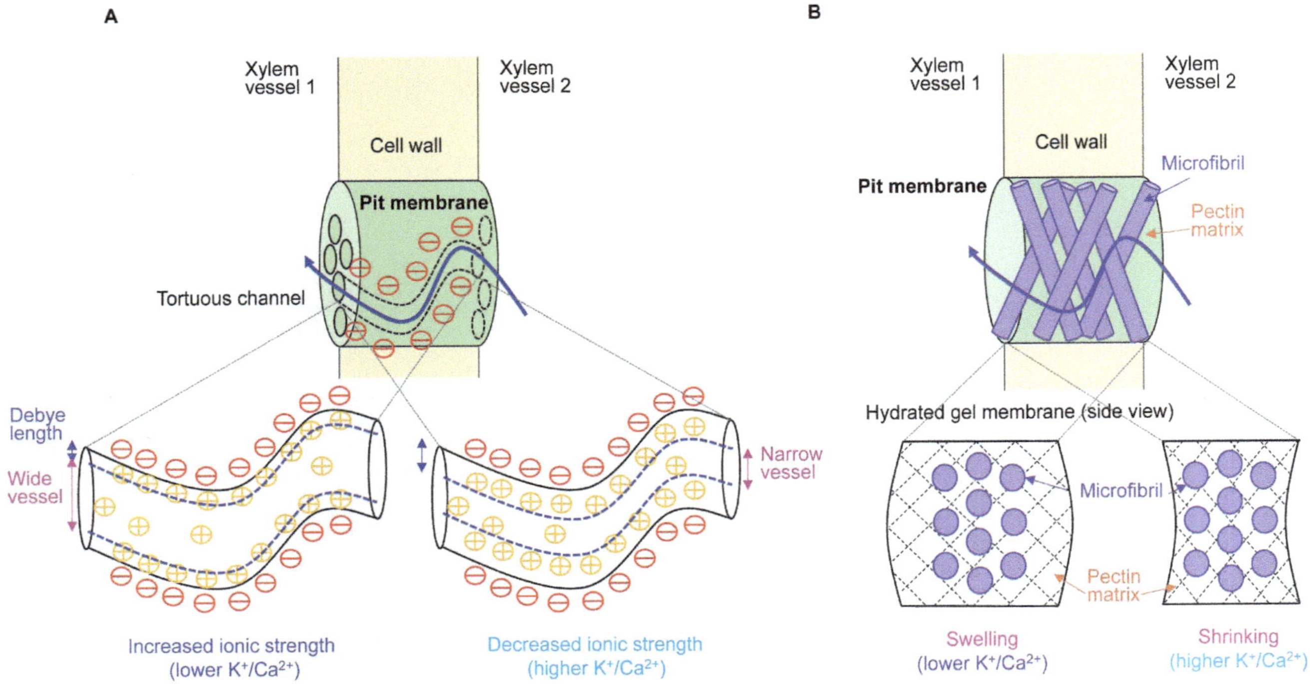

Figure 5. Putative physicochemical models for ion-mediated sap flow regulation in vascular plants. Schematic illustrations of **A**) the electrostatically induced hydrodynamic layer formation model and **B**) the ion-responsive hydrogel model to explain ion-mediated sap flow regulation in vascular plants. In the electrostatically induced hydrodynamic layer formation model, the ionic ratios affect the effective porous structure for control of water transport via the pit membrane. A relatively thin Debye layer formed at lower K^+/Ca^{2+} ratios, making a relatively wider flow path in the pit membrane, while a relatively thick Debye layer induced a narrow flow path at higher ionic ratios. In the hydrogel model and at lower K^+/Ca^{2+} ratios, pectins are swollen in the pit membrane with increased porosity based on Hofmeister series. This ion-mediated structural change seems to contribute to the increased flow rate through xylem vessels. At higher ionic ratios, pectins shrunk in the pit membrane with relatively decreased porosity. The effective structural changes may reduce the flow rate.

Temporal characteristic variations in ionic D_2O thickness ($\Delta\delta_{D_2O}$) affected by the K^+/Ca^{2+} ratio in the laurel stem at the field of view quantitatively show the interactive role of monovalent and divalent cations during the uptake of ionic solutions (Fig. 2B). The ionic D_2O thickness ($\Delta\delta_{D_2O}$) was estimated from the ratio of the neutron absorption intensity at time $t=t_1$ of each image to that of the first image at $t=0$ (Eq. (5)), which corresponded to ionic D_2O uptake. The contribution of K^+/Ca^{2+} ratios on the uptake of ionic solution in laurel stems was insignificant during the initial 5 hr. However, the $\Delta\delta_{D_2O}$ increased significantly over time at lower K^+/Ca^{2+} ratios. The ionic solution uptake rate was in the order of the K^+/Ca^{2+} ratio of 0.01>1>100. In particular, when the K^+/Ca^{2+} ratio decreased by 100-fold, the uptake rate of the ionic solutions in the laurel stems increased by approximately twofold. Changes in sap water uptake efficiency according to K^+/Ca^{2+} based on neutron imaging for an extended time (up to 60-h time scale) was similar to the results obtained from synchrotron X-ray imaging for a short time (50-min time scale). The interactive effect of different ionic compositions (K^+/Ca^{2+}) at a fixed concentration (50 mM) strongly affected the water uptake process irrespective of plant species and time scale.

To determine whether ion-mediated water flow modulation was independent of that driven by transpiration in leaves, the effects of different K^+/Ca^{2+} ratios were investigated in laurel stems with and without leaves. Fig. 3 shows temporal variations in ionic D_2O thickness ($\Delta\delta_{D_2O}$) along the excised stems of laurel samples with and without leaves for 65 h. The thickness $\Delta\delta_{D_2O}$ corresponded to ionic D_2O uptake (see Materials and Methods). On average, the uptake rates of the ionic solutions through leafless stems were twofold lower compared with stems with leaves that transpire under relatively high humidity conditions (95±1%). In addition, the ascent of ionic D_2O was more significant and faster at the lowest ionic ratio (K^+/Ca^{2+} =0.01). The uptake rate of ionic solution was in the order of the K^+/Ca^{2+} ratio of 0.01>1>100 for both systems with and without plant leaves. The varying cationic ratios synergistically regulated sap water transport in plants, irrespective of the existence of leaves.

The increase in ionic solution (h) was measured by consistently applying the same threshold value corresponding to a specific neutron absorption intensity for the neutron images (see Material and Methods). Changes in h with time for other ionic solutions of different K^+/Ca^{2+} ratios were then compared quantitatively (Fig. 4). The ionic effect is localized at pit membranes [3,17], which limit hydraulic conductance in xylem [41–43]. Thus, we assumed that the axial transport of ionic solution corresponded to radial transport through pit membranes in xylem.

The uptake of ionic solutions in our experiments was due to the convective flow under hydrostatic pressure differences driven by leaf transpiration and the diffusion driven by concentration differences between the ionic solutions and sap water already present in plants. Therefore, this can be modeled using two-dimensional diffusion-convection, which can be expressed as the following Eq. (6) [44].

$$h=\sqrt{4D_{eff}t}+V_0t+c, \tag{6}$$

where D_{eff}, V_0, and c are the effective diffusion coefficient, the convective velocity, and a constant, respectively. The water level h of an ionic solution was curve-fitted by Eq. (6), and the fitted curves (dotted lines in Fig. 4) can be used to determine D_{eff}, V_0, and c in each case. The diffusion coefficients D_{eff} were determined to be 4.7×10^{-5}cm^2/sec, 4.2×10^{-5}cm^2/sec, and 1.49×10^{-6}cm^2/sec when the K^+/Ca^{2+} ratios were 0.01, 1, and 100, respectively. The value of V_0 was in the order of 10^{-5} cm/s and the Péclet number was $Pe = LV_0/D_{eff} << 1$, where L is the characteristic length. This suggested that diffusion was dominant over convection for all K^+/Ca^{2+} ratios tested in this study. We can assume that the difference in initial water potential in all stem samples was negligible. The values of h were well-matched using curve-fitting with adjusted R^2 values of 0.98, 0.97, and 0.94, respectively.

The diffusion through pit membranes differed from that through homogeneous solution because it was influenced by the structural features of pores, such as size, shape, and connectivity. The D_{eff} for diffusion through a porous media was estimated based on the diffusion coefficient of ions in a dilute solution (D_0), the porosity (ε), and the tortuosity (τ), as follows [44]:

$$D_{eff} = \varepsilon D_0/\tau \tag{7}$$

The change in porous structure used for water transport can be estimated from D_{eff} obtained using the aforementioned curve-fitting. The change in D_{eff} at different K^+/Ca^{2+} ratios corresponded to the ratio of porosity to tortuosity (ε/τ) of the pit membrane. From the fitted curves, the ε/τ ratio of the pit membrane was observed to increase by approximately 12% at the ionic ratio of $K^+/Ca^{2+} = 0.01$, compared with that at $K^+/Ca^{2+} = 1$. Conversely, the ratio ε/τ decreased by 96% at $K^+/Ca^{2+} = 100$, compared with that at $K^+/Ca^{2+} = 1$. These results suggested that the effective porosity of pit membranes decreased sap flow as the K^+/Ca^{2+} ratio increased. Since the water flow through pit membrane plays a major role in determining the overall water transport through xylem conduits [43], we hypothesized that dynamic changes in the morphological structure of pit membrane induced by ions would be important for active water flow regulation in vascular plants.

To characterize the mechanism of interactive ionic effects on effective structural changes of pit membranes, we should consider the chemical compositions of pit membranes and the ion-structure interaction. Pit membranes are composed of coextensive cellulose-hemicellulose networks forming a fiber composite material as a primary cell wall structure [45]. Pectic polysaccharide is a water-retentive, shear-resistant matrix in a primary cell wall structure, but whether this hydrogel-like constituent is present in intervessel pit membranes and its function on the ionic effect remain unclear.

Taking into account the controversy over the existence of pectins in pit membranes of plants [46–49], two scenarios can explain ion-mediated variations in the effective porosity of pit membranes (Fig. 5). First, the effective porosity of pit membranes can be affected by electrostatically induced hydrodynamic layers on the pit wall [50,51]. The negatively charged surface of hydrated pit membranes [8] attracts cations from ionic solutions, creating the Debye layer near the surface. Since the concentrated cations in the Debye layer give rise to drag, the Debye length (κ^{-1}) affects the effective pore size through which sap water passes. The flux density (q) can be expressed as follows:

$$q = -\frac{n\pi r_0^2}{8\eta}\left(r_o - \kappa^{-1}\right)^2 \Delta P \tag{8}$$

where n is the number of pores per unit surface area, r_0 is the intrinsic radius of pore, η is fluid viscosity, and ΔP is the pressure difference per unit pore length. The Debye length κ^{-1} is reciprocally proportional to the root of ionic strength (I_c), and can be obtained as follows:

$$I_c = \frac{1}{2}\sum c_i z_i^2 \tag{9}$$

where c_i is the molar concentration of ion i and z_i is the ion valence. Therefore, even at the same concentration, the κ^{-1} decreases and q of sap water increases as the K^+/Ca^{2+} ratio decreases (Fig. 5A). This mechanism based on electrostatic interactions suggests that ion types and ionic compositions are important factors in ion-mediated flow regulation in vascular plants.

Second, by assuming that pit membranes are composed of a pectin-based hydrogel, the swelling and shrinking phenomena of hydrogels [1,3,13] can be used to characterize the interactive ion-mediated variation in the pore size of pit membranes, and thus flow regulation in vascular plants. In particular, the ion-specific Hofmeister series [52] can be used to explain the effects of different ion types and ionic ratios. According to the series, salting-out K^+ causes shrinking of the hydrogel, while salting-in Ca^{2+} induces swelling. Thus, a lower K^+/Ca^{2+} ratio is expected to induce swelling in the hydrogel structure, whereas a higher K^+/Ca^{2+} ratio causes relatively less swelling or shrinking (Fig. 5B). Shrinking of the hydrogel structure could decrease the porosity of pit membranes. Conversely, the swelling of hydrogel increases the porosity of pit membranes. Therefore, the flow rate of ionic solutions increased at lower K^+/Ca^{2+} ratios. The effects of structural variation in a hydrated gel matrix on the ion-responsive flow regulation in vascular plants can be used to characterize ionic effects.

In conclusion, we examined the ion-responsiveness of water transport in olive and laurel stems to increase our understanding of the mechanism of active water flow regulation in two representative vascular plants. Different ion types significantly affected water transport in xylem conduits. Sap flow rate decreased with an increasing K^+/Ca^{2+} ratio, while a decrease in the K^+/Ca^{2+} ratio accelerated the ascent of ionic solution. This interactive ionic effect is a common type of systematic flow regulation in vascular plants, irrespective of the plant species. The active ion-mediated flow regulation in the stem of a vascular plant may result from structural changes in pit membranes. The effective structural changes mediated by ions can be explained by the formation of electrostatically induced hydrodynamic layers and the ion-responsiveness of hydrogel structure based on Hofmeister series. The interactive ionic effects from a physicochemical standpoint describe the role of ion-responsiveness during water flow regulation in vascular plants.

Acknowledgments

We acknowledge the neutron source HANARO (High-Flux Advanced Neutron Application Reactor) at the KAERI for providing beam time and thank Hwasuk Oh (KAERI) for providing technical assistance with the neutron radiography experiments. X-ray imaging experiments were performed at the beamline 14C of the Photon Factory (PF), KEK (High Energy Accelerator Organization; Tsukuba, Japan).

The English in this document has been checked by at least two professional editors, both native speakers of English. For a certificate, please see:

http://www.textcheck.com/certificate/a2RJHA

Author Contributions

Conceived and designed the experiments: JR SA SK SL. Performed the experiments: JR SA SK TK. Analyzed the data: JR SK. Wrote the paper: JR SA SL.

References

1. Zimmermann MH (1978) Hydraulic architecture of some diffuse-porous trees. Can J Bot 56: 2286–2295.
2. Van Ieperen W, Van Meeteren U, Van Gelder H (2000) Fluid ionic composition influences hydraulic conductance of xylem conduits. J Exp Bot 51: 769–776.
3. Zwieniecki MA, Melcher PJ, Holbrook NM (2001) Hydrogel control of xylem hydraulic resistance in plants. Science 291: 1059–1062.
4. Domec JC, Meinzer FC, Lachenbrunch B, Housset J (2007) Dynamic variation in sapwood specific conductivity in six woody species. Tree Physiol 27: 1389–1400.
5. Jansen S, Gortan E, Lens F, Lo Gullo MA, Salleo S, et al. (2011) Do quantitative vessel and pit characters account for ion-mediated changes in the hydraulic conductance of angiosperm xylem? New Phytol 189: 218–228.
6. López-Portillo J, Ewers FW, Angeles G (2005) Sap salinity effects on xylem conductivity in two mangrove species. Plant Cell Environ 28: 1285–1292.
7. Gortan E, Nardini A, Salleo S, Jansen S (2011) Pit membrane chemistry influences the magnitude of ion-mediated enhancement of xylem hydraulic conductance in four Lauraceae species. Tree Physiol 31: 48–58.
8. Nardini A, Salleo S, Jansen S (2011) More than just a vulnerable pipeline: xylem physiology in the light of ion-mediated regulation of plant water transport. J Exp Bot 62: 4701–4718.
9. Trifilò P, Lo Gullo MA, Salleo S, Callea K, Nardini A (2008) Xylem embolism alleviated by ion-mediated increase in hydraulic conductivity of functional xylem: insights from field measurements. Tree Physiol 28: 1505–1512.
10. Gascó A, Salleo S, Gortan E, Nardini A (2007) Seasonal changes in the ion-mediated increase of xylem hydraulic conductivity in stems of three evergreens: any functional role? Physiol Plant 129: 597–606.
11. Gascó A, Nardini A, Gortan E, Salleo S (2006) Ion-mediated increase in the hydraulic conductivity of Laurel stems: role of pits and consequences for the impact of cavitation on water transport. Plant Cell Environ 29: 1946–1955.
12. Nardini A, Gascó A, Trifilo P, Lo Gullo MA, Salleo S (2007) Ion-mediated enhancement of xylem hydraulic conductivity is not always suppressed by the presence of Ca^{2+} in the sap. J Exp Bot 58: 2609–2615.
13. Lee J, Holbrook NM, Zwieniecki MA (2012) Ion induced changes in the structure of bordered pit membranes. Front Plant Sci 3: 55.
14. Van Ieperen W, Van Gelder A (2006) Ion-mediated flow changes suppressed by minimal calcium presence in xylem sap in Chrysanthemum and Prunus laurocerasus. J Exp Bot 57: 2743–2750.
15. Van Ieperen W (2007) Ion-mediated changes of xylem hydraulic resistance in planta: fact or fiction? Trends Plant Sci 12: 137–142.
16. Cochard H, Herbette S, Hernandez E, Holtta T, Mencuccini M (2010) The effects of sap ionic composition on xylem vulnerability to cavitation. J Exp Bot 61: 275–285.
17. Zwieniecki MA, Orians CM, Melcher PJ, Holbrook NM (2003) Ionic control of the lateral exchange of water between vascular bundles in tomato. J Exp Bot 54: 1399–1405.
18. Siebrecht S, Herdel K, Schurr U, Tischner R (2003) Nutrient translocation in the xylem of poplar-diurnal variations and spatial distribution along the shoot axis. Planta 217: 783–793.
19. Goodger JQ, Sharp RE, Marsh EL, Schachtman DP (2005) Relationships between xylem sap constituents and leaf conductance of well-watered and water-stressed maize across three xylem sap sampling techniques. J Exp Bot 56: 2389–2400.
20. Nardini A, Grego F, Trifilo P, Salleo S (2010) Changes of xylem sap ionic content and stem hydraulics in response to irradiance in *Laurus nobilis*. Tree Physiol 30: 628–635.
21. Chérel I (2004) Regulation of K^+ channel activities in plants: from physiological to molecular aspects. J Exp Bot 55: 337–351.
22. Smith KT, Shortle WC (2013) Calcium amendment may increase hydraulic efficiency and forest evapotranspiration. Proc Natl Acad Sci USA 110: E3739.
23. Gilliham M, Dayod M, Hocking BJ, Xu B, Conn SJ, et al. (2011) Calcium delivery and storage in plant leaves: exploring the link with water flow. J Exp Bot 62: 2233–2250.
24. Melcher PJ, Holbrook NM, Burns MJ, Zwieniecki MA, Cobb AR, et al. (2012) Measurements of stem xylem hydraulic conductivity in the laboratory and field. Methods Ecol Evol 3: 685–694.
25. Kim HK, Lee SJ (2010) Synchrotron X-ray imaging for nondestructive monitoring of sap flow dynamics through xylem vessel elements in rice leaves. New Phytol 188: 1085–1098.
26. Lee SJ, Kim Y (2008) In vivo visualization of the water-refilling process in xylem vessels using X-ray micro-imaging. Ann Bot 101: 595–602.
27. Brodersen CR, McElrone AJ, Choat B, Matthews MA, Shackel KA (2010) The dynamics of embolism repair in xylem: in vivo visualizations using high-resolution computed tomography. Plant Physiol 154: 1088–1095.
28. Nakanishi TM (2009) Neutron imaging applied to plant physiology. In: Bilheux HZ, McGreevy R, Anderson IS, editors. Neutron Imaging and Applications pp.305–317.
29. Nakanishi TM, Okuni Y, Furukawa J, Tanoi K, Yokota H, et al. (2003) Water movement in a plant sample by neutron beam analysis as well as positron emission tracer imaging system. J Radioanal Nucl Chem 255: 149–153.
30. Matsushima U, Kawabata Y, Hino M, Geltenbort P, Nicolai B (2005) Measurement of changes in water thickness in plant materials using very low-energy neutron radiography. Nucl Instrum Meth A 542: 76–80.
31. Menon M, Robinson B, Oswald SE, Kaestner A, Abbaspour KC, et al. (2007) Visualization of root growth in heterogeneously contaminated soil using neutron radiography. Eur J Soil Sci 58: 802–810.
32. Moradi AB, Conesa HM, Robinson B, Lehmann E, Kuehne G, et al. (2008) Neutron radiography as a tool for revealing root development in soil: capabilities and limitations. Plant Soil 318: 243–255.
33. Oswald SE, Menon M, Carminati A, Vontobel P, Lehmann E, et al. (2008) Quantitative imaging of infiltration, root growth, and root water uptake via neutron radiography. Vadose Zone J 7: 1035.
34. Tyree MT, Salleo S, Nardini A, Gullo MAL, Mosca R (1999) Refilling of embolized vessels in young stems of Laurel. Do we need a new paradigm? Plant Physiol 120: 11–21.
35. Matsushima U, Kardjilov N, Hilger A, Graf W, Herppich WB (2008) Application potential of cold neutron radiography in plant science research. J Appl Bot Food Qual 82: 90–98.
36. Matsushima U, Herppich WB, Kardjilov N, Graf W, Hilger A, et al. (2009) Estimation of water flow velocity in small plants using cold neutron imaging with D_2O tracer. Nucl Instrum Meth A 605: 146–149.
37. Strobl M, Manke I, Kardjilov N, Hilger A, Dawson M, et al. (2009) Advances in neutron radiography and tomography. J Phys D: Appl Phys 42: 243001.
38. Guizar-Sicairos M, Thurman ST, Fienup JR (2008) Efficient subpixel image registration algorithms. Opt Lett 33: 156–158.
39. Totzke C, Miranda T, Konrad W, Gout J, Kardjilov N, et al. (2013) Visualization of embolism formation in the xylem of liana stems using neutron radiography. Ann Bot 111: 723–730.
40. Kim T, Sim C, Kim M (2008) Research on water discharge characteristics of PEM fuel cells by using neutron imaging technology at the NRF, HANARO. Appl Radiat Isot 66: 593–605.
41. Wheeler JK, Sperry JS, Hacke UG, Hoang N (2005) Inter-vessel pitting and cavitation in woody Rosaceae and other vesselled plants: a basis for a safety versus efficiency trade-off in xylem transport. Plant Cell Environ 28: 800–812.
42. Choat B, Brodie TW, Cobb AR, Zwieniecki MA, Holbrook NM (2006) Direct measurements of intervessel pit membrane hydraulic resistance in two angiosperm tree species. Am J Bot 93: 993–1000.
43. Choat B, Cobb AR, Jansen S (2008) Structure and function of bordered pits: new discoveries and impacts on whole-plant hydraulic function. New Phytol 177: 608–626.
44. Cussler EL (1997) Diffusion: mass transfer in fluid systems. New York: Cambridge University Press.
45. Albersheim P, Darvill A, Roberts K, Sederoff R, Staehelin A (2010) Plant cell walls. New York: Garland Science.
46. Boyce CK, Zwieniecki MA, Cody GD, Jacobsen C, Wirick S, et al. (2004) Evolution of xylem lignification and hydrogel transport regulation. Proc Natl Acad Sci USA 101: 17555–17558.
47. Plavcová L, Hacke UG, Sperry JS (2011) Linking irradiance-induced changes in pit membrane ultrastructure with xylem vulnerability to cavitation. Plant Cell Environ 34: 501–513.
48. O'Brien TP, Thimann KV (1967) Observation of fine structure of oat coleoptile: III. correlated light and electron microscopy of the vascular tissues. Protoplasma 63: 443–478.
49. O'Brien TP (1970) Further observations on hydrolysis of cell wall in xylem. Protoplasma 69: 1–14.
50. Van Doorn WG, Hiemstra T, Fanourakis D (2011) Hydrogel regulation of xylem water flow: an alternative hypothesis. Plant Physiol 157: 1642–1649.
51. Santiago M, Pagay V, Stroock AD (2013) Impact of electroviscosity on the hydraulic conductance of the bordered pit membrane: a theoretical investigation. Plant Physiol 163: 999–1011.
52. Hofmeister F (1888) Zur Lehre von der Wirkung der Salze. Arch Exp Pathol Pharmakol 24: 247–260.

2

Assessment of Prosthesis Alignment after Revision Total Knee Arthroplasty Using EOS 2D and 3D Imaging

Marrigje F. Meijer[1]*, Alexander L. Boerboom[1], Martin Stevens[1], Sjoerd K. Bulstra[1], Inge H. F. Reininga[2]

1 Department of Orthopaedics, University of Groningen, University Medical Center Groningen, Gronigen, The Netherlands, **2** Department of Trauma Surgery, University of Groningen, University Medical Center Groningen, Groningen, The Netherlands

Abstract

Introduction: A new low-dose X-ray device, called EOS, has been introduced for determining lower-limb alignment in 2D and 3D. Reliability has not yet been assessed when using EOS on lower limbs containing a knee prosthesis. Therefore purpose of this study was to determine intraobserver and interobserver reliability of EOS 2D and 3D knee prosthesis alignment measurements after revision total knee arthroplasty (rTKA).

Methods: Forty anteroposterior and lateral images of 37 rTKA patients were included. Two observers independently performed measurements on these images twice. Varus/valgus angles were measured in 2D (VV2D) and 3D (VV3D). Intraclass correlation coefficients and the Bland and Altman method were used to determine reliability. T-tests were used to test potential differences.

Results: Intraobserver and interobserver reliability were excellent for VV2D and VV3D. No significant difference or bias between the first and second measurements or the two observers was found. A significant mean and absolute difference of respectively 1.00° and 1.61° existed between 2D and 3D measurements.

Conclusions: EOS provides reliable varus/valgus measurements in 2D and 3D for the alignment of the knee joint with a knee prosthesis. However, significant differences exist between varus/valgus measurements in 2D and 3D.

Editor: Matej Oresic, Steno Diabetes Center, Denmark

Funding: The authors have no support or funding to report.

Competing Interests: One of the authors will be and has been paid as a consultant by Zimmer (Warsaw, IN, USA) for purposes of education and training in knee arthroplasty. The department receives research institutional support from Inspine (Schiedam, NL), Stryker (Kalamazoo, Mich. USA) and Zimmer (Warsaw, IN, USA). Nevertheless there has not been any direct funding related to this study.

* Email: M.F.Meijer@umcg.nl

Introduction

Achieving optimal prosthetic alignment during total knee arthroplasty (TKA) is an essential part of the surgical procedure. Malpositioning of a knee prosthesis in the coronal plane causes earlier loosening and revision surgery [1]. Revision TKA (rTKA) has to be prevented, as this is associated with worse functional outcome and prosthesis survival [2,3]. Proper alignment in the coronal plane is associated with less pain, better knee function, faster rehabilitation and improved quality of life [4,5]. Optimal coronal alignment is considered ≤3° varus or valgus [6].

Conventional weight-bearing radiographs are generally used to measure alignment in the coronal and sagittal planes. Proportions and angles may not be correct though, given the divergence in the vertical and horizontal planes. A computed tomography (CT) scanogram can also be used to evaluate prosthetic alignment in the coronal, sagittal and rotational planes. However, due to high levels of radiation and high costs it cannot be used routinely. Moreover, with a CT-scan it is not possible to obtain images of the leg in weight-bearing position.

The EOS system has been developed for the evaluation of prosthetic alignment (EOS Imaging, Paris, France) [7]. With this biplanar low-dose X-ray technique, orthogonally made long-leg 2D radiographs and 3D reconstructions can be obtained. Major advantages are that images of the leg are obtained on a 1:1 scale with an amount of radiation 800–1000 times lower than CT-scans and 10 times lower than conventional X-rays [7,8]. However, the EOS software for creating 3D reconstructions is developed for lower limbs without knee prosthetic material. When a knee prosthesis is *in situ*, several anatomical reference points have disappeared or changed, making it difficult to mark reference points as described by the measurement protocol. Therefore, the measurement protocol was adjusted. Reliability of this protocol have not been investigated yet.

Purpose of this study was to determine intraobserver and interobserver reliability of 2D and 3D knee prosthesis alignment measurements after rTKA using EOS. As a secondary outcome we assessed whether significant differences existed between 2D and 3D measurements.

Materials and Methods

Fifty-four patients who underwent rTKA between January 1998 and November 2009 and who were available for the acquisition of EOS images between November 2009 and May 2010 were included. An anteroposterior (AP) and lateral (LAT) image of the operated leg was made with the EOS stereography system at the Radiology Department of our hospital as part of the standard follow-up protocol for rTKA. In accordance to regulations of the Medical Ethical Review Board of University Medical Center Groningen, patients were informed about the fact that data of their radiographs could be used for scientific research. If patients had objections to the use of their data these data were not included in the study.

Patients were positioned on the EOS platform in standing position with the right foot 10 cm in front of the left foot. SterEOS software (Biospace Imaging, Paris) was used to take 2D measurements of the AP images and 3D measurements of the AP and LAT images. The images were anonymized by removing names, patient numbers and birth dates. The guidelines for taking measurements as provided by the manufacturer were followed [9]. Since several landmarks disappear or change when a knee prosthesis is *in situ*, the observers made the following agreements on marking the landmarks:

- Instead of the center of tibial spines, the center of the tibial plateau is chosen;
- Instead of marking the distal femoral notch, the center of the femoral component is marked;
- Instead of marking the anatomic femoral condyles, the condyles of the femoral component are marked.

In order to calculate coronal and sagittal alignment parameters of the lower limb in 2D and 3D, the "lower limb alignment" mode is used. The first step is to define the left or right lower limb and to choose the modeling "lower limb alignment" mode. Next, identification of the lower limb on the AP and LAT images is done in 10 steps (Figure 1 and Figure 2):

Femur:

- Center of femoral head (points 1 and 4);
- Center of the distal femoral notch (points 2 and 5);
- Center of the diaphysis in its distal third (points 3 and 6).

Tibia:

- Center of the tibial spines. When a knee prosthesis is in situ the tibial spines disappear, therefore the center of the tibial plateau is chosen and the axis from the center of the ankle to the center of the tibial plateau represents the anatomical axis of the tibia (points 7 and 9);
- Center of the distal articular surface in the upper ankle joint (points 8 and 10).

The next step is adjustment of the landmarks in four steps (Figure 3):

1. Adjustment of the position of the sphere of the femoral head in both views. It is possible to enlarge or minimize the size of the sphere according to the size and shape of the femoral head, in order to mark the center of the femoral head as precisely as possible;
2. Adjustment of the point in the center of the distal third of the diaphysis of the femur;

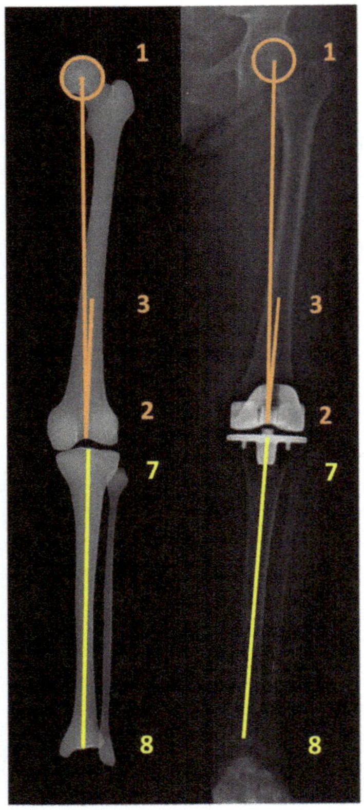

Figure 1. Identification of the lower limb on the frontal image.

3. Adjustment of the position of the point in the center of the femoral notch and tibial plateau, and marking of the femoral condyles. The condyles have to be identified on the AP and LAT images using the two spheres. It is possible to adjust the

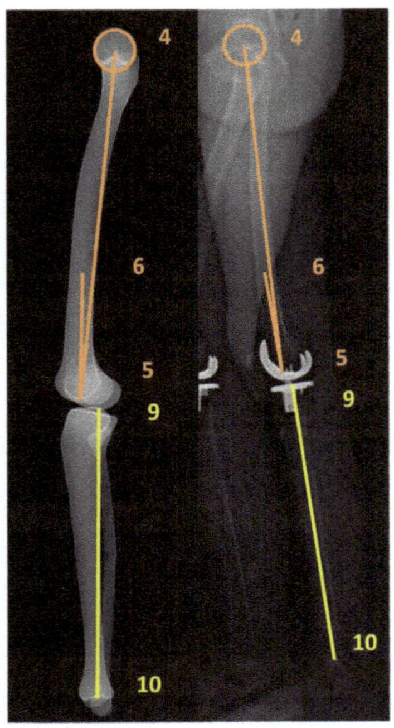

Figure 2. Identification of the lower limb on the lateral image.

size of the spheres, according to the size of the condyles. On the AP image the center of the spheres has to be located in the center of each condyle. On the LAT image the spheres have to be tangent to the posterior part of the condyles. It is important not to confuse the medial with the lateral condyles. In order to identify the right condyle, the epipolar line is used to differentiate between the two condyles by observing the correspondence of condylar height on both the AP and the LAT image;

4. Adjustment of the reference point in the center of the distal articular surface on the AP and LAT images.

VV2D is the angle between the mechanical axis of the femur (axis between points 1 and 2) and the tibia (axis between points 7 and 8) on the AP image (Figure 1). For the 3D measurement, the points marked on the AP (Figure 1) and LAT (Figure 2) images as described above are combined to generate the mechanical axes of femur and tibia. VV3D is the angle between the three-dimensional mechanical axis of the femur (axis between points 1–4 and 2–5) and tibia (axis between point 7–9 and 8–10).

Primary outcome measurement is the varus/valgus angle (VV) (angle between the mechanical axes of femur and tibia) in 2D (VV2D) and 3D (VV3D) because of its clinical importance. A positive value indicates valgus and a negative value indicates varus.

An independent researcher randomly numbered all images twice. In this way, two blinded sets of 40 AP and LAT images each were composed. Two observers (observer A and observer B) separately analyzed both sets of 40 images twice. Both observers were experienced in taking the measurements in 2D and 3D prior to the study.

Statistical analyses

Statistical analyses were performed using the PASW software package (version 18, SPSS, Chicago). Intraobserver and interobserver reliability were investigated by determining relative and absolute reliability [10]. Relative and absolute intraobserver reliability were investigated by respectively calculating intraclass correlation coefficients (ICCs) and using the Bland & Altman method [10]. The ICCs with 95% confidence interval (CI) for each 2D and 3D measurement were calculated and interpreted according to the benchmarks described by Fleiss. An ICC >0.75 represents an excellent correlation, 0.40–0.75 a moderate-to-good correlation and <0.40 represents a poor correlation [11].

Absolute intraobserver and interobserver reliability were calculated by the Bland & Altman method [12]. For intraobserver reliability the mean difference and 95% CI between measurement set 1 (M1) and measurement set 2 (M2) were calculated for both observers separately. For interobserver reliability the mean difference and 95% CI between the two observers were calculated. When intraobserver reliability was good for both observers, the means of M1 and M2 of observer A (n = 40) were compared with the means of both sets of observer B (n = 40).

To investigate agreement on the number of outliers between M1 and M2, as well as the two observers, Cohen's κ coefficients were calculated [13]. Angles with a deviation >3° varus or valgus from the neutral axis were considered outliers [6]. The κ values were interpreted according to Landis and Koch [14]: <0 represents less than chance agreement, 0.01–0.20 represents slight agreement, 0.21–0.40 fair agreement, 0.41–0.60 moderate agreement, 0.61–0.80 substantial agreement and 0.81–0.99 represents almost perfect agreement. χ^2 tests were performed to assess statistically significant differences in the number of outliers.

To identify significant differences between M1 and M2, a paired Student T-test was performed and the standard error of measurement (SEM) and smallest detectable change (SDC) were calculated. The formulas used to calculate the SEM and SDC are respectively SEM = standard error of difference/$\sqrt{2}$ and SDC = 1.96×$\sqrt{2}$× SEM. [15–17] A Student T-test for independent samples was performed to assess significant differences between the means of the measurements of the two observers, and the SEM and SDC were calculated.

Potential differences between VV2D and VV3D measurements were assessed using T-tests. First, the means of M1 and M2 of each observer for both VV2D and VV3D were calculated, creating a VV2D and VV3D set (n = 40/n = 40) for each observer. Next, the means of the mean of observer A and observer B for both VV2D and VV3D were calculated. In this way, one set of VV2D and one set of VV3D measurements was generated (n = 40/n = 40). A Paired-samples T-test was performed to detect any significant differences between both sets. The absolute difference between VV2D and VV3D was calculated for each subject. Meaning, the deviation of the neutral axis was stated as a positive value, regardless of the deviation being varus or valgus. The absolute differences were compared with the value 0 using a One-sample T-test, since a zero value indicates no absolute difference between VV2D and VV3D. Additionally, Cohen's κ was calculated to determine agreement on the number of outliers between measurements of VV2D and VV3D, with an outlier defined as >3° varus or valgus. A χ^2 test was performed to assess statistically significant differences in the number of outliers between VV2D and VV3D. For all statistical analyses, a p-value of <0.05 was considered to indicate statistical significance.

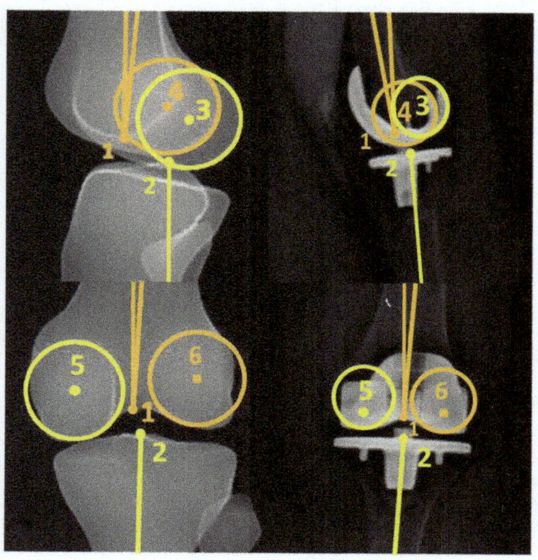

Figure 3. Adjustment of the landmarks on the frontal and lateral images.

Results

On 14 of the 54 images it was not possible to identify medial and lateral condyles of the femoral component on the LAT X-ray and were excluded from further analysis. Eventually, 40 AP and LAT images were available for final analysis. The patient population consisted of 21 men and 16 women, with a mean age of 64.5 years (range 32–83). Of the 40 sets of images, 23 images were made of the left lower limb and 17 of the right lower limb.

Relative intraobserver reliability was excellent when measuring VV2D and VV3D, with ICCs ≥0.98 (Table 1). There was no significant difference between the means of M1 and M2 for any angles. Absolute intraobserver reliability showed no significant bias between for VV2D and VV3D. The SEM was 0.20° and the SDC 0.55° for VV2D. For VV3D, the SEM was 0.43° and the SDC 1.20°. The calculated κ coefficient was 0.94 for both VV2D and VV3D.

Relative interobserver reliability was excellent for both angles, with ICCs ≥0.96 (Table 1). There was no significant difference between the measurements of observer A and observer B. Absolute interobserver reliability of VV2D and VV3D showed no significant bias between the measurements of the two observers. The SEM was 0.41° and the SDC 1.14° for VV2D. For VV3D, the SEM was 0.64° with an SDC of 1.77°. The κ coefficient was 0.78 for VV2D and 0.88 for VV3D.

There was a significant mean and absolute difference between VV2D and VV3D measurements. The mean difference between VV2D and VV3D was 1.00° (1.66–0.34) ($p = 0.004$) and the mean absolute difference was 1.61° (1.09–2.13), with a p-value of < 0.001 (Table 2). The κ coefficient for the agreement between the outliers as determined on 2D and 3D was 0.50.

Scatter graphs of the Bland & Altman method are presented in Figure S1, Figure S2, Figure S3, and Figure S4. Tables of the distribution of outliers are reported in Table S1.

Discussion

A new low-dose X-ray device, called EOS, was recently introduced for determining lower-limb alignment in 2D and 3D [7]. Reliability has not yet been assessed when performing EOS measurements on lower limbs containing a knee prosthesis. Purpose of this study was to determine intraobserver and interobserver reliability of 2D and 3D knee prosthesis alignment measurements after rTKA. Potential differences between 2D and 3D measurements were assessed as a secondary outcome.

Intraobserver and interobserver reliability were excellent for VV2D and VV3D, with no significant differences or systematic bias between the measurements of the two measurement sessions or observers. SEM and SDC of both VV2D and VV3D were small, but larger for VV3D. The κ coefficients showed substantial to almost-perfect intraobserver and interobserver reliability for determining outliers, for both 2D and 3D measurements. A significant mean and absolute difference existed between the angles measured in 2D and 3D.

Results of this study are comparable to other studies investigating reliability of EOS. Intraobserver and interobserver reliability were excellent when measuring VV2D and VV3D (with ICCs $>$ 0.99) on lower limbs containing no knee prostheses [18]. Interobserver reliability was good for EOS 3D varus/valgus measurements on lower limbs of children containing no knee prostheses (Pearson correlation coefficient (Pr) 0.82) [19]. Reliability studies on measurements of vertebrae [20], sagittal balance and spine curves (Pr ≥0.85 and ICCs ≥0.85) [21], spinal curve measurements (ICCs ≥0.84) [22], scoliosis (ICCs ≥0.97) [23], shoulder bony landmarks [24], pelvic and acetabular morphology (ICCs ≥0.80) [25], and pelvic tilt and acetabular cup orientation (ICCs 0.69–0.98) [26], also showed good overall reliability.

SEM and SDC for VV3D were greater than VV2D for both intraobserver and interobserver reliability. A smaller SEM and SDC means that measurements are more precise, but that doesn't indicate which of the two measurement types is more accurate or valid. In this study the SEM and SDC were larger for VV3D than for VV2D. This can be explained by the way in which 2D and 3D measurements are calculated. Since a 3D measurement is calculated through a combination of two planes (coronal and

Table 1. Reported intraobserver and interobserver reliability of varus/valgus angle measured in 2D and 3D.

Intraobserver reliability									
	M1*	M2*	Difference M1–M2 (95% CI)	Range of differenceM1–M2	P-value	ICC (95% CI)	SDΔ	SEM	SDC
VV2D	−1.0 (3.7)	−1.0 (3.8)	−0.02 (−0.11, 0.07)	−0.7, 0.6	0.66	1.00 (1.00, 1.00)	0.28	0.20	0.55
VV3D	−1.9 (3.2)	−2.0 (3.4)	0.08 (−0.11, 0.28)	−1.3, 2.7	0.39	0.98 (0.97, 0.99)	0.61	0.43	1.20
Interobserver reliability									
	Obs. A*	Obs. B*	Difference Obs. A–B (95% CI)	Range of difference obs. A–B	P-value	ICC 95% CI	SDΔ	SEM	SDC
VV2D	−1.1 (3.8)	−0.9 (3.7)	−0.16 (−0.34, 0.03)	−1.5, 0.8	0.85	0.99 (0.98, 0.99)	0.58	0.41	1.14
VV3D	−2.0 (3.4)	−1.9 (3.2)	−0.10 (−0.39, 0.19)	−2.5, 2.2	0.90	0.96 (0.93, 0.98)	0.91	0.64	1.77

*Results are given as mean (sd). Abbreviations: VV2D: varus/valgus angle in 2D, VV3D: varus/valgus angle in 3D, M1: measurement session 1, M2: measurement session 2, sd: standard deviation, CI: confidence interval, ICC: intraclass correlation coefficient, SDΔ: standard error of difference, SEM: standard error of measurement, SDC: smallest detectable change, Obs: observer. Angles are expressed in degrees (°).

Table 2. Difference between 2D and 3D varus/valgus angle measurements.

	Mean	SD	Mean difference	95% CI	P-value
VV2D	−.98	3.75	1.00	1.66–0.34	0.004
VV3D	−1.97	3.28			
Diff	1.61	1.62		1.09–2.13	<0.001

Abbreviations: VV2D: varus/valgus angle in 2D, VV3D: varus/valgus angle in 3D, sd: standard deviation, CI: confidence interval, SDΔ: standard error of difference, SEM: standard error of measurement, SDC: smallest detectable change. Results are given as mean (sd). Angles are expressed in degrees (°).

sagittal) and a 2D measurement is measured in the coronal plane only, slightly more variation can be expected in the 3D measurements and thus a higher SEM and SDC.

One could debate whether the significant differences between 2D and 3D measurements are of clinical importance. Both the mean and absolute difference were small (1.00° (1.66–0.34) and 1.61° (1.09–2.13), respectively). The mean difference is smaller than the absolute difference. For the absolute difference, we stated the deviation of the neutral axis as a positive value, regardless of the deviation being varus or valgus. For the mean difference, varus was stated as a negative value and valgus as a positive value. Calculating the mean difference using both positive and negative values, the deviation may be underestimated. There was only a moderate agreement between 2D and 3D measurements for assessment of outliers — meaning that in 2D different lower limbs are defined as outliers than in 3D.

The influence of lower-limb positioning on 2D measurements has been shown in previous studies. Varus or valgus deformity, axial rotation and flexion of the lower limb at the time of assessment of the radiographs alter coronal measurements of knee alignment [27–30]. When a measurement is taken in 3D, the system mathematically corrects for potential malpositioning during acquisition. EOS VV3D measurements of legs that not contain a knee prosthesis are more accurate than VV2D measurements, eliminating bias due to wrong lower-limb positioning [31]. Validity of EOS VV3D on legs not containing prosthetic material was also investigated in a cadaveric study [19] that measured varus/valgus angle three times using CT-scanning and EOS 3D with each specimen in three different positions: neutral, 10° external rotation and 10° internal rotation. No significant differences between CT and EOS 3D measurements were observed. To gain more insight into validity, additional research has to be conducted in which the accuracy of VV2D and VV3D EOS measurements on lower limbs containing a knee prosthesis are investigated.

This study has some limitations. First of all, when generating a 3D reconstruction of the lower limb with the EOS software it is possible to use the full 3D mode or the lower-limb alignment mode. When using the full 3D mode more angles can be calculated for knee prosthesis alignment, but even more landmarks that have disappeared or changed have to be identified. Hence it was decided not to use the full 3D mode because of a greater chance of errors. Secondly, when it was not possible to identify the medial and lateral condyles on the lateral images, the patient was excluded. In order to identify them on both the AP and the LAT image the condyles have to differ in height on the EOS images. To prevent this in the future, whether the condyles differ in height has to be checked directly after acquisition, otherwise acquisition has to be repeated. Finally, no generally accepted measurement protocol exists for 3D reconstructions of limbs with knee prosthesis material *in situ*. To tackle this issue, the two observers drew up a measurement protocol.

Our study showed that EOS provides reliable varus/valgus measurements of lower limbs containing a revision knee prosthesis in 2D and 3D. There is however a significant difference between varus/valgus measurements in 2D and 3D.

Supporting Information

Figure S1 Bland-Altman plot of intraobserver reliability for VV2D. The dotted line represents the mean difference and the dark lines represent the borders of the 95% confidence intervals.

Figure S2 Bland-Altman plot of intraobserver reliability for VV3D.

Figure S3 Bland-Altman plot of interobserver reliability for VV2D.

Figure S4 Bland-Altman plot of interobserver reliability for VV3D.

Table S1 Tables of the distribution of outliers.

Author Contributions

Conceived and designed the experiments: MFM ALB MS SKB IHFR. Performed the experiments: MFM ALB. Analyzed the data: MFM IHFR. Contributed reagents/materials/analysis tools: MFM ALB SKB. Wrote the paper: MFM. Critically revised the manuscript: ALB MS SKB IHFR. Approved the final version of this manuscript: MFM ALB MS SKB IHFR.

References

1. Ritter MA, Faris PM, Keating EM, Meding JB (1994) Postoperative alignment of total knee replacement. its effect on survival. Clin Orthop Relat Res 299: 153–156.
2. Baker P, Cowling P, Kurtz S, Jameson S, Gregg P, et al. (2012) Reason for revision influences early patient outcomes after aseptic knee revision. Clin Orthop Relat Res 470: 2244–2252.
3. Sheng PY, Konttinen L, Lehto M, Ogino D, Jamsen E, et al. (2006) Revision total knee arthroplasty: 1990 through 2002. A review of the finnish arthroplasty registry. J Bone Joint Surg Am 88: 1425–1430.
4. Choong PF, Dowsey MM, Stoney JD (2009) Does accurate anatomical alignment result in better function and quality of life? comparing conventional and computer-assisted total knee arthroplasty. J Arthroplasty 24: 560–569.
5. Longstaff L, Sloan K, Stamp N, Scaddan M, Beaver R (2009) Good alignment after total knee arthroplasty leads to faster rehabilitation and better function. J Arthroplasty 24: 570–578.
6. Jeffery RS, Morris RW, Denham RA (1991) Coronal alignment after total knee replacement. J Bone Joint Surg Br 73: 709–714.

7. Dubousset J, Charpak G, Dorion I, Skalli W, Lavaste F, et al. (2005) A new 2D and 3D imaging approach to musculoskeletal physiology and pathology with low-dose radiation and the standing position: The EOS system. Bull Acad Natl Med 189: 287–300.
8. Kalifa G, Charpak Y, Maccia C, Fery-Lemonnier E, Bloch J, et al. (1998) Evaluation of a new low-dose digital x-ray device: First dosimetric and clinical results in children. Pediatr Radiol 28: 557–561.
9. EOS-imaging (2011) sterEOS workstation operator manual.
10. Rankin G, Stokes M (1998) Reliability of assessment tools in rehabilitation: An illustration of appropriate statistical analyses. Clin Rehabil 12: 187–199.
11. Fleiss J (1986) The design and analysis of clinical experiments. new york: John whiley.
12. Bland JM, Altman DG (1986) Statistical methods for assessing agreement between two methods of clinical measurement. Lancet 1: 307–310.
13. Cohen JA (1960) A coefficient of agreement for nominal scales. Educational and Psychological Measurement 33: 159–174.
14. Landis JR, Koch GG (1977) The measurement of observer agreement for categorical data. Biometrics 33: 159–174.
15. Beckerman H, Roebroeck M, Lankhorst G, Becher J, Bezemer P, et al. (2001) Smallest real change, a link between reproductibility and responsiveness. Qual Life Res 10: 571–578.
16. Stratford P (1989) Reliability: Consistency or differentiating among subjects? Phys Ther 69: 299–300.
17. de Vet H, Bouter L, Bezemer P, Beurskens A (2001) Reproductibility and responsiveness of evaluative outcome measures. theoretical considerations illustrated by an empirical example. Int J Technol Assess Health Care 17: 479–487.
18. Guenoun B, Zadegan F, Aim F, Hannouche D, Nizard R (2012) Reliability of a new method for lower-extremity measurements based on stereoradiographic three-dimensional reconstruction. Orthop Traumatol Surg Res 98: 506–513.
19. Gheno R, Nectoux E, Herbaux B, Baldisserotto M, Glock L, et al. (2012) Three-dimensional measurements of the lower extremity in children and adolescents using a low-dose biplanar X-ray device. Eur Radiol 22: 765–771.
20. Rousseau MA, Laporte S, Chavary-Bernier E, Lazennec JY, Skalli W (2007) Reproducibility of measuring the shape and three-dimensional position of cervical vertebrae in upright position using the EOS stereoradiography system. Spine 32: 2569–2572.
21. Vidal C, Ilharreborde B, Azoulay R, Sebag G, Mazda K (2013) Reliability of cervical lordosis and global sagittal spinal balance measurements in adolescent idiopathic scoliosis. Eur Spine J 22: 1362–1367.
22. Somoskeoy S, Tunyogi-Csapo M, Bogyo C, Illes T (2012) Accuracy and reliability of coronal and sagittal spinal curvature data based on patient-specific three-dimensional models created by the EOS 2D/3D imaging system. Spine J 12: 1052–1059.
23. Ilharreborde B, Steffen JS, Nectoux E, Vital JM, Mazda K, et al. (2011) Angle measurement reproducibility using EOS three-dimensional reconstructions in adolescent idiopathic scoliosis treated by posterior instrumentation. Spine 36: 1306–1313.
24. Ohl X, Stanchina C, Billuart F, Skalli W (2010) Shoulder bony landmarks location using the EOS low-dose stereoradiography system: A reproducibility study. Surg Radiol Anat 32: 153–158.
25. Bittersohl B, Freitas J, Zaps D, Schmitz MR, Bomar JD, et al. (2013) EOS imaging of the human pelvis: Reliability, validity, and controlled comparison with radiography. J Bone Joint Surg Am 95: 581–589.
26. Lazennec JY, Rousseau MA, Rangel A, Gorin M, Belicourt C, et al. (2011) Pelvis and total hip arthroplasty acetabular component orientations in sitting and standing positions: Measurements reproductibility with EOS imaging system versus conventional radiographies. Orthop Traumatol Surg Res 97: 373–380.
27. Lonner JH, Laird MT, Stuchin SA (1996) Effect of rotation and knee flexion on radiographic alignment in total knee arthroplasties. Clin Orthop Relat Res 331: 102–106.
28. Radtke K, Becher C, Noll Y, Ostermeier S (2010) Effect of limb rotation on radiographic alignment in total knee arthroplasties. Arch Orthop Trauma Surg 130: 451–457.
29. Swanson KE, Stocks GW, Warren PD, Hazel MR, Janssen HF (2000) Does axial limb rotation affect the alignment measurements in deformed limbs? Clin Orthop Relat Res 371: 246–252.
30. Brouwer RW, Jakma TS, Brouwer KH, Verhaar JA (2007) Pitfalls in determining knee alignment: A radiographic cadaver study. J Knee Surg 20: 210–215.
31. Thelen P, Delin C, Folinais D, Radier C (2012) Evaluation of a new low-dose biplanar system to assess lower-limb alignment in 3D: A phantom study. Skeletal Radiol 41: 1287–1293.

3

A Proton Beam Therapy System Dedicated to Spot-Scanning Increases Accuracy with Moving Tumors by Real-Time Imaging and Gating and Reduces Equipment Size

Shinichi Shimizu[1], Naoki Miyamoto[2], Taeko Matsuura[3]*, Yusuke Fujii[4], Masumi Umezawa[4], Kikuo Umegaki[5], Kazuo Hiramoto[6], Hiroki Shirato[1]

1 Department of Radiation Oncology, Hokkaido University Graduate School of Medicine, Sapporo, Hokkaido, Japan, **2** Department of Medical Physics, Hokkaido University Graduate School of Medicine, Sapporo, Hokkaido, Japan, **3** Section of Medical Physics, Hokkaido University Hospital Proton Beam Therapy Center, Sapporo, Hokkaido, Japan, **4** Hitachi, Ltd., Hitachi Research Laboratory, Omika, Ibaraki, Japan, **5** Division of Quantum Science and Engineering, Hokkaido University Graduate School of Engineering, Sapporo, Hokkaido, Japan, **6** Hitachi, Ltd., Research & Development Group, Omika, Ibaraki, Japan

Abstract

Purpose: A proton beam therapy (PBT) system has been designed which dedicates to spot-scanning and has a gating function employing the fluoroscopy-based real-time-imaging of internal fiducial markers near tumors. The dose distribution and treatment time of the newly designed real-time-image gated, spot-scanning proton beam therapy (RGPT) were compared with free-breathing spot-scanning proton beam therapy (FBPT) in a simulation.

Materials and Methods: In-house simulation tools and treatment planning system VQA (Hitachi, Ltd., Japan) were used for estimating the dose distribution and treatment time. Simulations were performed for 48 motion parameters (including 8 respiratory patterns and 6 initial breathing timings) on CT data from two patients, A and B, with hepatocellular carcinoma and with clinical target volumes 14.6 cc and 63.1 cc. The respiratory patterns were derived from the actual trajectory of internal fiducial markers taken in X-ray real-time tumor-tracking radiotherapy (RTRT).

Results: With FBPT, 9/48 motion parameters achieved the criteria of successful delivery for patient A and 0/48 for B. With RGPT 48/48 and 42/48 achieved the criteria. Compared with FBPT, the mean liver dose was smaller with RGPT with statistical significance ($p<0.001$); it decreased from 27% to 13% and 28% to 23% of the prescribed doses for patients A and B, respectively. The relative lengthening of treatment time to administer 3 Gy (RBE) was estimated to be 1.22 (RGPT/FBPT: 138 s/113 s) and 1.72 (207 s/120 s) for patients A and B, respectively.

Conclusions: This simulation study demonstrated that the RGPT was able to improve the dose distribution markedly for moving tumors without very large treatment time extension. The proton beam therapy system dedicated to spot-scanning with a gating function for real-time imaging increases accuracy with moving tumors and reduces the physical size, and subsequently the cost of the equipment as well as of the building housing the equipment.

Editor: Jonathan A. Coles, Glasgow University, United Kingdom

Funding: This research was supported by the Japan Society for the Promotion of Science (JSPS) through the "Funding Program for World-Leading Innovative R&D on Science and Technology (FIRST Program)," initiated by the Council for Science and Technology Policy (CSTP). The funders had no role in study design, data collection and analysis, decision to publish, or preparation of the manuscript.

Competing Interests: The following is the patent relating to material pertinent to this article: "Moving body pursuit irradiating device and positioning method using this device"; Number: US6307914 B1; Issue Date: 2001-10-23; Inventors: Tatsuya Kunieda, Hiroki Shirato. Yusuke Fujii, Masumi Umezawa, and Kazuo Hiramoto are the permanent employees of Hitachi, Ltd. Their affiliation is as follows: Yusuke Fujii Hitachi, Ltd., Hitachi Research Laboratory. Masumi Umezawa Hitachi, Ltd., Hitachi Research Laboratory. Kazuo Hiramoto Hitachi, Ltd., Research & Development Group.

* E-mail: matsuura@med.hokudai.ac.jp

Introduction

Proton beam therapy (PBT) has the potential to create better dose distributions than X-ray therapy in many situations. There are two different types of PBT, passive scattering PBT and spot-scanning PBT [1,2]. Spot-scanning proton beam therapy (SSPT) is expected to be more suitable to create complex dose distributions and to be safer than the conventional passive scattering method because it reduces neutron contamination [3]. However, there is a larger uncertainty in the dose distribution for tumors in motion due to interplay effects between the time-dependent scanning beam delivery and tumor motion, and this is a disadvantage of the spot-scanning method when compared with passive scattering [4].

The precision of passive scattering proton beam delivery for tumors in motion has been estimated using the motion signals of

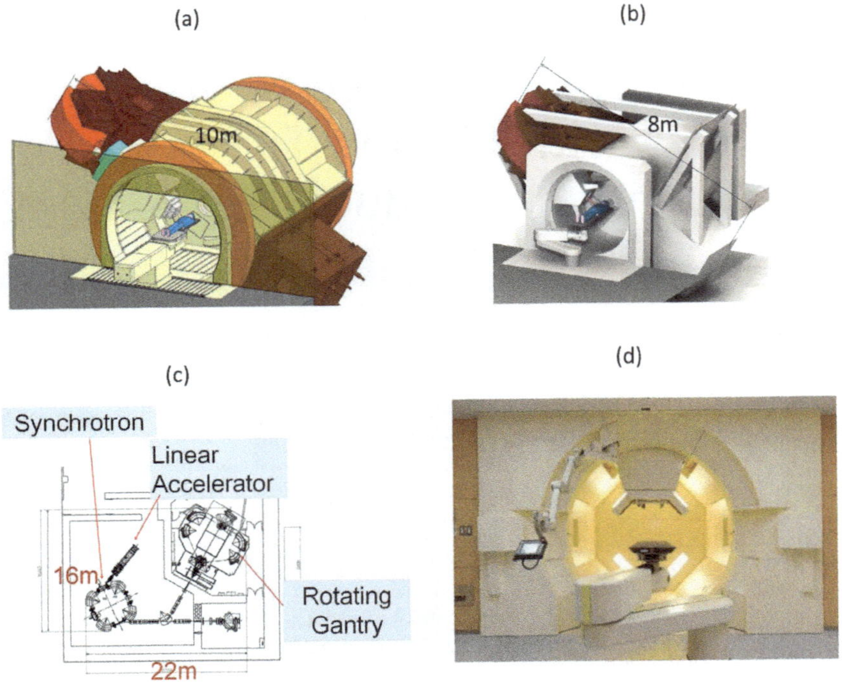

Figure 1. RGPT system at Hokkaido University. (a) The gantry of the passive scattering PBT system. (b) The gantry of the RGPT system. (c) The footprint for one gantry and one fixed beam system with a linear accelerator and synchrotron, and (d) The actual RGPT system installed.

surface skin markers in Tsunashima et al [5,6]. It was shown that the synchrotron magnet excitation pattern is an important factor to improve the precision of PBT. However, in clinical situations, it is difficult to achieve dose distributions that closely match the static irradiation, when gating is employed by using the motion of the skin surface, because the internal motion of lung and liver tumors is usually different from the surface motion of the chest wall [7,8]. This difference may be critical in the case of SSPT. Analysis of the internal motion of fiducial markers near a tumor can be expected to be useful in the evaluation of interplay effects [9]. Also, the cost and size of the SSPT equipment with its advanced technology are further concerns for potential users of SSPT.

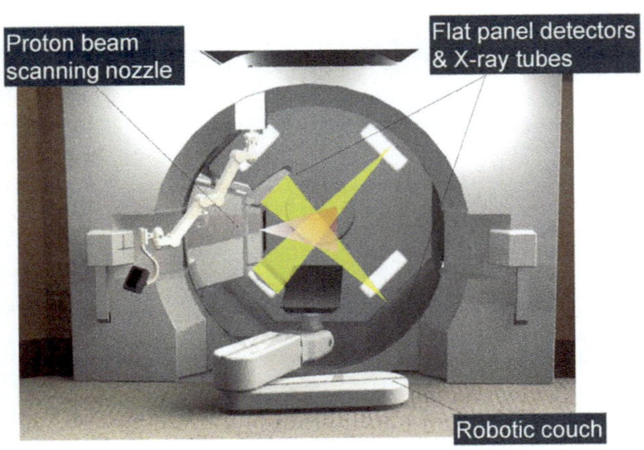

Figure 2. Design of a spot-scanning proton beam therapy-dedicated system with X-ray fluoroscopy. Two orthogonal sets of X-ray fluoroscopic generators and flat panels can be mounted in the gantry.

We have investigated gated PBT systems dedicated to the spot-scanning method as one solution to improve on these drawbacks. In a previous study, we investigated the dose distribution in a water phantom for a gated SSPT with a gating window of ± 2 mm [9]. The three-dimensional (3D) trajectory of a fiducial marker near a lung tumor, which was derived from actual data of internal fiducial markers in real-time tumor-tracking radiotherapy (RTRT), was used in the simulation. That study showed that gated SSPT for a moving target achieved a dose distribution similar to SSPT for a static target. However, it is not obvious whether this result is also satisfied in the human body. There are also concerns about the lengthening of treatment time due to the gating. The 3D motion of tumors is often irregular, involving baseline shifting, and it is also influenced by cardiac as well as respiratory motion, as we have reported elsewhere [7,10]. If a synchrotron is used without careful attention to these characteristics of tumor motion, on-off signals from internal fiducial markers will change irregularly and sporadically and the treatment time with gated SSPT may become considerably prolonged.

In this study, we investigate the impact of the gated spot-scanning method on proton dose distributions and the lengthening of treatment times in a clinical setting using actual patient computed tomography and recorded data of internal tumor motion.

Materials and Methods

We have been developing an RGPT system since 2009 (Figure 1). We have found that the cost for the system and related buildings are decreased, not increased, by dedicating to SSPT. This is possible because we can avoid the scattering components in the nozzle and reduce the size of the equipment and the overall footprint. The radius of the gantry can be shortened from 5 m to 4 m and the weight reduced from 160 tons to 100 tons. Since there is no energy loss with the absent of scattering components, the

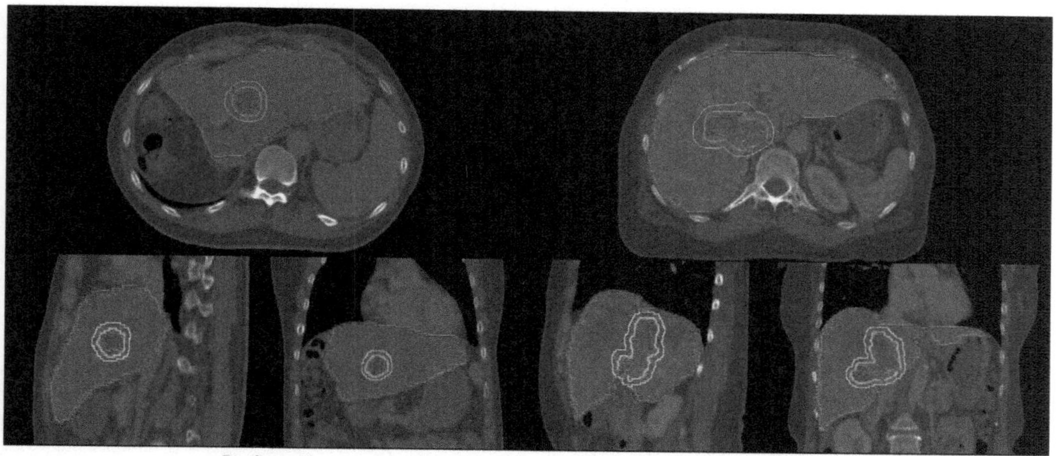

Figure 3. CT images and target delineations. Computed tomography for the patients with hepatocellular carcinoma included in this study. Gross tumor volumes (red), clinical target volumes (green), liver (blue), and planning target volumes for the RGPT (white) for patient A (left) and patient B (right).

maximum energy to treat tumors at 30 cm depth in a human body can be reduced from 250 MeV to 220 MeV. The efficiency of the proton beam increases from about 20% to about 100%, and thus the accelerated proton current can be reduced from 10 nC to 2 nC. Consequently, the size of the synchrotron becomes more compact than with passive scattering systems, its circumference being reduced from 23 m to 18 m. A 35% reduction, from 546 m^2 to 352 m^2, was achieved in the footprint for a system with one gantry and one fixed beam with the capacity to expand to a system with multiple gantries. The total cost was reduced accordingly. Acceptance tests are in progress, and clinical use of the system is to be started from March 2014.

As an SSPT-dedicated system does not require compensators and collimators, in principle, we are able to install two orthogonal sets of X-ray fluoroscopes in the gantry (Figure 2). The X-ray images can be acquired simultaneously with proton beam irradiation, and their fields of view will not be narrowed by these field-shaping devices. Cone-beam computed tomography, which is useful to reduce inter-fractional set-up errors, can be created by rotating the gantry using the X-ray fluoroscope [11]. By using simultaneous orthogonal fluoroscopic real-time images, fiducial markers near the tumor can be detected every 0.033 s with a delay of about 0.05 s and with an accuracy of 1 mm during the delivery of the SSPT, as in RTRT with X-ray therapy [12]. The tumor is irradiated only when its location corresponds to the planned position within an accuracy of ± 1–2 mm by gating the proton beam using the real-time-images. This function can reduce random errors, as is well known from the use of RTRT in X-ray therapy. In this study, the SSPT system is termed a real-time-image gated proton beam therapy (RGPT) since the proton beam is gated with the real-time-images of fiducial markers in the patient being treated.

The study investigates the efficacy of RGPT, comparing it to non-gated free-breathing SSPT (FBPT). CT data sets of two patients with hepatic carcinomas were used for the comparison, and CT images were taken at the end of the exhale phase with a 2.5-mm slice interval using a 64 multi-detector CT scan. The total liver volumes were 1105 cc and 1688 cc, respectively (Figure 3). The two tumors had clinical target volumes (CTV) of 14.6 cc and 63.1 cc, respectively. We assumed administration of 3.0 Gy (RBE (relative biological effectiveness) = 1.1) at the isocenter of the CTV. We further selected 8 representative patterns of tumor motion derived from the actual data of internal fiducial markers near hepatocellular carcinomas in X-ray RTRT (Figure 4). The amplitude and data acquisition time for each fiducial marker are shown in Table 1. As we have reported elsewhere [8], the 3D coordinates of the internal fiducial markers were detected and recorded every 0.033 s using two sets of fluoroscopes in the X-ray RTRT. The shift of the marker positions from the planned (original) positions was assumed to represent the shift of the tumor in this study. For simplicity, we have not included the deformable nature of patient body in the simulation, which would lead to the additional range changes in the beam path. The 8 patterns of tumor motion were applied to the 2 hepatic tumors in the following simulation, and for each pattern, 6 different initial breathing timings were considered at 1 s intervals.

The static plans were generated in a treatment planning system, VQA (Hitachi, Ltd., Japan). Parameters used in the treatment planning for each patient are shown in Table 2. Using the beam scanning sequence of a PROBEAT series proton accelerator (Hitachi, Ltd., Japan), each beam position was translocated by the values of the tumor motion at the moment of the spot irradiation using in-house simulation tools. Then, the dose distributions were calculated using the actual spot positions. In the treatment planning, the planning target volume (PTV) was drawn as the geometric expansion of CTV as in the photon planning. For RGPT, PTV was defined as PTV_{rg} = CTV + an internal margin (3 mm) + a residual margin (2 mm) and for FBPT, PTV_{fb} = CTV + an internal margin (5 mm LR, 5 mm AP, 10 mm SI) + a residual margin (2 mm). Here, the internal margin is added to compensate for the target motion, which mainly results from respiration and cardiac motion, while the residual margin is added to compensate for the various set-up uncertainties.

The synchrotron operation pattern and beam waiting function are schematically drawn in Fig. 5. The synchrotron operation in gating mode has the operation phases of injection, acceleration, wait for first gate, extraction, and deceleration. The operation cycle of the synchrotron varies approximately from 2 to 7 s. The acceleration and deceleration both require about 1 s. The flat top length, which consists of wait for first gate and extraction time, has a maximum of 5 s. Beam waiting function was installed to this system in order to improve irradiation efficiency. This function

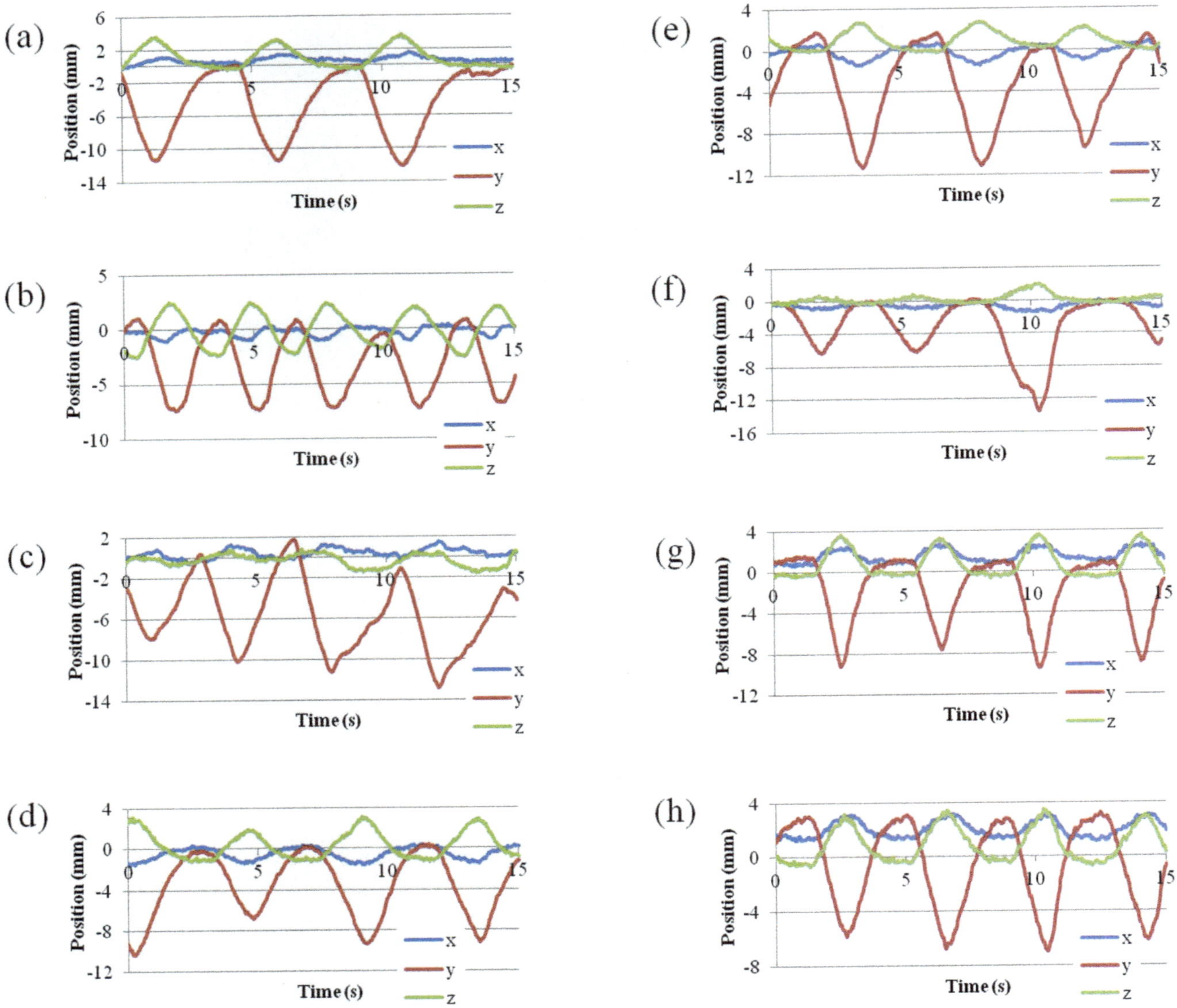

Figure 4. Tumor motions obtained with RTRT system. Eight patterns of tumor motion derived from actual data of internal fiducial markers near hepatocellular carcinomas in the X-ray RTRT of 8 patients.

enables to multiple gate irradiations per synchrotron operation cycle. In this function, waiting timer limit 200 ms has been applied from the view point of stability of circulating proton in the synchrotron and beam irradiation efficiency [13].

Table 1. x, y, and z components of the amplitude of movement of a fiducial marker near the tumor, and data acquisition time, in 8 patients with hepatocellular carcinomas.

Motion ID	x(LR) (mm)	y(SI) (mm)	z(AP) (mm)	Data acquisition time (s)
a	2	15.5	5.7	128
b	2.1	10.7	6.1	133
c	2.4	18	2.8	104
d	2.7	20	7.7	160
e	2.8	17.6	3.9	155
f	1.7	14	2.6	85
g	3.1	12.1	4.8	77
h	2.4	10.2	4.3	47

Data were taken by a X-ray real-time tumor-tracking radiotherapy (RTRT) system.

Table 2. Parameters used in the treatment planning.

Patient ID	A	B
Gantry angle	0°	270°
PTV (cm3)	38.7(RGPT), 123.3(FBPT)	134.3(RGPT), 204.2(FBPT)
Energy (MeV)	89–123(RGPT), 82–128(FBPT)	97–152(RGPT), 93–155(FBPT)
Number of layers	29(RGPT), 41(FBPT)	36(RGPT), 41(FBPT)
Spot interval (mm)	6	6
Max. MU/spot	0.04	0.04
Number of spots	2015(RGPT), 4638(FBPT)	4025(RGPT), 5314(FBPT)

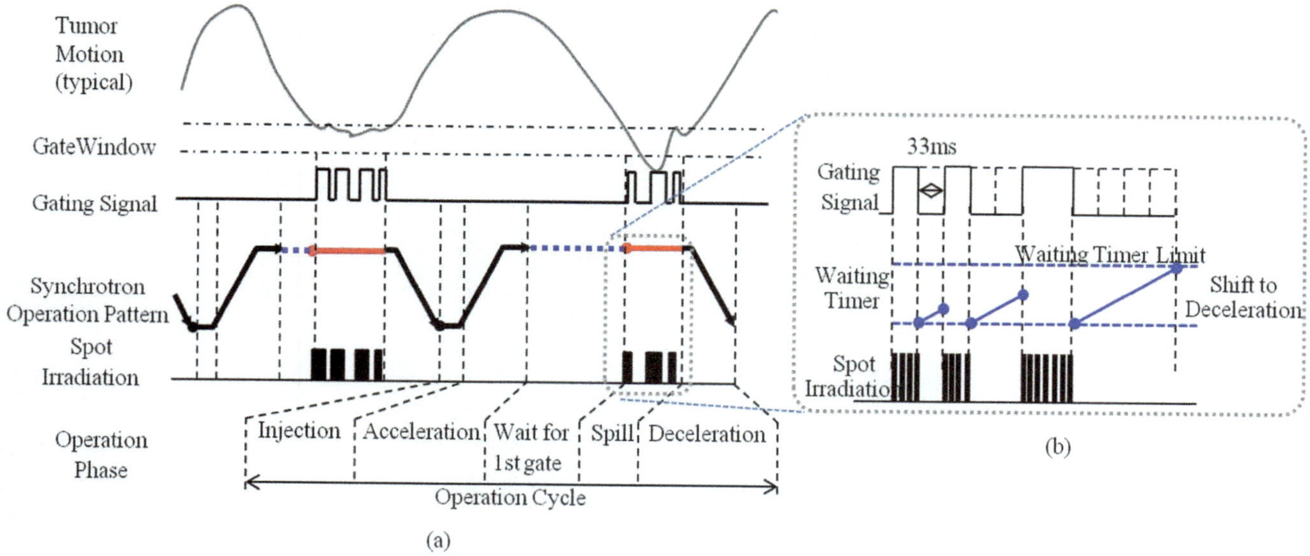

Figure 5. Diagram of the (a) synchrotron operation and (b) beam waiting function. The operation cycle of the synchrotron varies approximately from 2 to 7 s. The flat top length which consists of wait for the first gate and extraction time has a maximum of 5 s. During extraction, beam waiting function enables to irradiate proton beam to the multiple gates per operation cycle.

In this simulation, the maximum flat top and extraction time were set to 5 s and 4.4 s, respectively. The beam delivery started from the deepest layer to the shallowest layer and each iso-energy layer was individually rescanned. From the viewpoint of safety, the maximum deliverable dose per spot is limited to 0.04 in the monitor unit (MU) and the delivered dose is checked spot by spot, where the definition of MU is the same as that described in Gillin et al [14]. When the planned MU for a spot exceeds the pre-defined value under the limit of 0.04, the spot is revisited. We set the pre-defined value to 0.04, which indicates the minimum number of repeated deliveries is performed. Note that although a larger number of rescanning is expected to wash out the hot and cold spots that may occur as a result of the interplay effect, it should also lengthen the irradiation time. The scanning speed, the beam current, and the gating window were set to 10 m/s, 7.5 MU/s, and ±2 mm, respectively. The latency of the system is defined as the duration between the generation of the pulsed x-ray beam of the fluoroscope and the resultant proton beam-on/off, including the image acquisition/procession; it was set to 66 ms.

The mean of mean live dose (MLD) among 8 patterns of tumor motion in FBPT was compared with the mean of MLD in RGPT using paired t-test in each patient. The Ansari-Bradley test was used for comparisons between RGPT and FBPT on the maximum and minimum doses in the CTV.

This study has been approved by the institutional review board of Hokkaido University Hospital (011-0124). The requirement for written consent was waived by our institutional board according to the Ethical Guidelines for Clinical Studies of the Japanese Ministry of Health, Labour and Welfare.

Table 3. Treatment times for FBPT and RGPT.

Patient ID		A	B
FBRT for PTVfb		113	120
RGPT for PTVrg	static (s)*	74	101
	mean (s)	138	207
	max (s)	185	314
	min (s)	96	126

Mean, maximum, and minimum values are those of 8 respiratory patterns and 6 initial timings of motion data.

*: Treatment time required for static irradiation for PTV_{rg}, which is smaller than PTV_{fb}.

Results

The total irradiation time in RGPT and FBPT for each patient was estimated to irradiate 3.0 Gy (RBE) at the isocenter (Table 3). In RGPT, the mean treatment times for PTV_{rg} of patient A and patient B were 138 (96–185) s and 207 (126–314) s, respectively, where the range of values is shown in parentheses. If we irradiate the PTV_{rg} to a static target, the treatment time is estimated to be 74 s and 101 s, respectively. Thus, the physical ratios of lengthening of the treatment time due to the gating were 1.87 (138/74) and 2.05 (207/101) for patients A and B, respectively. However, the PTV_{rg} does not include internal margins in the free-breathing mode and is too small for actual irradiation with free-breathing. Treatment times for PTV_{fb}, the PTV including the internal margin in free-breathing, were 113 s and 120 s for patients A and B, respectively. Therefore, the clinical ratios of lengthening of the treatment time were estimated to be 1.22 (138/113) and 1.72 (207/120), respectively. The minimum treatment time with RGPT for PTV_{rg} (96s) was shorter than the treatment time with FBPT for PTV_{fb} (113s) due to the differences in the volumes of PTV_{rg} and PTV_{fb} (Table 3).

Table 4 details the maximum and the minimum doses in the CTV relative to the prescribed dose at the isocenter of the CTV for the combination of the 2 targets, 8 respiratory patterns, and 6 initial breathing timings. Based on the recommended dose homogeneity in ICRU (1999) [15], we considered that the dose was successfully delivered to the CTV if the dose in CTV was within the range between 95% and 107%. In the FBPT, 9 of 48 (9/48) and 0/48 motion parameters (including respiratory patterns and initial breathing timings) achieved the criteria for successful delivery, whereas in the RGPT, 48/48 and 42/48 achieved the

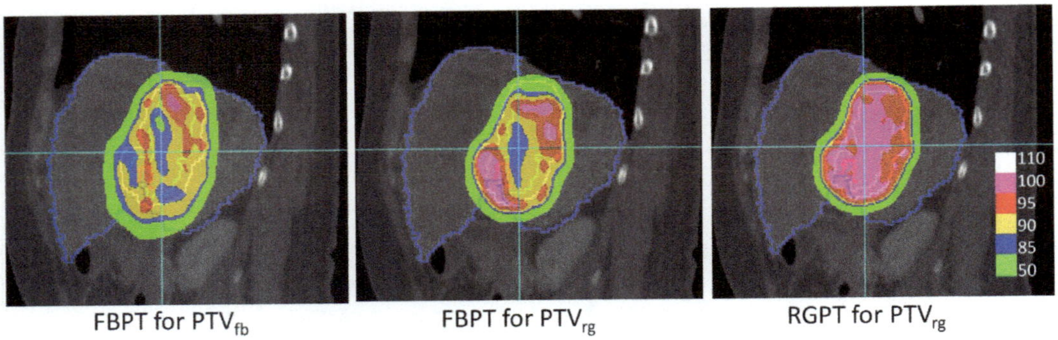

Figure 6. Comparison of dose distribution between FBPT and RGPT. Images of the dose distributions with FBPT for PTV_{fb}(left), FBPT for PTV_{rg} (center), and RGPT for PTV_{rg} (right) for the CT images of patient B with tumor motion ID of b.

criteria for patients A and B, respectively (Figure 6). The improvement in success rate was more pronounced in patient B, with a larger PTV. As shown in Table 4, the maximum to minimum range of 6 initial breathing timings was apparent in FBPT but was quite small in RGPT. The Ansari-Bradley test were applied and showed that RGPT reduced the variances in either maximum or minimum doses in 7 of 8 respiratory patterns in patient A and 6 of 8 in patient B with statistical significance ($p<0.05$) (Table 4). It reduced the variances in both maximum and minimum doses compared with the FBPT in 6 of 8 respiratory patterns in patient A and 4 of 8 respiratory patters in patient B with statistical significance ($p<0.05$). These facts suggest that the influence of the initial breathing timing on the dose homogeneity can be reduced in RGPT compared with free breathing in the

Table 4. Maximum and minimum doses in CTV scaled by the prescribed dose, and mean liver doses in FBPT and in RGPT, averaged over 6 initial timings of motion data.

FBPT						
Motion ID	Patient A			Patient B		
	Max	Min	MLD	Max	Min	MLD
static	1.01	0.98	0.27	1.02	0.98	0.28
a	1.11(1.20–1.06)	0.93(0.96–0.81)	0.27	1.18(1.26–1.09)	0.78(0.83–0.72)	0.28
b	1.05(1.11–1.01)	0.94(0.98–0.90)	0.27	1.11(1.14–1.08)	0.86(0.91–0.82)	0.28
c	1.08(1.15–1.03)	0.95(0.98–0.89)	0.27	1.13(1.26–1.08)	0.79(0.87–0.70)	0.28
d	1.06(1.10–1.03)	0.94(0.98–0.91)	0.27	1.19(1.26–1.11)	0.85(0.91–0.76)	0.28
e	1.07(1.11–1.03)	0.92(0.98–0.89)	0.27	1.15(1.20–1.11)	0.81(0.88–0.75)	0.28
f	1.05(1.07–1.00)	0.92(0.98–0.80)	0.27	1.09(1.10–1.07)	0.90(0.97–0.79)	0.28
g	1.05(1.11–1.03)	0.95(0.98–0.93)	0.27	1.16(1.29–1.09)	0.85(0.91–0.80)	0.28
h	1.05(1.11–1.01)	0.94(0.99–0.89)	0.27	1.19(1.29–1.06)	0.87(0.93–0.76)	0.28
RGPT						
Motion ID	Patient A			Patient B		
	Max	Min	MLD	Max	Min	MLD
static	1.02	0.99	0.13	1.03	0.98	0.23
a	1.02(1.03–1.02)	0.98(0.98–0.98)	0.13	1.03(1.03–1.03)	0.97(0.97–0.96)	0.22
b	1.02(1.03–1.02)	0.98(0.99–0.98)	0.13	1.05(1.05–1.03)	0.96(0.97–0.95)	0.22
c	1.03(1.04–1.02)	0.98(0.98–0.96)	0.13	1.03(1.03–1.03)	0.96(0.96–0.96)	0.23
d	1.02(1.02–1.02)	0.98(0.99–0.98)	0.13	1.05(1.06–1.04)	0.97(0.98–0.96)	0.22
e	1.03(1.03–1.03)	0.97(0.97–0.96)	0.13	1.06(1.06–1.05)	0.95(0.96–0.94)	0.23
f	1.02(1.02–1.01)	0.98(0.99–0.97)	0.13	1.04(1.04–1.04)	0.98(0.98–0.98)	0.22
g	1.03(1.03–1.03)	0.98(0.99–0.97)	0.13	1.05(1.08–1.03)	0.96(0.98–0.96)	0.23
h	1.03(1.03–1.02)	0.98(0.98–0.98)	0.13	1.03(1.04–1.02)	0.97(0.97–0.96)	0.23

The range of values are shown in brackets.

majority of situations. The mean liver dose for the liver volume minus the gross tumor volume (MLD) was also estimated and is shown in Table 4. Compared to FBPT, MLD was reduced in RGPT with statistical significance, from 0.27 to 0.13 ($p<0.001$) and from 0.28 to 0.22–0.23 ($p<0.001$) for patients A and B, respectively. The reduction rates of MLD were 51.9% and 17.9% for patient A and patient B, respectively. There was no apparent difference in the ratio of reduction in MLD between the 8 patterns of tumor motion in the 2 patients (Table 4).

Discussion

The present study found that the dose distribution with hepatic carcinomas can be improved in MLD by using RGPT with statistical significance, when compared with FBPT, based on a comparison using actual data sets of the internal motion of fiducial markers. It is notable that RGPT was able to provide 95–107% coverage of CTV even with the minimum number of repaintings. In addition to the better dose distribution in CTV for RGPT, the MLD can be reduced by about 50% in patient A, who had a small tumor, and by about 20% in patient B, who had a large tumor. We also found that the reduction rate of MLD did not depend on the patterns of tumor motion but on the size of the target. The large reduction rate for patient A with the small tumor suggests that RGPT would be suitable for patients with poor hepatic function and with small tumors, and it is worth noting in this context that patients with small tumors could be adequately treated with X-ray stereotactic radiotherapy in our previous study [16].

Another important finding here is that the treatment times were not prominently lengthened when using RGPT. From our clinical experience through X-ray treatment, the lengthening ratios of 1.22 and 1.72 that we observed in this study would be manageable. With respect to the evaluated treatment time, the additional dose due to real-time imaging is estimated to be less than 50 mGy, assuming the typical imaging conditions used in a conventional real-time imaging system. An accumulated imaging dose would be clinically acceptable. It must be noted that reductions in the PTV can greatly shorten the treatment time in SSPT. Adding to this difference due to the size of the target volume, a further developed gating function will reduce the estimated treatment time [13]. The new function enables multiple gated irradiations per synchrotron cycle, to improve the irradiation efficiency and reduce treatment times.

A shortcoming of this study is the use of a rigid motion model in the simulation; the scanning beam was assumed to change position relative to the static CTV in the human body. The dose distribution would change if the changes in the water-equivalent path length along the beam path were correctly included in the simulation. The number of fields also can affect the results. A precise analysis of these effects should be performed using 4D computed tomography or 4D magnetic resonance images, and the verification by actual measurements has to be done in future [17]. Also, it is important to note that to confirm this new system delivers the treatment as expected, we have to examine patient outcomes over time.

The effect of gold markers on the dose distribution has been known to be a potential hazard in particle therapy. Since SSPT does not require compensators and collimators, SSPT is suitable for multiple beam treatment. In a previous study, the effect of gold markers was found to be biologically negligible if multiple beams were used to irradiate the target [18].

In conclusion, spot-scanning proton beam therapy can improve dose distribution with real-time imaging and gating. There is no serious lengthening of treatment times with the real-time-image gating because of the smaller internal margin and new developments in gating functions. The results and considerations here allow the conclusion that a proton beam therapy system dedicated to spot-scanning and incorporating the capability for real-time imaging and gating can reduce the total size and cost of the equipment and facilities.

Author Contributions

Conceived and designed the experiments: MU KU KH HS. Analyzed the data: SS NM TM. Contributed reagents/materials/analysis tools: SS NM YF. Wrote the paper: TM HS.

References

1. Kawachi K, Kanai T, Matsuzawa H, Inada T (1983) Three dimensional spot beam scanning method for proton conformation radiation therapy. Acta Radiol Suppl. 364: 81–8.
2. Smith A, Gillin M, Bues M, Zhu XR, Suzuki K, et al. (2009) The M. D. Anderson proton therapy system. Med Phys. 36: 4068–83.
3. Hall EJ (2006) Intensity-modulated radiation therapy, protons, and the risk of second cancers. Int J Radiat Oncol Biol Phys. 65: 1–7.
4. Rietzel E, Bert C (2010) Respiratory motion management in particle therapy. Med Phys. 37: 449–460.
5. Tsunashima Y, Vedam S, Dong L, Umezawa M, Sakae T, et al. (2008) Efficiency of respiratory-gated delivery of synchrotron-based pulsed proton irradiation. Phys Med Biol. 53: 1947–59.
6. Tsunashima Y, Vedam S, Dong L, Umezawa M, Balter P, et al. (2010) The precision of respiratory-gated delivery of synchrotron-based pulsed beam proton therapy. Phys Med Biol. 55: 7633–47.
7. Seppenwoolde Y, Shirato H, Kitamura K, Shimizu S, van Herk M, et al. (2002) Precise and real-time measurement of 3D tumor motion in lung due to breathing and heartbeat, measured during radiotherapy. Int J Radiat Oncol Biol Phys. 53: 822–34.
8. Shirato H, Onimaru R, Ishikawa M, Kaneko J, Takeshima T, et al. (2012) Real-time 4-D radiotherapy for lung cancer. Cancer Sci. 103: 1–6.
9. Matsuura T, Miyamoto N, Shimizu S, Fujii Y, Umezawa M, et al. (2013) Integration of a real-time tumor monitoring system into gated proton spot-scanning beam therapy: an initial phantom study using patient tumor trajectory data. Med Phys. 40: 071729.
10. Shirato H, Suzuki K, Sharp GC, Fujita K, Onimaru R, et al. (2006) Speed and amplitude of lung tumor motion precisely detected in four-dimensional setup and in real-time tumor-tracking radiotherapy. Int J Radiat Oncol Biol Phys. 64: 1229–36.
11. Jaffray DA (2012) Image-guided radiotherapy: from current concept to future perspectives. Nat Rev Clin Oncol. 9: 688–99.
12. Shirato H, Shimizu S, Shimizu T, Nishioka T, Miyasaka K, et al. (1999) Real-time tumour-tracking radiotherapy. Lancet Oncol.353: 1331–2.
13. Umezawa M, Fujimoto R, Umekawa T, Fujii Y, Takayanagi T, et al. (2012) Development of the compact proton beam therapy system dedicated to spot-scanning with real-time tumor-tracking technology. AIP Conf. Proc. 1525: 360–363.
14. Gillin M, Sahoo N, Bues M, Ciangaru G, Sawakuchi G, et al. (2010) Commissioning of the discrete spot scanning proton beam delivery system at The University of Texas M. D. Anderson Cancer Center, Proton Therapy Center Houston. Med Phys. 37, 154–163.
15. ICRU (1999) Prescribing, recording and reporting photon beam therapy (supplement to ICRU Report 50) ICRU Report No 62 (Bethesda, MD: ICRU).
16. Toramatsu C, Katoh N, Shimizu S, Nihongi H, Matsuura T, et al. (2013) What is the appropriate size criterion for proton radiotherapy for hepatocellular carcinoma? A dosimetric comparison of spot-scanning proton therapy versus intensity-modulated radiation therapy. Radiat Oncol. 8: 48.
17. Schätti A, Zakova M, Meer D and Lomax AJ (2013) Experimental verification of motion mitigation of discrete proton spot scanning by re-scanning. Phys Med Biol. 58: 8555–72.
18. Matsuura T, Maeda K, Sutherland K, Takayanagi T, Shimizu S, et al. (2012) Biological effect of dose distortion by fiducial markers in spot-scanning proton therapy with a limited number of fields: a simulation study. Med Phys. 39: 5584–91.

4

Evaluation of Anterior Cervical Reconstruction with Titanium Mesh Cages versus Nano-Hydroxyapatite/Polyamide66 Cages after 1- or 2-Level Corpectomy for Multilevel Cervical Spondylotic Myelopathy: A Retrospective Study of 117 Patients

Yuan Zhang, Zhengxue Quan*, Zenghui Zhao, Xiaoji Luo, Ke Tang, Jie Li, Xu Zhou, Dianming Jiang

Department of Orthopedic Surgery, The First Affiliated Hospital of Chongqing Medical University, Chongqing, China

Abstract

Objective: To retrospectively compare the efficacy of the titanium mesh cage (TMC) and the nano-hydroxyapatite/polyamide66 cage (n-HA/PA66 cage) for 1- or 2-level anterior cervical corpectomy and fusion (ACCF) to treat multilevel cervical spondylotic myelopathy (MCSM).

Methods: A total of 117 consecutive patients with MCSM who underwent 1- or 2-level ACCF using a TMC or an n-HA/PA66 cage were studied retrospectively at a mean follow-up of 45.28±12.83 months. The patients were divided into four groups according to the level of corpectomy (1- or 2-level corpectomy) and cage type used (TMC or n-HA/PA66 cage). Clinical and radiological parameters were used to evaluate outcomes.

Results: At the one-year follow-up, the fusion rate in the n-HA/PA66 group was higher, albeit non-significantly, than that in the TMC group for both 1- and 2-level ACCF, but the fusion rates of the procedures were almost equal at the final follow-up. The incidence of cage subsidence at the final follow-up was significantly higher in the TMC group than in the n-HA/PA66 group for the 1-level ACCF (24% vs. 4%, $p = 0.01$), and the difference was greater for the 2-level ACCF between the TMC group and the n-HA/PA66 group (38% vs. 5%, $p = 0.01$). Meanwhile, a much greater loss of fused height was observed in the TMC group compared with the n-HA/PA66 group for both the 1- and 2-level ACCF. All four groups demonstrated increases in C2-C7 Cobb angle and JOA scores and decreases in VAS at the final follow-up compared with preoperative values.

Conclusion: The lower incidence of cage subsidence, better maintenance of the height of the fused segment and similar excellent bony fusion indicate that the n-HA/PA66 cage may be a superior alternative to the TMC for cervical reconstruction after cervical corpectomy, in particular for 2-level ACCF.

Editor: Mohammed Shamji, Toronto Western Hospital, Canada

Funding: This research was supported by the National Natural Science Foundation of China (Grant No. 81272039). URL:http://www.nsfc.gov.cn. The funders had no role in study design, data collection and analysis, decision to publish, or preparation of the manuscript.

Competing Interests: The authors have declared that no competing interests exist.

* E-mail: quanzx18@126.com

Introduction

Several surgical techniques have been suggested for the treatment of multilevel cervical spondylotic myelopathy (MCSM). However, the optimal surgical procedure remains controversial [1,2,3,4]. Both anterior and posterior approaches have been reported with satisfactory clinical outcomes [5,6,7]. Full decompression of the spinal cord and stable reconstruction of cervical alignment are the two critical aims of this surgery [5]. Based on increased etiological data, recent reports have proposed that the compression of the spinal cord in MCSM most likely originates from anterior regions, such as cervical discs and osteophytes [8,9], suggesting that anterior procedures may be more reasonable for MCSM. Without the limitation of the disc levels, anterior cervical corpectomy and fusion (ACCF) is considered a favorable option compared with anterior cervical discectomy and fusion (ACDF) among the anterior techniques [10]. More importantly, ACCF can remove almost all pathologies that cause spinal cord compression, such as prolapsed discs, osteophytes and ossified posterior longitudinal ligament (OPLL) [11].

The reconstruction of the cervical spine is relatively important following corpectomy-mediated decompression. Using auto-grafts harvested from the iliac crest or fibula for fusion has been considered the "gold standard" for anterior cervical column reconstruction. Unfortunately, donor-site complications remain [12]. Allografts can be used to avoid the morbidity associated with autograft harvest, but this technique decreases the rate of arthrodesis and increases the rate of graft collapse [13]. Titanium mesh cages (TMCs) filled with local cancellous bone autografts have been used for decades for cervical reconstruction after corpectomy [9,14], with advantages including few donor-site complications, early biomechanical stabilization, a short operation duration and high fusion rates (range: 97%–100%); however, the inevitable complication of subsidence and other disadvantages, including stress shielding and radiopacity also occur [15,16,17,18,19]. The nano-hydroxyapatite/polyamide66 cage (nano-HA/PA66 cage) is a hollow cylinder manufactured of the n-HA/PA66 composite (Figure 1). The use of this cage filled with autograft has been reported for anterior cervical reconstruction in recent years, with satisfactory clinical outcomes [20,21]. Few studies have compared the outcomes of TMCs and n-HA/PA66 cages. The aim of the present study was to comparatively assess the clinical outcomes of TMCs vs. n-HA/PA66 cages for MCSM after 1- or 2-level corpectomy to provide a basis for selecting the appropriate method for reconstructing the cervical spine.

Materials and Methods

This study was approved by the Institutional Review Board of the First Affiliated Hospital of Chongqing Medical University, and all aspects of the study comply with the Declaration of Helsinki. The Institutional Review Board of the First Affiliated Hospital of Chongqing Medical University also waived the requirement for patient consent because this study was retrospective, the data were analyzed anonymously and patient care was not affected by the study. Between June 2006 and December 2010, a total of 117 consecutive patients (65 males and 52 females) who underwent ACCF for MCSM by a senior surgeon (QUAN) were evaluated retrospectively. All patients presented with myelopathy prior to the operation, and magnetic resonance images confirmed MCSM diagnoses. Patients with cervical trauma, infections, tumors, rheumatoid arthritis, congenital deformities, severe osteoporosis or previous cervical spine surgery were excluded from our study.

All patients underwent a 1- or 2-level corpectomy, based on the level of the lesion, followed by cervical reconstruction with a TMC (Medtronic Sofamor Danek, Memphis, TN, USA) or an n-HA/PA66 cage (Sichuan National Nanotechnology Co., Ltd., Chengdu, China). The n-HA/PA66 cages were designed and fabricated by the Institute of Materials Science and Technology, Sichuan University, and our department, and they have been approved for clinical use since 2005 by the State Drug and Food Administration of China. The n-HA/PA66 cages have an 8- to 14-mm outer diameter and a 3- to 8-mm inner diameter and are of appropriate length for clinical utilization; each cage has grooves at each end to increase the friction between the cage and vertebral endplates and several 2-mm holes in the wall of the cage [20,22]. We divided the patients into four groups based on the number of levels fused (1- or 2-level ACCF) and cage selection (TMC or n-HA/PA66 cage).

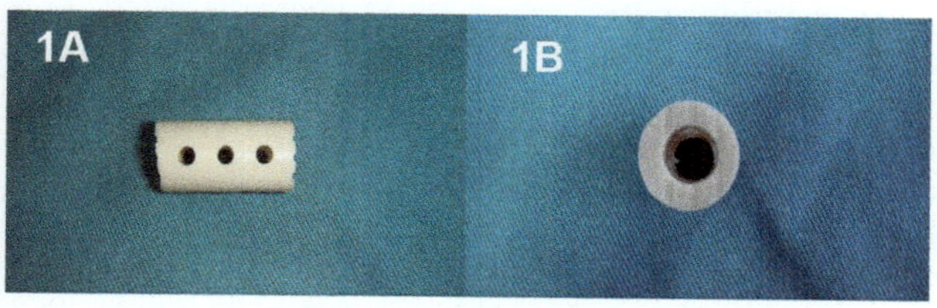

Figure 1. Photographs of lateral (1A) and superior (1B) views of the nano-hydroxyapatite/polyamide66 cage.

All surgeries were performed using a right-sided anterior cervical approach. After accurate exposure of the surgical region, a Caspar screw distraction was used for adequate distraction. Following the discectomy at the cephalic and caudal level of the lesion segment, 1- or 2-level corpectomies were performed using a Kerrison rongeur. Hypertrophic osteophytes and the posterior longitudinal ligament were removed in every case to ensure that the dura mater was widely exposed. The adjacent cartilage endplates were removed as fully as possible, and the bony endplates were preserved. An appropriately sized TMC or n-HA/PA66 cage was then prepared, filled with autogenous cancellous bone from the resected vertebra and then implanted into the intervertebral space after corpectomy using a titanium anterior cervical plate for internal fixation. All patients were instructed to wear a cervical collar for six weeks postoperatively.

The surgery time, blood loss and hospital stay were recorded. Clinical and radiological follow-ups were conducted immediately and at three months, six months and one year after surgery and then annually thereafter. The Japanese Orthopedic Association (JOA) score was used to assess neurologic status, and a 10-point visual analogue scale (VAS) was used to grade neck pain. The anteroposterior, neutral lateral and flexion/extension lateral cervical plain radiographs at preoperative, immediate postoperative, 1-year follow-up and the final follow-up were examined to assess radiologic parameters, including the height of the fused segment, the loss of height of the fused segment, cervical sagittal alignment and fusion status. The distance between the midpoint of the cephalic endplate and the caudal endplate of the fused segment was measured in millimeter (mm) and used as the height of the fused segment using Carestream software (Carestream Health, Inc. Toronto, Canada). Loss of height of the fused segment was defined as a reduction in height of the fused segment from the immediate postoperative period to follow-ups, and subsidence was defined as a loss of height of greater than 3 mm [23]. Cervical sagittal alignment was defined as the Cobb angle formed between the lower endplates of C2 and C7 on neutral lateral cervical plain film [24]. Bony fusion was defined as the trabeculation and bridging between the cage and adjacent endplates and the absence of motion between spinous processes upon flexion/extension in the fused segments. Three-dimensional computed tomography (3D-CT) scans were taken to further confirm the fusion status by observing the trabeculation between the autogenous cancellous graft and adjacent endplates [25].

Statistical analyses were performed using SPSS (version 16.0, SPSS Inc., Chicago, IL). Quantitative data are presented as the mean ± standard deviation. Repeated measures ANOVA was used for statistical analyses of differences in mean values, and the Chi-squared test was used for categorical data. The threshold for statistical significance was set to $p<0.05$.

Results

A total of 117 patients (65 males and 52 females) were included in this study, with a mean follow-up of 45.28±12.83 months (range: 25 to 70 months). Based on the number of corpectomies (1- or 2-level) and cage selection (TMC or n-HA/PA66 cage), the patients were divided into four groups. 52 patients underwent 1-level ACCF (Figure 2) and 19 patients underwent 2-level ACCF (Figure 3) with n-HA/PA66 cages. 25 patients underwent 1-level ACCF (Figure 4) and 21 patients underwent 2-level ACCF (Figure 5) with TMCs. The demographics of the patients are shown in Table 1. No significant differences were detected in gender, age, hospital stay, surgery time, blood loss or follow-up

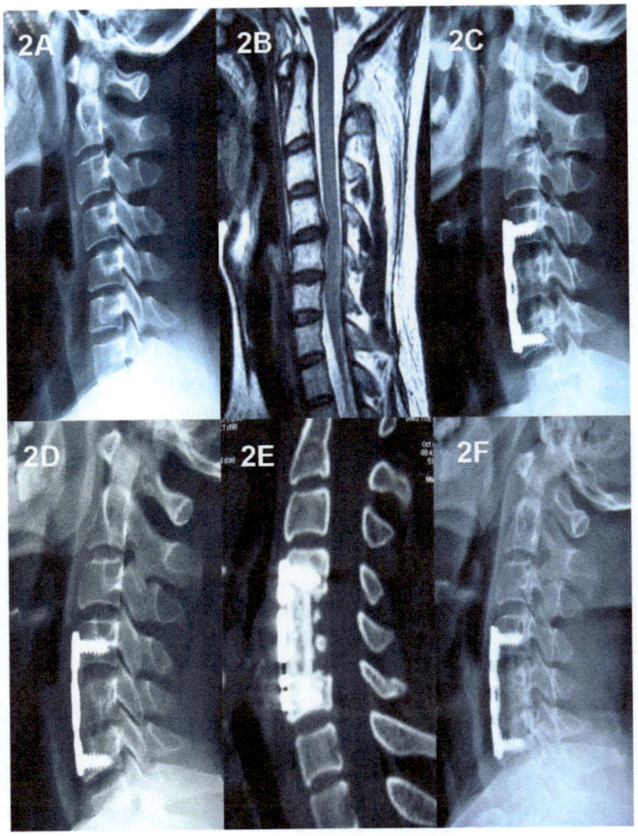

Figure 2. A 36-year-old male who underwent 1-level corpectomy with a nano-hydroxyapatite/polyamide66 cage used for cervical reconstruction. The preoperative cervical X-ray film (2A) and MRI scan (2B) show the spinal cord compression resulting from C4/5 and C5/6 disc herniations. The immediately postoperative lateral X-ray (2C) shows C5 corpectomy and the n-HA/PA66 cage used for reconstruction, and an obvious radiolucent gap can be observed between the cage and the endplates. The lateral X-ray film (2D) shows no obvious radiolucent gap, and the 3D-CT (2E) scan shows the autogenous bone granules filling the cage and achieving bony fusion with adjacent endplates at the 1-year follow-up. A lateral X-ray film (2F) at the final follow-up (four years and eight months) shows satisfying bony fusion and no obvious migration or subsidence.

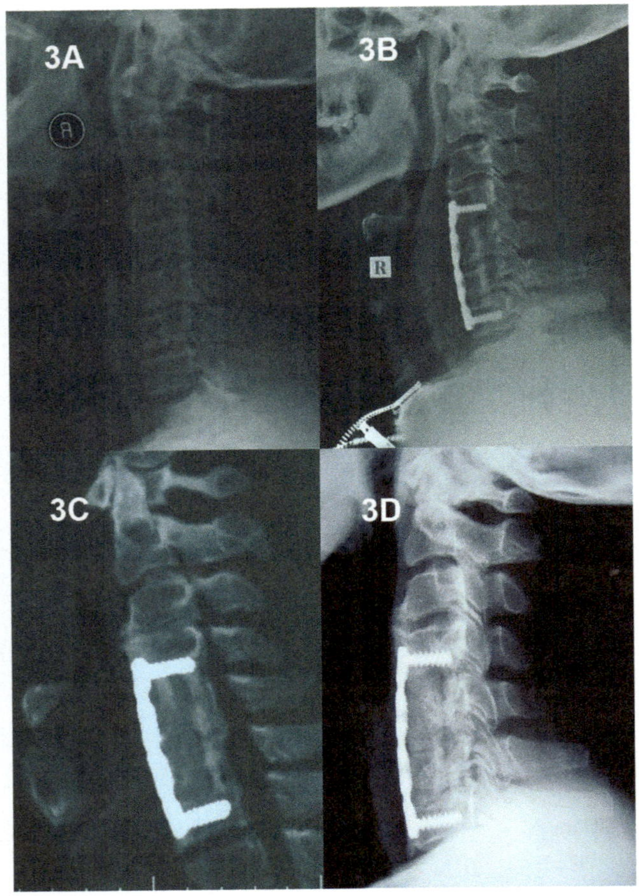

Figure 3. A 61-year-old male who underwent 2-level corpectomy with a nano-hydroxyapatite/polyamide66 cage used for cervical reconstruction. A preoperative cervical X-ray film (3A) shows a loss of cervical lordosis. The immediately postoperative lateral X-ray (3B) shows C5 and C6 corpectomy and the n-HA/PA66 cage used for reconstruction. The 3D-CT (3C) and lateral X-ray (3D) show obvious bony fusion and restoration of cervical alignment at the final follow-up (four years and four months).

(months) between the TMC group and the n-HA/PA66 group for either 1- or 2-level ACCF.

Radiological and clinical parameters are shown in Table 2. For 1-level ACCF, the mean height of the fused segment improved in the TMC group from 52.03±4.35 mm preoperatively to 59.52±4.36 mm immediately postoperative, and it improved from 53.55±6.20 mm to 61.84±6.86 mm in the n-HA/PA66 cage group. Similar results were observed for 2-level ACCF, with heights of 71.71±6.16 mm preoperatively improving to 80.04±6.00 mm immediately post-operative in the TMC group, whereas the heights were 70.30±8.08 mm in the n-HA/PA66 group preoperatively and improved to 77.28±7.56 mm immediately postoperative. Preoperative or immediately postoperative fused segment heights did not differ significantly for either 1- or 2-level ACCF between the TMC and n-HA/PA66 groups.

However, the loss in height of the fused segment in the TMC group was greater than that in the n-HA/PA66 group at the one-year follow-up (2.13±0.68 mm vs. 1.18±0.58 mm, $p<0.01$) and at the final follow-up (2.62±0.82 mm vs. 1.56±0.61 mm, $p<0.01$) for the 1-level ACCF, with similar results observed for 2-level ACCF (2.63±0.61 mm vs. 1.57±0.58 mm, $p<0.01$) at the one-year follow-up and (3.05±0.59 mm vs. 1.88±0.57 mm, $p<0.01$) at the final follow-up. The TMC group also showed a significantly greater rate of subsidence for 1-level ACCF than the n-HA/PA66 group at one year (16% vs. 2%; $p = 0.02$) and at the final follow-up (24% vs. 4%; $p = 0.01$). Furthermore, for 2-level ACCF, the TMC group suffered a more marked incidence of subsidence than the n-HA/PA66 group at one year (33% vs. 5%; $p = 0.03$) and at the final follow-up (38% vs. 5%; $p = 0.01$). The majority of cases with cage subsidence showed bony fusion at the final follow-up; moreover, no progression to neurological manifestations arose. No case with subsidence received revisional surgery. Bony fusions of the grafts were similar at the final follow-up, with 96% (24/25) of patients in the TMC group exhibiting them vs. 98% (51/52) in the n-HA/PA66 group for 1-level ACCF, whereas for 2-level ACCF, 95% (20/21) of patients developed bony fusions in the TMC group vs. 95% (18/19) in the n-HA/PA66 group. However, at the one-year follow-up, the TMC group exhibited a lower rate of bony fusion, although not statistically significant, than the n-HA/PA66 group (22/25 (88%) vs. 49/52 (94%) for 1-level ACCF; 16/21 (76%) vs. 17/19 (90%) for 2-level ACCF). No revisional surgery was required for patients who did not exhibit bony fusion at the

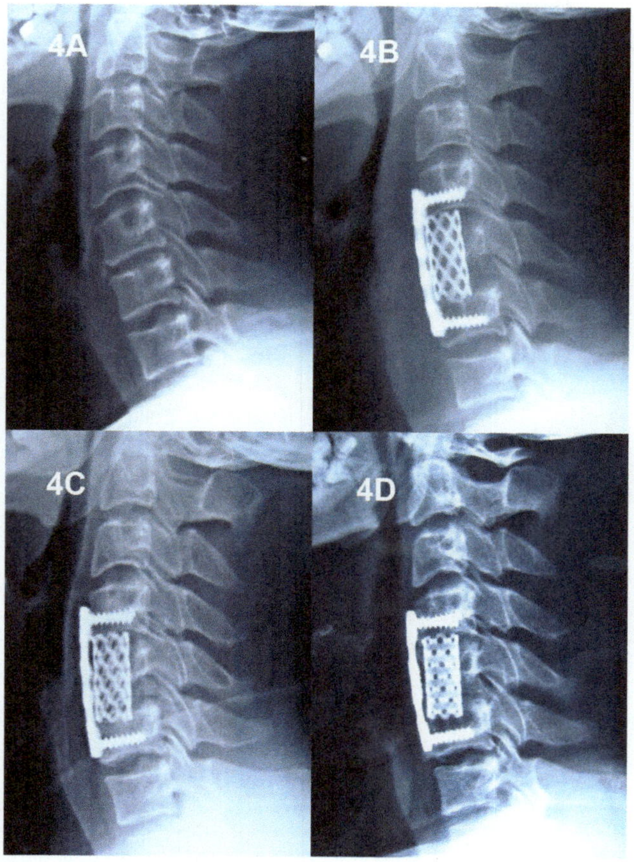

Figure 4. A 53-year-old male who underwent 1-level corpectomy with a titanium mesh cage used for cervical reconstruction. The preoperative cervical X-ray film (4A) and immediately postoperative lateral X-ray (4B) show C5 corpectomy and the titanium mesh cage used for reconstruction. The lateral X-ray one year postoperative (4C) and at the final follow-up (two years and six months; 4D) shows bony fusion between the graft and the adjacent endplates; nevertheless, marked cage subsidence was observed.

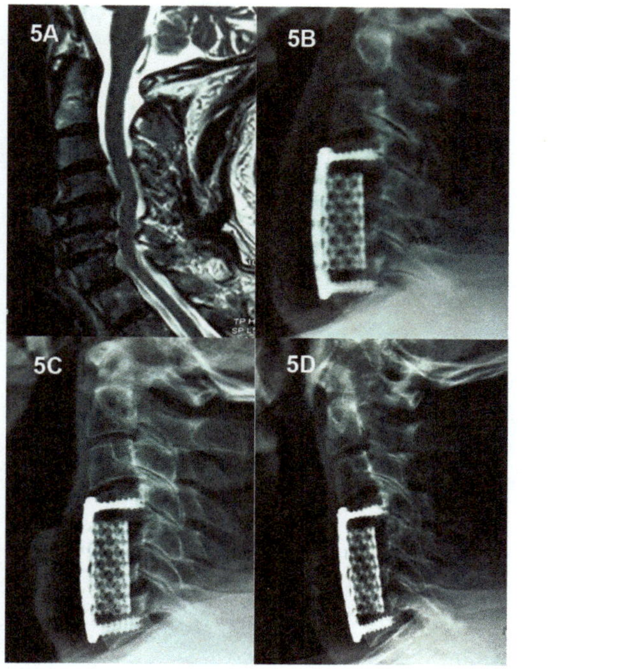

Figure 5. A 46-year-old male who underwent 2-level corpectomy with a titanium mesh cage used for cervical reconstruction. A cervical MRI scan (5A) shows multi-level disc herniations (C4/5, C5/6, C6/7) and oppression of the spinal cord. The immediately postoperative lateral X-ray (5B) shows C5 and C6 corpectomy and the titanium mesh cage used for reconstruction in which the cervical alignment was marginally restored. A lateral X-ray at the one-year follow-up (5C) shows subsidence. A lateral X-ray at the final follow-up (5D) shows increased subsidence and a loss of cervical alignment.

final follow-up because the anterior cervical plate and screws remained in position and the patients did not complain of discomfort. For all four groups, there was a slight improvement in the mean C2–C7 Cobb angle when preoperative values were compared with the final follow-up measurements. When preoperative or final follow-up postoperative measurements were compared, no significant differences were detected in Cobb angle between the TMC and n-HA/PA66 groups either for 1- or 2- level ACCF.

The preoperative JOA scores did not differ between the TMC and n-HA/PA66 groups regardless of the number of levels fused. At the final follow-up, JOA scores had improved significantly in all four groups. No significant differences were detected between the TMC and n-HA/PA66 groups for either 1-or 2-level ACCF at the final follow-up. The mean preoperative VAS score was similar between the two kinds of cage groups for both 1- and 2-level ACCF. However, at the last follow-up, the mean VAS score in the TMC group was higher, albeit insignificantly, than that of the n-HA/PA66 group (1.44 ± 1.08 vs. 1.17 ± 1.25 ($p = 0.42$) for 1-level ACCF; 2.33 ± 1.06 vs. 1.58 ± 1.12 ($p = 0.06$) for 2-level ACCF).

Discussion

In recent years, ACCF has been recognized as a reliable and effective procedure for the treatment of MCSM. The advantage of the direct decompression resulting from the resection of the object causing oppression of the spinal cord from the anterior column is supported by the many reports of successful clinical outcomes in treating MCSM [26,27]. In addition to decompression, reconstruction of the cervical spine is a critical procedure. TMC has been used widely for years. Packed with autogenous graft from the removed vertebra, this apparatus can provide early biomechanical stabilization of the anterior column, restoration and maintenance of the intervertebral height and cervical alignment and enlargement of the stenotic neural foramen and can avoid the potential complications caused by autogenous graft collection [28]. However, implant-related complications cannot be ignored. TMC subsidence, the typical hardware-related complication, has been reported to range from 0% to 30% [29]. Although the relevance of TMC subsidence remains controversial, the subsidence can have serious consequences, such as the buckling of the cervical ligamentum flavum, foraminal stenosis and re-compression of the cervical spinal cord and nerve roots [16,17,28,29].

The n-HA/PA66 is a composite made by infiltrating nano-HA into PA66; it mimics natural bone in that apatite is distributed within a collagen matrix. Thus, the composite possesses both the mechanical strength of HA and the elastic properties of PA66. A previous study documented that the n-HA/PA66 composite was safe and that its mechanical properties complement natural bone well [22]. The n-HA/PA66 cage is a biomimetic implant fabricated from n-HA/PA66 composite. This device has been

Table 1. Demographic and clinical data of patients.

Parameters	1-level ACCF		2-level ACCF	
	TMC	n-HA/PA66 cage	TMC	n-HA/PA66 cage
No.of patients (n)	25	52	21	19
Male/female (n)	11/14	29/23	13/8	12/7
Mean age (years)	55.04±11.09	56.56±12.13	57.81±11.50	57.00±10.95
Hospital stay (days)	16.04±3.67	14.90±3.73	16.76±4.04	15.42±2.39
Surgery time (minutes)	148.40±24.82	143.65±30.50	186.19±28.54	184.74±26.32
Blood loss (ml)	145.20±61.85	133.46±68.57	189.52±90.30	173.68±58.61
Follow-up (months)	49.80±13.06	44.06±13.60	43.42±12.18	44.74±10.33
Involved segments				
1-level corpectomy C4/C5/C6	6/16/3	7/36/9		
2-level corpectomy C4-C5/C5-C6			10/11	11/8

used for spinal reconstruction for several years, and considerable clinical results have been reported [20,21,30]. Our previous research showed a 94.3% bony fusion rate in 35 patients and a 2.9% subsidence rate with n-HA/PA66 cages in reconstructions following cervical corpectomy [20]. Yang et al. [30] reported using n-HA/PA66 cages for anterior reconstruction after thoracolumbar corpectomy in 51 patients and achieved a 90.2% bony fusion rate with a low incidence of cage subsidence. Yang et al. [21] achieved a 97% fusion rate and a 6% subsidence rate in 35 patients with n-HA/PA66 cages for single-level cervical corpectomy and fusion.

Subsidence was typically observed when TMC was used for cervical reconstruction after corpectomy. Daubs et al. [31]

Table 2. Radiographic and clinical outcomes in each group.

Parameter	1-level ACCF			2-level ACCF		
	TMC	n-HA/PA66 cage	P	TMC	n-HA/PA66 cage	P
Height of fused segments (mm)						
Pre-operation	52.03±4.35	53.55±6.20	0.29	71.71±6.16	70.30±8.08	0.52
Immediately post-op	59.52±4.36	61.84±6.86	0.11	80.04±6.00	77.28±7.56	0.21
Loss of height of fused segments (mm)						
One year follow-up	2.13±0.68	1.18±0.58	<0.01	2.63±0.61	1.57±0.58	<0.01
Last follow-up	2.62±0.82	1.56±0.61	<0.01	3.05±0.59	1.88±0.57	<0.01
Fusion rate						
One year follow-up	(22/25) 88%	(49/52) 94%	0.34	(16/21) 76%	(17/19) 90%	0.27
Last follow-up	(24/25) 96%	(51/52) 98%	0.59	(20/21) 95%	(18/19) 95%	0.44
Subsidence rate						
One year follow-up	(4/25)16%	(1/52) 2%	0.02	(7/21) 33%	(1/19) 5%	0.03
Last follow-up	(6/25) 24%	(2/52) 4%	0.01	(8/21) 38%	(1/19) 5%	0.01
C2-C7 Cobb angle (°)						
Pre-op	8.60±5.77	9.69±6.14	0.41	9.33±6.34	9.16±6.81	0.93
Immediately post-op	12.76±5.10	13.15±5.13	0.77	13.10±5.02	13.89±6.39	0.68
Last follow-up	9.96±5.29	10.98±5.20	0.44	9.81±5.81	12.16±6.18	0.23
JOA score (points)						
Pre-operation	12.24±2.18	12.17±2.26	0.87	11.10±2.53	11.63±1.86	0.42
Immediately post-op	14.40±1.63	14.75±1.37	0.41	13.48±2.23	14.26±1.33	0.23
Last follow-up	14.88±1.59	15.37±1.24	0.25	13.76±2.34	14.84±1.83	0.1
VAS of neck pain (points)						
Pre-operation	4.76±1.85	4.37±1.66	0.23	5.14±1.24	5.26±1.59	0.76
Immediately post-op	2.04±1.02	1.85±1.07	0.56	3.00±1.22	2.63±1.16	0.35
Last follow-up	1.44±1.08	1.17±1.25	0.42	2.33±1.06	1.58±1.12	0.06

described an early subsidence in 30% (7 of 27) of cases with ACCF. In our series, by the final follow-up, for 1-level ACCF, we observed that the n-HA/PA66 group exhibited a significantly lower rate of subsidence than the TMC group (4% vs. 24%; p = 0.01). Moreover, the difference in subsidence rates was much greater when compared for 2-level ACCF, we observed subsidence in 8 of 21 cases (38%) in the TMC group vs. 1 of 19 cases (5%) in the n-HA/PA66 group (p = 0.01). Increased patient age, severe osteoporosis, excessive endplate removal and intra-operative over-distraction have been demonstrated to be risk factors of TMC subsidence [17]. However, the metal attributes and the shape of the TMC are likely the most important factors. The sharp teeth at both ends of the TMC are beneficial to early stabilization by embedding the cage into adjacent endplates. Unfortunately, the contact interface between the TMC and endplates is small (we describe this pattern as a "point-to-surface contact"), and the intensity of pressure at the contact surface is so great that it may result in excessive insertion of the cage into the vertebra. In contrast, the n-HA/PA66 cage has a broader surface at both ends with which to contact the endplates. We describe this pattern as "surface-to-surface contact," and it distributes the loads on the interface and decreases incidences of cage subsidence. Unlike the sharp teeth that the TMC possesses, the n-HA/PA66 cage has grooves at the terminal faces that can increase the friction between the cage and endplates and that is sufficient to prevent cage migration. In our study, even in the case of 2-level ACCF, we did not observe n-HA/PA66 cage migration or extrusion.

Majd ME et al. [32] reported a fusion rate of 97% in cervical reconstructions with TMC, and a fusion rate of 100% was observed by Rieger et al. [33] using the same technique. In our study, for both 1- and 2-level ACCF, the fusion rates in the TMC group and the n-HA/PA66 group were almost equivalent at the final follow-up. However, the n-HA/PA66 group showed higher fusion rates, albeit insignificantly, than the TMC group at the 1-year follow-up (94% vs. 88% (p = 0.34) for 1-level ACCF; 90% vs. 76% (p = 0.27) for 2-level ACCF). Previous reports have demonstrated that the difference in fusion conditions was primarily due to the different elastic moduli between the two struts [20,22]. Compared with TMC, the n-HA/PA66 cage possesses an elastic modulus similar to that of the autogenous graft inside the cage [22,34]. As described by Wolff's law, bone grows in response to applied stress and is resorbed when mechanical stimulus is absent. Due to the appropriate elastic modulus, n-HA/PA66 cages may reduce stress shielding and promote fusion effectively. In addition, the n-HA/PA66 cage exhibits excellent biocompatibility and osteoconductive ability in vivo. Animal experiments demonstrated that when implanted, the cage can release Ca^{2+} and PO_4^{3-} from its surface, which gradually forms a crystal layer on the cage surface that bridges the graft and implant bed to provide a trestle for osteogenesis [35]. Moreover, the holes in the n-HA/PA66 cage wall may enable blood circulation between the implant bed and the autograft within the cage, which would aid in the growth of the bone graft. Previous studies have reported that subsidence occurs in up to 80% of patients during the early postoperative period prior to bony fusion [36]. In the present study, similar results were observed in all four groups, with the majority of height loss in the fused segment occurring during the 1st postoperative year and heights remaining almost identical to these levels at the final follow-up. Considering the reduced loss of fused segmental height and earlier bony fusion in the n-HA/PA66 group compared with the TMC group, the data indicate that the earlier bony fusion in the n-HA/PA66 group may contribute to the decrease in the loss of fused segmental height. However, the differences in present study are still insignificantly. In the future, larger samples and longer follow-ups should be required to demonstrate this conclusion.

Some studies have demonstrated that the number of corpectomy levels is a risk factor for TMC subsidence. The increase in ACCF levels may eventually cause not only a higher incidence of subsidence but also more severe subsidence when TMC cages are used [31,37]. We observed similar outcomes in our TMC groups. As a result of these published data, previous reports have suggested that 2-level ACCF using TMC cages may not be appropriate therapeutic options for treating MCSM. However, in this study, even for 2-level corpectomy, we observed that the amount of subsidence was much lower in the n-HA/PA66 group compared with the TMC group. Furthermore, we did not observe a high incidence of subsidence. These observations suggest that the n-HA/PA66 cage may provide greater stability than the TMC and may more effectively maintain fused segmental height. The data also indicate that the n-HA/PA66 cage may be a better therapeutic choice for 2-level ACCF.

With the utilization of TMC in cervical reconstruction after corpectomy, restoration of cervical alignment is possible [24]. In the present study, we employed the C2–C7 Cobb angle to evaluate cervical sagittal alignment, the preoperative Cobb angle were similar in four groups, and we observed an improvement in the Cobb angle at the final follow-up compared with preoperative values in all four groups, respectively. There were no significant differences in the Cobb angle at the final follow-up between the TMC and n-HA/PA66 groups in both the 1- and 2-level ACCF; however, we noted that the n-HA/PA66 groups showed little better improvements of C2–C7 Cobb angles. These differences may be due to the greater loss in segmental height when using TMC for cervical reconstructions.

The JOA and VAS scales were used to assess clinical efficacy in our study. We noted improvements in these two parameters in all four groups. At the final follow-up, the mean JOA score was similar between the TMC and n-HA/PA66 groups for both the 1- and 2-level ACCF. However, we observed that the patients in the TMC group presented with higher, albeit non-significant, VAS scores than those in the n-HA/PA66 group, particularly in the 2-level ACCF group. Previous studies [9,31,36,37] showed that subsidence was strongly correlated with neck pain. Although no significant difference was detected in this outcome in our study, these results nevertheless indicate that patients treated with n-HA/PA66 cage for ACCF may suffer less axial neck pain than patients treated with TMC. In our view, the increased loss in segmental height in the TMC group may underlie these differences, and we will pay close attention to this issue in future follow-ups.

Conclusion

This retrospective study demonstrated that both the TMC and n-HA/PA66 cage resulted in effective clinical and radiographic outcomes when used to treat MCSM with cervical reconstruction after corpectomy. However, with its optimized biomechanical characteristics and unique shape, the n-HA/PA66 cage achieves similar bony fusion rates but lower rates of subsidence. Furthermore, even in the case of 2-level ACCF, the n-HA/PA66 cage can maintain fused segment height better and lower incidences of subsidence compared with TMC. The n-HA/PA66 cage may be a better alternative for cervical reconstruction than TMC after corpectomy, particularly for 2-level ACCF.

Author Contributions

Conceived and designed the experiments: YZ ZQ. Performed the experiments: YZ ZQ XL ZZ DJ KT. Analyzed the data: YZ JL XZ ZZ. Contributed reagents/materials/analysis tools: ZQ DJ. Wrote the paper: YZ.

References

1. Lin Q, Zhou X, Wang X, Cao P, Tsai N, et al. (2012) A comparison of anterior cervical discectomy and corpectomy in patients with multilevel cervical spondylotic myelopathy. Eur Spine J 21: 474–481.
2. Song KJ, Lee KB, Song JH (2012) Efficacy of multilevel anterior cervical discectomy and fusion versus corpectomy and fusion for multilevel cervical spondylotic myelopathy: a minimum 5-year follow-up study. Eur Spine J 21: 1551–1557.
3. Edwards CC 2nd, Heller JG, Murakami H (2002) Corpectomy versus laminoplasty for multilevel cervical myelopathy: an independent matched-cohort analysis. Spine (Phila Pa 1976) 27: 1168–1175.
4. Tani T, Ushida T, Ishida K, Iai H, Noguchi T, et al. (2002) Relative safety of anterior microsurgical decompression versus laminoplasty for cervical myelopathy with a massive ossified posterior longitudinal ligament. Spine (Phila Pa 1976) 27: 2491–2498.
5. Lian XF, Xu JG, Zeng BF, Zhou W, Kong WQ, et al. (2010) Noncontiguous anterior decompression and fusion for multilevel cervical spondylotic myelopathy: a prospective randomized control clinical study. Eur Spine J 19: 713–719.
6. Herkowitz HN (1988) A comparison of anterior cervical fusion, cervical laminectomy, and cervical laminoplasty for the surgical management of multiple level spondylotic radiculopathy. Spine (Phila Pa 1976) 13: 774–780.
7. Matz PG, Anderson PA, Groff MW, Heary RF, Holly LT, et al. (2009) Cervical laminoplasty for the treatment of cervical degenerative myelopathy. J Neurosurg Spine 11: 157–169.
8. Lu J, Wu X, Li Y, Kong X (2008) Surgical results of anterior corpectomy in the aged patients.with cervical myelopathy. Eur Spine J 17: 129–135.
9. Dorai Z, Morgan H, Coimbra C (2003) Titanium cage reconstruction after cervical corpectomy. J Neurosurg Spine 99: 3–7.
10. Oh MC, Zhang HY, Park JY, Kim KS (2009) Two-level anterior cervical discectomy versus one-level corpectomy in cervical spondylotic myelopathy. Spine (Phila Pa 1976) 34: 692–696.
11. Hilibrand AS, Fye MA, Emery SE, Palumbo MA, Bohlman HH (2002) Increased rate of arthrodesis with strut grafting after multilevel anterior cervical decompression. Spine (Phila Pa 1976) 27: 146–151.
12. Wittenberg RH, Moeller J, Shea M, White AA 3rd, Hayes WC (1990) Compressive strength of autologous and allogenous bone grafts for thoracolumbar and cervical spine fusion. Spine (Phila Pa 1976) 15: 1073–1078.
13. Kotil K, Tari R (2011) Two level cervical corpectomy with iliac crest fusion and rigid plate fixation: a retrospective study with a three-year follow-up. Turk Neurosurg 21: 606–612.
14. Kinoshita A, Kataoka K, Taneda M (1999) Multilevel vertebral body replacement with a titanium mesh spacer for aneurysmal bone cyst: technical note. Minim Invasive Neurosurg 42: 156–158.
15. Yan D, Wang Z, Deng S, Li J, Soo C (2011) Anterior corpectomy and reconstruction with titanium mesh cage and dynamic cervical plate forcervical spondylotic myelopathy in elderly osteoporosis patients. Arch Orthop Trauma Surg 131:1369–1374.
16. Hee HT, Madj ME, Holt RT, Whitecloud TS 3rd, Pienkowski D (2003) Complications of multilevel cervical corpectomies and reconstruction with titanium cages and anterior plating. J Spinal Disord 16: 1–8.
17. Lim TH, Kwon H, Jeon CH, Kim JG, Sokolowski M, Natarajan R, et al. (2001) Effect of endplate conditions and bone mineral density on the compressive strength of the graft-endplate interface in anterior cervical spine fusion. Spine (Phila Pa 1976) 26: 951–956.
18. Lee SH, Sung JK (2008) Anterior cervical stabilization using a semi-constrained cervical plate and titanium. J Clin Neurosci 15: 1227–1234.
19. Ying Z, Xinwei W, Jing Z, Shengming X, Bitao L, et al. (2007) Cervical corpectomy with preserved posterior vertebral wall for cervical spondylotic myelopathy: a randomized control clinical study. Spine (Phila Pa 1976) 32: 1482–1487.
20. Zhao Z, Jiang D, Ou Y, Tang K, Luo X, et al. (2012) A hollow cylindrical nanohydroxyapatite/polyamide composite strut for cervical reconstruction after cervical corpectomy. J Clin Neurosci 19: 536–540.
21. Yang X, Chen Q, Liu L, Song Y, Kong Q, et al. (2013) Comparison of anterior cervical fusion by titanium mesh cage versus nano-hydroxyapatite/polyamide cage following single-level corpectomy. Int Orthop 37: 2421–2427.
22. Wang X, Li Y, Wei J, de Groot K (2002) Development of biomimetic nano-hydroxyapatite/poly(hexamethylene adipamide) composites. Biomaterials 23: 4787–4791.
23. Gercek E, Arlet V, Delisle J, Marchesi D (2003) Subsidence of stand-alone cervical cages in anterior interbody fusion: warning. Eur Spine J 12: 513–516.
24. Andaluz N, Zuccarello M, Kuntz C (2012) Long-term follow-up of cervical radiographic sagittal spinal alignment after 1- and 2-level cervical corpectomy for the treatment of spondylosis of the subaxial cervical spine causing radiculomyelopathy or myelopathy: a retrospective study. J Neurosurg Spine 16: 2–7.
25. Liu Y, Qi M, Chen H, Yang L, Wang X, et al. (2012) Comparative analysis of complications of different reconstructive techniques following anterior decompression for multilevel cervical spondylotic myelopathy. Eur Spine J 21: 2428–2435.
26. Kirkpatric JS, Levy JA, Carillo J, Moeini SR (1999) Reconstruction after multilevel corpectomy in the cervical spine. A sagittal plane biomechanical study. Spine (Phila Pa 1976) 24: 1186–1191.
27. Sevki K, Mehmet T, Ufuk T, Azmi H, Mercan S, et al. (2004) Results of surgical treatment for degenerative cervical myelopathy: anterior cervical corpectomy and stabilization. Spine (Phila Pa 1976) 29: 2493–2500.
28. Chibbaro S, Benvenuti L, Carnesecchi S, Marsella M, Pulera F, et al. (2006) Anterior cervical corpectomy for cervical spondylotic myelopathy: experience and surgical results in a series of 70 consecutive patients. J Clin Neurosci 13: 233–238.
29. Bilbao G, Duart M, Aurrecoechea JJ, Pomposo I, Igartua A, et al. (2010) Surgical results and complications in a series of 71 consecutive cervical spondylotic corpectomies. Acta Neurochir (Wien) 152: 1155–1163.
30. Yang X, Song Y, Liu L, Liu H, Zeng J, et al. (2012) Anterior reconstruction with nano-hydroxyapatite/polyamide-66 cage after thoracic and lumbar corpectomy. Orthopedics 35: e66–73.
31. Daubs MD (2005) Early failures following cervical corpectomy reconstruction with titanium mesh cages and anterior plating. Spine (Phila Pa 1976) 30: 1402–1406.
32. Majd ME, Vadhva M, Holt RT (1999) Anterior cervical reconstruction using titanium cages with anterior plating. Spine (Phila Pa 1976) 24: 1604–1610.
33. Rieger A, Holz C, Marx T, Sanchin L, Menzel M (2003) Vertebral autograft used as bone transplant for anterior cervical corpectomy: technical note. Neurosurgery 52: 449–453.
34. HuangM, Feng J, Wang J, Zhang X, Li Y, et al. (2003) Synthesis and characterization of nano-HA/PA66 composites. J Mater Sci Mater Med 14: 655–660.
35. Xu Q, Lu H, Zhang J, Li G, Deng Z, et al. (2010) Tissue engineering scaffold material of porous nanohydroxyapatite/polyamide66. Int J Nanomedicine 13: 331–5.
36. Fengbin Y, Jinhao M, Xinyuan L, Xinwei W, Yu C, et al. (2013) Evaluation of a new type of titanium mesh cage versus the traditional titanium mesh cage for single-level, anterior cervical corpectomy and fusion. Eur Spine J 22: 2891–2896.
37. Chen Y, Chen D, Guo Y, Wang X, Lu X, et al. (2008) Subsidence of titanium mesh cage: a study based on 300 cases. J Spinal Disord Tech 21:489–492.

5

Low-Dose X-Ray Irradiation Promotes Osteoblast Proliferation, Differentiation and Fracture Healing

Ming Chen[1]◑, Qun Huang[2]◑, Wei Xu[2], Chang She[2], Zong-Gang Xie[2], Yong-Tao Mao[2], Qi-Rong Dong[2]*, Ming Ling[1]*

1 Department of Orthopedics, Shaanxi Provincial Peoples Hospital, Xi'an, Shaanxi, China, **2** Department of Orthopedics, Second Affiliated Hospital of Soochow University, Suzhou, Jiangsu, China

Abstract

Great controversy exists regarding the biologic responses of osteoblasts to X-ray irradiation, and the mechanisms are poorly understood. In this study, the biological effects of low-dose radiation on stimulating osteoblast proliferation, differentiation and fracture healing were identified using in vitro cell culture and in vivo animal studies. First, low-dose (0.5 Gy) X-ray irradiation induced the cell viability and proliferation of MC3T3-E1 cells. However, high-dose (5 Gy) X-ray irradiation inhibited the viability and proliferation of osteoblasts. In addition, dynamic variations in osteoblast differentiation markers, including type I collagen, alkaline phosphatase, Runx2, Osterix and osteocalcin, were observed after both low-dose and high-dose irradiation by Western blot analysis. Second, fracture healing was evaluated via histology and gene expression after single-dose X-ray irradiation, and low-dose X-ray irradiation accelerates fracture healing of closed femoral fractures in rats. In low-dose X-ray irradiated fractures, an increase in proliferating cell nuclear antigen (PCNA)-positive cells, cartilage formation and fracture calluses was observed. In addition, we observed more rapid completion of endochondral and intramembranous ossification, which was accompanied by altered expression of genes involved in bone remodeling and fracture callus mineralization. Although the expression level of several osteoblast differentiation genes was increased in the fracture calluses of high-dose irradiated rats, the callus formation and fracture union were delayed compared with the control and low-dose irradiated fractures. These results reveal beneficial effects of low-dose irradiation, including the stimulation of osteoblast proliferation, differentiation and fracture healing, and highlight its potential translational application in novel therapies against bone-related diseases.

Editor: Jan Peter Tuckermann, University of Ulm, Germany

Funding: This work was supported by the National Natural Science Foundation of China (81171730) and the Plans for Graduate Research and Innovation in Colleges and Universities of Jiangsu Province (CXZZ12_0841). The funders had no role in study design, data collection and analysis, decision to publish, or preparation of the manuscript.

Competing Interests: The authors have declared that no competing interests exist.

* Email: dongqirong@hotmail.com (QRD); lingming029@163.com (ML)

◑ These authors contributed equally to this work.

Introduction

Bone development and homeostasis are maintained through the balance between bone-forming osteoblasts and bone-resorbing osteoclasts. Osteoblasts are the chief bone-making cells that are responsible for the production of bone extracellular matrix during bone remodeling or healing [1]. During the process of bone formation, osteoblasts must proliferate, differentiate and induce mineralization of the bone extracellular matrix. A variety of genes in osteoblasts, including fluctuations in type I collagen (Col1), alkaline phosphatase (ALP), osteopontin (OPN), osteonectin (ON), osteocalcin (OCN) and others, undergo characteristic sequential changes in phenotypic gene expression during this series of events [2].

It is well known that high-dose irradiation delivers deleterious effects to bone tissue, including osteoradionecrosis, sclerosis, loss of bone mass and bone fracture, in a dose- and time-dependent manner [3–6]. Damage to osteoblasts and osteocytes is thought to be a primary contributor to the reduced bone mineral density that is observed following irradiation. Previous studies have suggested that irradiation can impair bone formation by impeding osteoblast proliferation and differentiation, inducing cell-cycle arrest, reducing collagen production and increasing the sensitivity to apoptotic agents [7,8]. However, the effects of low-dose irradiation, especially at levels less than 1Gy, on bone responses and healing have rarely been described in the literature. Orthopedic patients are more often subjected to radiation exposure, such as radiography, computed tomography or fluoroscopy during surgery, where the exposure to ionizing radiation is typically at low-dose levels (<1 Gy) [9,10]. In addition, several studies have revealed the detrimental effects of low-dose irradiation (<1 Gy) through various molecular mechanisms, including increases in reactive oxygen species formation, DNA double-strand breaks and chromosomal breakage [11–13]. Conversely, other studies have reported contrasting results concerning low-dose irradiation. For example, Li *et al.* reported that 75 mGy X-ray irradiation induced maximal stimulation of bone marrow hematopoietic progenitor cell proliferation and a significant increase in the mobilization of these cells to the peripheral blood post-irradiation [14]. In addition, Liang *et al.* reported that the proliferative capacity of bone marrow-derived mesenchymal stem cells (BM-MSCs) exposed to low-dose X-rays was significantly enhanced compared with the non-irradiated control group [15]. Nevertheless, the biological response of osteoblast lineage cells to low-dose X-ray irradiation remains controversial. Recently, the study performed by Pramojanee *et al.* showed that 1.5 mGy X-ray irradiation decreased oxidative stress in osteoblasts and did not alter cell viability, cellular proliferation or cellular apoptosis [11]. A previous study demonstrated that 2 Gy X-ray ionizing radiation induced time-dependent cell cycle arrest and had no significant effects on osteoblast proliferation and differentiation in an osteoblastic cell line [16,17]. However, Park *et al.* [18] reported that 2 Gy X-ray irradiation not only increased differentiation and mineralization of the cells but also upregulated the expression of ALP, Col1, OPN and OCN in the early stage of differentiation.

It is generally considered that sequential proliferation and differentiation of osteoblasts is indispensable for bone remodeling and healing. Our preliminary studies surprisingly demonstrated that 1 Gy X-ray irradiation promoted callus formation and mineralization in a rat model [19], and this type of radiation was also shown to have different effects on the proliferation and differentiation of osteoblasts in vitro (0.5–1 Gy) [20]. However, the underlying mechanism has not been evaluated in osteoblasts exposed to low-dose irradiation. In this study, we investigated the mechanism by which low-dose X-ray irradiation (0.5 Gy) influences the proliferation and differentiation of osteoblasts and promotes fracture healing. Osteogenic gene expression patterns were evaluated to explore the possible mechanisms involved in irradiation-stimulated osteoblast differentiation *in vivo* and *in vitro*. Our findings provide a greater understanding of the biological responses of osteoblasts exposed to low-dose X-ray irradiation and highlight the potential positive effects of this treatment.

Methods

Cell culture and irradiation

MC3T3-E1 subclone 14 cells were purchased from the Chinese Academy of Sciences Cell Bank. The same procedures, such as seeding time, cell numbers and replacing osteogenic medium, were performed during our study. Cells were cultured in α-MEM (HyClone, USA) containing 10% fetal bovine serum (Gibco, USA), 100 U/ml penicillin and 100 μg/ml streptomycin. In the osteoblast differentiation experiments, the culture media was replaced with osteogenic medium supplemented with 50 μg/ml ascorbic acid (Sigma-Aldrich, USA) and 10 mM β-glycerophosphate (Sigma-Aldrich, USA) after the cells had achieved 70–80% confluence. The cells were exposed to a single 0.5 Gy (low-dose) or 5 Gy (high-dose) dose of X-ray irradiation at a rate of 200 cGy/min using a medical linear accelerator with a 6 MV radiation source (Siemens Primus, Concord, CA, USA). All irradiations were performed at room temperature, and the control samples were treated similarly but were not irradiated. The time at irradiation was termed day 0. The cells were maintained in a 5% CO_2 atmosphere at 37°C, and the medium was exchanged every 3 days.

Fracture model establishment and irradiation

All animal studies were performed in strict accordance with the recommendations in the Guide for the Care and Use of Laboratory Animals of the National Institutes of Health. The protocol was approved by the Committee on the Ethics of Animal Experiments of the Second Affiliated Hospital of Soochow University. All surgeries were performed under chloral hydrate anesthesia, and all efforts were made to minimize suffering.

Male Sprague-Dawley rats (body weight 220±20 g) were obtained from the Animal Unit Center of Soochow University. A total of 96 rats were used in our *in vivo* studies. The animals were acclimated for 7 days prior to the experiments and were administered food and water ad libitum. Closed femur fractures were created as described previously [19]. Briefly, the rats were anesthetized with 3.6% chloral hydrate (360 mg/kg, intraperitoneal injection). A lateral parapatellar knee incision was made to expose the distal femoral condyles. A 1.2-mm diameter K-wire was inserted into the length of the medullary canal of the femur from the trochlear groove until the wire exited through the greater trochanter and the skin. The distal end was positioned deeply into the articular surface of the knee, and a mid-diaphyseal fracture was created via three-point bending with a custom-made guillotine-like fracture apparatus. Clear oblique fracture lines or comminuted fractures were excluded based on radiography performed after the surgery. Then, the established fracture animal models were randomized into the irradiation and control groups. The animals in the irradiation group were administered a single dose (0.5 or 5 Gy) of X-ray irradiation locally to the operated thigh using a linear accelerator with a 6 MV radiation source. Control rats were treated in the same manner as the irradiation groups; however, these rates were not exposed to X-ray irradiation.

CCK-8 assay for cell viability

MC3T3-E1 cells after irradiation were seeded in 96-well plates at a density of 3000 cells/well and cultured in an incubator for 1- to 7-day periods. The Cell Counting Kit-8 (CCK-8; Dojindo, Japan) was employed to quantitatively evaluate cell viability. Briefly, α-MEM (100 μl) with 10 μl CCK-8 was added to each pre-cultured well, and the plates were then incubated for 2 h at 37°C. The absorbance was determined at a wavelength of 450 nm using a TECAN Infinite M200 microplate reader (Tecan Group Ltd., Switzerland).

Bromodeoxyuridine (BrdU) incorporation for cell proliferation

The cells were plated and treated as described above for 2, 4 or 6 days. A BrdU ELISA kit (Roche, Germany) was used to determine cell proliferation according to the manufacturer's instructions. First, BrdU was added to the medium, and the plates were incubated for 2 h at 37°C. Then, the cells were fixed, and the DNA was denatured for 30 min at room temperature after removal of the culture medium. The anti-BrdU antibody was then added to bind to the BrdU that had been incorporated into the newly synthesized cellular DNA. Finally, the immune complexes were detected by the subsequent substrate reaction, and the absorbance of each well was measured using a TECAN Infinite M200 microplate reader at 370 nm (492 nm reference wavelength).

Flow cytometric analysis

The cell cycle progression of MC3T3-E1 cells was analyzed by flow cytometry. After irradiation, the cells were incubated for 3 days. The harvested cells were washed twice with PBS, fixed with ice-cold 70% ethanol and stored at 4°C overnight. The fixed cells were then washed with PBS again and incubated in 100 μl RNase A/PBS (200 μg/ml) at 37°C for 30 min. Intracellular DNA was labeled with 300 μl propidium iodide (PI, 10 μg/ml) at 4°C for 15 min, and the stained cells were analyzed on a flow cytometer for relative DNA content based on increased red fluorescence. The data were presented as percentages of the total population.

Table 1. List of Oligonucleotide Primer Sequences for Real-Time PCR.

Gene	Primer Sequences
β-actin	Forward: 5′- GAGAGGGAA ATCGTGCGTGAC-3′
	Reverser: 5′- CATCTGCTGGAAGGTGGACA-3′
Col1α1	Forward: 5′-AAGGCCCACGGGGACCTGTT-3′
	Reverser: 5′-GGGCCAGGCACGGAA ACTCC-3′
Col2α1	Forward: 5′-CTACGGCGACGGCAACCTGG-3′
	Reverser: 5′-TGCCCTCGGCCCTCATCTCC-3′
OCN	Forward: 5′-GCGCATCTATGGCACCACCGT-3′
	Reverser: 5′-TTTGGA GCAGCTGTGCCGTCC-3′
ALP	Forward: 5′-GCCCAGGCA ACCTCGAGCAG-3′
	Reverser: 5′-TCCGACCCACGGAGGGTTCC-3′
Runx2	Forward: 5′-TCCAGGAGGACAGCAAGGAGGC-3′
	Reverser: 5′-TCGGTTGGTCTCGGTGGCTGG-3′
Osterix	Forward: 5′- AGAAGATCCCTCCCAGCGCCC-3′
	Reverser: 5′- GGGTTGGCTGTCCCGTCTCC-3′
OPG	Forward: 5′-ATCGGCCACGCGAACCTCAC-3′
	Reverser: 5′-GCTGCTCGCTGGGTTTGCAG-3′
RANKL	Forward: 5′-GGGCCA ACCGAGACTACGGC-3′
	Reverser: 5′-GGATGCAGCGGACCCTCGTG-3′

Greater than 1×10^4 cells were analyzed per sample, and 3 independent experiments were conducted.

Alizarin Red staining

The degree of mineralization in MC3T3-E1 cells was determined in 24-well plates by Alizarin Red staining. Irradiated osteoblasts were fixed for 1 h in ice cold 70% ethanol 21 days after irradiation. The cells were then washed thoroughly with deionized H_2O, and mineralization was detected with 40 mM Alizarin red (pH 4.2) for 15 min. Following staining, cells were washed thoroughly with deionized H_2O to remove non-specific Alizarin red staining. After air-drying, the cell culture plates were evaluated by light microscopy.

Western blot analysis

The cells were homogenized in RIPA lysis buffer (Beyotime, China) using a sonic dismembrator containing protease and phosphatase inhibitors (Roche, Switzerland). Freshly isolated cell homogenates were centrifuged for 10 min at 12,000×g and 4°C. The supernatant was collected, and the protein concentration was determined using a bicinchoninic acid (BCA) protein assay kit (Beyotime, China). All samples were then diluted to an equal concentration in PBS and boiled for 5 min. Equal amounts of protein (30 μg) were subjected to 8–15% SDS-PAGE and then transferred onto polyvinylidene fluoride (PVDF) membranes. After blocking with 5% w/v non-fat dry milk for 1 h at room temperature, the membranes were incubated overnight with primary antibodies against β-actin (ab133626, Abcam, USA; dilution 1:3000), Col1α (ab34710, Abcam, USA; dilution 1:5000), ALP (ab95462, Abcam, USA; dilution 1:2000), OCN (AB10911, Millipore, USA; dilution 1:1000), Runx2 (sc-10758, Santa Cruz, USA; dilution 1:500) and Osterix (ab22552, Abcam, USA; dilution 1:2000) at 4°C with gentle shaking. After washing thrice in PBST, the blots were incubated with a 1:2000 dilution of goat anti-rabbit IgG horseradish peroxidase (HRP)-conjugated secondary antibody (ab97200, Abcam, USA) for 2 h at room temperature. The blots were washed thrice and visualized using a chemiluminescence kit (BioInd, Israel). Images were then captured with a chemiluminescence imaging system (Syegene, UK). Given that protein levels differ in relative abundance, exposure times or image intensities were varied to produce linear stain-to-background ratios.

Real-time quantitative PCR analysis

Rats were euthanized at 7, 14, 21 and 28 days after irradiation (4 rats per group). The fracture callus and 1–2 mm of the normal bone margin were carefully excised from the soft tissue using a scalpel. The samples were frozen in liquid N_2, pulverized using a nitrogen-cooled mortar and pestle apparatus and purified for total RNA using the Trizol system (Invitrogen, USA) according to the manufacturer's instructions. First-strand cDNA was obtained from the total RNA (1 μg) using RevertAid M-MuLV reverse transcriptase and oligo (dT) primer (Fermentas, Lithuania). Real-time PCR was performed in a total volume of 20 μl, which consisted of 1 μl of cDNA (500 ng), 1 μl of gene-specific 10 μM PCR primer-pair stock and 10 μl of SsoFast EvaGreen Mix (Bio-Rad, USA), using the Bio-Rad CFX96 system according to the manufacturer's protocol. The primer sequences for β-actin, Col1a1, Col2α1, OCN, ALP, Runx2 and Osterix are presented in Table 1. The PCR conditions consisted of an initial step at 95°C for 30 s to activate the DNA polymerase followed by 40 cycles of 5 s at 95°C and 5 s at 60°C, which were subsequently followed by the melting curve test. The relative amount of mRNA expression normalized to β-actin was expressed as a fold change, which was calculated using the comparative Ct ($2^{-\Delta\Delta Ct}$) method using the control group as a reference with $2^{-\Delta\Delta Ct}=1$. Each sample was assayed in triplicate, and each experiment was independently repeated thrice.

Histology and analysis

The fractured femurs were harvested on days 7, 14, 21 and 28 post-irradiation (4 rats per group). Excess muscle and soft tissue were excised and fractured femurs were assessed by radiography. Four specimens from each group were fixed in 10% neutral buffered formalin. The specimens were decalcified for 4–5 weeks in 10% EDTA (pH 7.2), embedded in paraffin and sectioned at a thickness of 3 μm. The sections were cut through the long axis of each femur in the sagittal plane and stained with Masson's trichrome stain and TRAP stain (three levels per animal). Osteoclast counts were obtained from the number of TRAP-positive cells. The total callus area, total cartilage area and total woven bone area were quantified using Image Pro Plus 6.0 software as described previously [21].

Immunohistochemistry was also performed on these sections using a previously described method [22]. The sections were mounted on poly-L-lysine-coated glass slides and then air-dried overnight at room temperature. The sections were then deparaffinized with xylene and hydrated with serial concentrations of 100, 95, 80 and 70% alcohol. Endogenous peroxidase activity was blocked with 0.5% hydrogen peroxide in methanol for 60 min. Following a Tris-buffered saline (TBS)/0.1% bovine serum albumin (BSA) wash, hyaluronidase treatment (hyaluronidase 1 mg/ml in sodium acetate buffer, pH 5.5, 0.85% NaCl) was performed for 30 min at 37°C. After washing with TBS/0.1% BSA, the sections were incubated with blocking solutions (fresh 10 ml of TBS/0.5% BSA containing 130 μl of normal horse serum) at room temperature for 15 min. The sections were then incubated with the proliferating cell nuclear antigen (PCNA) monoclonal antibody (PC10; sc-56, Santa Cruz, USA) and OCN polyclonal antibody (AB10911, Millipore, USA) at a 1:100 dilution. A subsequent reaction was performed using a Vectastain avidin/biotin-peroxidase complex (ABC) kit. The sections were reacted with diaminobenzidine (DAB) solution and were then counterstained with methyl green. We identified the cell type in the histological analyses based on tissue types, callus areas and cellular morphology [23]. Briefly, in the early stages after fracture, the calluses were mainly composed of soft tissue, including cell debris and mesenchymal cells, which exhibited a high proliferation activity. Chondrocytes were detected in the cartilage island. The premature cells were located in the margin of the cartilage adjacent to the soft tissue and were small and round in shape. The hypertrophic or mature chondrocytes were located in the center of the cartilage tissue or adjoined to the woven bone and displayed vacuole morphology. The vessel located in the soft tissue presented a cavity structure, which was encircled by flat endothelial cells.

Statistical analysis

Statistical analyses were performed using SPSS version 17.0 (IBM SPSS, USA). All data are expressed as the means ± SD. One-way or two-way analysis of variance (ANOVA) and post-hoc multiple comparisons were used for statistical analyses. A difference was considered significant if the p-value was <0.05.

Results

Low-dose X-ray irradiation increases the cell viability and proliferation of osteoblastic MC3T3-E1 cells

We performed cell viability CCK-8 assays at days 1 through 7 following irradiation. As shown in Fig. 1, no statistically significant differences in CCK-8 activity in MC3T3-E1 cells were noted between the individually irradiated groups and the non-irradiated controls at day 1 post-irradiation. However, cells irradiated with a single, low dose (0.5 Gy) exhibited an increased in cell viability at days 2 to 6 ($p<0.05$), whereas high-dose (5 Gy) X-ray irradiation significantly reduced cell viability at days 2 to 7 ($p<0.05$). In addition, 0.5 Gy of irradiation exhibited no significant effect by day 7, and this result might be attributed to the notion that MC3T3-E1 cell growth had plateaued in both the control and the low-dose irradiation cultures. To determine whether this variation in cell viability was due to cell proliferation, BrdU incorporation was measured after irradiation. The results indicated that low-dose (0.5 Gy) X-ray irradiation promoted cell proliferation on days 2, 4 and 6 post-irradiation compared with the 0 Gy control ($p<0.05$), whereas high-dose (5 Gy) irradiation inhibited MC3T3-E1 cell proliferation (Fig. 2A). Cell cycle analysis by flow cytometry revealed that single, low-dose (0.5 Gy) X-ray irradiation induced a decrease in the proportion of cells at the sub-G1 phase, which indicates active apoptosis (6.75%±0.21%, $p<0.05$ *vs.* control), whereas increasing levels of cell death by apoptosis were observed in the high-dose irradiation group (14.26%±0.41%, $p<0.05$ *vs.* control). Moreover, our results indicated that low-dose irradiation caused a 5.85% increase in the S+G2/M phases of the cell cycle in osteoblasts compared with control ($p<0.05$), whereas high-dose irradiation had no effect (Fig. 2B). These results indicated that low-dose X-ray irradiation potentially promotes osteoblast survival and renewal.

Low-dose X-ray irradiation promotes osteoblasts differentiation and mineralization in *vitro*

After X-ray irradiation, MC3T3-E1 cells were further cultured in osteogenic medium, and the expression levels of proteins associated with osteoblast differentiation were examined by Western blot at 4, 7, 10 and 14 days after irradiation. The statistical analysis histograms are presented in Fig. 3A–F. Osteoblast differentiation markers, such as OCN, Runx2 and Osterix, were inhibited temporarily at 4 days post-irradiation in both the low- and high-dose groups, with the levels of Runx2 and Osterix demonstrating the most prominent decreases in the low-dose group (Fig. 3A, D–F). The levels of Col1α were decreased at 4 and 14 days but were elevated at 10 days post-irradiation in the low-dose group, whereas a continual decrease in Col1α levels was observed in the high-dose group from days 4 to 14 after irradiation (Fig. 3A, B). Irradiation-stimulated increases in alkaline ALP levels occurred at 7 and 10 days after 0.5 Gy and 5 Gy X-ray irradiation (Fig. 3A, C). In addition, both the 0.5 Gy and 5 Gy radiation doses led to significant increases in OCN levels at 10 days, with the increases in the 0.5 Gy group continuing through 14 days post-irradiation (Fig. 3A, F). Decreased Runx2 levels were detected in the high-dose group at 7 days and in the low-dose group at 10 days; however, both low- and high-dose irradiation stimulated increases in Runx2 protein levels at 14 days after irradiation (Fig. 3A, D). In addition, the expression of Osterix in the low-dose group was significantly increased at 7, 10 and 14 days compared with the non-irradiated control group (Fig. 3A, E). These findings indicate that X-ray irradiation induced dynamic variations in the differentiation of pre-osteoblastic cells. Although we observed temporary reductions in osteogenic markers of early osteoblast differentiation after single-dose X-ray irradiation, dramatic increases in the related differentiation markers occurred at the medium differentiation. In addition, Alizarin Red staining demonstrated that low-dose irradiation promoted mineralization in MC3T3-E1 cells. For cells irradiated with high-dose irradiation, the mineralized bone nodules decreased in number (Fig. 2C). Together, low-dose X-ray irradiation promoted osteoblasts differentiation and mineralization in *vitro*.

Low-dose X-ray irradiation accelerates endochondral and intramembranous ossification in fracture healing

A rat femur fracture model was employed to study fracture healing after irradiation. Fracture calluses from irradiated and non-irradiated rats, which were age- and sex-matched, were examined by radiography assessment and Masson's trichrome staining at days 7, 14, 21 and 28 following irradiation (Fig. 4). The radiographs indicate that 0.5 Gy X-ray irradiation accelerated callus mineralization and fractures repair, whereas 5 Gy X-ray irradiation delayed fracture healing (Fig. 4B). Histology sections of the calluses confirmed accelerated fracture healing and remodeling in low-dose (0.5 Gy) irradiated rats compared with the non-irradiated control group. However, the fractures in high-dose (5 Gy) animals demonstrated delayed healing. On day 7 following irradiation, low-dose irradiated rats presented increased callus areas and cartilage formation compared with non-irradiated rats. In contrast, decreased callus areas and less bone and cartilage formation were detected in high-dose irradiation rats (Fig. 4A, C–D). By day 14, the calluses in the high-dose group were also composed of less cartilage and woven bone area compared with the control group (Fig. 4A, D, E). On days 21 to 28, fractures in the low-dose irradiated and control rats were healed, and cartilage tissue was essentially absent in the calluses. However, healing was incomplete in the fractures of high-dose irradiated rats where a central area of cartilage tissue persisted (Fig. 4A, D). In addition to the accelerated osteogenesis, the fractures in the low-dose group underwent more rapid remodeling. In particular, low-dose irradiated rats exhibited abundant woven bone formation that peaked at 14 days; this event occurred earlier than the bone formation observed in the non-irradiated group, in which peak bone area was measured at 21 days. Subsequently, the bone areas

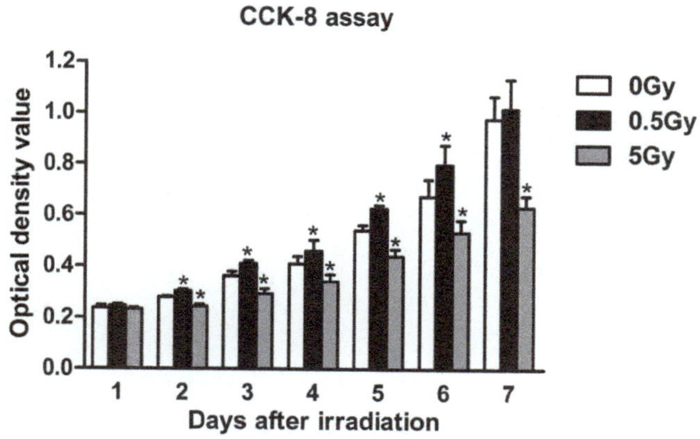

Figure 1. MC3T3-E1 cell viability as determined by the CCK-8 assay. Compared with the control cells (0 Gy), single low-dose (0.5 Gy) irradiation significantly increased cell viability from days 2 to 6, whereas high-dose (5 Gy) irradiation significantly reduced cell viability from days 2 to 7. *$p<0.05$ *vs.* the control group.

of both groups progressively decreased (Fig. 4A, E). Beginning on day 21, low-dose-irradiated rats demonstrated decreased callus area, and most of the initial woven bone within the calluses had been remodeled with lamellar bone, which persisted through 28 days post-irradiation (Fig. 4A, C). By 28 days, the fractures in the low-dose irradiated rats had essentially undergone complete remodeling, and the femurs exhibited a similar morphology to non-fractured bone. In the control group, extensive remodeling was not observed until 28 days post-irradiation. Moreover, abnormal mineralization and remodeling were involved in fracture healing after high-dose irradiation. Fracture calluses in high-dose irradiated rats remained enlarged and contained areas of woven bone where greater amounts of mature collagen (red stained) were deposited at 28 days (Fig. 4A).

Immunohistochemistry revealed increased numbers of proliferating cells during fracture repair in low-dose (0.5 Gy) irradiated rats. This increase in proliferating cells included periosteal cells, osteoblasts and mesenchymal cells or chondrocytes, which are known to contribute to intramembranous ossification, chondrogenesis and endochondral ossification during fracture repair. On day 7, near the fracture site, the periosteal cells stained by PCNA antibodies in the fibrous layer were increased in the low-dose group compared with the non-irradiated group. In contrast, the high-dose irradiated group displayed significantly decreased numbers of PCNA-positive periosteal cells (Fig. 5A, B). In soft calluses, greater chondrogenesis was observed in the 0.5 Gy group on day 7; small, round, premature chondrocytes and mesenchymal cells were detected near the cartilage tissue. The proliferating

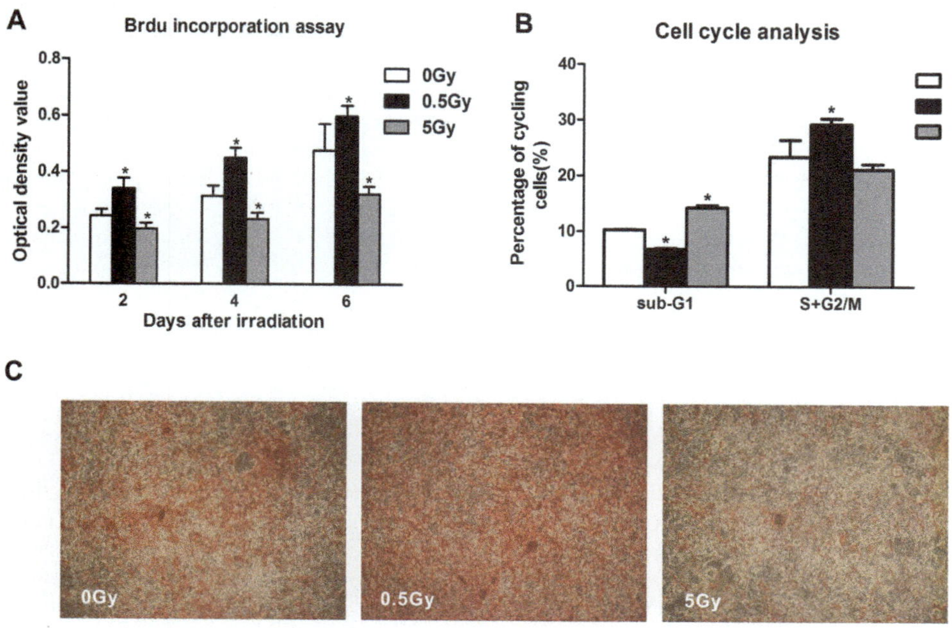

Figure 2. MC3T3-E1 cell proliferation and mineralization after irradiation. Low-dose (0.5 Gy) irradiation significantly promoted cell proliferation from days 2 to 6 compared with control cells (0 Gy), whereas high-dose (5 Gy) irradiation inhibited cell proliferation (A). Low-dose (0.5 Gy) irradiation resulted in an approximate 6.75% decrease in the percentage of cells in the sub-G1 phase, whereas high-dose (5 Gy) irradiation elicited an approximate 14.26% increase in the percentage of cells in the sub-G1 phase (B). Low-dose (0.5 Gy) irradiation accelerated osteoblasts mineralization 21 days after irradiation, and high-dose (5 Gy) irradiation decreased alizarin red staining (C). *$p<0.05$ *vs.* the control group.

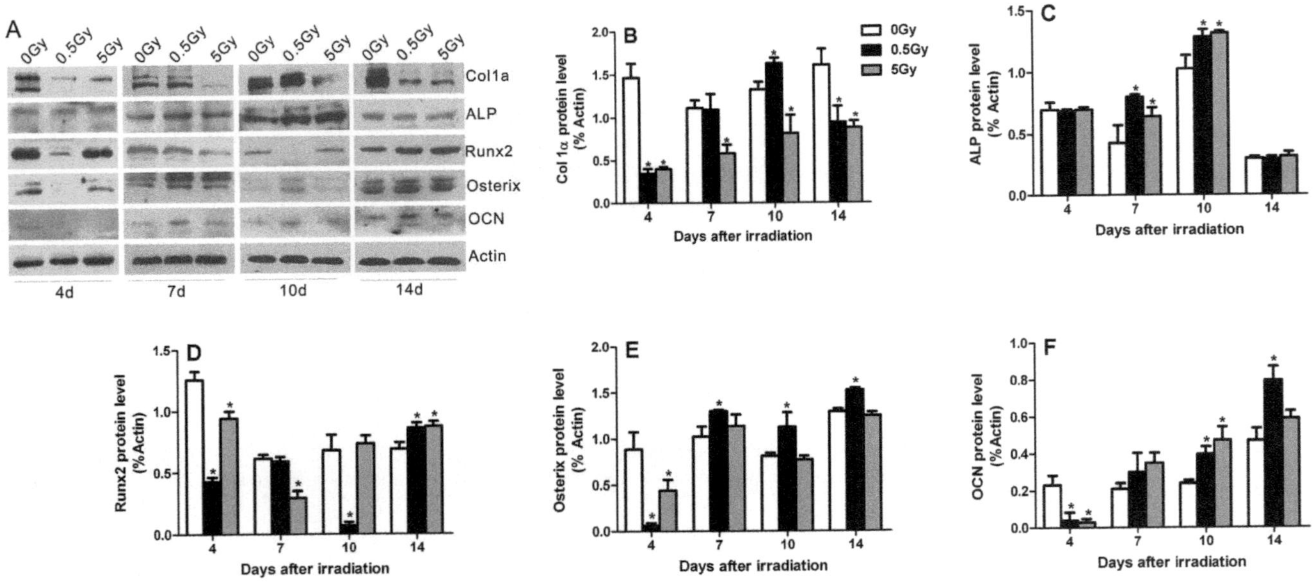

Figure 3. The effects of irradiation on the expression of osteoblast differentiation markers *in vitro*. The expression of Col1α, ALP, Runx2, Osterix and OCN proteins was assessed by Western blot on post-irradiation days 4, 7, 10 and 14 (A). The Col1α (B), ALP (C), Runx2 (D), Osterix (E) and OCN (F) protein levels were normalized to β-actin expression. *$p<0.05$ *vs.* the control group.

premature chondrocytes stained by PCNA antibodies were significantly increased in the low-dose group compared with the non-irradiated group. In contrast, deceased PCNA-positive cells, of which mesenchymal cells were predominant, were observed in the high-dose group (Fig. 5C, D). On day 14, a greater reduction in PCNA-positive cells was detected in each group compared with the early phase. The proliferating chondrocytes in the non-irradiated control were more numerous compared with the irradiated groups (Fig. 5C, D). In addition, vascularization was observed in the fibrous calluses, and fewer PCNA-positive mesenchymal cells were noted in the low-dose and control groups. Furthermore, the majority cells in the soft callus area differed in appearance from the hypertrophic chondrocytes observed in the high-dose group, and fibrous tissue was observed in a criss-cross pattern in the cartilage calluses on day 14 (Fig. 5C). In addition, immunohistochemistry demonstrated that low-dose irradiation also increased the expression of OCN protein among proliferating cells on day 14 after irradiation (Fig. 6A, B). PCNA is a protein involved in the major DNA replication repair machinery of cells. When not engaged in DNA replication, PCNA (most often under the control of p53) commits cells to cell cycle arrest and repair of DNA damage. Alternatively, when repair is not possible, absent or low levels of functional PCNA may drive cells to apoptosis [24]. On the one hand, the suppression of PCNA signaling promotes cellular apoptosis [25]. In contrast, PCNA activation suppresses osteoblast apoptosis during *in vitro* culture [26]. These facts reveal that PCNA is also related to cellular apoptosis. Our results indicate that low-dose irradiation increased PCNA protein expression in the calluses. To some degree, this that low-dose irradiation protects cells against apoptosis during fracture repair.

Osteoblast differentiation was accelerated in the fractures of low-dose irradiated rats

The expression of genes involved in osteoblast differentiation was also examined in the callus tissue of fractures from irradiated and non-irradiated rats (Fig. 7). Col2a1 expression was elevated earlier in fractures from low-dose irradiated rats compared with non-irradiated control rats. This observation was consistent with the increase in cartilage observed in low-dose irradiated rats by histomorphometry at day 7, signifying the acceleration of the endochondral phase of fracture repair (Fig. 7B). Moreover, Col2a1 expression was absent in low-dose irradiated and non-irradiated rats by day 21, whereas Col2a1 expression persisted until day 28 in high-dose irradiated rats. Additionally, the expression of the osteoblast-specific transcription factors Runx2 and Osterix was elevated in fracture calluses from low-dose irradiated rats, whereas Runx2 and Osterix expression in the fracture calluses appeared to be not effected by high-dose irradiation (Fig. 7D, E). Furthermore, the expression of the osteoblast differentiation markers ALP and OCN was elevated earlier in fractures from irradiated rats (both low- and high-dose), which is consistent with accelerated osteoblast differentiation (Fig. 7C, F). In the fractures from low-dose irradiated rats, Col1a1 expression appeared earlier, and peak levels were observed by days 14–21 compared with the maximal expression observed at day 28 in non-irradiated control rats (Fig. 7A). ALP expression in fractures from irradiated rats was significantly increased compared with non-irradiated rats on day 14 (Fig. 7C). Furthermore, OCN expression levels were also elevated earlier in fractures from irradiated rats compared with non-irradiated rats, and this increase persisted to 28 days post-irradiation (Fig. 7F). These findings suggest that osteoblasts undergo more rapid differentiation in low-dose irradiated rats; in contrast, high-dose irradiation results in unnatural osteoblast differentiation that is characterized by delayed collagen expression and collagen maturation. Furthermore, this type of rapid osteoblast differentiation in low-dose irradiated rats is consistent with the more rapid completion of endochondral and intramembranous ossification.

Low-dose irradiation accelerates callus remodeling via enhanced osteoclast-induced signals

The fracture calluses were stained for TRAP expression, which is an osteoclast marker. In day 14, 0.5 Gy X-ray irradiation increased the number of osteoclasts in the fracture calluses by

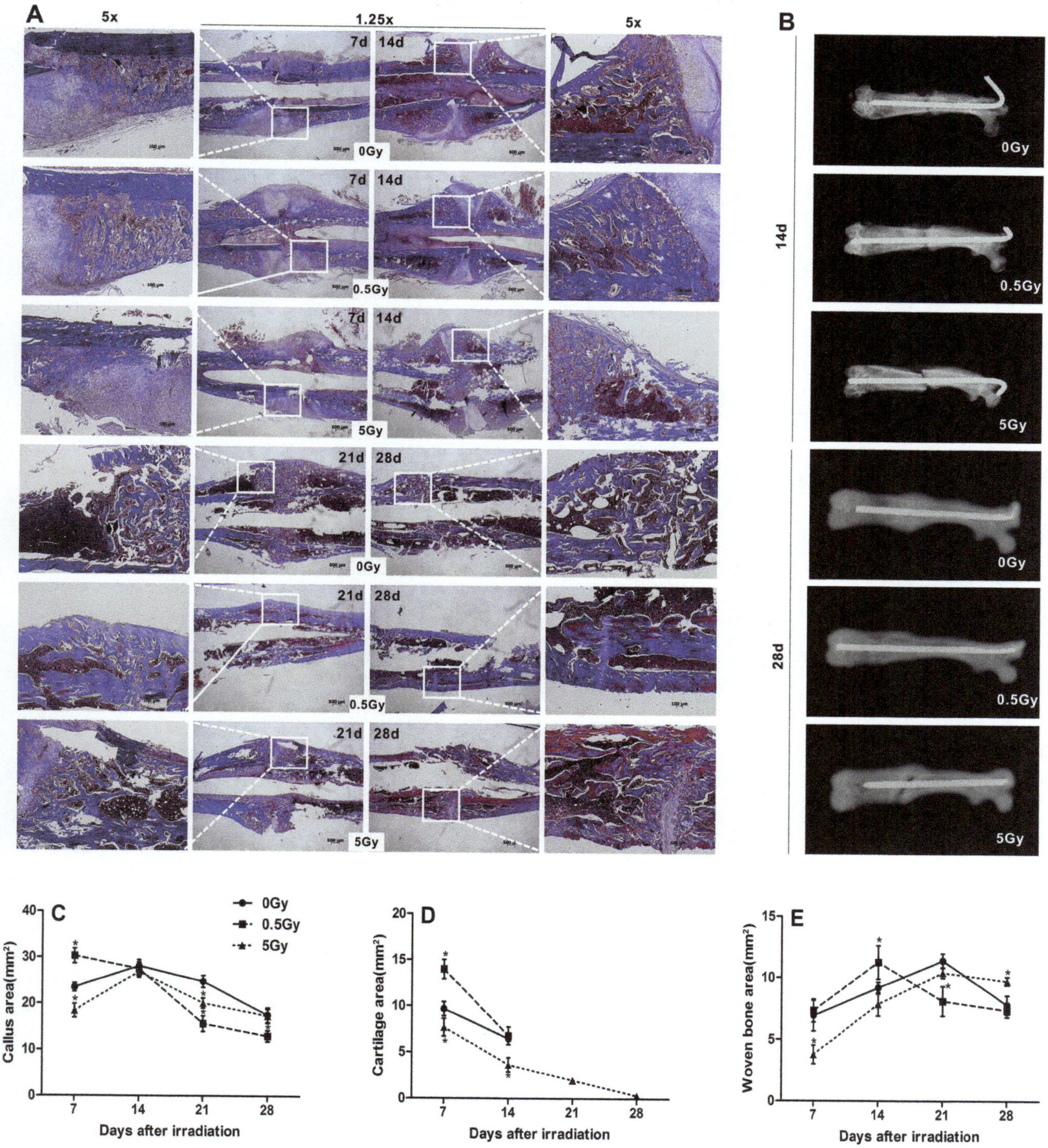

Figure 4. The effects of irradiation on fracture healing. Fractured femurs were harvested and immediately assessed by radiography. Representative histologies of fractured femurs stained with Masson's trichrome staining is depicted at 7, 14, 21 and 28 days after X-ray irradiation; accelerated remodeling on day 21 in fractures irradiated with low-dose X-ray irradiation was evident comparing the contracted calluses to the broad calluses that remained in the control fractures, whereas non-union on day 28 was observed in fractures that received high-dose X-ray irradiation (A). Radiographs demonstrated the accelerated callus mineralization and fracture repair (B). Histomorphometric measurements (total callus area, cartilage area, woven bone area) were performed, and the results are presented as a diagram (C, D, E). n = 4 rats/group, *$p<0.05$ *vs.* the control group.

61.9% ($p<0.01$) compared with non-irradiated fractures. This observation was consistent with accelerated bone remodeling. By day 21, fractures in the non-irradiated rats contained a certain number of osteoclasts. Surprisingly, few osteoclasts were observed in 21 day-old fractures from 0.5 Gy X-ray irradiated rats. However, high-dose (5 Gy) X-ray irradiation decreased osteoclast numbers at each time-point (Fig. 8A, B). Real-time PCR was performed to measure the expression of the osteoclast-inducing

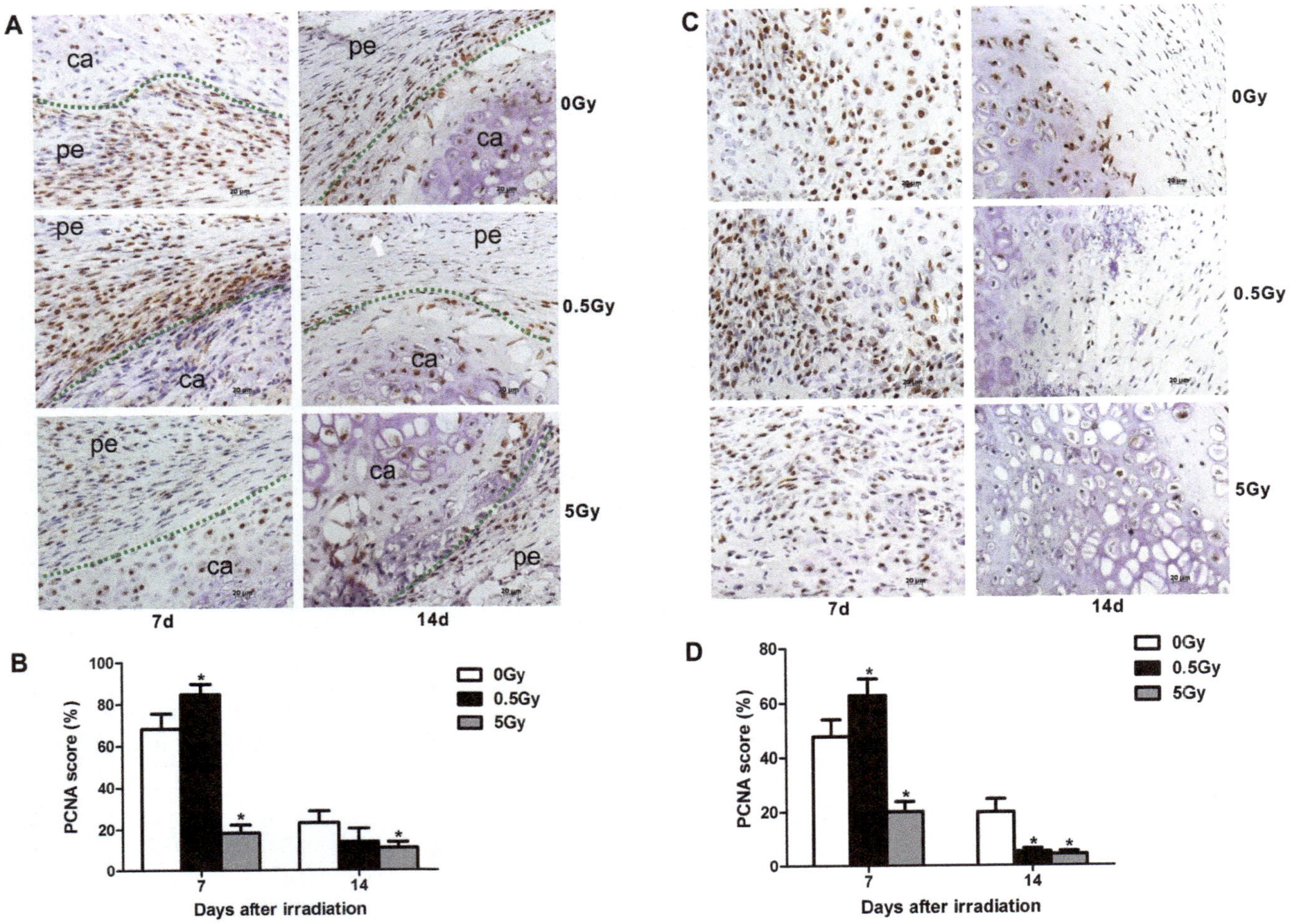

Figure 5. Cell proliferation during intramembranous osteogenesis and chondrogenesis. PCNA immunostaining was performed at 7 and 14 days after X-ray irradiation. Low-dose X-ray irradiation promoted the proliferation of periosteum cells and chondrocytes at day 7 after irradiation in fracture sites, whereas high-dose X-ray irradiation inhibited the proliferation of these cells at both days 7 and 14 post-irradiation (A, C). Quantification of cell proliferation in each group (B, D). The green dot represents the demarcation between the soft tissue and cartilage, and the white arrow denotes a vessel. pe: periosteum, ca: cartilage, n = 4 rats/group,*$p<0.05$ *vs.* the control group.

gene RANKL and its receptor antagonist OPG. The fracture calluses from 0.5 Gy irradiated rats exhibited an increased overall expression of both RANKL and OPG, and both genes were elevated earlier in fractures in 0.5 Gy irradiated rats compared with non-irradiated rats (Fig. 8C, D). The maximum expression levels of RANKL occurred at 14 days in the fracture tissue from the 0.5 Gy X-ray group and at 21 days in the control. RANKL expression exhibited a sharp peak in facture tissues from the 0.5 Gy X-ray group, whereas the control group exhibited a lower order of magnitude of expression that was more sustained. The RANKL/OPG radio in 0.5 Gy group was significantly increased compared with non-irradiated group at 14 days. However, the ratio of RANKL/OPG was reduced during fracture repair in the 5 Gy irradiated rats (Fig. 8E). These data were consistent with the differences observed in osteoclast numbers in the fracture calluses. Thus, our results suggest that 0.5 Gy irradiation accelerates callus remodeling by enhanced osteoclast-induced signals.

Discussion

In this study, we observed increased proliferation and differentiation among osteoblasts in cell culture and fracture healing models stimulated by low-dose irradiation. Given that osteoblasts exhibit a developmental sequence of events, including distinct proliferative, differentiating and mineralizing stages, we selected different time points for the proliferation and differentiation analyses in our study. After single-dose 0.5 Gy X-ray irradiation, osteoblastic cell activity was enhanced, consistent with increased osteoblast proliferation. Similarly, increased numbers of PCNA-positive cells were detected in calluses early during the fracture-healing process. In addition, low-dose (0.5 Gy) X-ray irradiation promoted osteoblastic cell survival and reduced apoptotic cell death based on the sub-G1 cell cycle analysis of cultured cells. Furthermore, low-dose irradiation induced accelerated osteoblast differentiation and fracture healing by triggering the expression of osteoblast-specific differentiation markers and inhibiting apoptosis. These results demonstrated the stimulatory effect of low-dose irradiation on osteogenesis, which was mediated through increased osteoblast proliferation and differentiation.

Despite accumulating evidence highlighting the biological effects of irradiation on bone, a series of controversies remain in this field. For example, although previous researchers have demonstrated the detrimental effects of irradiation on bone [7,27–29], other reports demonstated positive effects of irradiation on osteoblastic differentiation and bone-specific gene expression [16,18,20,30]. Furthermore, a few studies have reported stimula-

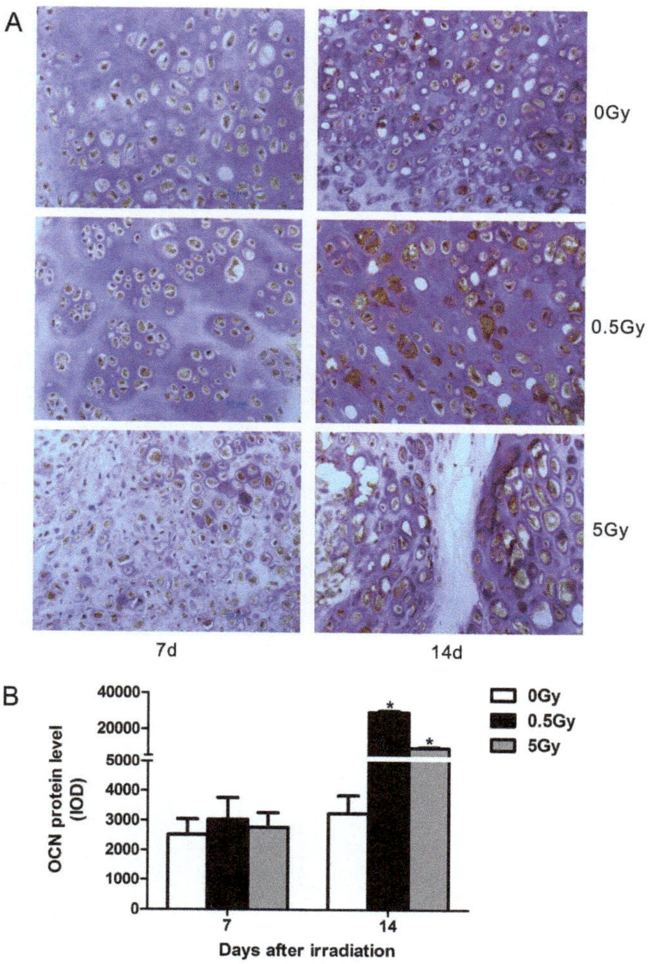

Figure 6. Irradiation increased OCN-positive cells in calluses on day 14 after irradiation. Representative immunohistochemistry of the calluses stained with OCN antibody at 7 and 14 days after X-ray irradiation (A). Quantification of OCN protein expression in each group (B). n = 4 rats/group,*$p<0.05$ *vs.* the control group.

tory effects of low-dose X-ray irradiation (<0.2 Gy) on the proliferation of BM-MSCs, which are osteoblast progenitors and may undergo osteoblastic differentiation in osteogenic medium [16]. These contradictory conclusions may be due to differences in cell lines, irradiation doses and time points used in the gene expression analyses. Our study primarily focused on the effects of low-dose X-ray irradiation on osteoblast proliferation and differentiation both *in vivo* and *in vitro*. Given that the radiosensitivity of cells differs according to cell type and differentiation stage, the relatively low dose of 0.5 Gy was used in our experiments. After 0.5 Gy irradiation, Osteoblast proliferation increased for increased BrdU incorporation and PCNA-positive cells were detected *in vivo* and *in vitro*. The consistent inhibitory effect of high-dose (5 Gy) irradiation on osteoblast proliferation was also reported in this study. A variety of types of DNA damage, including single-strand breaks, double-strand breaks and base damage, occur in response to radiation, and the DNA repair process is activated to address such damage. However, high-dose radiation can induce extensive DNA damage that is difficult to repair and might interfere with cell cycle progression, at which point cells undergo programmed cell death [16,17,31]. Adaptive protection against DNA damage and bystander effects might also occur in response to low-dose radiation, generally in terms of the protective mechanisms associated with hormesis [11,15,32,33]. Our results indicate that low-dose irradiation elicited DNA synthesis in osteoblastic cells with an increase in proliferation activity and apoptosis suppression. Although the effect of 0.5 Gy irradiation on osteoblast viability and proliferation was mild, the differences between the control and 0.5 Gy groups were statistically significant. At a minimum, this result indicates that osteoblasts can complete DNA repair at the early stage in response to 0.5 Gy irradiation and that osteoblast proliferation is not inhibited. As demonstrated in our previous study, ≤1.0 Gy irradiation had no significant effect on cell proliferation, viability and apoptosis [20]. This contradiction was attributed to the modulation of the irradiation procedure. In the previous experiment, osteoblasts were irradiated the day after seeding. However, in the present study, we performed an irradiation schedule whereby the irradiated osteoblasts in the logarithmic phase of growth were immediately seeded onto a plate. It is known that different cell types and stages of differentiation exhibit varying susceptibility and responses to radiation exposure.

The osteoblast differentiation process is tightly controlled by bone-specific regulatory factors. Col1 is the main structural component of bone matrix. ALP is important in stabilizing the matrix. OCN is another non-collagenous protein that is almost exclusively expressed in bone and is upregulated during matrix mineralization [34,35]. In the case of bone, the dynamic and well-

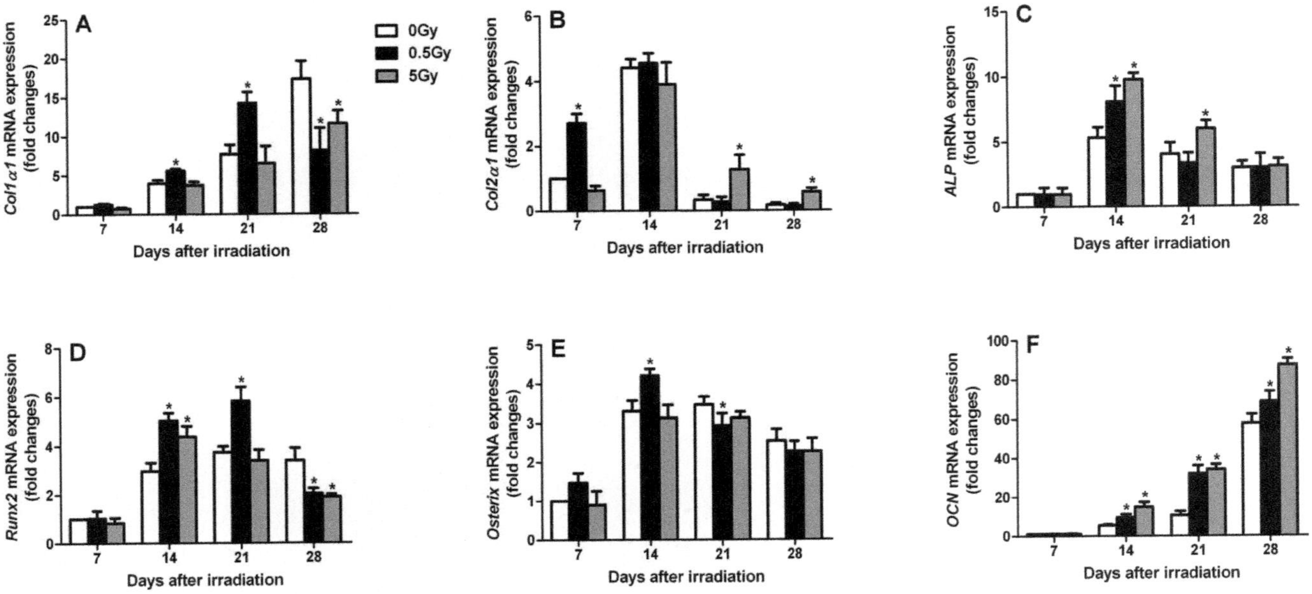

Figure 7. Irradiation-stimulated changes in mRNA expression patterns of osteoblast differentiation-related genes in fracture callus tissues. Real-time PCR was performed at various time points after X-ray irradiation. The following primer sets were used: Col1a1 (A), Col2a1 (B), ALP (C), Runx2 (D), Osterix (E) and OCN (F). n = 4 rats/group,*$p<0.05$ *vs.* the control group.

regulated expression patterns of these marker genes depend on the differentiation stage of the osteoblasts [18,35]. For example, Col1 is expressed from the beginning of osteoblast differentiation, whereas only mature osteoblasts in the matrix calcification stage secrete OCN. From our experiments, X-ray irradiation induced significant differentiation effects on osteoblasts. For example, after relatively low-dose irradiation, Col1, ALP and OCN expression was increased in the mature stage of osteoblast differentiation. Similarly, high-dose irradiation also enhanced the expression of osteoblastic differentiation markers with the exception of Col1, which was clearly decreased at all time points. Interestingly, a temporary decline in the expression of several differentiation markers at 4 days after both low-dose and high-dose irradiation *in vitro* was noted, and the following reasons might contribute to this dynamic tendency. First, this decline in expression might represent a cellular survival strategy when radiation damage is present [17]. The major trigger of the cellular response to irradiation is the destruction of genome integrity, and cells can mount a coordinated response to genotoxic stresses, including irradiation, by activating a network of interacting signaling pathways collectively known as the DNA damage response [32]. In response to irradiation, osteoblasts immediately initiate DNA repair mechanisms. Lau et al. [17] reported that discrete γ-H2AX foci that reflect DNA damage were detected as early as 30 min after irradiation in osteoblasts, and approximately all double-strand breaks were effectively rejoined after a repair period of 24 h. As a survival strategy, osteoblasts either retain their proliferative capability and repair DNA damage or are programmed to die (or become senescent or prematurely terminally differentiated) if DNA is heavily damaged [17,32,33]. Therefore, cells primarily focus on DNA repair during the early stages after irradiation, whereas the differentiation potential is inhibited. Second, the progressive development of the osteoblastic phenotype, which requires precise coordination between cellular proliferation and differentiation, might play a critical role in the early stages after irradiation [17]. Cell fate is decided according to the balance between self-renewal and differentiation, where cell self-renewal blocks differentiation and supports cell division [36]. Our results revealed that low-dose irradiation stimulated pre-osteoblast proliferation, which may be related to the decreased expression of differentiation markers in the early stage after irradiation. Consistently, following low-dose irradiation, the expression of the transcription factors Runx2 and Osterix, which are key regulators in osteoblast differentiation, was significantly high-dose irradiation. In other words, the increased proliferation observed following low-dose irradiation may constrain the differentiation potentiality in the early stages after irradiation. Although high-dose irradiation increased terminal differentiation among osteoblasts, it inhibited cell proliferation and reduced production of the extracellular matrix. Thus, the cells' bone forming capacity was weakened in response to high-dose irradiation. However, low-dose irradiation enhanced osteoblast proliferation in the early stages, increased the expression of osteogenic markers and promoted the terminal differentiation process. This result demonstrates that low-dose X-ray increases the osteogenic potential of osteoblast.

Fracture healing is a complex process during which mesenchymal stem cells are recruited to the site of injury and subsequently undergo proliferation and differentiation into bone-forming cells [37]. The present study reveals that low-dose irradiation acts as a positive factor in the fracture-healing process given that it promoted cell proliferation, differentiation and fracture healing in animal models. Accelerated intramembranous bone formation and endochondral bone formation were observed in low-dose irradiated fractures. Low-dose irradiation also accelerated callus remodeling by enhanced osteoclast-induced signals. Furthermore, low-dose irradiation enhanced the expression of osteoblast differentiation genes in the fracture calluses. Our *in vivo* experimental results were consistent with the results of osteoblast culture *in vitro*. For example, the number of proliferating cells increased in calluses from fractures irradiated with low-dose X-ray radiation, and gene expression studies from fracture callus tissues demonstrated an enhanced rate of chondrocyte and osteoblast differentiation after low-dose irradiation. Maximal expression of Col2a1 occurred early after low-dose irradiation, demonstrating

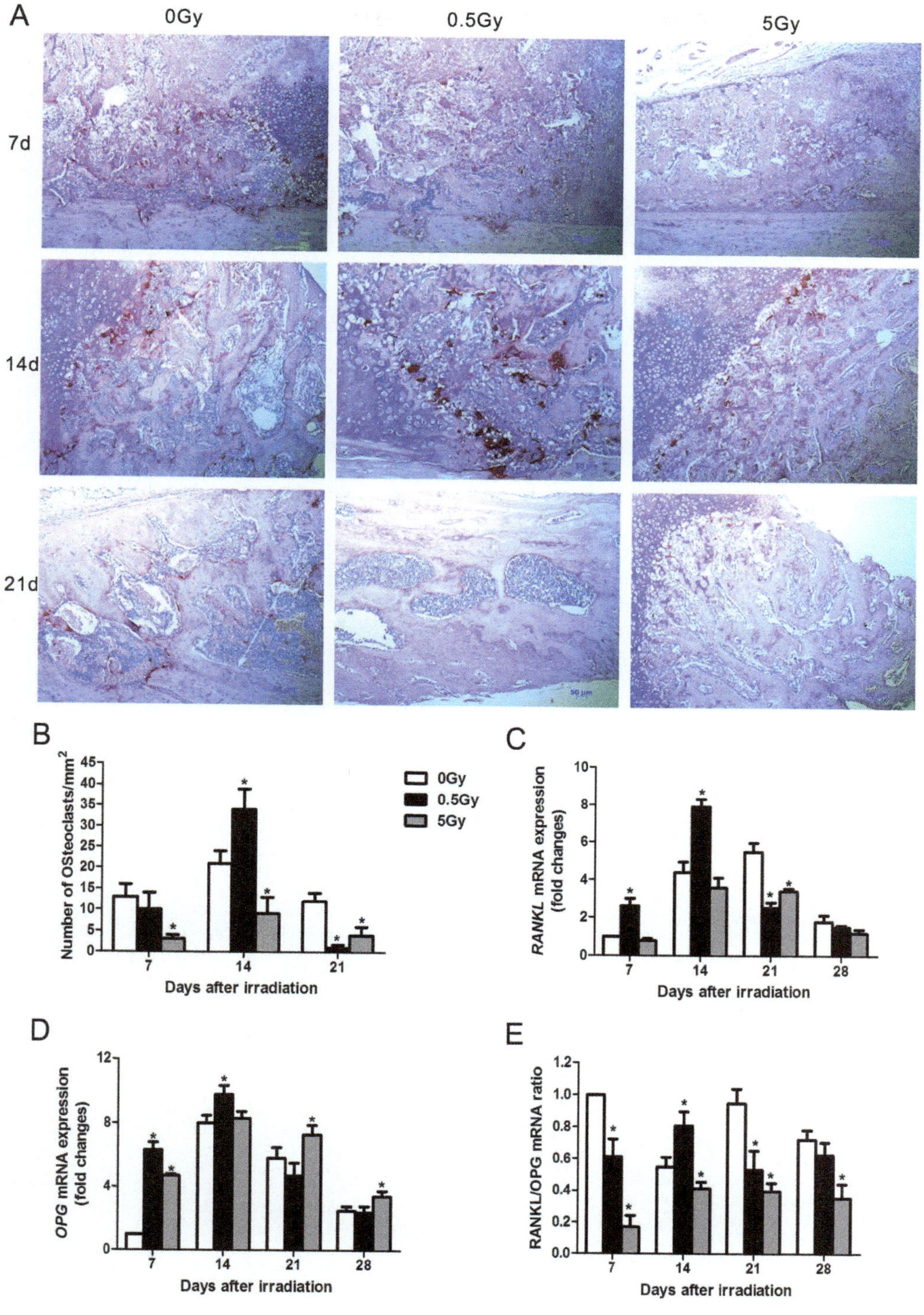

Figure 8. Low-dose X-ray irradiation accelerated bone remodeling. TRAP staining was performed on callus sections at 7, 14 and 21 days after X-ray irradiation (A). Osteoclast numbers were counted in sections per group (B). RANKL and OPG mRNA levels in the fracture callus were examined by real-time PCR (C, D).The RANKL/OPG ratio was calculated (E). n = 4 rats/group,*$p<0.05$ *vs.* the control group.

the acceleration of complete endochondral ossification. These mature, calcified cartilage tissues may act as a template for bone formation and remodeling. Consistent with the acceleration of the cartilage phase of fracture repair, the expression of osteogenic genes, such as ALP, OCN, Col1a1, Runx2 and Osterix, peaked early or were increased in the low-dose irradiated callus tissues. These results document that low-dose X-ray irradiation enhances the bone formation potential of osteoblast in *vitro* and *vivo*. In addition to enhanced bone formation, our findings also suggest that callus remodeling was accelerated upon low-dose irradiation. We performed TRAP staining to determine whether low-dose X-ray irradiation-induced callus remolding was associated with the potential for accelerated osteoclast formation. Our study reveals that the calluses from the rats irradiated by low-dose X-ray irradiation had more osteoclastogenesis. The RANKL/OPG ratio was consistently increased in the fractures after low-dose X-ray radiation. Finally, fracture union was rapid, and the rate of remodeling was enhanced in low-dose irradiated fractures. Our findings are consistent with previous descriptions indicating that low-dose X-ray irradiation promotes the mineralization of fracture callus tissue in rats [19]. However, callus formation and fracture union were delayed in high-dose X-ray-irradiated fractures, and greater collagenous fiber senescence occurred in high-dose irradiated fracture callus tissue. The following reasons contributed to this observation. On one hand, the discoordination between reduced proliferation and abnormal expression of osteogenic genes might result from decreased bone formation. On the other hand, the reduced number of osteoclasts affected callus remodeling, leading to bone matrix aging or sclerosis.

One limitation of this study was that over-active cell proliferation and tumorigenicity should be addressed for all low-dose irradiation interventions. In fact, because current hospital medical imaging procedures may increase patient exposure to low-dose radiation, the risk of cancer development represents a serious concern. Additionally, human epidemiological data warn that irradiation might trigger abnormal cell proliferation and thus promote tumor growth [10]. Nevertheless, our data show that low-dose X-ray irradiation may induce middle and late osteoblast differentiation simultaneously. Another limitation was that we exclusively focused on the effects of radiation on the fracture healing process using a rat fracture model *in vivo* in the present study. However, we failed to detect changes in the distinct regions or non-fractured sites. Irradiation affects bone tissues by both cellular and physicochemical processes, including bone metabolism and fracture healing. The altered compositions of bone tissues lead to differential response to irradiation [38]. Different local environments and components were noted in the fracture or non-fractured sites. In other words, irradiation had different effects on distinct regions of bone. Given the lack of investigations focused on non-fractured bones, the generalization of our conclusion should be interpreted with caution. In addition, low-dose irradiation appeared to accelerate age-related changes in skeletal micro-architecture [39]. In this study, limited passages of osteoblasts and adult animals were employed for *in vitro* and *in vivo* studies. However, it remains unclear whether the stimulatory effects of low-dose irradiation on osteoblasts and fracture healing represent an age-related phenomenon.

Conclusion

In summary, our experiments revealed that X-ray irradiation at low- or high-doses exhibited opposing effects on osteogenesis. Low-dose (0.5 Gy) X-ray irradiation presented certain beneficial effects on osteoblast proliferation, differentiation and fracture repair. Although high-dose (5 Gy) X-ray irradiation increased terminal differentiation among osteoblasts, it weakened the bone formation capacity of osteoblasts by inhibiting cell proliferation and reducing extracellular matrix production. These findings provide a better understanding of low-dose irradiation-induced biological responses during bone formation and might lead to the development of improved strategies with translational applications for bone-related diseases in humans.

Author Contributions

Performed the experiments: MC QH. Wrote the paper: MC QH QRD ML. Designed and led the study: QRD. Conducted irradiation: MC WX CS. Conducted statistical analysis: WX ML CS. Contributed reagents and fracture model establishment: ZGX YTM.

References

1. Matsumura S, Hiranuma H, Deguchi A, Maeda T, Jikko A, et al. (1998) Changes in phenotypic expression of osteoblasts after X irradiation. Radiat Res 149: 463–471.
2. Long F (2012) Building strong bones: molecular regulation of the osteoblast lineage. Nat Rev Mol Cell Biol 13: 27–38.
3. Phulpin B, Dolivet G, Marie PY, Poussier S, Gallet P, et al. (2010) Re-assessment of chronic radio-induced tissue damage in a rat hindlimb model. Exp Ther Med 1: 553–560.
4. Takahashi S, Sugimoto M, Kotoura Y, Sasai K, Oka M, et al. (1994) Long-term changes in the haversian systems following high-dose irradiation. An ultrastructural and quantitative histomorphological study. J Bone Joint Surg Am 76: 722–738.
5. Peyre HM, Coffigny H, Reillaudou M, Beaumatin J, Morin M, et al. (2000) Transformation by radiation of rat foetal glial cells. Int J Radiat Biol 76: 87–94.
6. Jia D, Gaddy D, Suva LJ, Corry PM (2011) Rapid loss of bone mass and strength in mice after abdominal irradiation. Radiat Res 176: 624–635.
7. Szymczyk KH, Shapiro IM, Adams CS (2004) Ionizing radiation sensitizes bone cells to apoptosis. Bone 34: 148–156.
8. Sakurai T, Sawada Y, Yoshimoto M, Kawai M, Miyakoshi J (2007) Radiation-induced reduction of osteoblast differentiation in C2C12 cells. J Radiat Res 48: 515–521.
9. Theocharopoulos N, Perisinakis K, Damilakis J, Papadokostakis G, Hadjipavlou A, et al. (2003) Occupational exposure from common fluoroscopic projections used in orthopaedic surgery. J Bone Joint Surg Am 85-A: 1698–1703.
10. Fazel R, Krumholz HM, Wang Y, Ross JS, Chen J, et al. (2009) Exposure to low-dose ionizing radiation from medical imaging procedures. N Engl J Med 361: 849–857.
11. Pramojanee SN, Pratchayasakul W, Chattipakorn N, Chattipakorn SC (2012) Low-dose dental irradiation decreases oxidative stress in osteoblastic MC3T3-E1 cells without any changes in cell viability, cellular proliferation and cellular apoptosis. Arch Oral Biol 57: 252–256.
12. Sangsuwan T, Haghdoost S (2008) The nucleotide pool, a target for low-dose gamma-ray-induced oxidative stress. Radiat Res 170: 776–783.
13. Asaithamby A, Chen DJ (2009) Cellular responses to DNA double-strand breaks after low-dose gamma-irradiation. Nucleic Acids Res 37: 3912–3923.
14. Li W, Wang G, Cui J, Xue L, Cai L (2004) Low-dose radiation (LDR) induces hematopoietic hormesis: LDR-induced mobilization of hematopoietic progenitor cells into peripheral blood circulation. Exp Hematol 32: 1088–1096.
15. Liang X, So YH, Cui J, Ma K, Xu X, et al. (2011) The low-dose ionizing radiation stimulates cell proliferation via activation of the MAPK/ERK pathway in rat cultured mesenchymal stem cells. J Radiat Res 52: 380–386.
16. He J, Qiu W, Zhang Z, Wang Z, Zhang X, et al. (2011) Effects of irradiation on growth and differentiation-related gene expression in osteoblasts. J Craniofac Surg 22: 1635–1640.
17. Lau P, Baumstark-Khan C, Hellweg CE, Reitz G (2010) X-irradiation-induced cell cycle delay and DNA double-strand breaks in the murine osteoblastic cell line OCT-1. Radiat Environ Biophys 49: 271–280.
18. Park SS, Kim KA, Lee SY, Lim SS, Jeon YM, et al. (2012) X-ray radiation at low doses stimulates differentiation and mineralization of mouse calvarial osteoblasts. BMB Rep 45: 571–576.
19. Zhou XZ, Zhang G, Dong QR, Chan CW, Liu CF, et al. (2009) Low-dose X-irradiation promotes mineralization of fracture callus in a rat model. Arch Orthop Trauma Surg 129: 125–132.
20. Xu W, Xu L, Chen M, Mao YT, Xie ZG, et al. (2012) The effects of low dose X-irradiation on osteoblastic MC3T3-E1 cells in vitro. BMC Musculoskelet Disord 13: 94.
21. Naik AA, Xie C, Zuscik MJ, Kingsley P, Schwarz EM, et al. (2009) Reduced COX-2 expression in aged mice is associated with impaired fracture healing. J Bone Miner Res 24: 251–264.
22. Iwaki A, Jingushi S, Oda Y, Izumi T, Shida JI, et al. (1997) Localization and quantification of proliferating cells during rat fracture repair: detection of proliferating cell nuclear antigen by immunohistochemistry. J Bone Miner Res 12: 96–102.
23. Srivastava UK, Srivastava SR, Guru PY (1989) Rat luteal cells in tissue culture: a technique for obtaining primary cell culture without enzymatic dissociation. Indian J Exp Biol 27: 602–606.
24. Paunesku T, Mittal S, Protic M, Oryhon J, Korolev SV, et al. (2001) Proliferating cell nuclear antigen (PCNA): ringmaster of the genome. International journal of radiation biology 77: 1007–1021.
25. Yu YL, Chou RH, Liang JH, Chang WJ, Su KJ, et al. (2013) Targeting the EGFR/PCNA signaling suppresses tumor growth of triple-negative breast cancer cells with cell-penetrating PCNA peptides. PloS One 8: e61362.
26. Schnoke M, Midura SB, Midura RJ (2009) Parathyroid hormone suppresses osteoblast apoptosis by augmenting DNA repair. Bone 45: 590–602.
27. Tsai CJ, Hofstede TM, Sturgis EM, Garden AS, Lindberg ME, et al. (2013) Osteoradionecrosis and radiation dose to the mandible in patients with oropharyngeal cancer. Int J Radiat Oncol Biol Phys 85: 415–420.

28. Lee IJ, Koom WS, Lee CG, Kim YB, Yoo SW, et al. (2009) Risk factors and dose-effect relationship for mandibular osteoradionecrosis in oral and oropharyngeal cancer patients. Int J Radiat Oncol Biol Phys 75: 1084–1091.
29. Williams HJ, Davies AM (2006) The effect of X-rays on bone: a pictorial review. Eur Radiol 16: 619–633.
30. Chae HJ, Chae SW, Kang JS, Bang BG, Han JI, et al. (1999) Effect of ionizing radiation on the differentiation of ROS 17/2.8 osteoblasts through free radicals. J Radiat Res 40: 323–335.
31. Smialek MA, Moore SA, Mason NJ, Shuker DE (2009) Quantification of radiation-induced single-strand breaks in plasmid DNA using a TUNEL/ELISA-based assay. Radiat Res 172: 529–536.
32. Sugrue T, Brown JA, Lowndes NF, Ceredig R (2013) Multiple facets of the DNA damage response contribute to the radioresistance of mouse mesenchymal stromal cell lines. Stem Cells 31: 137–145.
33. Feinendegen LE (2005) Evidence for beneficial low level radiation effects and radiation hormesis. Br J Radiol 78: 3–7.
34. Caetano-Lopes J, Canhao H, Fonseca JE (2007) Osteoblasts and bone formation. Acta Reumatol Port 32: 103–110.
35. Choi JY, Lee BH, Song KB, Park RW, Kim IS, et al. (1996) Expression patterns of bone-related proteins during osteoblastic differentiation in MC3T3-E1 cells. J Cell Biochem 61: 609–618.
36. Singh AM, Reynolds D, Cliff T, Ohtsuka S, Mattheyses AL, et al. (2012) Signaling network crosstalk in human pluripotent cells: a Smad2/3-regulated switch that controls the balance between self-renewal and differentiation. Cell Stem Cell 10: 312–326.
37. Zhang M, Ho HC, Sheu TJ, Breyer MD, Flick LM, et al. (2011) EP1(−/−) mice have enhanced osteoblast differentiation and accelerated fracture repair. J Bone Miner Res 26: 792–802.
38. Green DE, Adler BJ, Chan ME, Lennon JJ, Acerbo AS, et al. (2013) Altered composition of bone as triggered by irradiation facilitates the rapid erosion of the matrix by both cellular and physicochemical processes. PloS One 8: e64952.
39. Alwood JS, Kumar A, Tran LH, Wang A, Limoli CL, et al. (2012) Low-dose, ionizing radiation and age-related changes in skeletal microarchitecture. J Aging Res 2012: 481983.

Clinical, Radiological and Ultrasonographic Findings Related to Knee Pain in Osteoarthritis

Keith K. W. Chan[1]*, Regina W. S. Sit[2], Ricky W. K. Wu[3], Allen H. Y. Ngai[3]

1 School of Public Health and Primary Care, Faculty of Medicine, The Chinese University of Hong Kong, Hong Kong, 2 Jockey Club School of Public Health and Primary Care, Faculty of Medicine, The Chinese University of Hong Kong, Hong Kong, 3 The Hong Kong Institute of Musculoskeletal Medicine, Hong Kong

Abstract

Background: Pain is the predominant symptom of knee osteoarthritis (OA) and the main reason of disability. Ultrasound is now one of the new imaging modality in Musculoskeletal medicine and its role in assessing the pain severity in the knee osteoarthritis is evaluated in this study.

Objectives: (1) To study the correlation between ultrasonographic (US) findings and pain score and (2) whether ultrasonographic findings show a better association of pain level than conventional X-rays in patients suffering from primary knee osteoarthritis.

Methods: In this multi-center study, 193 patients with primary knee OA were asked to score their average knee pain using the Western Ontario and McMaster Universities Arthritis (WOMAC) questionnaire;patients would then go for a radiological and an US evaluation of their painful knee. Findings from both imaging modalities will be studied with the associated pain score.

Results: Ultrasound showed that knee effusion has positive correlation with pain score upon walking ($r = 0.217$) and stair climbing ($r = 0.194$). Presence of suprapatellar synovitis had higher pain score on sitting (Spearman's Rank correlation $= 0.355$). The medial($r = 0.170$) and lateral meniscus protrusion ($r = 0.201$) were associated with pain score upon stair climbing.

Conclusions: Our study found that both imaging modalities shown some significant association with the aspect of pain; neither one is clearly better but rather complementary to each other. A trend is found in both modalities: walking pain is related to pathologies of the either the lateral or medial tibiofemoral joint(TFJ)while stair climbing pain is related to both tibiofemoral joint pathologies and also to the patellofemoral joint (PFJ) pathology. This suggested that biomechanical derangement is an important aspect in OA knee pain.

Editor: Wang Zhan, University of Maryland, College Park, United States of America

Funding: The authors have no support or funding to report.

Competing Interests: The authors have declared that no competing interests exist.

* E-mail: drkeithchan@gmail.com

Introduction

Osteoarthritis (OA) is one of the most common medical conditions in elderly people.[1] Worldwide estimates suggested that 9.6% of men and 18.0% of women aged 60 years have symptomatic OA of the hips or knees.[2] It is also the most common reason for restricted daily activity [3] with significantly impact on the quality of life among affected people.[4]

Pain is the predominant symptom of OA knee and is the main reason for medical consultation; besides, it the main reason of disability especially during painful episodes.[5–7].

Conventional X-rays were used traditionally in diagnosing OA knee by demonstrating the presence of osteophytes, bone deformities and joint space narrowing. However, studies on OA knee had demonstrated that there was not much correlation between the X-rays findings and the severity of OA knee pain.[8–12] Recent concept on osteoarthritis is that OA knee is a whole joint disease involving not only the bones and cartilages; but also involves pathologies in the intra and periarticular soft tissues.[13] One possible reason for the weak correlation is that while conventional X-rays is good at picking up bony lesions, they are falling short in giving accounts on the whole joint by its inability to directly visualize articular cartilage, synovial recesses, menisci and other soft tissues involved in the pathophysiology of OA knee.

Ultrasound (US) imaging is a non-invasive, widely available and relatively inexpensive technique that can be used to image soft tissues. With the advancement of technology, the newer US machine models can be equipped with high frequency probes that are very useful for musculoskeletal imaging to study the periarticular and intraarticular structures.[14–17] A study on OA knee had showed that US findings of knee effusion and protrusion of medial meniscus with displacement of the medial collateral ligament are associated with pain in OA knee.[18] Clinicians can now use musculoskeletal US to detect soft tissue pathologies in OA knee to supplement clinical and/or radiological diagnoses.

This study looks at the intraarticular and peri-articular soft tissue changes found among OA knee patients using real-time musculoskeletal US imaging. We aim to investigate (1) the probable correlation between ultrasonographic findings and pain score and (2) whether ultrasonographic findings show a better association of pain level than conventional X-rays in patients suffering from primary knee osteoarthritis. The pain score under the section of Western Ontario and McMaster Universities Arthritis (WOMAC) Index will be used in this study.[19]

The Study

Setting and patients

The study is a multicenter study undertaken in Hong Kong at the primary health care level in three different clinical settings: two private general practice clinics, two public primary care outpatient clinics and one primary care clinic of a private hospital. These three settings cover most of the primary health care consultations in Hong Kong.

Convenient sampling was used in this study. Adult patients over 40 years of age attending one of the five primary health care clinics were asked for presence of knee pain in one or both knees for the more than one month. Those patients with a positive answer were screened for presence of OA knee using the ACR clinical criteria of OA knee.[20] (Appendix S1) All patients identified to have OA knees were included in the study. Patients were excluded if he or she (1) had a gouty or pseudo-gouty attack over the knee with the week prior the study; (2) had direct trauma to the knee within the past month prior to the study; (3) had intra-articular injection or aspiration within the month prior to the study; (4) had previous knee operation; (5) declined to undergo either the US or X-ray knee examinations or (6) declined to be included in the study.

Methods

Ethics approval had been sought and endorsed from the Kowloon West Cluster, Clinical Research Ethics Committee (KWC-CRE), Hong Kong. Written consent was obtained from patients who agreed to participate in the study; the content of the consent form was approved by the ethics committee.

Patients were asked to score their average knee pain during the past month as a baseline on a 10 cm visual analogue scale (VAS) from 0 to 100 mm. If both knees were painful, the most symptomatic knee was used for study. (Appendix S2)

Demographic data obtained from patient included age, sex, height and weight, and body mass index. Patients would then self-complete the pain subscale section of the Chinese version of the WOMAC questionnaire. (Appendix S3) A nurse was available for help if patients needed assistance. Patients would then go for a radiological and an US evaluation of their more painful knee.

Radiological Evaluation

All patients would have X-rays of their more painful knee. A standing weight bearing anterior-posterior (AP)[21] view was used to assess the medial and the lateral tibial femoral joints (TFJs) and a skyline view of the knee to assess the patello-femoral joint (PFJ). The X-rays were then assessed independently using a standardized scoring sheet and also be graded according to the Kellgren and Lawrence (K/L) method of classification[22] from grades 0 to 4 by two fellow radiologists blinded to the clinical and US results and to each other. (Appendix S4)

Ultrasound Evaluation

All patients then underwent an US examination on the same knee using a standardized protocol with Esoate (MyLab 25 model) with a linear probe (model LA435 12–18 Mhz) and a centre frequency 13 MHz. (Appendix S5) Gray-scale were used during the screening procedure. Power Colour Doppler was used to check for blood flow in the synovium. To avoid examiner bias, all US examiners had to attend, prior to the study, a standardization workshop under the guidance of an expert specialized in musculoskeletal US scanning. All ultrasound examiners were blinded from the X-ray results during the ultrasound examination and all relevant ultrasound findings as stated in the protocol were saved for an independent reassessment later if necessary by a second examiner.

Statistical analysis

Statistical analyses were performed using the statistical package PASW Statistics 18. Pearson's correlation and Spearman's Rank correlation were used to examine the association among pain scores, ultrasound and X-ray findings where appropriate. Difference of pain scores in X-ray grading as well as trend were examined by Analysis of variance (ANOVA). Two tailed p-values at level of 0.05 or less were considered to be of statistical significance.

Results

A total of 193 patients were recruited in this study. Table 1 summarized the demographic data as well as the characteristics of all subjects with pain scores, ultrasound and X-ray findings. Patients answered zero mark in pain score were assigned as no pain in such aspect. The distribution of the five pain scores in relation to walking, stair climbing, lying, sitting and standing were studied. Comparison of pain scores on walking and stair climbing with different ultrasound and X-ray findings were presented in Table 2 with significant figures highlighted. Other significant findings not shown in these 2 tables include (1) presence of suprapatellar synovitis had a moderate strong correlation with higher pain score on sitting (Spearman's Rank correlation = 0.355); (2) knee effusion has positive correlation with pain score upon walking (0.217) and climbing (0.194) but not with sitting; (3) the narrower the minimal joint width of the medial TFJ ($r = -0.175$) and the wider the joint width at the lateral point of the lateral TFJ ($r = 0.236$) on the standing X-rays, the stronger the pain score on standing.

Discussion

In our study, the higher the KL grading was associated with more pain in general. The finding is in line with a recent systematic review that higher grade of osteoarthritis (K/L 3 or above) is a stronger predictor of pain than lower grades (K/L 2 or less).[8] This study is so designed that the patients recruited should include at least 30 patients from each of the 5 K/L gradings (Grades 0–4) so that the results of the present study is more representative of OA knee in general with different grades of severities.

Our study showed that the presence of suprapatellar synovitis had a moderate strong correlation with higher pain score on sitting whereas such correlation was not found upon walking and standing. This could be explained by a previous study conducted by the author that there exist two types of pain among OA knee patients: a mechanical pain and an inflammatory pain. The former, being biomechanical in nature, is associated with joint

Table 1. Characteristics of the study subjects (N = 193).

	Women (n = 143)		Men (n = 50)		Total (n = 193)	
Age (year)	58.9	±13.5	59.3	±15.1	59.0	±13.9
Weight (kg)	60.4	±10.0	70.4	±10.1	63.0	±10.9
Height (m)	1.56	±0.06	1.67	±0.05	1.59	±0.08
BMI (kg/m^2)	24.9	±4.1	25.2	±3.1	25.0	±3.9
Pain score (non-zero)					n	mean± sd
Walking					154	4.1±2.3
Stair climbing					186	5.6±2.5
Lying					97	3.5±2.6
Sitting					87	2.6±2.2
Standing					130	3.4±2.2
Ultrasound (Front)						
Patient supine with knee flexed to 30°						
Knee effusion in supra-patella recess (mm)					125	6.73±4.36
Supra-patella Synovitis, synovial thickness (mm)					73	4.36±2.21
Sky view with patient supine and knee fully flexed, cartilage thickness at						
Lateral femoral condyle (maximal thickness, mm)					193	2.35±0.67
Lateral femoral condyle (minimal thickness, mm)					193	1.31±0.58
Medial femoral condyle (maximal thickness, mm)					193	2.28±0.76
Medial femoral condyle (minimal thickness, mm)					193	1.15±0.61
Ultrasound (Medial) - Patient supine with external rotation of leg and knee flexed to 10°						
Medical meniscus extrusion(mm)					144	4.57±2.33
Maximum length of osteophyte from level of cortical bone(mm)					152	3.77±2.27
Ultrasound (Lateral) - Patient supine with internal rotation of leg and knee flexed to 10°						
Lateral meniscus extrusion (mm)					137	4.01±1.85
Maximum length of osteophyte from cortical bone (mm)					149	3.19±1.73
X-ray						
Joint width of the medial TFJ compartment						
Minimal joint					193	2.1±1.5
Medial point					193	8.5±2.9
Mid-point					193	4.6±1.9
Joint width of the lateral TFJ compartment						
Minimal joint					193	1.4±1.1
Medial point					193	11.3±3.9
Mid-point					193	4.9±1.6
Joint width of the PFJ at						
Medial facet					193	3.7±1.5
Lateral facet					193	3.0±1.4
KL grading					Grade	n(%)
					0	42(21.8%)
					1	33(17.1%)
					2	43(22.3%)
					3	43(22.3%)
					4	32(16.6%)

movements such as walking and stair claiming whereas the latter is caused by flares of joint inflammation.[23] Synovitis is a sign of joint inflammation and its association with pain when sitting and not with walking or stair climbing suggests that the resting OA knee pain during sitting is more likely inflammatory pain. This finding is also consistent with the EULAR study, which showed no correlation between US inflammatory signs and pain intensity during physical activity.[24]

This study showed that knee effusion has positive correlation with pain score upon walking and climbing, but not with sitting.

Table 2. Association among pain score (non-zero) on Walking and Stair Climbing, Ultrasound and X-Ray readings.

Ultrasound readings						
	Front					
	Knee effusion in supra-patella recess	Supra-patella Synovitis	Lateral femoral condyle cartilage		Medical femoral condyle cartilage	
			Maximal thickness	Minimal thickness	Maximal thickness	Minimal thickness
Walking	**0.217***	0.151	−0.024	**−0.181***	−0.051	−0.143
Stair Climbing	**0.194***	0.107	0.055	−0.060	0.005	−0.131
	Medial		**Lateral**			
	Meniscus extrusion	Max length of osteophyte from level of cortical bone	Meniscus extrusion	Max length of osteophyte from cortical bone		
Walking	0.177	0.136	**0.217***	0.171		
Stair Climbing	**0.170***	**0.162***	**0.201***	0.127		
X-Ray readings						
	Joint width of the medial TFJ compartment			Joint width of the lateral TFJ compartment		
	Minimal joint	Medial point	Mid-point	Minimal joint	Lateral point	Mid-point
Walking	−0.146	−0.093	**−0.192***	−0.068	−0.009	−0.021
Stair Climbing	**−0.175***	−0.070	**−0.179***	0.043	−0.001	**0.149***
	Joint width of the PFJ					
	Medial facet	Lateral facet				
Walking	−0.087	−0.155				
Stair Climbing	0.010	**−0.166***				
	Pain score on walking (non-zero)			Pain score on stair climbing (non-zero)		
KL grading on X-rays	N	Mean±SD	p-value of ANOVA	N	Mean±SD	p-value of ANOVA
0	31	3.3±2.5	**0.002**	41	4.9±2.5	**0.001**
1	22	3.3±2.1	(linear trend<**0.001**)	30	5.1±2.6	(linear trend<**0.001**)
2	30	3.9±2.0		42	5.2±2.2	
3	40	4.3±2.4		43	5.7±2.4	
4	31	5.3±1.9		30	7.2±2.0	
KL grading on X-rays			p-value of t-test			p-value of t-test
0–1	53	3.3±2.3	0.001	71	5.0±2.5	0.009
2–4	101	4.5±2.2		115	5.9±2.3	

*P<0.05; Data presented as Pearson correlation coefficient.

Similar findings are found in other overseas studies.[17,19,24] This suggests that the knee effusion among OA knee patients relates more to mechanical rather than inflammatory pain. Knee effusion has been shown to affect knee mechanics and muscle activity during gait in individuals with knee osteoarthritis and therefore can be a cause of the mechanical pain by itself.[25]

The knee joint is a complex joint consisting of a patellofemoral joint (PFJ) articulating the patella with the femoral condyle and two tibiofemoral joints, one medial and one lateral (medial and lateral TFJs), articulating the medial and lateral tibial plateau with the corresponding femoral condyles.Although X-rays measure mainly bony pathologies and ultrasound on soft tissue pathologies, both the X-ray and ultrasound findings in our study showed two trends in common(1) walking pain is related to pathologies of the either the lateral or medial TFJ;(2) stair climbing pain is related to both TFJ pathologies and also to the PFJ pathology.

Meniscus subluxation was highly associated with painful OA knee.[26] Our US studies showed that lateral meniscal extrusion was associated with increased pain score on walking. X-ray studies, on the other hand, showed pain on walking was associated with the narrowing of the medial TFJ at mid-point. When stair climbing, pathologies from both the medial and lateral TFJ are implicated. The US findings showed that stair climbing pain has a positive correlation to both medial meniscal protrusion and lateral meniscus protrusion; whereas on X-rays, the narrower the medial TFJ at midpoint and the wider the lateral TFJ at midpoint,more the pain. Both of these X-rays findings are commonly found among bow knees (Genu Varus) which are commonly found among OA knee patients.

Pain with stair climbing, especially on descending stairs is a well known feature with OA knee involving the PFJs.[27] Our X-ray studies found that the narrower the lateral facet joint, the more the pain on stair climbing. However, our US finding showed that the thickness of the lateral femoral condyle cartilage, which is a measurement of the lateral PFJ, has no association with stair climbing. Such finding is expected because ultrasound can only measure, through the sky view, the cartilage of the upper part of the femoral condyle. Level walking involves only 15° to 20° of flexion of the femoral condyle during which the lower part of the patella facet is in opposition with the upper part of the femoral condyle,[28] and it is where the ultrasound is measuring. Stair climbing involved 30° to 60° of flexion which is beyond the US measurements.

Some limitations of our study should be mentioned. Although all the ultrasounds were performed by musculoskeletal physicians who are Registrants in Musculoskeletal Ultrasound (RMSK) of the American Registry for Diagnostic Medical Sonography and that all of them had undergone a standardization workshop prior to the study, the US inter-observer reliability was not studied. Recent studies had revealed that there still can be high inter-observer reliability.[29,30] Secondly, as there is still no widely agreed standardized definition of USG findings or widely acquisition protocols on OA knee US screening, we therefore produce definitions of pathological findings based on some published report.[31–34] We employed a conservative "cut off point" for all pathological definitions. This may potentially lead to underestimation of the association of ultrasound finding and pain score. Thirdly, the study design is to recruit equal numbers of OA knee patient from all K/L grading. Such inclusion of mild cases of OA may undermine the pain association and hence may account for the overall low association score.

Conclusions

Although X-rays and musculoskeletal ultrasound measure different structural tissues of the osteoarthritic knee, our study found that both imaging modalities shown some significant association with the aspect of pain. However, neither one is clearly better, but they rather complementary to each other. Walking pain is related to pathologies of the either the lateral or medial TFJ. Stair climbing pain is related to both TFJ pathologies and also to the PFJ pathology. This suggests that biomechanical derangement is an important aspect that is often overlooked, but needed to be addressed by physicians in the management of OA knee pain. Future research concerning the prognostic value of the different findings from both modalities in planning treatment or intervention can be conducted in order to improve clinical outcomes of patients suffering chronic OA knee.

Supporting Information

Appendix S1

Appendix S2

Appendix S3

Appendix S4

Appendix S5

Acknowledgments

The authors are grateful to the Hong Kong Institute of Musculoskeletal Medicine (HKIMM) for sponsoring the X-ray films and for providing statistical support for the study. We also have to thank Esoate China Limited for providing the US machines for all the five centers during the study period. Last but not list to the team of musculoskeletal physicians and radiologists who had scarified many working hours to get US and X-rays done.

US Team:
Dr. Keith KW Chan
Dr. Ricky WK Wu
Dr. Andrew KK Ip
Dr. Stanley KW Lam
Dr. Allen HY Ngai
Dr. Mark WW Lai
Dr. Paco WY Lee
X-ray team:
Dr. CH Tang
Dr. KS Lam
Dr. John Lo

Author Contributions

Conceived and designed the experiments: KKWC RWSS RWKW AHYN. Performed the experiments: KKWC RWSS RWKW AHYN. Analyzed the data: KKWC RWSS RWKW AHYN. Contributed reagents/materials/analysis tools: KKWC RWSS RWKW AHYN. Wrote the paper: KKWC RWSS RWKW AHYN.

References

1. Lawrence RC, Hochberg MC, Kelsey JL, McDuffie FC, Medsger TA Jr, et al. (1989) Estimates of the prevalesnce of selected arthritic and musculoskeletal diseases in the United states. J Rheumatol 16: 427–441.
2. Murray CJL, Lopez AD, eds. (1996) The global burden of disease. A comprehensive assessment of mortality and disability from diseases, injuries, and risk factors in 1990 and projected to 2020. Cambridge (MA): Harvard School of Public Health on behalf of the World Health Organization and The World Bank.
3. Martin J, Meltzer H, Elliot D (1988) The prevalence of disability among adults. OPCS survery of disability in general practice (Report 1). London: HMSO.
4. Woo J, Lau E, Lee P, Kwok T, Lau WC, et al.(2004) Impact of osteoarthritis on quality of life in a Hong Kong Chinese population. J Rheumatol 31: 2433–2438.
5. Hopman-Rock M, Odding E, Hofman A, Kraaimaat FW, Bijlsma JW (1996) Physical and psychosocial disability in elderly subjects in relation to pain in the hip and/or knee. *J Rheumatol* 23:1037–1044.
6. Jordan JM, Luta G, Renner J, Dragomir A, Hochberg M, et al. (1997) Knee pain and knee osteoarthritis severity in self-reported task specific disability: the Johnstone County Osteoarthritis Project. J Rheumatol 24:1344–1349.
7. Davis MA, Ettinger W, Neuhaus J, Mallon KP (1991) Knee osteoarthritis and physical functioning: evidence from the NHANES I epidemiological follow up study. J Rheumatol 18: 591–598.
8. Bedson J, Croft PR (2008) The discordance between clinical and radiographic knee osteoarthritis: a systematic search and summary of the literature. BMC Musculoskeletal Disorders 9: 116.
9. Claessens AA, Schouten JS, van den Ouweland FA, Valkenburg HA (1990) Do clinical findings associate with radiographic osteoarthritis of the knee? Ann Rheum Dis 49: 771–774.
10. Hart DJ, Spector TD, Brown P, Wilson P, Doyle DV, et al. (1991) Clinical signs of early osteoarthritis: reproducibility and relation to x ray changes in 541 women in the general population. Ann Rheum Dis 50: 467–470.
11. Lawrence JS, Bremner JM, Bier F (1966) Osteo-arthrosis. Prevalence in the population and relationships between symptoms and x-ray changes. Ann Rheum Dis 25: 1–24.
12. Davis MA, Ettinger WH, Neuhaus JM, Barclay JD, Segal MR (1992) Correlates of knee pain among US adults with and without radiographic knee osteoarthritis. J Rheumatol 19: 1943–1949.
13. Felson DT, Lawrence RC, Dieppe PA, Hirsch R, Helmick CG, et al. (2000) Osteoarthritis: new insights. Part 1: the disease and its risk factors. Ann Intern Med 133: 635–646.
14. Grassi W, Filipucci E, Busilacchi P. (2004) Musculoskeletal ultrasound. Best Practice & Research Clinical Rhematology 18: 813–826.
15. Gibbon WW. (2004) Applications of ultrasound in arthritis. Semin Musculoskelet Radiol 8: 313–328.
16. Monteforte P, Sessarego P, Rovetta G. (2008) Sonographic assessment of soft tissue alternations in osteoarthritis of the knee. G Ital Med Lav Ergon 30: 75–77.
17. de Miguel Mendieta E, Cobo Ibanez T, Uson Jaeger J, Bonilla Hermán G, Martín Mola E (2006) Clinical and ultrasonographic findings related to knee pain in osteoarthritis. Osteoarthritis Cartilage 14: 540–544.
18. Naredo E, Cabero F, Palop MJ, Collado P, Cruz A, et al. (2005) Ultrasonographic findings in knee osteoarthritis: a comparative study with clinical and radiographic assessment. Osteoarthritis Cartilage 13: 568–574.
19. Bellamy N, Buchanan WW, Goldsmith CH, Campbell J, Stitt LW (1988) Validation study of WOMAC: a health status instrument for measuring clinically important patient relevant outcomes to antirheumatic drug therapy in patients with osteoarthritis of the hip or knee. J Rheumatol 15: 1833–1840.

20. Altman R, Asch E, Bloch D, Bole G, Borenstein D, et al. (1986) Development of criteria for the classification and reporting of osteoarthritis. Classification of osteoarthritis of the knee. Arthritis Rheum 29: 1039–1049.
21. Guermazi A, Burstein D, Conaghan P, Eckstein F, Hellio Le Graverand-Gastineau MP, et al. (2008) Imaging in osteoarthritis. Rheum Dis Clin North Am 34: 645–687.
22. Kellgren JH, Lawrence JS (1957) Radiological assessment of osteoarthritis. Ann Rheum Dis 16: 494–501.
23. Chan KKW, Chan LWY (2011) A qualitative study on patients with knee osteoarthritis to evaluate the influence of different pain patterns on patients' quality of life and to find out patients' interpretation and coping strategies for the disease. Rheumatology Reports **3** (e3):9–15.
24. Conaghan P, D'agostino MA, Ravaud P, Baron G, Le Bars M, et al. (2005) EULAR report on the use of ultrasonography in painful knee osteoarthritis. Part 2: exploring decision rules for clinical utility. Ann Rheum Dis 64: 1710–1714.
25. Rutherford DJ, Hubley-Kozey CL, Stanish WD (2012) Knee effusion affects knee mechanics and muscle activity during gait in individuals with knee osteoarthritis. Osteoarthritis Cartilage 20: 974–981.
26. Gale DR, Chaisson CE, Totterman SM, Schwartz RK, Gale ME, et al. (1999) Meniscal subluxation: association with osteoarthritis and joint space narrowing. Osteoarthritis Cartilage 7: 526–532.
27. Peat G, Duncan RC, Wood LR, Thomas E, Muller S (2012) Clinical features of symptomatic patellofemoral joint osteoarthritis. Arthritis Res Ther 14: R63.
28. Kapandji IA. (2007) The Physiology of the Joints. Edinburgh: Churchill Livingstone.
29. Abraham AM, Goff I, Pearce MS, Francis RM, Birrell F (2011) Reliability and validity of ultrasound imaging of features of knee osteoarthritis in the community. BMC Musculoskeletal Disorders 12: 70.
30. Iagnocco A, Perricone C, Scirocco C, Ceccarelli F, Modesti M, et al. (2012) The interobserver reliability of ultrasound in knee osteoarthritis. Rheumatology (Oxford) 51: 2013–2019.
31. Kristoffersen H, Torp-Pedersen S, Terslev L, Qvistgaard E, Holm CC, et al. (2006) Indications of inflammation visualized by ultrasound in osteoarthritis of the knee. *Acta Radiol* 47: 281–286.
32. D'Agostino MA, Conaghan P, Le Bars M, Baron G, Grassi W, et al. (2005) EULAR report on the use of ultrasonography in painful knee osteoarthritis. Part 1: prevalence of inflammation in osteoarthritis. Ann Rheum Dis 64: 1703–1709.
33. Grassi W, Lamanna G, Farina A, Cervini C (1999) Sonographic imaging of normal and osteoarthritic cartilage. Semin Arthritis Rheum 28: 398–403.
34. Chhem RK, Cardinal E. (1999) Guidelines and gamuts in musculoskeletal ultrasound. New York: Wiley-Liss.

7

Optimal Iodine Staining of Cardiac Tissue for X-Ray Computed Tomography

Timothy D. Butters[1¶], Simon J. Castro[1¶], Tristan Lowe[2¶], Yanmin Zhang[3,4], Ming Lei[3,4], Philip J. Withers[2], Henggui Zhang[1*]

1 School of Physics and Astronomy, The University of Manchester, Manchester, Greater Manchester, United Kingdom, **2** School of Materials Science, The University of Manchester, Manchester, Greater Manchester, United Kingdom, **3** Institute of Cardiovascular Sciences, Faculty of Medical and Human Sciences, The University of Manchester, Manchester, Greater Manchester, United Kingdom, **4** Department of Pharmacology, University of Oxford, Oxford, Oxfordshire, United Kingdom

Abstract

X-ray computed tomography (XCT) has been shown to be an effective imaging technique for a variety of materials. Due to the relatively low differential attenuation of X-rays in biological tissue, a high density contrast agent is often required to obtain optimal contrast. The contrast agent, iodine potassium iodide (I_2KI), has been used in several biological studies to augment the use of XCT scanning. Recently I_2KI was used in XCT scans of animal hearts to study cardiac structure and to generate 3D anatomical computer models. However, to date there has been no thorough study into the optimal use of I_2KI as a contrast agent in cardiac muscle with respect to the staining times required, which has been shown to impact significantly upon the quality of results. In this study we address this issue by systematically scanning samples at various stages of the staining process. To achieve this, mouse hearts were stained for up to 58 hours and scanned at regular intervals of 6–7 hours throughout this process. Optimal staining was found to depend upon the thickness of the tissue; a simple empirical exponential relationship was derived to allow calculation of the required staining time for cardiac samples of an arbitrary size.

Editor: Joseph P. R. O. Orgel, Illinois Institute of Technology, United States of America

Funding: This work was supported by an EPSRC project grant (EP/J00958X/1) and The Manchester Henry Moseley X-ray Imaging Facility was funded in part by the EPSRC (grants EP/F007906/1, EP/F001452/1, and EP/I02249X/1). The funders had no role in study design, data collection and analysis, decision to publish, or preparation of the manuscript.

Competing Interests: The authors have declared that no competing interests exist.

* Email: henggui.zhang@manchester.ac.uk

¶ These authors contributed equally to this work.

Introduction

Imaging the heart is of vital importance to the study of cardiac anatomy and the role of structural remodelling in various pathologies, including heart failure. Cardiac imaging also lends itself to investigating the role of structure in excitation wave conduction, and it's contribution to arrhythmogenesis. Over the years various techniques have been used to map cardiac structures at a range of spatial scales. These vary from magnetic resonance imaging (MRI) for whole organ and tissue section scanning, to scanning electron microscopy (SEM) to elucidate sub-cellular structures of cardiac myocytes [1,2]. At the whole organ and tissue section level the reconstructions can be used to study structural differences between healthy and diseased organs, as well as for computational simulation studies in which the electrical activation of the heart is modelled in a realistic geometry [3–6]. For both of these applications a high resolution reconstruction with a fine level of detail is required to resolve structures that play a role in the development of cardiac disease [7,8].

For many years MRI has been the 'gold standard' for heart imaging, especially when reconstructing the whole organ. However, due to the limitations of sample size within large magnetic field systems it has only been possible to scan the hearts of small animals such as mice, rats and rabbits at a high resolution (~50 μm) [9]. Reconstructions of larger samples, such as those from humans, have been limited to a voxel size of 1–5 mm for 1.5–3.0 T clinical systems [10].

X-ray computed tomography (XCT) has many advantages over MRI for cardiac reconstructions. The sample size is limited only by the bay in which the scanner is housed; it is therefore possible to scan hearts from large mammals as well as those from small animals such as mice with the same machine. Voxel sizes of ~40 μm and ~36 μm have previously been obtained in rat [11] and dog [12] hearts respectively; since resolution scales with sample size, we would expect a resolution of ~100 μm could be obtained for the human heart. The scan times are also typically much shorter with XCT, taking anywhere from a few minutes [13,14] to ~2 hours, compared to ~10 hours for a comparable MRI scan [15].

Unfortunately, XCT images of biological tissue tend to be of low contrast, greatly limiting the use and application of standard XCT results. Several studies have shown however, that by using a suitable contrast agent there is an increase in differential attenuation of X-rays and contrast is improved. Metscher has

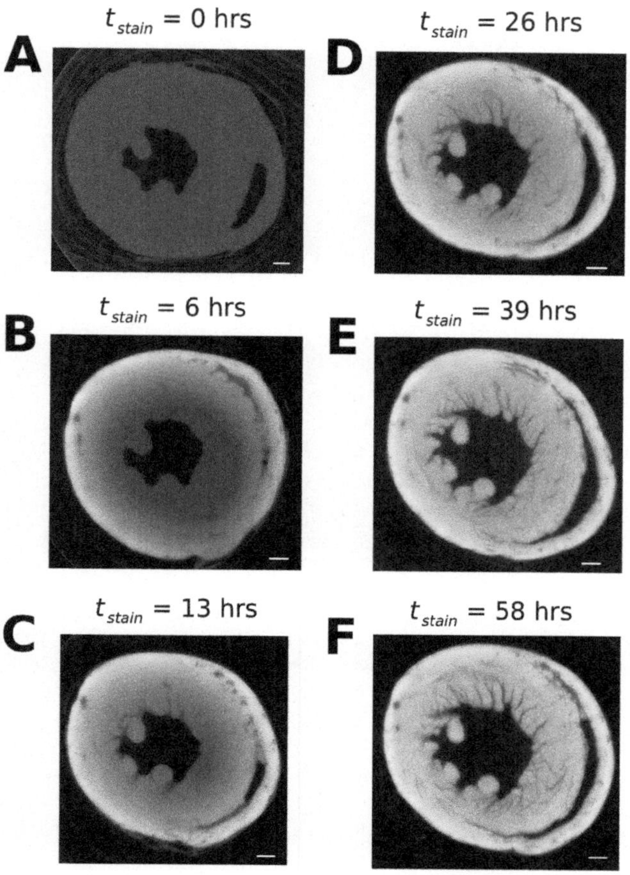

Figure 1. Reconstructed virtual XCT transverse slices of the mouse ventricles at varying staining times. A) 0 hours; B) 6 hours; C) 13 hours; D) 26 hours; E) 39 hours; F) 58 hours. The scale bars in the bottom right of each panel are representative of 1 mm. The polythene wrapping and bijou tube, clearly visible in the periphery of panel A, are shown to be of low contrast compared to the stained tissue (panels B–F).

highlighted several contrast agents for use in biological samples, including iodine potassium iodide (I_2KI) and phosphotungstic acid, all of which improve contrast and allow various structures to be easily identified [16]. More recently, Jeffery *et al.* were able to resolve the arrangement of muscle fibres in rodent heads with application of I_2KI [17]. In a similar study, Stephenson *et al.* were able to obtain sufficient contrast in rat and rabbit hearts with I_2KI so as to segment the cardiac conduction system [11,12].

The staining procedure is essential in order to achieve feature definition during the reconstruction and segmentation stages. The amount of time the tissue is incubated in the staining solution is a key factor for contrast, as both under- and over-staining have negative consequences. If the tissue is prematurely removed from the solution the staining will be incomplete and parts of the tissue will retain their low contrast properties when imaged. This can complicate analysis; for example, automated methods of segmentation, such as region-growing, often rely on each distinct region having consistent intensity. Automatic methods of segmentation fail as a result of incomplete staining, increasing the need for manual segmentation. Conversely, staining tissue with I_2KI for prolonged periods of time has been shown to cause tissue shrinkage; whilst the extent of shrinkage can be reduced using a suitable fixative, it cannot be completely eliminated [18].

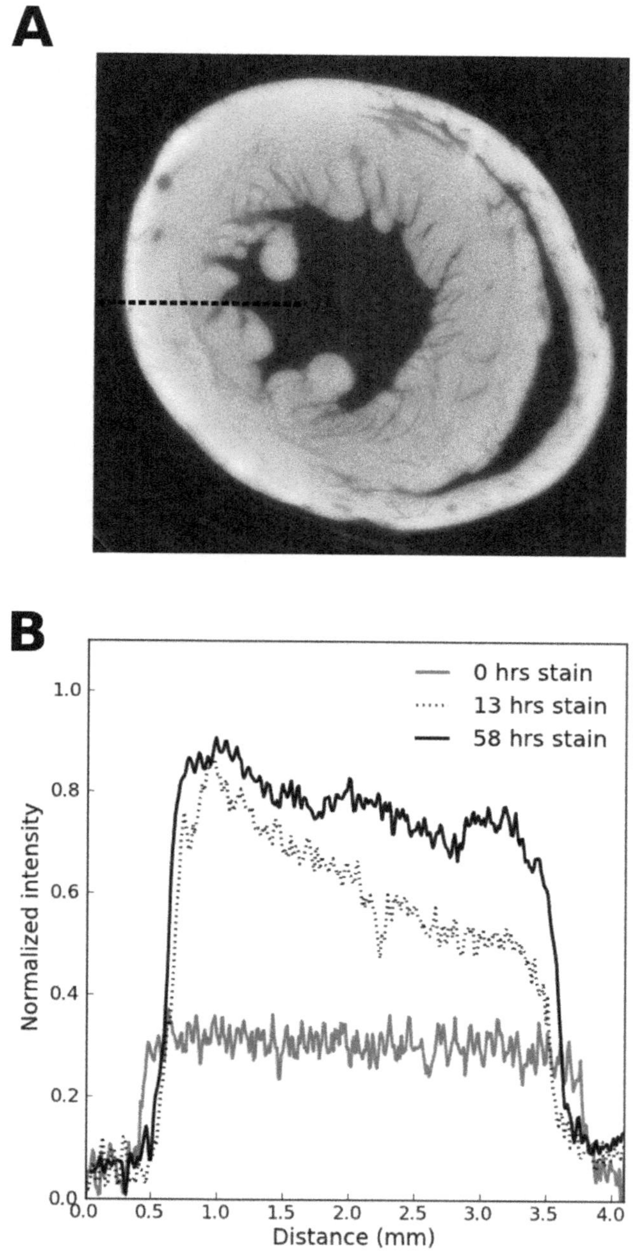

Figure 2. Example tomographic slice with intensity profile across the ventricular wall. A) Transverse tomographic slice through the ventricles with dashed line indicating the sampling location for the intensity line profile. B) Intensity line profiles for 0 hours, 13 hours and 58 hours incubation time.

Therefore, an optimal staining time would be the minimum time required to completely stain the sample, reducing the effects of shrinkage as much as possible. However, this can only be determined by trial and error, and, to the best of our knowledge, there is no study which quantifies the staining process and its relationship to sample size.

This study aims to address this issue by quantifying the staining process and identifying the optimal incubation time for cardiac tissue in I_2KI solution for XCT imaging. To achieve this, mouse hearts were scanned at a series of staining stages to track the saturation of solution within the tissue. From the resulting data it

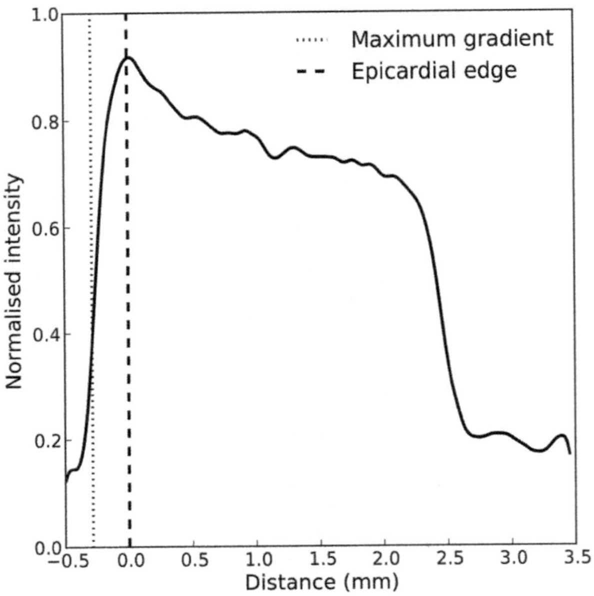

Figure 3. Adopted method for locating the epicardial edge. First the line profile is filtered with a Gaussian kernel (black line; $\sigma = 4$) in order to reduce noise. The maximum intensity gradient is subsequently detected (dotted line). The epicardial edge is then defined as the next point (towards the endocardium) at which $dI/dx = 0$ (dashed line).

was possible to deduce a relationship between the tissue thickness and required staining time, which will allow one to determine the optimal staining time for a given sample size.

Materials and Methods

Ethics Statement

This study was approved by the University Research Ethics Committee, University of Manchester. The animals from which samples were obtained were euthanized in accordance with directive 2010/63/EU of the European Parliament and in compliance with the ethical standards of the University of Manchester and the UK Home Office Animals (Scientific Procedures) Act 1986.

Mouse Hearts

Whole hearts were excised from four adult mice and fixed in phosphate buffered formal saline (4% formaldehyde made up in phosphate buffered saline) for a period of 48 hours. The use of a fixative such as phosphate buffered formal saline allows for sample storage, and reduces the extent of tissue shrinkage associated with the use of contrast agent [18]. The tissue was stained using the procedure outlined in Stephenson *et al.* [11]. The contrast agent was a 3.75% I_2KI solution made up using 10% neutral buffered formalin. The four samples were placed in the I_2KI solution at room temperature. After allowing a period of 6–7 hours to stain, the samples were removed in stages from the staining agent and blotted to remove excess solution. Each sample was then wrapped in polythene and inserted into a plastic bijou tube to ensure stability during the scanning process whilst minimising beam attenuation by the sample holder (Fig. 1).

Scanning Procedure

The specimens were analysed using a Nikon Metris 225/320 kV XCT system in conjunction with a 2K×2K Perkin Elmer detector (1621-16-bit amorphous silicon flat-panel detector with 200 μm pixel pitch). This is housed in a customised bay at the Henry Moseley X-ray Imaging Facility at The University of Manchester.

The sample tube containing the plastic-wrapped specimen was fixed to the rotating stage of the XCT system. During the XCT analysis the specimen was rotated over a 360° rotation range for a time period of approximately 24 minutes, collecting 2001 projections per scan with a voxel size 11 μm. An accelerating voltage of

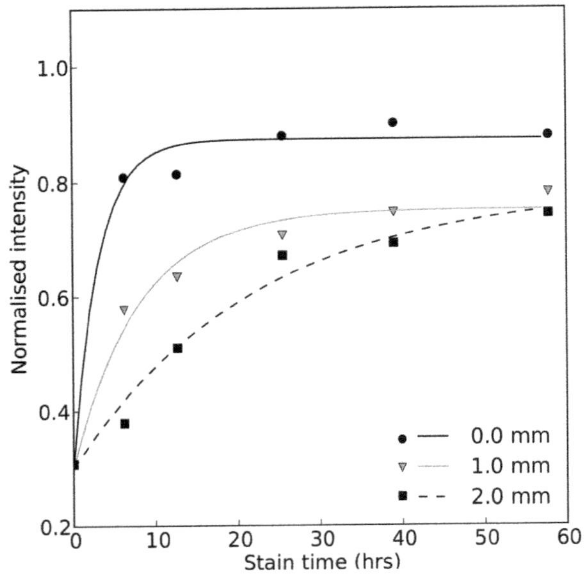

Figure 4. Time course of intensity during the staining process for different points within the tissue. The experimental data is represented by the data points, with fitted curves of the form given in equation 1.

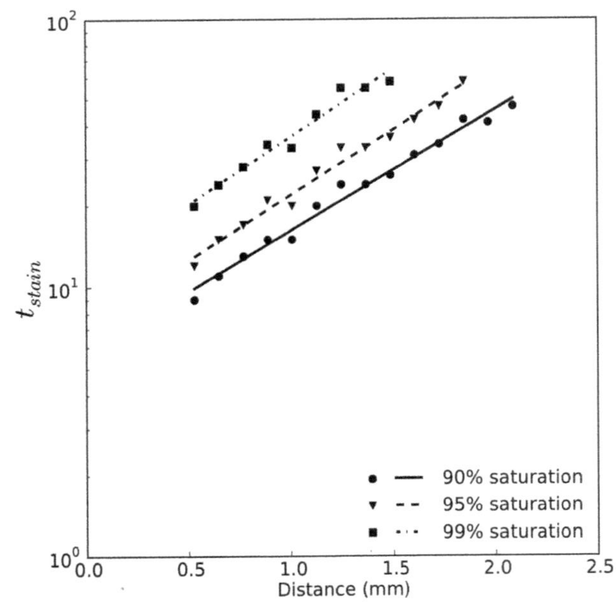

Figure 5. Semi-logarithmic plot of the required staining time for different levels I_2KI saturation as a function of distance. Curves are fitted according to equation 2 and with fitted coefficients given in Table 1.

Table 1. Fitted coefficients for calculating staining times for a given saturation level.

Saturation Level	A	k
90%	5.72	1.04
95%	7.17	1.12
99%	11.3	1.16

Coefficients A and k can be used in conjunction with equation 2 to obtain optimal staining time for an arbitrary location within the tissue.

50 kV was used, along with a current of 285 μA, and an exposure time of 708 ms per projection. In addition the focus was optimized for the low energy spectrum and the system alignment was rechecked in order to optimize resolution.

Analysis

After image acquisition the data sets were reconstructed using the Nikon Metris XCT-Pro reconstruction software (Metris XT 1.6, version 2.1.3509.24 387, 10 August 2009). No beam hardening correction [19] or noise reduction was applied in order to maintain consistency during our analysis. The reasoning behind this is two-fold: firstly, beam hardening correction is based on the grey level of the image [19]. Since the intensity level varies with staining throughout the study, the correction would be inconsistent between scans. Secondly, the intensity profile through the sample is affected by the uneven staining of the tissue: attempting to obtain a flat intensity profile by applying beam hardening correction therefore defeats the purpose of quantifying the accumulation of contrast agent over time.

Following reconstruction, datasets were partially aligned in 3D such that the apico-basal axis lay parallel with the z-axis (i.e. perpendicular to the transverse plane). 2D transverse slices were then extracted midway through the ventricles for analysis. Due to varying sample placement between scans, it was necessary to ensure that the same region was compared in each dataset. Slice location was noted with respect to the top of the atria and bottom of the ventricles; using this information we were able to identify approximately the same slice in each dataset. This approximation was then verified by identifying distinguishing features (e.g. papillary muscles) to ensure the same region was compared.

Once alignment was complete, a line profile of intensity was measured with a width of 5 pixels (taking an average to reduce the effects of noise) from epicardium to endocardium, as Fig. 2 illustrates. The epicardial edge was detected using a three step process, as shown in Fig. 3. 1) The line profile was filtered with a Gaussian kernel ($\sigma=4$) in order to reduce noise, 2) the maximal change in intensity of the line profile ($\mathrm{d}I/\mathrm{d}x|_{max}$) was located, 3) the epicardial edge was defined as the next point towards the endocardium where $\mathrm{d}I/\mathrm{d}x=0$. The line profile was then discretized into twenty 0.1 mm segments starting from the epicardial edge. Each segment was assigned an intensity value I based on the average value of the pixels within the segment, and a value of distance x corresponding to the distance between the epicardial edge (0 mm) and each segment and finally a value of t which corresponded to incubation time.

These values were used to analyse the time required to adequately stain tissue at various locations within the ventricular wall. Intensity was plotted against time for various locations (see Fig. 4) within the tissue and fitted with curves of the form:

$$I=I_0+(I_{max}-I_0)(1-e^{-kt}), \quad (1)$$

using MatLab's *fminsearch* function. This formulation assumes that the unstained tissue (i.e. $t=0$) had an initial intensity I_0 which exponentially tended towards a maximal value of intensity I_{max} with stain time. We defined optimal staining time as the minimum time required for the tissue to reach its saturated value of intensity. The desirable level of saturation is likely to depend upon the intended application; therefore, we defined three levels of saturation in the ventricles based upon the ratio of I/I_{max} (90%, 95%, 99%) and calculated the optimal staining time accordingly.

Results

Fig 1. shows the reconstructed slices of the ventricles throughout the staining process. The intensity level of the grey-scale images is shown to increase quicker in the epicardium than the endocar-

Table 2. Summary of controllable factors and their values used in the study.

Controlled variable	
Species	Mouse
Fixative	Phosphate buffered formal saline
Contrast agent	I_2KI
Contrast agent concentration	3.75%
Contrast agent solvent	Formalin (10%)
Temperature	Room temperature
X-ray target	Tungsten
X-ray accelerating voltage	50 kV
Projections	2001

dium; since the intensity is related to the amount of I_2KI accumulation, this indicates the epicardium accumulates I_2KI quicker than the endocardium. This is likely due to the fact that the epicardium is in direct contact with the contrast agent and thus stains quicker than other areas. Whilst it is possible that I_2KI solution could enter the chambers of the heart and stain the endocardium directly, the results indicate that the endocardium took longer to stain, suggesting that contrast agent reached this area primarily by diffusion through the myocardium.

The intensity of each segment was plotted over time and a curve was fitted according to equation 1, as shown in Fig. 4. Representing the data in this way illustrates how the increase in intensity, and thus the accumulation of I_2KI, is slower at more distant points within the tissue. The time required to optimally stain each segment of tissue therefore increases with distance into the sample.

Based on the fitted curves, we measured the points at which I/I_{max} was equal to 90%, 95% and 99%, giving an indication of the optimal staining time throughout the myocardium. Due to the effects of beam hardening, I_{max} is highest at the epicardium and decreases towards the endocardium. Therefore, taking the ratio of I/I_{max} as a marker of tissue stain saturation removed bias due to beam hardening. Having measured these quantities for all values of x we fitted an equation of the form:

$$t_{stain} = Ae^{kx}, \qquad (2)$$

where t_{stain} is the required staining time and A and k are constants to be fitted for the three saturation values. Fig. 5 shows the result of this fitting process in the form of a semi-logarithmic plot, with fitted values A and k given in Table 1.

Discussion

As shown in Fig. 2B, as the staining time increases, the line profile of intensity across the tissue becomes flatter. This indicates a more uniform optical density, which would be expected for homogeneous tissue. If the line profile is not flat, this would indicate an incomplete staining process, as parts of the tissue contain more contrast agent than others. As shown in Fig. 5, the required staining time is exponentially dependent on the distance into the tissue (since the scale is semi-logarithmic a straight line plot is obtained).

To calculate the optimum staining time the values shown in Table 1 can be used in conjunction with equation 2 to determine the time needed to achieve 90%, 95% and 99% saturation at an arbitrary distance into the tissue. For small tissue samples, such as the mouse hearts used in this study, it is possible to achieve a saturation of 99%. This is ideal for segmentation, as a uniform intensity is obtained which facilitates the use of automated algorithms, such as region-growing. For thicker tissue samples a saturation level of 99% may not be practically obtainable; therefore parameters for equation 2 have also been given for 95% and 90% saturation. As stated, it can be seen that in our experiments the diffusion process occurred from the epicardial surface towards the endocardium. Due to the exponential relationship between staining time and tissue thickness it may be necessary to stain larger samples from both the epicardial and endocardial surfaces simultaneously, which would allow twice the amount of tissue to be stained in the same amount of time.

Limitations

The effect of time upon contrast agent diffusion is one factor affecting contrast of XCT images; other controls such as the concentration of the contrast agent, species and specimen size need to be quantified in further studies to fully understand staining conditions for optimal XCT contrast. Other controllable factors include temperature, contrast agent and solvent used, and are summarised in Table 2.

It has been shown that I_2KI concentration significantly impacts upon scan results [11,12,17] and is also likely to affect the incubation time required to successfully stain a soft tissue sample. In our study we chose a constant concentration suitable for imaging smaller hearts [11]. Whilst this has been essential for maintaining a manageable sample size, the effect of concentration on the staining process remains to be fully evaluated.

This study also concentrates only on mouse tissue, with results being extrapolated to cardiac tissue of other animals. Since tissue structure [20–23] and density [24–26] have only a small amount of variation across species, I_2KI can be expected to stain cardiac tissue in a similar way across species.

Conclusions

Contrast-enhanced XCT is a technique which can be used to image the whole heart with high resolution compared with other imaging techniques such as MRI. The use of contrast agent allows for detailed structures such as the cardiac conduction system and fibre orientation to be resolved using XCT-based imaging analysis [27]. The quality of results from contrast-enhanced XCT depend greatly upon the staining process, in particular the length of time samples are stained. In this study we have characterised and quantified this process in mouse hearts, and derived an empirical relationship between required incubation time and sample thickness. This relationship can be used as a guide for future contrast enhanced XCT studies of cardiac tissue.

Acknowledgments

All scanning was performed at the EPSRC-funded Henry Moseley X-Ray imaging Facility, Manchester University. We are grateful to the staff at the facility for their co-operation.

Thanks to Robert Bradley for the use of HMtools software.

Thanks to Cassandra Smith for contributing to the data analysis.

Author Contributions

Conceived and designed the experiments: TDB SJC TL HZ. Performed the experiments: TDB SJC YZ. Analyzed the data: SJC. Contributed reagents/materials/analysis tools: ML PJW. Contributed to the writing of the manuscript: TDB SJC TL ML PJW HZ. Funding: HZ.

References

1. Schuster A, Chiribiri A, Ishida M, Morton G, Paul M, et al. (2012) Cardiovascular magnetic resonance imaging of isolated perfused pig hearts in a 3T clinical MR scanner. Interventional medicine & applied science 4: 186–192.
2. Laschi R, Govoni E (1986) Cell ultrastructure in disease. Scanning electron microscopy: 193–8.
3. Aslanidi OV, Colman MA, Varela M, Zhao J, Smaill BH, et al. (2013) Heterogeneous and anisotropic integrative model of pulmonary veins: computational study of arrhythmogenic substrate for atrial fibrillation. Interface Focus 3: 20120069–20120069.
4. Zhao J, Butters TD, Zhang H, LeGrice IJ, Sands GB, et al. (2013) Image-based model of atrial anatomy and electrical activation: a computational platform for investigating atrial arrhythmia. IEEE transactions on medical imaging 32: 18–27.

5. Colman MA, Aslanidi OV, Kharche S, Boyett MR, Garratt CJ, et al. (2013) Pro-arrhythmogenic Effects of Atrial Fibrillation Induced Electrical Remodelling- Insights from 3D Virtual Human Atria. The Journal of physiology.
6. Butters TD, Aslanidi OV, Zhao J, Smaill B, Zhang H (2013) A novel computational sheep atria model for the study of atrial fibrillation. Interface Focus 3: 20120067–20120067.
7. Zhao J, Krueger MW, Seemann G, Meng S, Zhang H, et al. (2012) Myofiber orientation and electrical activation in human and sheep atrial models. Conference proceedings: Annual International Conference of the IEEE Engineering in Medicine and Biology Society IEEE Engineering in Medicine and Biology Society Conference 2012: 6365–8.
8. Zhao J, Butters TD, Zhang H, Pullan AJ, LeGrice IJ, et al. (2012) An image-based model of atrial muscular architecture: effects of structural anisotropy on electrical activation. Circulation Arrhythmia and electrophysiology 5: 361–70.
9. Jelicks LA, Tanowitz HB (2011) Advances in imaging of animal models of Chagas disease. Advances in parasitology 75: 193–208.
10. Benson AP, Bernus O, Dierckx H, Gilbert SH, Greenwood JP, et al. (2011) Construction and validation of anisotropic and orthotropic ventricular geometries for quantitative predictive cardiac electrophysiology. Interface focus 1: 101–16.
11. Stephenson RS, Boyett MR, Hart G, Nikolaidou T, Cai X, et al. (2012) Contrast enhanced micro-computed tomography resolves the 3-dimensional morphology of the cardiac conduction system in mammalian hearts. PloS one 7: e35299.
12. Aslanidi OV, Nikolaidou T, Zhao J, Smaill BH, Gilbert SH, et al. (2013) Application of micro-computed tomography with iodine staining to cardiac imaging, segmentation, and computational model development. IEEE transactions on medical imaging 32: 8–17.
13. Trinh L, Lowe T, Campbell GM, Withers PJ, Martin PJ (2013) Bread dough aeration dynamics during pressure step-change mixing: Studies by X-ray tomography, dough density and population balance modelling. Chemical Engineering Science 101: 470–477.
14. Sun YL, Lowe T, McDonald SA, Li QM, Withers PJ (2013) In-situ investigation and image-based modelling of aluminium foam compression using micro X-ray computed tomography. 7th International Conference on Advanced Computational Engineering and Experimenting.
15. Ayache N, Delingette H, Sermesant M, editors (2009) Functional Imaging and Modeling of the Heart, volume 5528 of *Lecture Notes in Computer Science*. Berlin, Heidelberg: Springer Berlin Heidelberg. doi:10.1007/978-3-642-01932-6.
16. Metscher BD (2009) MicroCT for comparative morphology: simple staining methods allow high-contrast 3D imaging of diverse non-mineralized animal tissues. BMC physiology 9: 11.
17. Jeffery NS, Stephenson RS, Gallagher JA, Jarvis JC, Cox PG (2011) Micro-computed tomography with iodine staining resolves the arrangement of muscle fibres. Journal of biomechanics 44: 189–92.
18. Vickerton P, Jarvis J, Jeffery N (2013) Concentration-dependent specimen shrinkage in iodine-enhanced microCT. Journal of anatomy 223: 185–93.
19. Dewulf W, Tan Y, Kiekens K Sense and Non-Sense of Beam Hardening Correction in CT Metrology.
20. Guterl KA, Haggart CR, Janssen PM, Holmes JW (2007) Isometric contraction induces rapid myocyte remodeling in cultured rat right ventricular papillary muscles. American journal of physiology Heart and circulatory physiology 293: H3707–12.
21. Modesti PA, Vanni S, Bertolozzi I, Cecioni I, Lumachi C, et al. (2004) Different growth factor activation in the right and left ventricles in experimental volume overload. Hypertension 43: 101–8.
22. Kajstura J, Zhang X, Liu Y, Szoke E, Cheng W, et al. (1995) The Cellular Basis of Pacing-Induced Dilated Cardiomyopathy: Myocyte Cell Loss and Myocyte Cellular Reactive Hypertrophy. Circulation 92: 2306–2317.
23. Gerdes AM, Capasso JM (1995) Structural remodeling and mechanical dysfunction of cardiac myocytes in heart failure. Journal of molecular and cellular cardiology 27: 849–56.
24. Ford WR, Menon V, Bhambhani A, Liyanage R, Khan MI, et al. (1997) Changes in myocardial density during postinfarction healing: effect on estimation of in vivo left ventricular mass by echocardiographic imaging. Canadian journal of physiology and pharmacology 75: 1075–82.
25. Masugata H, Mizushige K, Senda S, Kinoshita A, Sakamoto H, et al. (1999) Relationship between myocardial tissue density measured by microgravimetry and sound speed measured by acoustic microscopy. Ultrasound in Medicine & Biology 25: 1459–1463.
26. Vinnakota KC, Bassingthwaighte JB (2004) Myocardial density and composition: a basis for calculating intracellular metabolite concentrations. American journal of physiology Heart and circulatory physiology 286: H1742–9.
27. Haibo Ni, Castro S, Stephenson R, Jarvis J, Lowe T, et al. (2013). Extracting myofibre orientation from micro-CT images: An optimisation study.

8

Dynamic Bowtie Filter for Cone-Beam/Multi-Slice CT

Fenglin Liu[1,2]*, Qingsong Yang[2], Wenxiang Cong[2], Ge Wang[2]

1 Key Lab of Optoelectronic Technology and System, Engineering Research Center of Industrial Computed Tomography Nondestructive Testing, Ministry of Education, Chongqing University, Chongqing, China, **2** Biomedical Imaging Center, Center for Biotechnology and Interdisciplinary Studies, Department of Biomedical Engineering, Rensselaer Polytechnic Institute, Troy, New York, United States of America

Abstract

A pre-patient attenuator ("bowtie filter" or "bowtie") is used to modulate an incoming x-ray beam as a function of the angle of the x-ray with respect to a patient to balance the photon flux on a detector array. While the current dynamic bowtie design is focused on fan-beam geometry, in this study we propose a methodology for dynamic bowtie design in multi-slice/cone-beam geometry. The proposed 3D dynamic bowtie is an extension of the 2D prior art. The 3D bowtie consists of a highly attenuating bowtie (HB) filled in with heavy liquid and a weakly attenuating bowtie (WB) immersed in the liquid of the HB. The HB targets a balanced flux distribution on a detector array when no object is in the field of view (FOV). The WB compensates for an object in the FOV, and hence is a scaled-down version of the object. The WB is rotated and translated in synchrony with the source rotation and patient translation so that the overall flux balance is maintained on the detector array. First, the mathematical models of different scanning modes are established for an elliptical water phantom. Then, a numerical simulation study is performed to compare the performance of the scanning modes in the cases of the water phantom and a patient cross-section without any bowtie and with a dynamic bowtie. The dynamic bowtie can equalize the numbers of detected photons in the case of the water phantom. In practical cases, the dynamic bowtie can effectively reduce the dynamic range of detected signals inside the FOV. Furthermore, the WB can be individualized using a 3D printing technique as the gold standard. We have extended the dynamic bowtie concept from 2D to 3D by using highly attenuating liquid and moving a scale-reduced negative copy of an object being scanned. Our methodology can be applied to reduce radiation dose and facilitate photon-counting detection.

Editor: Jie Tian, Institute of Automation, Chinese Academy of Sciences, China

Funding: This work was supported in part by the National Instrumentation Program (2013YQ030629), Chongqing Science and Technology Research Plan (cstc2012gg-yyjs70016) in China, and NIH R01 EB011785. The funders had no role in study design, data collection and analysis, decision to publish, or preparation of the manuscript.

Competing Interests: The authors have declared that no competing interests exist.

* Email: liufl@cqu.edu.cn

Introduction

X-ray computed tomography (CT) is a corner stone of modern hospitals and clinics, and still under rapid development. Two contemporary topics are radiation dose reduction and multi-energy imaging. These two topics are actually interconnected. Let us first review some background information, which will lead to the main point of this paper on a 3D dynamic bowtie design.

CT radiation dose is a public major concern, especially for children. A British study quantified the cancer risk associated with the use of diagnostic x-rays, arguably causing ~700 cases of cancer per year in Britain and >5,600 cases in US [1]. Hence, the well-known ALARA ("*As Low As Reasonably Achievable*") principle has been accepted. It is ideal to send x-ray photons along each path as less as possible.

CT contrast resolution is rather poor in the context of soft tissue imaging. X-ray detection technology has been almost exclusively based on energy-integration. On the other hand, the best photon-counting detectors recognize photons individually and spectrally. Photon-counting detectors can reveal elemental composition and support contrast-enhanced studies through K-edge imaging [2]. However, the dynamic range of the photon-counting detector is rather limited. When the flux on the detector is lower than the maximum count rate, the imaging performance is excellent, but if multiple photons arrive in temporal proximity, the detector may not be able to resolve them as separate events. This loss means spectral distortion [3]. Hence, it is highly desirable to prescribe the attenuated photon flux on a per-ray basis.

Over the past years, CT dose reduction and multi-energy CT have attracted a major attention. For that purpose, optimally balancing an attenuated x-ray flux distribution is a pre-requisite. Up to date, a pre-patient attenuator, which is called a "bowtie filter" or "bowtie", is already in use. Such a bowtie filter selectively attenuates photons emitted from an x-ray source as a function of the angle of an x-ray [4]. Thus, the bowtie compresses the dynamic range on the detector by increasing attenuation for x-rays further from the iso-center of a field of view (FOV), which typically travel through less tissue. Thus, the bowtie helps improve image quality, since readings of the detectors are substantially equalized, the dynamic range is reduced for more detailed information quantization [5]. Also, by blocking low-energy x-rays, the bowtie also works with an x-ray beam filter to reduce the beam-hardening effect [6]. Furthermore, by blocking radiation to the periphery of a patient where the attenuation path is the shortest, the radiation dose is reduced, so is the scatter-to-primary ratio [7–9]. The limitation of the current bowtie filter is that the attenuation profile it produces is fixed and cannot be adaptively changed with the gantry rotation. Although modern CT scanners employ a small number of bowtie filters for different applications, these filters are not personalized and must be fixed for an entire scan.

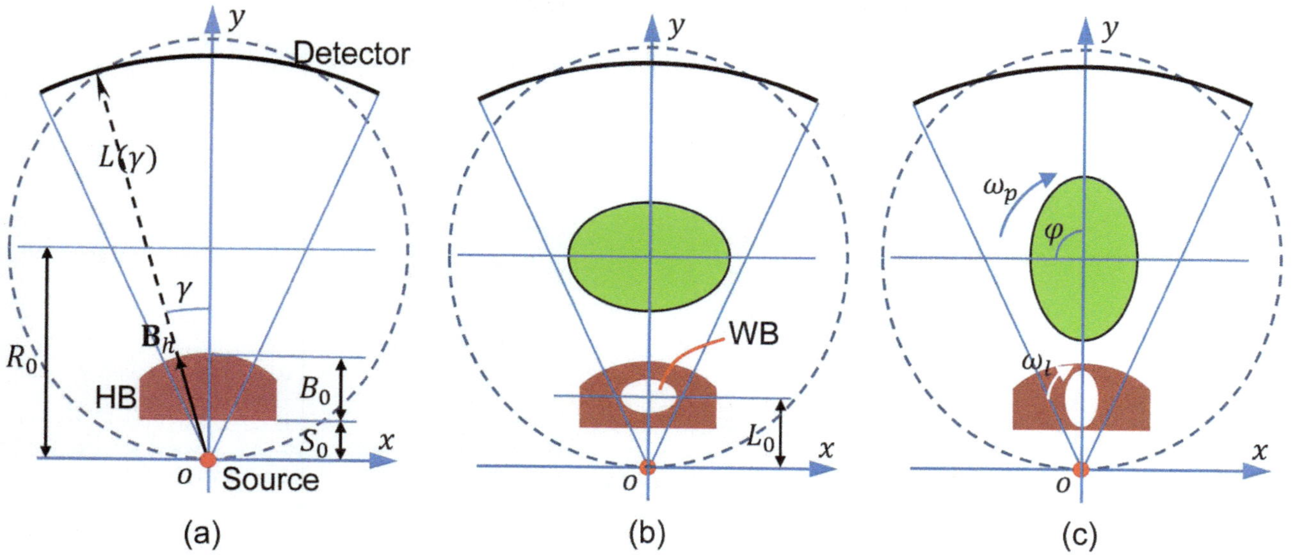

Figure 1. Dynamic bowtie in fan-beam geometry for a balanced flux distribution upon an equiangular detector array. (a) No object in the field of view (FOV) corresponds to a liquid highly attenuating bowtie (HB); (b) an elliptical phantom in the FOV corresponds to the HB containing a weakly attenuating bowtie (WB) that compensates for the attenuation due to the phantom; and (c) the WB is synchronously rotated with the gantry for dynamic compensation (for example, $\varphi = \pi/2$).

As a complementary method, an attenuation-based tube current modulation method was proposed to allow dose reduction [10,11]. This method modulates an incoming x-ray flux as a function of the view angle, instead of the angle of an individual x-ray. Hence, the tube current modulation can be customized on a per-patient basis. However, the problem is that this modulation changes neither the scatter to primary ratio nor the dynamic range for any given view angle.

Because the combination of a traditional bowtie filtration and a tube current modulation cannot meet the sophisticated needs for CT dose reduction and multi-energy imaging, a dynamic bowtie was proposed to smartly filter the radiation emitted towards a patient in synchrony with a data acquisition process. Along this direction, various beam-shaping filters were designed. The effects of the bowtie design on image quality and radiation dose were also reported [12–14]. Recently, the feasibility of a flexible piecewise-linear dynamic bowtie was studied [15], in which a set of triangular wedges were used as a basis to approximate any desirable attenuating profile. The initial simulation results showed a major reduction in the dynamic range of raw data. In an earlier study, we proposed a dynamic bowtie design for fan-beam CT, which uses a rotating bowtie filter for control within each fan-beam coupled with a tube current modulation for control across view angles [16]. However, these dynamic bowtie designs are fan-beam geometry oriented, and not intended for moderate or large cone angles.

Inspired by a dynamic beam-shaper report and a digitally controlled beam attenuator utilizing a highly attenuating fluid controlled with pistons [17,18], in this paper, we focus on a simple, general and easy-to-implement methodology for 3D bowtie design. The proposed 3D dynamic bowtie is an extension of the 2D prior art. The 3D bowtie consists of a highly attenuating bowtie (HB) filled in with heavy liquid and a weakly attenuating bowtie (WB) immersed in the liquid of the HB. The HB targets a balanced flux distribution on a detector array when no object is in the field of view (FOV). The WB compensates for an object in the FOV, and

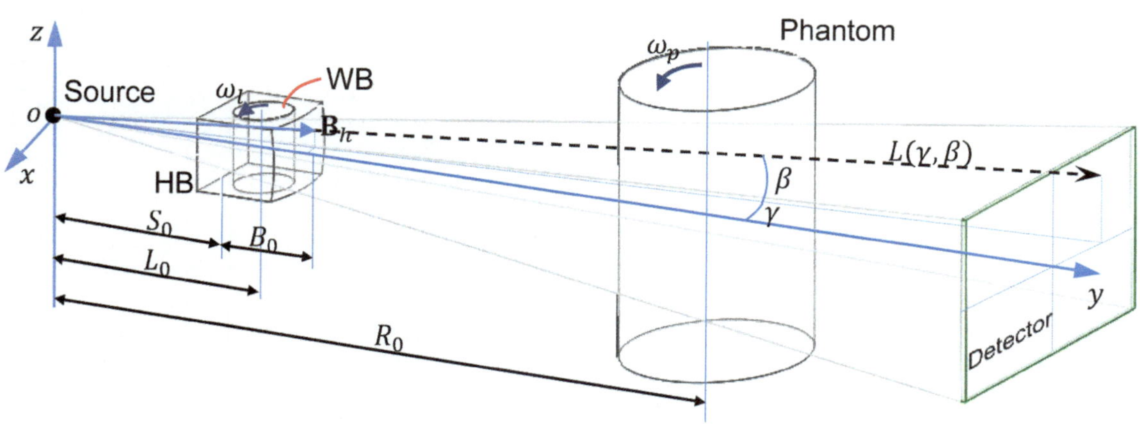

Figure 2. Dynamic bowtie in a cone-beam geometry with a flat panel detector plate.

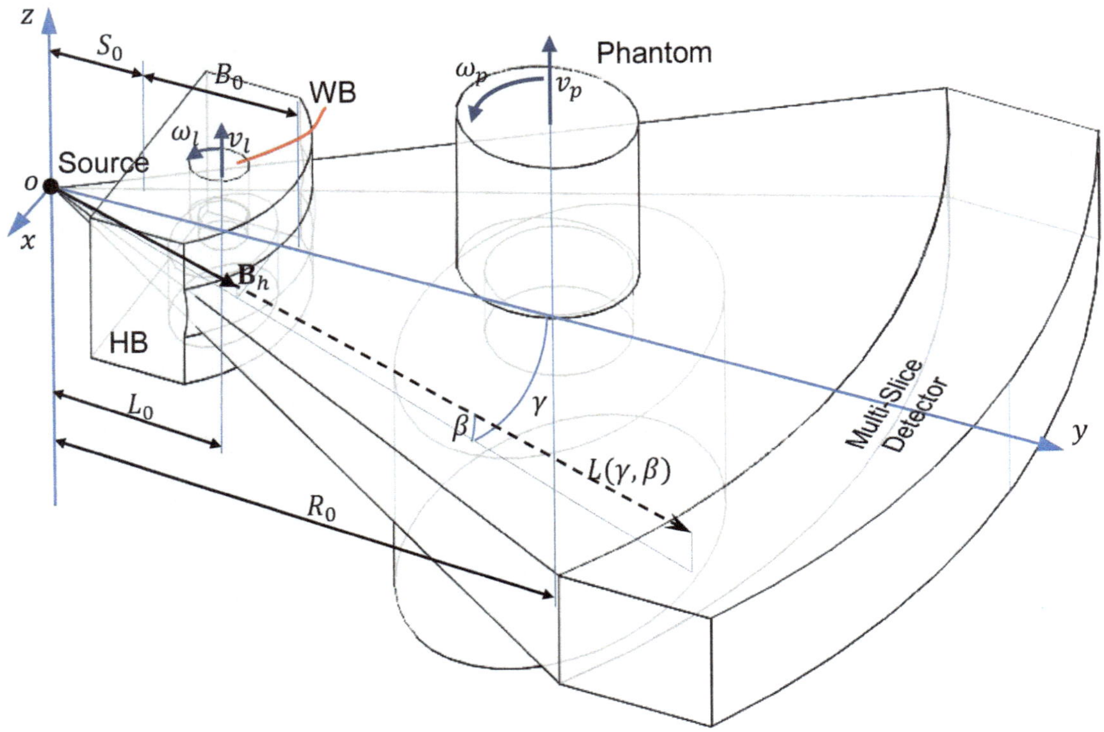

Figure 3. Dynamic bowtie in a spiral multi-slice geometry with a multi-slice detector array.

hence is a scaled-down version of the object. The WB is rotated and translated in synchrony with the source rotation and patient translation so that the overall flux balance is maintained on the detector array. In the next section, representative 3D bowties for different imaging modes are analyzed, and the HB contours are derived for fan-beam CT and multi-slice/cone-beam CT including helical CT. In the third section, numerical simulation results are reported to demonstrate the performance of the dynamic bowtie in cone-beam geometry. In the last section, relevant issues are discussed.

Methodology

When an x-ray beam irradiates an object in cone-beam geometry, the length of each x-ray path varies significantly as a function of the angular position of the ray within a tilted fan-beam, the tilting angle, and the object. If these variations are not effectively compensated, a large dynamic range will be required, or a data overflow problem will be generated in detectors. This is especially problematic for spectral detectors whose counting rates are much slower than the current integrating counterparts. To meet such a challenge, a smart bowtie can be used to optimally shape the x-ray beam so that the expected numbers of photons are equalized across detector channels. The major task of the dynamic bowtie design is to determine the bowtie shape and its dynamics to undo the path length changes during a CT scan. In this following, we first analyze the bowtie filter profile for the central beam plane in fan-beam geometry, and then extend the idea to cone-beam geometry. For convenience, we assume a monochromatic x-ray source without loss of generality.

Bowtie Filter for Fan-beam CT

On the central imaging plane, a multi-slice/cone-beam becomes a fan-beam. We assume a fan-beam geometry with detector cells equi-angularly distributed. An x-ray source is rotated along a circular trajectory of radius R_0. Let $L(\gamma)$ denotes a ray in the fan-beam, where the angle γ specifies the ray in the fan-beam. The coordinate systems are established in FIG. 1, where $\sigma := \{o; x,y,z=0\}$ is fixed with the source. We first require that when no object is in the field of view (FOV) data detected are uniform with a bowtie. Then, if we place a high attenuation liquid bowtie (HB) shown as FIG. 1 (a) for uniform detector readings, the profile $\mathbf{B}_h(\gamma)$ of the bowtie can be expressed in σ as

$$\mathbf{B}_h(\gamma)=\begin{bmatrix} x_h \\ y_h \end{bmatrix}=\begin{bmatrix} S_0\tan\gamma+B_0\sin\gamma+x(\gamma) \\ S_0+B_0\cos\gamma+y(\gamma) \end{bmatrix}, \quad (1)$$

where S_0 is the distance from the source to the HB, B_0 is the attenuation length of the HB. $x(\gamma)$ and $y(\gamma)$ define a bowtie layer to compensate for the inhomogeneous intensity distribution of x-rays from an x-ray source.

Since a cross-section of the human head, chest, and abdomen can be approximated to be elliptical, the bowtie filter can be analytically designed for such objects. As illustrated in FIG. 1 (b), when an elliptical water phantom with a semi-major axis A and a semi-minor axis B is placed within the fan-beam, the acquired data will vary according to different path lengths. Then, the fan-beam projection $P_w(\varphi,\gamma)$ through the homogenous elliptical object with an attenuation coefficient μ_w can be derived as [19]

$$P_w(\varphi,\gamma)=\begin{cases} \dfrac{2\mu_w AB}{S^2(\varphi+\gamma)}\sqrt{S^2(\varphi+\gamma)-(R_0\sin\gamma)^2}, & for\ |R_0\sin\gamma|\le S(\varphi+\gamma) \\ 0 & for\ |R_0\sin\gamma|>S(\varphi+\gamma) \end{cases} \quad (2)$$

where $S^2(\varphi+\gamma)=A^2\cos^2(\varphi+\gamma)+B^2\sin^2(\varphi+\gamma)$.

To make the acquired data uniform, we can insert an elliptical low attenuation chamber (the WB) with a semi-major axis a and a

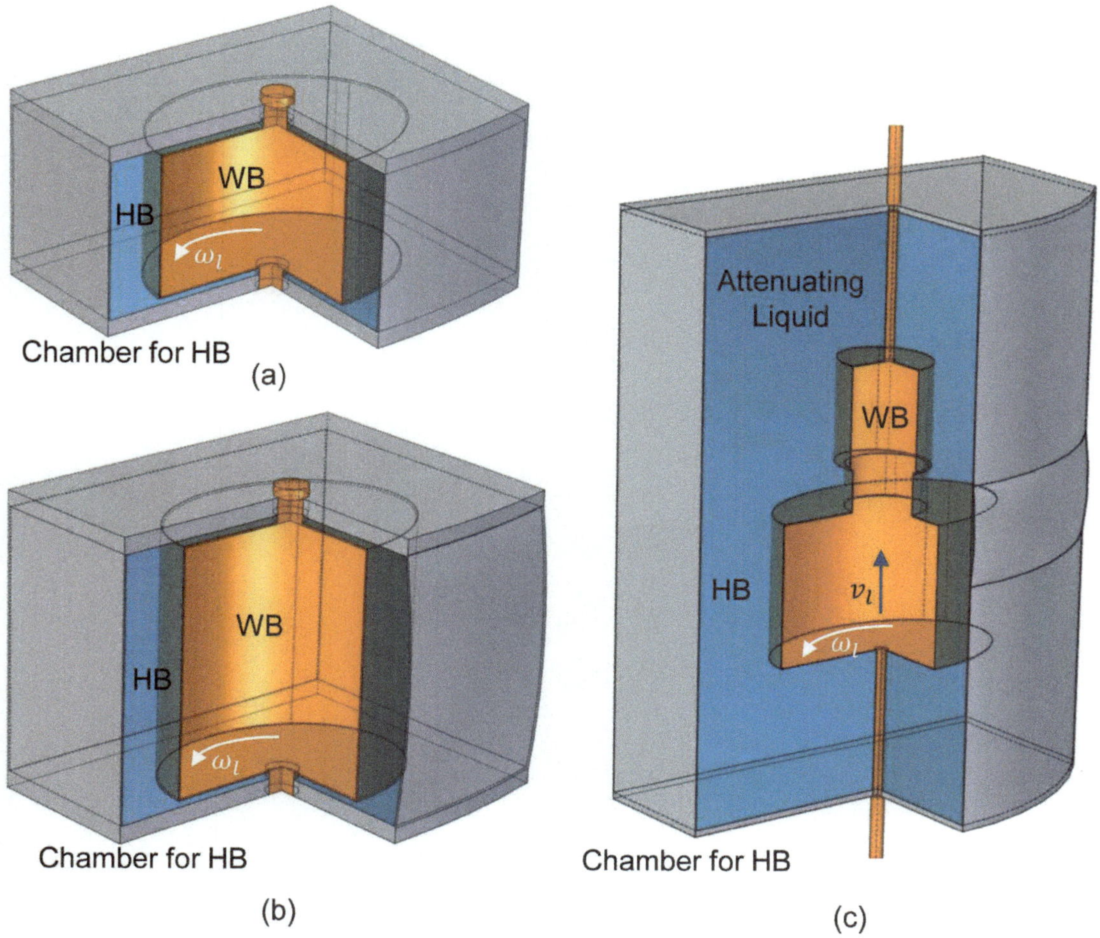

Figure 4. Exemplary designs of the dynamic bowtie without driving components. (a) A dynamic bowtie for fan-beam CT, (b) and (c) for cone-beam CT and spiral multi-slice CT respectively. The attenuating liquid for HB is $CeCl_3$ solution. The WB material is air. The containers for HB and WB are made of 0.5 mm thick aluminum and 0.2 mm thick plastic, respectively.

semi-minor axis b into the HB. When the WB is rotated synchronously with the source, the variation of projection $P_w(\varphi,\gamma)$ can be perfectly compensated for. For that purpose, we have the net projection expressed as

$$P(\varphi+\gamma)=P_h-P_l(\varphi,\gamma)+P_w(\varphi,\gamma), \tag{3}$$

Where P_h is the full projection only with the HB (without a WB) which yields uniform projection data by design, $P_l(\varphi,\gamma)$ is the differential projection of the high density liquid replaced by the WB. Let $L_0=S_0+B_0/2$, μ_h and μ_l be the attenuation coefficient of the HB and WB respectively. If

$$\frac{R_0}{L_0}=\frac{\mu_h-\mu_l}{\mu_w}=\frac{A}{a}=\frac{B}{b}, \tag{4}$$

we have

$$P_l(\varphi,\gamma)=P_w(\varphi,\gamma) \tag{5}$$

and

$$P(\varphi,\gamma)=P_h=\text{const.} \tag{6}$$

That is, we can have a constant projection profile during a full scan.

Our proposed dynamic bowtie for fan-beam CT is to have a rotating solid WB in a stationary liquid HB. An earlier dynamic beam shaper reported by Roessl et al. used a circular metal piece with a reduced elliptical patient inside, which is rotated in synchrony with the source to compensate for heterogeneous x-ray path lengths through the patient and a "pre-shaper" to equalize the x-ray flux [17]. Both the methods use a reduced version of the patient for the compensation purpose, and they both perform the flux normalization. The main differences between these methods lie in the following aspects. First, the attenuating materials are different. The key component for our design is the use of highly attenuating liquid, instead of rigid solid. Second, the main functionalities are different. Actually, our method covers the previously reported method as a special case (fan-beam geometry is a special case of cone-beam geometry). It is underlined that the key idea is to introduce a highly attenuating liquid as the background medium so that the dynamic compensation can be

Table 1. Parameters used for the design of a dynamic bowtie.

Parameter	Value
Source trajectory	Full circle
Scan radius (R_0)	57 cm
Source to detector distance (SDD)	114 cm
X-ray energy (keV)	100
Number of projections	1160
Number of detector pixels	672×100
Detector slice thickness (Δh)	2 mm
Detector angular aperture ($\Delta\gamma$)	1.354×10^{-3} radian
HB container material	Aluminum
HB container thickness (t_{hb})	0.05 cm
HB container attenuation (μ_{hb}) [27]	0.460 cm^{-1}
HB liquid attenuator	$CeCl_3$ solution
HB liquid attenuation (μ_h)	$3\mu_w$
HB attenuation length (B_0)	14 cm
WB attenuator	Air
WB container material	C-552 air-equivalent plastic
WB container thickness (t_{lb})	0.02 cm
WB container attenuation (μ_{lb}) [21]	0.112 cm^{-1}
Water attenuation coefficient (μ_w) [28]	0.171 cm^{-1}
Source to bowtie distance (S_0)	12 cm

realized in cone-beam geometry allowing circular and spiral multi-slice/cone-beam scanning modes.

Bowtie Filter for Multi-slice/Cone-Beam CT

Now, let us extend the dynamic bowtie design from fan-beam geometry to multi-slice/cone-beam geometry. The coordinate system for cone-beam CT is in FIG. 2, where $\sigma := \{o; x,y,z\}$ is fixed with the source. Let $L(\gamma,\beta)$ denote a ray within the cone-beam, where γ and β specifies the angle in reference to the two orthogonal central planes respectively. Similar to the fan-beam case, we want to define a surface for the HB to produce uniform detector data, the surface $\mathbf{B}_h(\gamma,\beta)$ of the HB can be expressed in σ as follows:

$$\mathbf{B}_h(\gamma,\beta)=\begin{bmatrix} x_h \\ y_h \\ z_h \end{bmatrix}=\begin{bmatrix} S_0\tan\gamma+B_0\cos\beta\sin\gamma+x(\gamma,\beta) \\ S_0+B_0\cos\beta\cos\gamma+y(\gamma,\beta) \\ \left(B_0+\dfrac{S_0}{\cos\beta\cos\gamma}\right)\sin\beta+z(\gamma,\beta) \end{bmatrix}, \quad (7)$$

where $x(\gamma,\beta)$, $y(\gamma,\beta)$, $z(\gamma,\beta)$ define a bowtie layer for x-ray flux normalization, similar to what we have formulated in the fan-beam case.

Let us use a cylindrical water phantom of an elliptical cross-section with a semi-major axis A and a semi-minor axis B in the cone-beam case, since a patient is quite similar to a cylinder. Then,

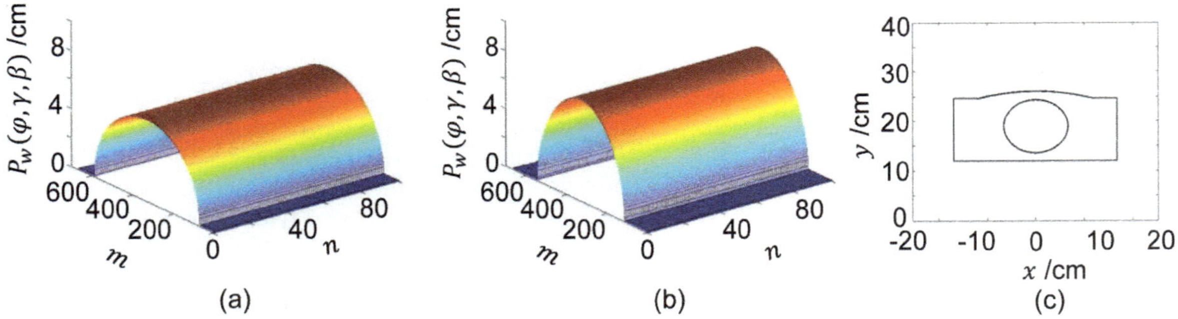

Figure 5. Projections of an elliptical water phantom and the bowtie profile. The projection angle φ is indexed by the projection number $i(0\le i\le1160)$, $\varphi=i\times\Delta\varphi$, $\Delta\varphi=2\pi/1160$. The ray angle γ is indexed by the horizontal detector number, $\gamma=(335-m)\times\Delta\gamma$, $(0\le m<672)$. The ray angle β is indexed by the vertical detector number, $\beta=(n-49)\times\mathrm{atan}(\frac{\Delta h}{SDD})$, $(0\le n<100)$. (a)–(b) Surface displays of the sinogram from a water phantom for $\varphi=0$ and $\varphi=\pi/2$ respectively, and (c) the bowtie profile for $\varphi=0$ and $\beta=0$.

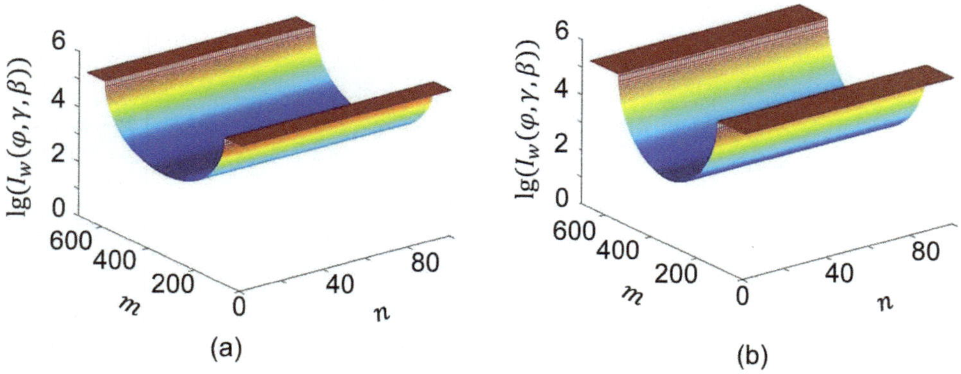

Figure 6. Numbers of detected photons along x-rays through the water phantom without any bowtie (on a log scale). (a) and (b) Surface displays for the numbers of detected photons for $\varphi=0$ and $\varphi=\pi/2$ respectively.

the acquired multi-slice/cone-beam data will have more variations than in the fan-beam case. Mathematically, the multi-slice/cone-beam projection $P_w(\varphi,\gamma,\beta)$ through the homogenous cylindrical phantom with an attenuation coefficient μ_w can be obtained as

$$P_w(\varphi,\gamma,\beta)=\begin{cases}\dfrac{\frac{2\mu_w AB}{S^2(\varphi+\gamma)}\sqrt{S^2(\varphi+\gamma)-(R_0 sin\gamma)^2}}{\cos\beta}, & for|R_0\sin\gamma|\le S(\varphi+\gamma),\\ 0 & for|R_0\sin\gamma|>S(\varphi+\gamma)\end{cases} \quad (8)$$

where $S^2(\varphi+\gamma)=A^2\cos^2(\varphi+\gamma)+B^2\sin^2(\varphi+\gamma)$.

Just like what we have done in the fan-beam case, to make the acquired data have identical expected values, we can insert a cylindrical WB with a semi-major axis a and a semi-minor axis b into the HB. When the WB and the source are rotated in synchrony, the variation in $P_w(\varphi,\gamma,\beta)$ can be appropriately canceled out. Specifically, we have the whole projection expressed as

$$P(\varphi,\gamma,\beta)=P_h-P_l(\varphi,\gamma,\beta)+P_w(\varphi,\gamma,\beta). \quad (9)$$

If we set the parameters according to Eq. (4), we have

$$P_l(\varphi,\gamma,\beta)=P_w(\varphi,\gamma,\beta) \quad (10)$$

and

$$P(\varphi,\gamma,\beta)=P_h=\text{const.} \quad (11)$$

Bowtie Filter for Helical CT

As illustrated in FIG. 3, we can also handle a helical multi-slice/cone-beam scan as well. The difference between such circular and helical scans will be significant only if a longitudinally non-uniform object is imaged, such as a patient. In this case, the WB should be a miniature of the object to be scanned, and the WB motion must be different from that for circular multi-slice/cone-beam scanning. In addition to the synchronized rotation of the WB and the source, the WB needs to be translated as well in synchrony with the object translation but at a slower speed. Let $p=L_0/R_0$, then we have

$$v_l=v_p\times p \quad (12)$$

where v_l and v_p are the translation speeds of the WB and the object respectively.

Bowtie Design

The dynamic bowtie is a purposely-shaped highly attenuating liquid container with a customized low attenuation bowtie inside that can be moved under precise control in synchrony with both the source rotation and the patient translation. When a bowtie is designed, there are two major factors to be taken into account.

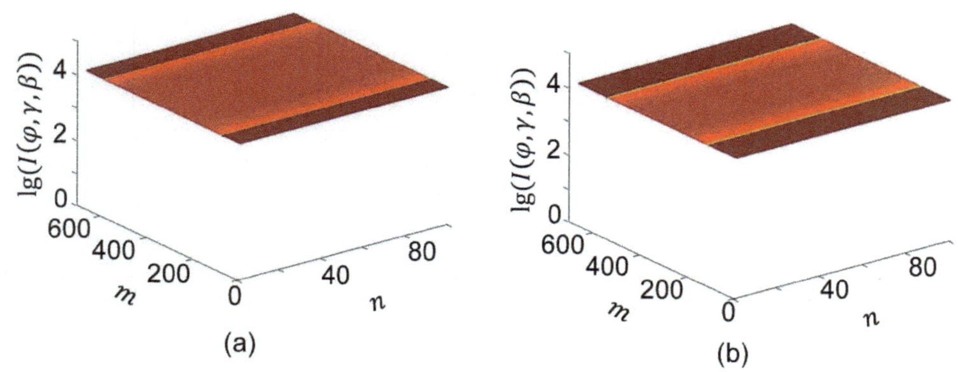

Figure 7. Numbers of detected photons along x-rays through the water phantom with the proposed dynamic bowtie (on a log scale). (a) and (b) Surface displays for the numbers of detected photons for $\varphi=0$ and $\varphi=\pi/2$ respectively.

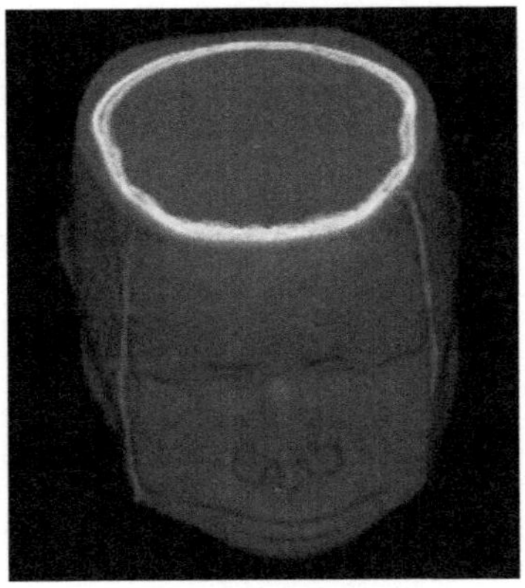

Figure 8. Head CT model approximated as an ellipse of semi-major axis $A=102$ mm and semi-minor axis $B=81$ mm.

The first factor is the selection of the highly attenuating liquid and weakly attenuating material, and the other one is the material to make the container for HB. Based on medical CT applications, our initial choice of the ideal attenuation coefficients for HB and WB are $\mu_h-\mu_l=(3\sim5)\mu_w$, which means the size of the WB is (1/3–1/5) of the object to be scanned. An ideal casing material of the HB should have the same attenuation characteristics as the liquid, while the attenuation coefficient of the WB should be as low as possible. Since air is an ideal WB material with almost zero attenuation, in the following design and simulation, we focus on the WB which is an air chamber with a thin-walled low attenuation container (an interesting point we want to point out is that we can use a 3D printing technique such as pseudo halftone [20] to produce an inhomogeneous weakly attenuating chamber to mimic a patient more realistically).

Some exemplary dynamic bowties are shown in FIG. 4, without driving components. In the designs, the highly attenuating liquid is cerous chloride ($CeCl_3$) because it is quite soluble, and we can have $\mu_h-\mu_l=(3\sim5)\mu_w$ by adjusting its concentration [18]. The HB container material can be 0.5 mm thick aluminum. The WB attenuator is air and its container material can be 0.2 mm thick C-552 air-equivalent plastic [21].

water cylinder of an elliptical cross-section of a semi-major axis $A=200$ mm and a semi-minor axis $B=160$ mm.

FIG. 5 (a) shows projection profiles $P_w(\varphi,\gamma,\beta)$ of the water phantom without any bowtie. Setting the projection angle $\varphi=0$ and the fan angle $\gamma=0$, the minimum projection value along the central ray $P_w(0,0,0)$ was obtained. Setting $\varphi=\pi/2$ and $\gamma=0$, the maximum value along the central ray $P_w(\pi/2,0,0)$ was obtained.

The side of the HB facing the source was assumed flat for convenience. Then, with Eq. (7), the surface of HB $\mathbf{B}_h(\gamma,\beta)$ was computed. The WB was rotated angularly around the axis perpendicularly through the bowtie center. By Eq. (4), the WB is an elliptical chamber scaled down from an object by a factor of 1/3 of the object, which means an elliptical cylinder chamber with a semi-major axis $a=66.67$ mm and a semi-minor axis $b=53.33$ mm. FIG. 5 (c) visualizes the bowtie for $\varphi=0$ and $\beta=0$.

Numerical Test

First, the numbers of detected photons without the dynamic bowtie were calculated for the water phantom of $A=200$ mm and $B=160$ mm over a full scan. By Beer's law,

$$I_w(\varphi,\gamma,\beta)=I_0e^{-P_w(\varphi,\gamma,\beta)}, \tag{13}$$

the numbers of projection data were synthesized, as plotted in FIG. 6 for $\varphi=0$ and $\varphi=\pi/2$ respectively, assuming the number of emitted photons per second $I_0=2\times10^5$ along each ray path.

Second, with the dynamic bowtie for the aforementioned phantom and $I_0=2\times10^7$ (the increment in the flux is to overcome the attenuation of the bowtie), the numbers of photons were simulated again for each ray path. Practically, the influence of the container materials of the HB and WB should not be ignored. Then, by Eq. (11) we have

$$I(\varphi,\gamma,\beta)=I_0e^{-(P_h(\gamma,\beta)+P_{lt}(\varphi,\gamma,\beta))}, \tag{14}$$

Where $P_h(\gamma,\beta)$ is the projection of the HB, $P_{lt}(\varphi,\gamma,\beta)$ is the projection of the WB container, and

$$P_h(\gamma,\beta)=B_0\times\mu_h+\left(1+\frac{1}{\cos\gamma\cos\beta}\right)t_{hb}(\mu_{hb}-\mu_h), \tag{15}$$

$$P_{lt}(\varphi,\gamma,\beta)=\begin{cases}0,\ for\ |L_0\sin\gamma|>s(\varphi+\gamma)\\ \dfrac{\frac{2ab}{s^2(\varphi+\gamma)}\sqrt{s^2(\varphi+\gamma)-(L_0\sin\gamma)^2}}{\cos\beta}\mu_{lb},\ for\ |L_0\sin\gamma|\le s(\varphi+\gamma)\text{ and }|L_0\sin\gamma|>s_l(\varphi+\gamma)\\ \dfrac{\frac{2ab}{s^2(\varphi+\gamma)}\sqrt{s^2(\varphi+\gamma)-(L_0\sin\gamma)^2}-\frac{2a_lb_l}{s_l^2(\varphi+\gamma)}\sqrt{s^2(\varphi+\gamma)-(L_0\sin\gamma)^2}}{\cos\beta}\mu_{lb},\ otherwise\end{cases}, \tag{16}$$

where $s^2(\varphi+\gamma)=a^2\cos^2(\varphi+\gamma)+b^2\sin^2(\varphi+\gamma)$, $s_l^2(\varphi+\gamma)=a_l^2\cos^2(\varphi+\gamma)+b_l^2\sin^2(\varphi+\gamma)$, $a_l=a-t_{lb}$, $b_l=b-t_{lb}$.

From Eqs. (14)–(16), when $\mu_{hb}\to\mu_h$, μ_{lb} and t_{lb} are small enough, we have $I(\varphi,\gamma,\beta)\approx\text{const}$, which means that we can effectively regulate the numbers of detected photons along each ray path through the water phantom.

FIG. 7 shows the numbers of detected photons $I(\varphi,\gamma,\beta)$ for $\varphi=0$ and $\varphi=\pi/2$ respectively. It is seen that the numbers of detected photons were made quite uniform with only slight variations mainly due to the container material for WB.

Numerical Simulation

Idealized Design

Table 1 lists the parameters used for the design of an exemplary dynamic bowtie. To simulate the dynamic range of detector readings, a mono-energetic x-ray tube was assumed to work at 100 keV, and the numbers of detected photon were the same I_0 without a bowtie for a blank scan. When the WB is an air chamber with attenuation coefficient μ_l, the bowtie was designed with the liquid of attenuation coefficient $\mu_h=3\mu_w$, as aforementioned, for a

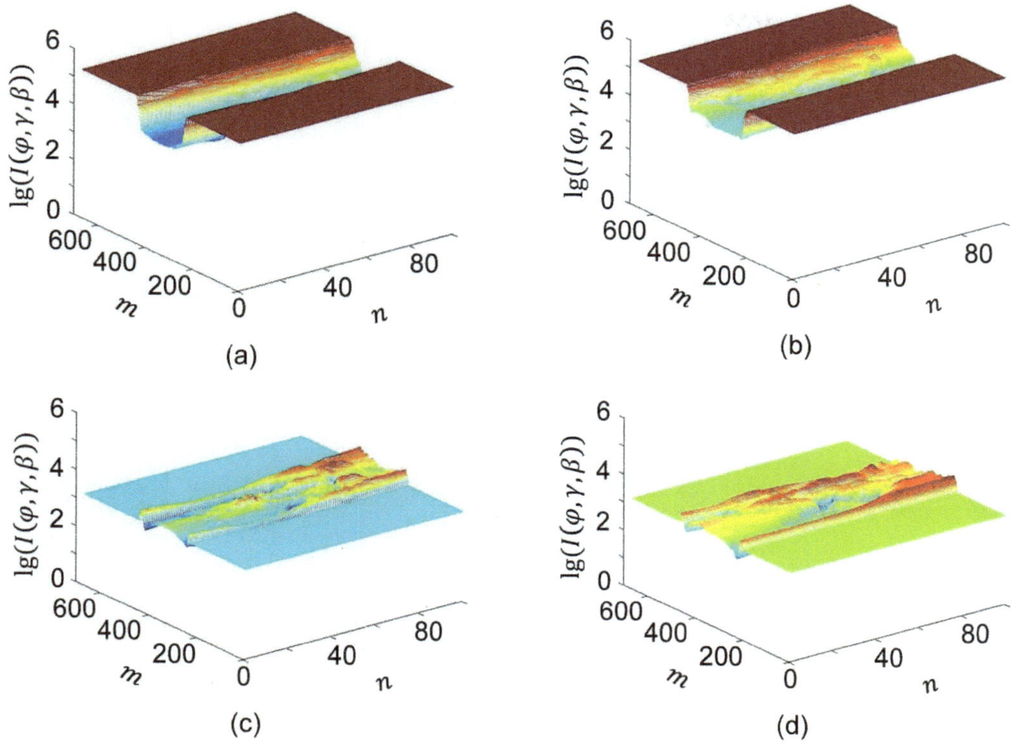

Figure 9. Numbers of detected photons along x-rays through the head CT volume without and with the proposed dynamic bowtie (on a log scale). (a) and (b) Numbers of detected photons assuming $I_0 = 2 \times 10^5$ without a bowtie for $\varphi = 0$ and $\varphi = \pi/2$ respectively. (c) and (d) Numbers of detected photons assuming $I_0 = 2 \times 10^6$ with a proposed bowtie for $\varphi = 0$ and $\varphi = \pi/2$ respectively.

Realistic Demonstration

To show the practical value of our 3D dynamic bowtie, we selected a 3D CT image volume to simulate the detected photons and compared the dynamic ranges of the signals with and without the dynamic bowtie respectively. FIG. 8 is a 3D head CT volume from the Visible Human project [22]. After scaling, the head was approximated as a cylinder with an elliptical cross-section of a semi-major axis $A = 102$ mm and a semi-minor axis $B = 81$ mm.

As mentioned earlier, we designed a dynamic bowtie for the cylindrical water phantom of $A = 102$ mm and $B = 81$ mm. FIG. 9 illustrates the numbers of detected photons for $\varphi = 0$ and $\varphi = \pi/2$ with and without the dynamic bowtie respectively. It is seen that the dynamic ranges of the signals differ greatly in the two cases, showing the advantage of the dynamic bowtie in FIG. 9(c) and (d).

Discussion and Conclusions

As demonstrated in FIG. 7, for a water phantom it is feasible to make the expected numbers of detected photons almost the same across all the detector elements with a dynamic bowtie. If a cross section of a patient can be well approximated in this way, the dynamic range of detectors can be optimally matched to that of projection data. As shown in FIG. 9, without a bowtie only a small portion of the detector dynamic range is utilized to depict the signal variation. With a dynamic bowtie, the dynamic range problem can be basically remedied, leading to a reduced radiation dose for a given image quality requirement.

Our proposed approach for the design of a dynamic bowtie is to fit a rotating or spiraling WB into a liquid HB. For a clinical CT scan, it is desirable that the WB should be individualized before imaging. With the progress of the 3D surface scanning of human body [23,24], and the popularization of 3D printing technology [25,26], it seems feasible to individualize dynamic bowties via rapid prototyping based on an individualized optical surface model. Furthermore, this process can be completely automatic in the future, and finished in less than a couple of minutes. Specifically, we could just capture the body surface of a patient, deform a digital atlas such as the visible human dataset into the surface model, and produce rotating patient-specific WB. FIG. 10 illustrates a dynamic bowtie design for full-body helical cone-beam scanning. As aforementioned, the WB is a reduced copy of the patient. During helical cone-beam scanning, the WB movement will be fully synchronized with the helical scanning trajectory from the beginning to the end. It is underlined that the geometrical adaptability and technical feasibility of the proposed 3D dynamic bowtie promises significant performance improvement and dose saving.

In addition to the similarities and differences we have already discussed above between our proposed liquid-based device and the rigid solid beam shaper [17], here we would like to mention more unique merits associated with our approach. First, it is convenient to change the density of liquid HB by adjusting the solution concentration to adapt the device for different applications. Also, proper solution elements can be selected for various attenuating needs; for example, the cerium with the K-edge at 40 keV provides a beam well matched to the attenuation characteristics of iodine [18]. Besides the reusability of the liquid HB, our scheme is mechanically cheaper and easier to print a thin-walled plastic WB than the idea to print a hollow rigid solid. Finally, the WB is placed within the liquid HB as a single unit which is compact and efficient for system integration.

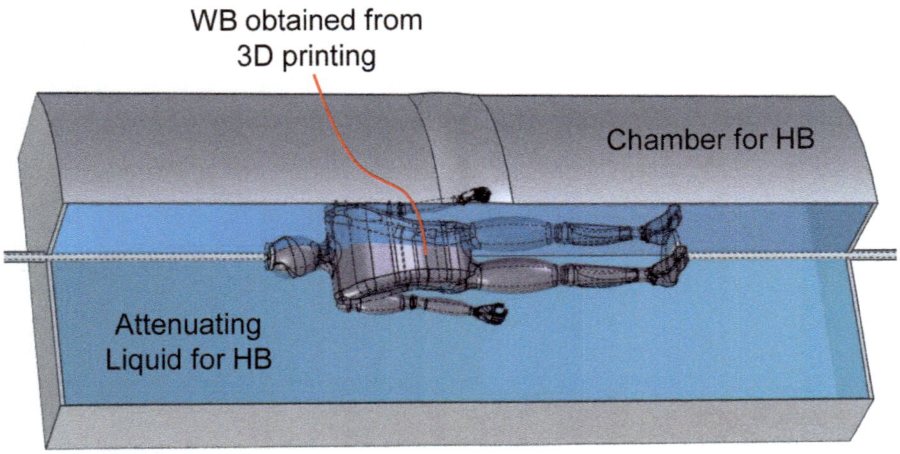

Figure 10. Dynamic bowtie for full body helical CT, in which the WB is rapidly prototyped according to an individualized patient contour obtained from surface scanning.

As explained above, the dynamic bowtie rotation and the helical scan are fully synchronized from the beginning to the end. In a typical CT system, a dynamic bowtie is a small part. Its control can be easily realized if the speed is not too rapid. When high speed is important for some applications, namely, cardiac imaging, we believe that our design should also work in principle but high precision engineering will be involved which could be expensive. In other words, other than cardiac imaging, the liquid bowtie design could be an interesting option.

It is acknowledged that in this initial study, a monochromatic x-ray source has been assumed. In practice, an x-ray source is polychromatic. The multi-energy spectrum introduces an additional layer of complexity. In this scenario, we need to match HB liquid and WB content with the x-ray spectrum being an additional key factor, augment the objective function in terms of numbers of detected photons and utilize the least square criterion for an overall optimization. In a follow-up study, we will perform the bowtie simulation for cone-beam and helical scan with a polychromatic spectrum, and analyze the dynamic range, noise and dose reduction with clinic datasets.

In conclusion, we have proposed a methodology for the design of dynamic bowties for multi-slice/cone-beam CT in either circular or helical scanning mode, and demonstrated its feasibility in a realistic numerical study. The main contribution is to embed a 3D WB as a miniature of a patient being scanned into a liquid HB, and coordinate their motions to compensate for any attenuation path differences. Further refinement of the current design is under way.

Author Contributions

Conceived and designed the experiments: FL GW. Performed the experiments: FL QY WC. Analyzed the data: FL QY WC. Contributed reagents/materials/analysis tools: FL WC GW. Wrote the paper: FL WC GW.

References

1. Berrington de Gonzalez A, Darby S (2004) Risk of cancer from diagnostic X-rays: estimates for the UK and 14 other countries. Lancet 363: 345–351.
2. Ballabriga R, Campbell M, Heijne E, Llopart X, Tlustos L, et al. (2011) Medipix3: A 64 k pixel detector readout chip working in single photon counting mode with improved spectrometric performance. Nuclear Instruments & Methods in Physics Research Section a-Accelerators Spectrometers Detectors and Associated Equipment 633: S15–S18.
3. Taguchi K, Frey EC, Wang XL, Iwanczyk JS, Barber WC (2010) An analytical model of the effects of pulse pileup on the energy spectrum recorded by energy resolved photon counting x-ray detectors. Medical Physics 37: 3957–3969.
4. Hsieh J (2009) Computed Tomography: Principles, Design, Artifacts, and Recent Advances, 2nd Edition: Society of Photo Optical Instrumentation Engineering.
5. Mutic S, Palta JR, Butker EK, Das IJ, Huq MS, et al. (2003) Quality assurance for computed-tomography simulators and the computedtomography-simulation process: Report of the AAPM radiation therapy committee task group no. 66. Medical Physics 30: 2762–2792.
6. Blessing M, Bhagwat MS, Lyatskaya Y, Bellon JR, Hesser J, et al. (2012) Kilovoltage beam model for flat panel imaging system with bow-tie filter for scatter prediction and correction. Physica Medica-European Journal of Medical Physics 28: 134–143.
7. Boone JM (2010) Method for evaluating bow tie filter angle-dependent attenuation in CT: Theory and simulation results. Medical Physics 37: 40–48.
8. Bartolac S, Graham S, Siewerdsen J, Jaffray D (2011) Fluence field optimization for noise and dose objectives in CT. Medical Physics 38: S2–S17.
9. McKenney SE, Nosratieh A, Gelskey D, Yang K, Huang S-y, et al. (2011) Experimental validation of a method characterizing bow tie filters in CT scanners using a real-time dose probe. Medical Physics 38: 1406–1415.
10. Gies M, Kalender WA, Wolf H, Suess C, Madsen MT (1999) Dose reduction in CT by anatomically adapted tube current modulation. I. Simulation studies. Medical physics 26: 2235.
11. Kalender WA, Wolf H, Suess C (1999) Dose reduction in CT by anatomically adapted tube current modulation. II. Phantom measurements. Medical physics 26: 2248.
12. Zeng GSL (2004) Nonuniform noise propagation by using the ramp filter in fan-beam computed tomography. Ieee Transactions on Medical Imaging 23: 690–695.
13. Toth T, Cesmeli E, Ikhlef A, Horiuchi T, Flynn M (2005) Image quality and dose optimization using novel x-ray source filters tailored to patient size. Medical Imaging 2005: Physics of Medical Imaging, Pts 1 and 2 5745: 283–291.
14. Mail N, Moseley DJ, Siewerdsen JH, Jaffray DA (2009) The influence of bowtie filtration on cone-beam CT image quality. Medical Physics 36: 22–32.
15. Hsieh SS, Pelc NJ (2013) The feasibility of a piecewise-linear dynamic bowtie filter. Medical Physics 40.
16. Liu F, Wang G, Cong W, Hsieh S, Pelc N (2013) Dynamic bowtie for fan-beam CT. Journal of X-Ray Science and Technology 21: 579–590.
17. Roessl E, Proksa R. Dynamic Beam-Shaper for High Flux Photon-Counting Computed Tomography 2013; Europe/Zurich.
18. Peppler W, Kudva B, Dobbins J, Lee C, Mistretta C (1982) A DIGITALLY CONTROLLED BEAM ATTENUATOR. American Journal of Roentgenology 139: 426–426.
19. Kak AC, Slaney M, Society for Industrial and Applied Mathematics. (2001) Principles of computerized tomographic imaging. Classics in applied mathematics 33. Philadelphia, Pa.: Society for Industrial and Applied Mathematics (SIAM, 3600 Market Street, Floor 6, Philadelphia, PA 19104). pp. 1 electronic text (xiv, 327 p.).

20. Google website. Available: http://www.google.com/patents/US6724499. Accessed 2014 June 30.
21. NIST website. Available: http://physics.nist.gov/PhysRefData/XrayMassCoef/ComTab/c552.html. Accessed 2014 June 30.
22. NTIS website. Available: http://www.ntis.gov/products/vishuman.aspx. Accessed 2014 June 30.
23. Mavroidis C, Ranky R, Sivak M, Patritti B, DiPisa J, et al. (2011) Patient specific ankle-foot orthoses using rapid prototyping. Journal of Neuroengineering and Rehabilitation 8.
24. Gaisberger C, Steininger P, Mitterlechner B, Huber S, Weichenberger H, et al. (2013) Three-dimensional surface scanning for accurate patient positioning and monitoring during breast cancer radiotherapy. Strahlentherapie Und Onkologie 189: 887–893.
25. Bogue R (2013) 3D printing: the dawn of a new era in manufacturing? Assembly Automation 33: 307–311.
26. Wang W, Wang T, Yang Z, Liu L, Tong X, et al. (2013) Cost-effective Printing of 3D Objects with Skin-Frame Structures. Acm Transactions on Graphics 32.
27. NIST website. Available: http://physics.nist.gov/PhysRefData/XrayMassCoef/ElemTab/z13.html. Accessed 2014 June 30.
28. NIST website. Available: http://physics.nist.gov/PhysRefData/XrayMassCoef/ElemTab/water.html. Accessed 2014 June 30.

Diagnostic Accuracy of Computer-Aided Detection of Pulmonary Tuberculosis in Chest Radiographs: A Validation Study from Sub-Saharan Africa

Marianne Breuninger[1,2,3]*, Bram van Ginneken[4], Rick H. H. M. Philipsen[4], Francis Mhimbira[2], Jerry J. Hella[2], Fred Lwilla[2], Jan van den Hombergh[5], Amanda Ross[1,6], Levan Jugheli[1,2,6], Dirk Wagner[3], Klaus Reither[1,2,6]

1 Swiss Tropical and Public Health Institute, Basel, Switzerland, **2** Ifakara Health Institute, Bagamoyo, United Republic of Tanzania, **3** Center for Infectious Diseases and Travel Medicine, University Hospital Freiburg, Freiburg, Germany, **4** Diagnostic Image Analysis Group, Radboud University Medical Center, Nijmegen, The Netherlands, **5** PharmAccess International, Dar es Salaam, United Republic of Tanzania, **6** University of Basel, Basel, Switzerland

Abstract

Background: Chest radiography to diagnose and screen for pulmonary tuberculosis has limitations, especially due to inter-reader variability. Automating the interpretation has the potential to overcome this drawback and to deliver objective and reproducible results. The CAD4TB software is a computer-aided detection system that has shown promising preliminary findings. Evaluation studies in different settings are needed to assess diagnostic accuracy and practicability of use.

Methods: CAD4TB was evaluated on chest radiographs of patients with symptoms suggestive of pulmonary tuberculosis enrolled in two cohort studies in Tanzania. All patients were characterized by sputum smear microscopy and culture including subsequent antigen or molecular confirmation of *Mycobacterium tuberculosis* (M.tb) to determine the reference standard. Chest radiographs were read by the software and two human readers, one expert reader and one clinical officer. The sensitivity and specificity of CAD4TB was depicted using receiver operating characteristic (ROC) curves, the area under the curve calculated and the performance of the software compared to the results of human readers.

Results: Of 861 study participants, 194 (23%) were culture-positive for M.tb. The area under the ROC curve of CAD4TB for the detection of culture-positive pulmonary tuberculosis was 0.84 (95% CI 0.80–0.88). CAD4TB was significantly more accurate for the discrimination of smear-positive cases against non TB patients than for smear-negative cases (p-value$<$ 0.01). It differentiated better between TB cases and non TB patients among HIV-negative compared to HIV-positive individuals ($p<0.01$). CAD4TB significantly outperformed the clinical officer, but did not reach the accuracy of the expert reader ($p=0.02$), for a tuberculosis specific reading threshold.

Conclusion: CAD4TB accurately distinguished between the chest radiographs of culture-positive TB cases and controls. Further studies on cost-effectiveness, operational and ethical aspects should determine its place in diagnostic and screening algorithms.

Editor: Yoshihiko Hoshino, National Institute of Infectious Diseases, Japan

Funding: This study was supported by the European and Developing Countries Clinical Trials Partnership (EDCTP) as part of the project "Evaluation of new and emerging diagnostics for childhood tuberculosis in high burden countries" (TB CHILD) [IP.2009.32040.007]. The development of the CAD4TB software was supported by the EDCTP as part of the project "Evaluation of Multiple Novel and Emerging Technologies for TB Diagnosis in Smear negative and HIV infected Persons in High-burden Countries" (TB NEAT study) [IP.09.32040.009]. Delft Imaging Systems (CAD4TBII, http://www.delftimagingsystems.com/tb-solutions/cad4tb) provided a research grant to Bram van Ginneken and Rick HHM Philipsen for the development of CAD4TB. The funders had no role in study design, data collection and analysis, decision to publish, or preparation of the manuscript.

Competing Interests: Delft Imaging Systems (CAD4TBII, http://www.delftimagingsystems.com/tb-solutions/cad4tb) provided a research grant to Bram van Ginneken and Rick HHM Philipsen for the development of CAD4TB. There are no patents, further products in development or marketed products to declare.

* Email: marianne.breuninger@venus.uni-freiburg.de

Introduction

The role and potential of chest radiography as a diagnostic and screening tool for pulmonary tuberculosis (PTB) has long been debated. As a rapid examination that can be interpreted on-site with a high sensitivity (between 74 and 90% for PTB related abnormalities, up to 97%, if any abnormality is considered [1–4]), it has a firm place in the diagnosis of pulmonary tuberculosis. However, the lower specificity, a lack of consistency in how results are reported and high levels of inter- and intra-reader variability are matters of concern. Interpreting chest radiographs is complex and subjective: it is a two dimensional representation of a three dimensional structure, and there are varied manifestations of PTB. The complexity of the interpretation code and the structure of the report form affect the result [5,6]. Different readers are also

Table 1. Classification of study population according to clinical and microbiological data.

Group	Description	Short form
A	Smear positive/culture positive, *Mycobacterium tuberculosis*	s+/c+ M.tb
B	Smear negative/culture positive, *Mycobacterium tuberculosis*	s−/c+ M.tb
C	Smear negative or positive/culture positive, nontuberculous mycobacteria (NTM), irrespective of clinical relevance	s ±/c+ NTM
D	All cultures negative, CXR and clinical symptoms very suspect for PTB (clinically diagnosed TB)	s−/c− clin.TB
E	Cytologically/histologically/microbiologically confirmed extrapulmonary TB	EPTB
F	All smears and cultures negative and sustained recovery up to 5 months (e.g. resolved bronchitis or pneumonia)	Controls
G	Loss to follow-up after recruitment or any other combination of results (e.g. still symptomatic after 5 months)	Indeterminate

influenced by experience and professional training [7,8] and momentary factors like distraction, focus and tiredness.

In contrast, the automated reading of radiographs by computers is devoid of inter- and intra-observer variability. Research in this field started fifty years ago. Although early optimistic goals such as "fully automating the chest exam" [9] are still far from being achieved, at least one application, the automatic detection of masses and micro-calcifications in mammograms, has been successfully integrated in clinical routine to support radiologists in their decision [10].

Most of the research on computer-aided diagnosis (CAD) of chest radiographs focuses on the detection of nodules, but there are a number of research groups also working on promoting CAD in PTB. Among these, the Diagnostic Image Analysis Group at Radboud University Medical Center, Nijmegen, The Netherlands introduced CAD4TB, a software to determine whether a chest X-ray (CXR) shows evidence of PTB. CAD4TB underwent field tests in 2010 and has been developed since then. Previous software versions were comparable to clinical officers for detecting culture confirmed tuberculosis (TB) among 166 presumptive TB patients at a Zambian clinic (v1.08; area (A_z) under the receiver operating characteristic (ROC) curve = 0.73) [11] and reached a sensitivity of 95% at a specificity of 57% in 95 CXRs of homeless people in London (texture abnormality detection system; $A_z = 0.86$) [12].

A recently published review article on automatic screening for tuberculosis in chest radiographs by Jaeger and colleagues [13] concludes that even though proposed CAD algorithms seem to perform reasonably well when tested individually, no fair comparison can be made without testing the systems on the same, preferably large and publicly available dataset of well characterized patients. The authors further emphasise that there are hardly any validation studies from clinical or screening situations so far and therefore a lack of evidence on how the systems perform in the practical field.

We conducted the first validation study to assess the diagnostic accuracy of the most recent CAD4TB software (v3.07, updated release) on a large set of well characterized adult presumptive PTB patients from sub-Saharan Africa. We compared the performance of the automated reading with the results of human observers of different experience levels.

Methods

Study Population

This validation study was done on chest radiographs of participants from two cohort studies (TB Cohort and TB CHILD study) which have been conducted at the TB Clinic of the Ifakara Health Institute (IHI) in Bagamoyo, Tanzania. Tanzania has a high burden of active TB: according to the first national Tuberculosis Prevalence Survey in 2013 the prevalence is 295 cases per 100,000 population [14]. Bagamoyo, a town of 35,000 inhabitants, is located on the coast, approximately 70 km from the commercial capital Dar es Salaam.

Individuals presenting with clinical signs and symptoms suggestive of pulmonary TB to surrounding primary health care facilities were referred to the IHI TB Clinic. Patients who met the inclusion criteria and gave informed consent were consecutively enrolled into either the TB Cohort or TB CHILD study. In both studies the patients were followed up for 5 to 18 months. The main objective of the TB Cohort study was to generate a sound understanding of TB epidemiology in the Bagamoyo region, while the TB CHILD study was conducted to assess performance characteristics of new TB diagnostics in adults and children. Written informed consent was obtained from all literate patients. In case of illiteracy, informed oral consent was attested by an impartial witness and documented with the patient's fingerprint according to ICH GCP guidelines as approved by the IHI Institutional Review Board and the Medical Research Coordinating Committee of the National Institute for Medical Research, Tanzania. Patients who received anti-TB treatment during the last year, were severely sick or did not reside within the study area were not included. All adult patients from both studies were eligible for the CAD4TB validation study if they initially presented with persistent cough of 2 weeks or more and at least one of the following TB associated findings: haemoptysis, chest pain, fever, night sweats, constant fatigue, recent unexplained weight loss, loss of appetite, malaise or contact with a known TB case.

Specimen collection & Laboratory methods

At enrolment, the participants answered a detailed questionnaire about their medical history, underwent a clinical examination, had a chest radiograph taken and sputum and blood samples were collected. All CXRs (resolution: 1760×2140 pixel) were taken with a Philips Cosmos BS radiography system, which operated combined with a Philips PCR System Eleva S processor. Two sputum specimens, one 'spot' and one early morning, were routinely obtained and used for acid-fast bacilli (AFB) smear and culture examination. All samples were decontaminated using the standard NALC-NaOH method, inoculated on both solid (Löwenstein-Jensen, LJ) and liquid (Mycobacterium Growth Identification Tube, MGIT) media and incubated at 37°C. Smears were performed from the decontaminated pellet, followed with Ziehl-Neelsen (ZN) staining. All positive cultures were tested by ZN microscopy for the presence of AFB, and *Mycobacterium tuberculosis* (M.tb) was confirmed by MPT64 antigen and/or molecular tests (Genotype MTBC, CM or AS; Hain Lifescience,

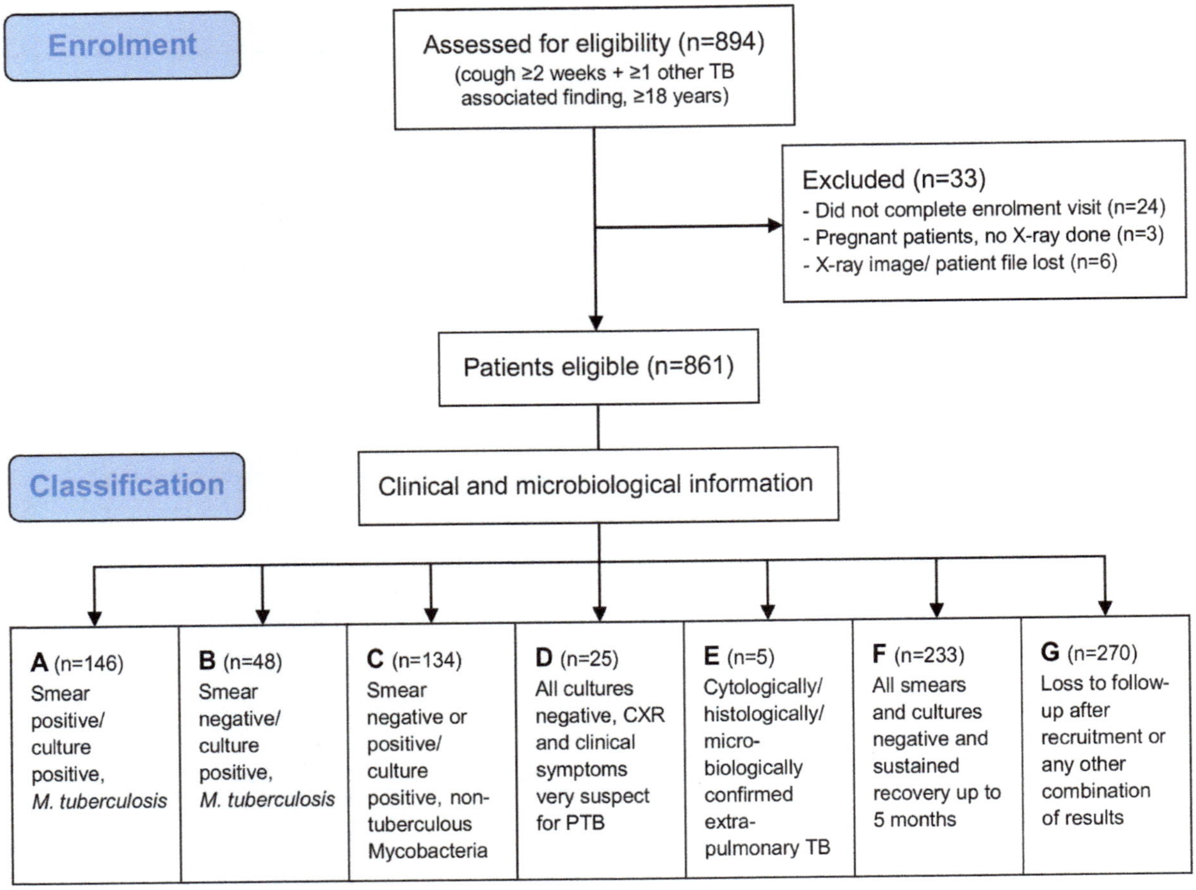

Figure 1. Flow chart of individuals taking part in the study.

Nehren). Interpretation of all microbiological tests was carried out blind to clinical information and radiological results. Voluntary HIV counselling and testing was offered to all participants. The laboratory work was carried out according to Good Clinical Laboratory Practice to guarantee objective standards, quality control and assurance.

Classification

All patients were classified by the study physicians (M.D., 1–3 years of clinical experience) in consultation with a senior physician (M.D., 20 years of clinical experience) into seven groups (table 1) according to all clinical and microbiological information available 5 months after enrolment. Allocation to the groups was not mutually exclusive. For the purpose of this analysis, it was agreed that classification to either group A (s+/c+ M.tb) or B (s−/c+ M.tb) supersedes classification to C (s ±/c+ NTM) or E (EPTB), and classification to either group G (Indeterminate) or D (s−/c− clin.TB) supersedes classification to group C (s ±/c+ NTM). Patients with resolved symptoms after 5 months and who were confirmed to be definitely free of TB (group F) will be referred to as 'Controls' in the following.

Reading of the chest radiographs

The computer-aided analysis of the CXRs was performed independently and blind to clinical information and radiological results by the Diagnostic Image Analysis Group at Radboud University Medical Center, Nijmegen, The Netherlands. The images were processed with the latest CAD4TB software version (v3.07, updated release). CAD4TB is a software framework in which various subsystems for the detection of textural and shape abnormalities, for symmetry and correlation analyses operate at pixel and image level [15].

In CAD, the analysis is broken down to several computable steps [16]: First, radiographs are pre-processed to normalise image features like resolution and grey scale. During segmentation, the next step, the software seeks the anatomical orientation of the image by demarcating structures like the lungs, clavicles and ribs. The defined lung fields are then analysed for their shape, global symmetry and local texture. In addition, a global correlation with a typical normal CXR is determined. Scores generated by these subsystems are combined to an overall score for each image which summarises the result of the automated analysis as an abnormality score for the presence of active disease between 0–100.

In addition, the same set of images was read by two human observers: one experienced chest physician as expert reader and one clinical officer who had practical experience in reading chest X-ray exams in his role as District Tuberculosis and Leprosy Coordinator and had completed a one week course on "X-ray interpretation of tuberculosis and HIV-related opportunistic infections among people living with HIV" [17]. The two readers rated the images using the 'Tanzanian X-ray score', a template for a structured CXR report. At the end of their report, the readers were asked to choose between four possible conclusions:

Table 2. Summary statistics of study population.

	No data	All	Group A	Group B	Group C	Group D	Group E	Group F	Group G
			s+/c+ M.tb	s−/c+ M.tb	s±/c+ NTM	s−/c− clin.TB	EPTB	Controls	Indeterminate
Characteristic									
n (%)	0	861 (100)	146 (17)	48 (6)	134 (16)	25 (3)	5 (1)	233 (27)	270 (31)
Mean age (SD[1])	0	42 (15)	37 (13)	41 (13)	42 (15)	46 (16)	37 (10)	42 (16)	44 (16)
Female sex n (%)	0	433 (50)	48 (33)	25 (52)	76 (57)	12 (48)	4 (80)	122 (52)	146 (54)
HIV positive n (%)	4	379 (44)	50 (34)	35 (73)	66 (49)	10 (40)	2 (40)	92 (39)	124 (46)
History of TB n (%)	0	144 (17)	17 (12)	6 (13)	27 (20)	12 (48)	0 (0)	26 (11)	56 (21)
Symptoms at first visit									
Cough ≥ 2 weeks n (%)	0	820 (95)	139 (95)	45 (94)	129 (96)	23 (92)	4 (80)	227 (97)	253 (94)
Night sweats n (%)	1	426 (50)	92 (63)	24 (50)	64 (48)	19 (76)	3 (60)	89 (38)	135 (50)
Haemoptysis n (%)	10	91 (11)	11 (8)	4 (8)	16 (12)	5 (20)	0 (0)	24 (10)	31 (12)
Fever n (%)	0	470 (55)	91 (62)	31 (65)	78 (58)	15 (60)	3 (60)	114 (49)	138 (51)
Weight loss n (%)	6	447 (52)	101 (70)	34 (71)	60 (45)	10 (40)	4 (80)	101 (44)	137 (51)

[1]standard deviation.

1. normal.
2. abnormal, findings not suggestive for active TB (TB sequel possible).
3. abnormal, findings consistent with active TB, but TB sequel or other lung pathology possible.
4. abnormal, findings highly suggestive for active TB.

Three different reading thresholds were defined correspondingly, ranging from considering only 'abnormalities highly suggestive for TB' (conclusion 4) to 'TB consistent abnormalities' (conclusion 3+4) to 'any abnormality' (conclusion 2–4) for a positive test result.

The readings of chest radiographs were carried out retrospectively for both, the automated and the human interpretation, and had no influence on the diagnosis of the study participants. The human readers were only aware of the inclusion criteria of the study and the age of the patients but blind to clinical information, bacteriological results as well as each other's results.

Data analysis

Culture-confirmed M.tb was used as a reference standard to assess the diagnostic accuracy of CAD4TB and the human readers for the diagnosis of PTB. Individuals whose state of disease could be definitely determined were included in the analyses: group A (s+/c+ M.tb) and B (s−/c+ M.tb) as true cases and group F (Controls) as definite non TB patients. Secondary performance analyses were carried out in which individuals of group C (s ±/c+ NTM) and E (EPTB) were considered additionally to group F (Controls) to be most likely free of pulmonary TB. Individuals of group D (s−/c− clin.TB) were classified partly due to an abnormal X-ray and were excluded from the analysis.

Receiver operating characteristic (ROC) curves and their areas under the curve (A_z) were calculated based on the output of the software. Their 95% confidence intervals (CI) and p-values were computed using the De Long method [18]. The performance of the human readers was summarised by calculating sensitivities, specificities, positive and negative predictive values as well as diagnostic likelihood ratios and their 95% confidence intervals for reporting 'abnormalities highly suggestive for TB' (conclusion 4), 'TB consistent abnormalities' (conclusion 3+4) or 'any abnormality' (conclusion 2–4). The same performance measures were calculated for several exemplary cut-offs of the CAD4TB software. Proportions in different groups were compared using the chi-squared test. McNemar's test was applied to compare the specificity of CAD and humans at assumed levels of sensitivity. Mann-Whitney-Wilcoxon test was used to compare the CAD scores between different groups. All calculations were done using the statistical package 'R', version 3.0.0 [19] together with the extension packages 'pROC' [20], 'epiR' [21], 'ggplot2' [22], 'reshape2' [23] and 'plotrix' [24]. All data used for the analyses is deposited in a public repository and can be accessed via http://dx.doi.org/10.6084/m9.figshare.936571.

Ethical considerations

The TB Cohort and TB CHILD studies were approved by the IHI Institutional Review Board and the Medical Research Coordinating Committee of the National Institute for Medical Research, Tanzania.

Results

A total of 894 patients were enrolled in the CAD4TB validation study. Thirty-three patients had to be excluded from analysis because of an incomplete enrolment visit, pregnancy or missing chest radiograph (figure 1). The final set of images for analysis

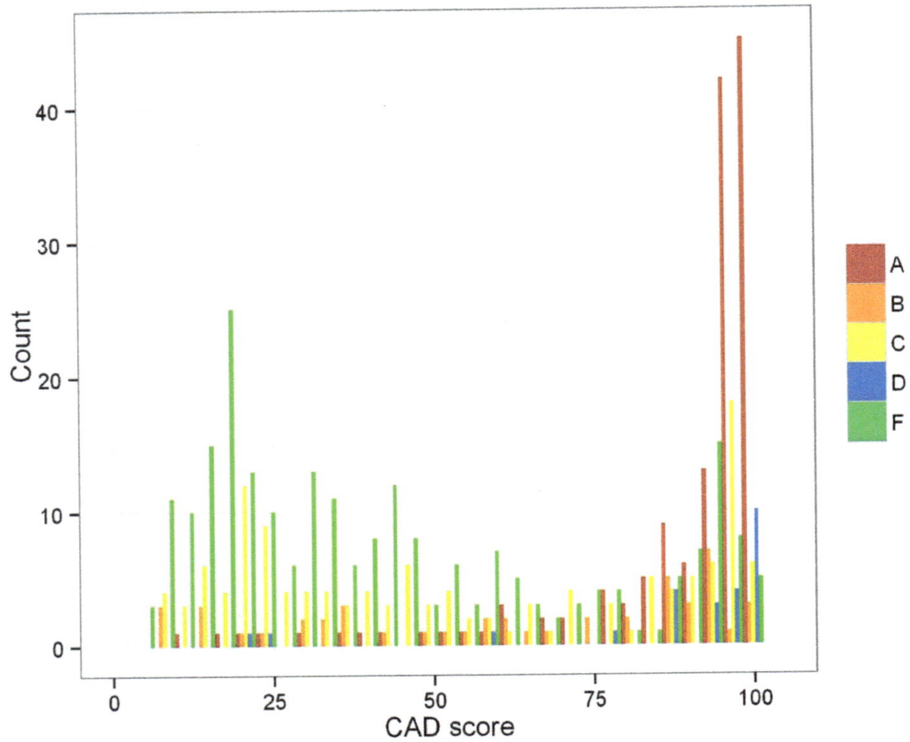

Figure 2. Distribution of CAD scores for patient groups A (s+/c+ M.tb), B (s−/c+ M.tb), C (s±/c+ NTM), D (s−/c− clin.TB) and F (Controls).

consisted of 861 digital, posterior-anterior (PA) chest radiographs. Six of these radiographs were originally in a conventional film format and later digitized.

Group A (s+/c+ M.tb) and B (s−/c+ M.tb) included 194 (23%) of the study participants who were culture-positive for *Mycobacterium tuberculosis*. A further 233 patients (27%) presented with TB consistent symptoms but proved to be culture-negative with a sustained recovery after 5 months and therefore were classified as group F (Controls) (figure 1).

Overall, the prevalence of HIV was 44%. There was a significant difference between groups ($p<0.01$) with the highest prevalence (73%, 95%CI 58–84%) in group B (s−/c+ M.tb) and the lowest (34%, 95%CI 27–43%) in group A (s+/c+ M.tb). The proportion of patients who reported a prior history of TB was 17% overall, but differed significantly ($p<0.01$) between classifications and was highest (48%, 95%CI 28–68%) among group D (s−/c− clin.TB) (table 2).

Culture-positive individuals (group A (s+/c+ M.tb) + B (s−/c+ M.tb)) were significantly more likely to suffer from night sweats (60 vs. 38%), fever (63 vs. 49%) and weight loss (70 vs. 44%) than individuals classified as group F (Controls) ($p<0.01$). There was no evidence of a difference in the frequency of haemoptysis between these groups ($p=0.33$).

The distribution of CAD scores (figure 2) for group A (s+/c+ M.tb) and D (s−/c− clin.TB) tends towards higher scores, this is less marked for group B (s−/c+ M.tb). The scores attained by individuals classified as group C (s±/c+ NTM) and F (Controls) are clustered around lower values but can be found across the whole range. Around one third of the individuals of group F (Controls) did attain a CAD score greater than 50. On the whole there is considerable overlap in the distribution of CAD scores (table 3). The CAD scores in group B (s−/c+ M.tb) are significantly lower than those of group A (s+/c+ M.tb) and higher than those of group F (Controls) ($p<0.01$).

The automated reading software was able to distinguish between culture positive PTB cases (group A (s+/c+ M.tb) + B (s−/c+ M.tb)) and non TB patients (group F (Controls)) with an area under the curve of 0.84 (95%CI 0.80–0.88). Including all M.tb culture-negative patients (group C (s±/c+ NTM), E (EPTB) and F (Controls)) as the negative reference standard, CAD4TB performed slightly, but not significantly, worse: $A_z=0.81$ (95%CI 0.77–0.85), $p=0.28$ (figure 3). CAD4TB displayed a greater ability to differentiate smear-positive (group A (s+/c+ M.tb)) than smear-negative (group B (s−/c+ M.tb)) diseased individuals against non TB patients (group F (Controls)): $A_z=0.90$ (95%CI 0.86–0.93) against $A_z=0.67$ (95%CI 0.58–0.75), $p<0.01$ (figure 4). Similarly, the software distinguished diseased individuals (group A (s+/c+ M.tb) + B (s−/c+ M.tb)) from non TB patients (group F (Controls)) significantly more accurately among the HIV negative than among the HIV positive patient population: $A_z=0.89$ (95%CI 0.85–0.94) against $A_z=0.79$ (95%CI 0.72–0.86), $p<0.01$ (figure 5). Among group A (s+/c+ M.tb), B (s−/c+ M.tb) and F (Controls) there was no evidence of a difference in the performance of CAD4TB in between patients with and without history of TB: $A_z=0.84$ (95%CI 0.80–0.89) against $A_z=0.79$ (95%CI 0.65–0.92), $p=0.42$. The area under the curve of CAD4TB for the discrimination of group B (s−/c+ M.tb) against C (s±/c+ NTM) was 0.56 (95%CI 0.46–0.65).

We calculated a set of cut-offs of the CAD4TB score for our patient population (table 4). For example, a cut-off of ≥74 leads to a sensitivity and specificity of CAD4TB of 77% (95%CI 71–83%) and 79% (95%CI 74–84%), respectively. Optimal values of sensitivity cannot be obtained without a considerable trade-off of specificity, and vice versa.

Table 3. Median CAD scores and 90% central range.

	All	Group A s+/c+ M.tb			Group B s−/c+ M.tb		
		All	HIV+	HIV-	**all**	HIV+	HIV-
Median CAD score	61	97	90	97	67	62	86
90% central range	11–100	44–100	33–100	60–100	11–99	13–98	12–96
	Group C s±/c+ NTM	**Group D s−/c− clin.TB**	**Group E EPTB**	**Group F Controls**	**Group G Indeterminate**		
Median CAD score	48	97	83	34	57		
90% central range	13–98	32–100	38–92	9–95	11–100		

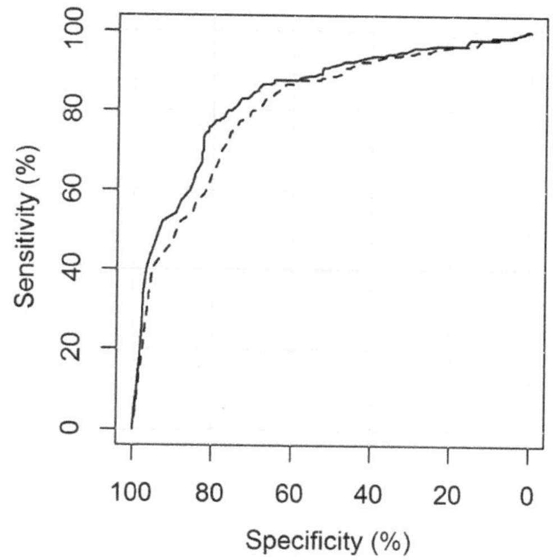

Figure 3: ROC analysis for the detection of M.tb culture-positive individuals. Legend. —A (s+/c+ M.tb), B (s−/c+ M.tb) vs. F (Controls): $A_z = 0.84$ (0.80–0.88), - - - A (s+/c+ M.tb), B (s−/c+ M.tb) vs. C (s±/c+ NTM), E (EPTB), F (Controls): $A_z = 0.81$ (0.77–0.85), p = 0.28.

Setting the CAD4TB cut-off to give sensitivity values achieved by human readers allowed us to compare the performance of automated and human readings (figure 6). There was no evidence of a difference between the specificities achieved by the software and both human readers reporting 'any abnormality' (p = 0.49, 0.88). This was different for tuberculosis specific reporting thresholds: CAD4TB was significantly more specific (p = 0.02) than the clinical officer reporting 'TB consistent abnormalities' but did not reach the accuracy level of the expert reader (p = 0.02).

A review, carried out by a third reader (senior radiologist with extensive experience in TB), of the images (n = 7) rated as false negative by CAD4TB at the exemplary cut-off (<74) but as true positive (conclusion 3+4) by both human readers did not reveal any obvious pattern of abnormalities missed by CAD4TB.

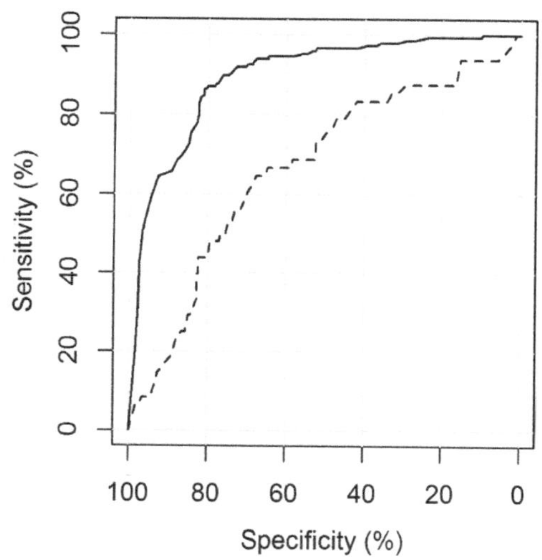

Figure 4. ROC analysis for the detection of M.tb culture-positive individuals by smear status. Legend. — A (s+/c+ M.tb) vs. F (Controls): $A_z = 0.90$ (0.86–0.93), - - - B (s−/c+ M.tb) vs. F (Controls): $A_z = 0.67$ (0.58–0.75), p<0.01.

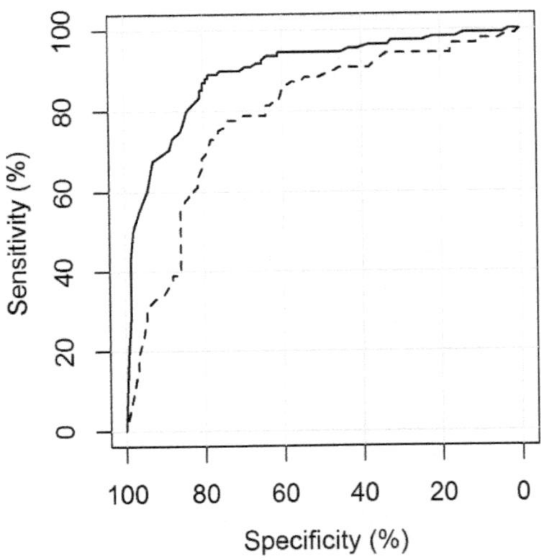

Figure 5. ROC analysis for the detection of M.tb culture-positive individuals by HIV Status. Legend. — HIV negative. A (s+/c+ M.tb), B (s−/c+ M.tb) vs. F (Controls): $A_z = 0.89$ (0.85–0.94), - - - HIV positive. A (s+/c+ M.tb), B (s−/c+ M.tb) vs. F (Controls): $A_z = 0.79$ (0.72–0.86), $p < 0.01$.

Discussion

Automating the interpretation of a chest radiograph for the detection of active pulmonary tuberculosis leads to objective, reproducible results and a standardized way of reporting. The main finding of our study is that the automated reading software CAD4TB (v3.07, updated release) achieved a good diagnostic accuracy ($A_z = 0.84$ (95%CI 0.80–0.88)) on a large set of CXRs of presumptive TB patients from sub-Saharan Africa. The accuracy of CAD4TB was slightly, but not significantly, worse in our secondary analysis using a binary classification of patients (M.tb culture-positive vs. negative) which we included for a better comparability with other diagnostic accuracy studies.

In our study, performance of automated and human reading was comparable when the observers considered 'any abnormality'. For a more TB specific reading threshold, however, the software outperformed the clinical officer significantly but did not reach the accuracy of the expert reader. The software identified a significantly higher proportion of smear-positive compared to smear-negative, culture-positive individuals - most likely because smear-negative PTB patients tend to have more discrete or atypical radiographic features, especially in combination with HIV infection [25]. This assumption is substantiated by the fact that CAD4TB detected PTB cases significantly more accurately among HIV negative than HIV positive individuals.

Identifying cases of active PTB among symptomatic individuals with abnormal CXRs due to other pulmonary conditions (e.g. pneumonia) or sequelae of tuberculosis remains challenging for both human and automated readers. This fact manifests itself in low specificity values as a consequence of the considerable overlap in the distribution of CAD scores for the defined groups and the far higher proportion of patients who reported a history of TB among group D (s−/c− clin.TB).

One of the strengths of our study is the direct comparison of automated and human reading on the same set of images. Due to inter-reader variability in the interpretation of chest radiographs and the ability to include only one clinical officer and expert reader, the degree to which this comparison can be generalized is strongly limited. It is possible that other clinical officers or expert

Table 4. Performance of CAD4TB and human readers.

	Threshold for test positivity	Sens.[1] [%] (95%CI)	Spec.[2] [%] (95%CI)	PPV[3] [%] (95%CI)	NPV[4] [%] (95%CI)	PLR[5] (95%CI)	NLR[6] (95%CI)
CAD4TB	≥23	95 (91–98)	33 (27–39)	54 (49–60)	89 (80–94)	1.42 (1.29–1.56)	0.16 (0.08–0.29)
	≥37	91 (86–94)	52 (46–59)	61 (55–67)	87 (80–92)	1.9 (1.65–2.19)	0.18 (0.11–0.28)
	≥56	85 (79–90)	69 (62–75)	69 (63–75)	85 (79–89)	2.71 (2.22–3.31)	0.22 (0.15–0.31)
	≥74	77 (71–83)	79 (74–84)	76 (69–82)	81 (75–86)	3.75 (2.88–4.88)	0.29 (0.22–0.37)
	≥89	62 (55–69)	85 (80–89)	77 (70–84)	73 (67–78)	4.12 (2.98–5.7)	0.45 (0.37–0.54)
	≥95	47 (40–54)	94 (91–97)	88 (80–93)	68 (63–73)	8.41 (4.86–14.56)	0.56 (0.49–0.64)
Expert reader	4	59 (52–66)	98 (95–99)	96 (91–99)	74 (69–79)	27.62 (11.52–66.26)	0.42 (0.35–0.49)
	3,4	78 (71–83)	85 (80–89)	81 (75–87)	82 (77–87)	5.18 (3.78–7.1)	0.26 (0.2–0.34)
	2,3,4	84 (78–89)	72 (65–77)	71 (65–77)	84 (79–89)	2.97 (2.4–3.67)	0.22 (0.16–0.31)
Clinical officer	4	7 (4–12)	97 (94–99)	70 (46–88)	56 (51–61)	2.8 (1.1–7.15)	0.95 (0.91–1)
	3,4	76 (69–82)	65 (58–71)	64 (58–70)	76 (70–82)	2.15 (1.78–2.61)	0.37 (0.29–0.49)
	2,3,4	97 (94–99)	18 (13–24)	50 (45–55)	89 (77–96)	1.19 (1.11–1.27)	0.14 (0.06–0.35)

[1]sensitivity [2]specificity [3]positive predictive value [4]negative predictive value [5]positive likelihood ratio [6]negative likelihood ratio. All parameters were assessed against group A and B as positive reference standard and group F as negative controls.

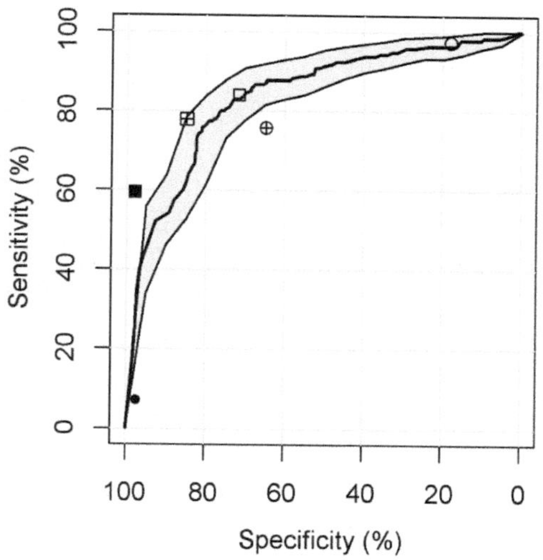

Figure 6. Comparison of automated and human reading. Legend. Sensitivity and specificity to distinguish group A (s+/c+ M.tb) and B (s−/c+ M.tb) vs. F (Controls). Line and shaded area: ROC curve and 95% CI for CAD4TB. The expert reader is represented by square symbols, the clinical officer by round symbols. The different fill of the symbols indicate different reading thresholds: empty symbols ='any abnormality', crossed symbols ='TB consistent abnormalities' and filled symbols ='abnormalities highly suggestive for TB'.

readers would have outperformed the software in our study. A second limitation of our study is the fact that it was conducted in only one high burden country and it would be preferable to repeat it in different settings to assess generalizability of the results.

HIV infection seems to influence the diagnostic accuracy of CAD4TB, so our findings cannot be readily generalized to populations that differ significantly in their HIV prevalence. A further constraint of the study is the high proportion (31%, group G) of patients who either could not be followed up sufficiently to comply with the precise classification criteria or that were still non TB patients but symptomatic after five months and therefore could not be classified as group F (Controls). However, since a heterogeneous patient group is concerned and the data can be most likely assumed to be missing at random, it can be postulated that study results were not substantially influenced.

The relatively high number of patients that were found to be culture-positive for NTMs (16%, group C) is not uncommon in the sub-Saharan African context [26–28]. This is probably largely due to contamination of culture samples either at patient level or from the environment as only few patients suffered from a pathogenetic relevant NTM infection that fulfilled the diagnostic criteria for a Nontuberculous Mycobacterial Lung Disease according to the American Thoracic Society [29]. The inability of CAD4TB to differentiate between patients of group B (s−/c+ M.tb) and C (s±/c+ NTM) might be due to the heterogeneity of group C (s±/c+ NTM).

Maduskar et al. evaluated the performance of a previous CAD4TB version and compared it to both, clinical officers rating the radiograph between 0–100 and the binary decision of an expert reader (as radiological reference) for the presence of TB consistent abnormalities [11]. We decided to use hierarchical reading thresholds as we believe that this reflects the common radiological practice in a setting like ours. The high accuracy achieved for the radiological reference (A_z = 0.91 (95%CI 0.86–0.95)) [11] is consistent with our finding that CAD4TB approaches values of sensitivity and specificity achieved by the expert reader.

The diagnostic accuracy of CAD4TB for the bacteriological reference was higher using the newer version in our study compared to previous CAD4TB versions used in the study of Maduskar and another small scale study [29]. This suggests advancement in the development of the software, which is especially encouraging as we evaluated its performance on images obtained from a different X-ray machine than the one it was originally developed for.

Current national diagnostic algorithms for presumptive adult TB patients in many sub-Saharan African countries request between two to six negative sputum smear examinations and a failed treatment with a broad-spectrum antibiotic for 7 days before a chest X-ray is ordered [31–38]. According to recommendations of the World Health Organization (WHO), the CXR exam should even precede an administration of antibiotics in settings where HIV is highly prevalent and resources are constrained [39]. In both cases a thorough X-ray report and its integration with clinical information by a medically trained person is needed for the final diagnosis of smear-negative PTB. Our findings indicate that in this situation the CAD4TB software could assist less experienced readers in their judgment. It could not entirely replace the human interpretation for radiographic questions beyond that of active tuberculosis as the software was not designed to detect other pathologies. Its output, a single number, does not reflect the presence of abnormalities unrelated to TB, whose detection might be not less important or even prompt immediate action (such as pneumothorax). In addition, the high proportion of patients of group F (Controls) who did attain a 'false positive' high CAD score due to other pulmonary pathologies as pneumonia have to be taken into consideration.

By contrast, the very condensed output of the automated reading might be preferable for the binary decision in screening situations of either conveying a screened individual to confirmatory testing or to declare the absence of PTB. A strong feature of CAD4TB in its current stage of development is its continuous output, which allows adjusting the reading threshold to the purpose of use, local epidemiology and availability of resources (such as the capacity to perform smear microscopy or the number of Xpert MTB/Rif cartridges).

It is not known whether active screening will have a positive effect on TB epidemiology [40]; however, the slow decline in incidence and case detection gap suggest that a more active approach could complement patient-initiated pathways [41] and enhance their efficacy. Among the broad spectrum of possible active case finding strategies, the new comprehensive WHO guidelines for the systematic screening for active tuberculosis among certain risk groups, in which chest radiography found its firm place, if available, as a first or second screening step [42]. A robust CAD has the potential to enhance and facilitate the implementation of these recommendations by ensuring high test standards of objectivity, reproducibility and accuracy without straining personnel resources. A prerequisite for the CAD application is the availability of digital radiography, which is not yet the case in most of resource-constrained high-burden settings. However, it has been identified as a key action point in a WHO Workshop to Scale Up the Implementation of Collaborative TB/HIV Activities in Africa earlier this year [43] as it has been shown to be feasible and to result in a significant better quality of chest radiography compared to conventional X-ray technology in countries with limited resources [44].

Prospective studies on cost-effectiveness, operational and ethical aspects of the use of CAD in different high burden countries are needed. Future research should also address the question whether the integration of a CAD output with clinical variables like symptoms and risk factors could result in a more accurate screening step.

In conclusion, the computer-aided diagnosis system CAD4TB is a reproducible and accurate test for the detection of pulmonary tuberculosis on radiographs in symptomatic patients. This prompts additional research on how its potential, both as assistance for clinical officers in the diagnostic interpretation of radiographs and as standalone triage test in systematic screening settings, can be exploited.

Acknowledgments

We would like to acknowledge the contribution of Mwinyikambi Salum to this study by reading the radiographs. We wish to thank all participants of the TB cohort and TB CHILD projects.

Author Contributions

Conceived and designed the experiments: MB KR LJ DW JVDH FL. Performed the experiments: MB RP BVG FM JJH JVDH KR. Analyzed the data: MB AR KR LJ. Wrote the paper: MB KR AR. Critical review of the manuscript for important intellectual content: BVG RP FM JJH FL JVDH DW LJ.

References

1. Story A, Aldridge RW, Abubakar I, Stagg HR, Lipman M, et al. (2012) Active case finding for pulmonary tuberculosis using mobile digital chest radiography: an observational study. Int J Tuberc Lung Dis 16: 1461–1467. Available: http://www.ncbi.nlm.nih.gov/pubmed/22981252.
2. Van't Hoog AH, Meme HK, Van Deutekom H, Mithika AM, Olunga C, et al. (2011) High sensitivity of chest radiograph reading by clinical officers in a tuberculosis prevalence survey. Int J Tuberc Lung Dis 15: 1308–1314. Available: http://www.ingentaconnect.com/content/iuatld/ijtld/2011/00000015/00000010/art00007.
3. Den Boon S, White NW, Van Lill SWP, Borgdorff MW, Verver S, et al. (2006) An evaluation of symptom and chest radiographic screening in tuberculosis prevalence surveys. Int J Tuberc Lung Dis 10: 876–882.
4. Van Cleeff M, Kivihya-Ndugga L, Meme H, Odhiambo J, Klatser P (2005) The role and performance of chest X-ray for the diagnosis of tuberculosis: a cost-effectiveness analysis in Nairobi, Kenya. BMC Infect Dis 5: 111. Available: http://www.pubmedcentral.nih.gov/articlerender.fcgi?artid = 1326228&tool = pmcentrez&rendertype = abstract. Accessed 2012 Nov 7.
5. Graham S, Das GK, Hidvegi RJ, Hanson R, Kosiuk J, et al. (2002) Chest radiograph abnormalities associated with tuberculosis: reproducibility and yield of active cases. Int J Tuberc Lung Dis 6: 137–142. Available: http://www.ncbi.nlm.nih.gov/pubmed/11931412. Accessed 2012 Oct 2.
6. Den Boon S, Bateman ED, Enarson D a, Borgdorff MW, Verver S, et al. (2005) Development and evaluation of a new chest radiograph reading and recording system for epidemiological surveys of tuberculosis and lung disease. Int J Tuberc Lung Dis 9: 1088–1096. Available: http://www.ncbi.nlm.nih.gov/pubmed/16229219.
7. Zellweger JP, Heinzer R, Touray M, Vidondo B, Altpeter E (2006) Intra-observer and overall agreement in the radiological assessment of tuberculosis. Int J Tuberc Lung Dis 10: 1123–1126. Available: http://www.ncbi.nlm.nih.gov/pubmed/17044205.
8. Balabanova Y, Coker R, Fedorin I, Zakharova S, Plavinskij S, et al. (2005) Variability in interpretation of chest radiographs among Russian study. BMJ 331: 379–382.
9. Conners R, Harlow C, Dwyer S (1982) Radiographic image analysis: past and present. Proceedings of the 6th international conference on pattern recognition. IEEE Computer Society Press. pp. 1152–1168.
10. Samulski M, Hupse R, Boetes C, Mus RDM, den Heeten GJ, et al. (2010) Using computer-aided detection in mammography as a decision support. Eur Radiol 20: 2323–2330. Available: http://www.pubmedcentral.nih.gov/articlerender.fcgi?artid = 2940044&tool = pmcentrez&rendertype = abstract. Accessed 2014 Jan 9.
11. Maduskar P, Muyoyeta M, Ayles H, Hogeweg L, Peters-Bax L, et al. (2013) Detection of tuberculosis using digital chest radiography: automated reading vs. interpretation by clinical officers. Int J Tuberc Lung Dis 17: 1613–1620(8). Available: http://www.ingentaconnect.com/content/iuatld/ijtld/2013/00000017/00000012/art00020. Accessed 2013 Nov 22.
12. Hogeweg L, Story A, Hayward A, Aldridge R, Abubakar I, et al. (2011) Computer-aided detection of tuberculosis among high risk groups: potential for automated triage. at: Annual Meeting of the Radiological Society of North America 2011.
13. Jaeger S, Karargyris A, Candemir S, Siegelman J, Folio L, et al. (2013) Automatic screening for tuberculosis in chest radiographs: a survey. Quant Imaging Med Surg 3: 89–99. Available: http://www.pubmedcentral.nih.gov/articlerender.fcgi?artid = 3636475&tool = pmcentrez&rendertype = abstract. Accessed 2013 Sep 3.
14. Leth F van (2013) First Tuberculosis Prevalence Survey in the United Republic of Tanzania. Primary Analysis. Final Report.
15. Hogeweg L, Mol C, de Jong PA, Dawson R, Ayles H, et al. (2010) Fusion of local and global detection systems to detect tuberculosis in chest radiographs. Med Image Comput Comput Assist Interv 13: 650–657. Available: http://www.ncbi.nlm.nih.gov/pubmed/20879456.
16. Ginneken B van, Schaefer-Prokop C, Prokop M (2011) Computer-aided diagnosis: How to Move from the Laboratory to the Clinic. Radiology 261: 719–732. Available: http://radiology.rsna.org/content/261/3/719.short. Accessed 2013 Nov 26.
17. ICAP Columbia University (2014) Resources. Available: http://icap.columbia.edu/resources/. Accessed 2014 May 9.
18. DeLong ER, DeLong DM, Clarke-Pearson DL (1988) Comparing the areas under two or more correlated receiver operating characteristic curves: a nonparametric approach. Biometrics Sep: 837–845.
19. R Core Team (2013) R: A language and environment for statistical computing. R Foundation for Statistical Computing, Vienna, Austria. Available: http://www.r-project.org/.
20. Robin X, Turck N, Hainard A, Tiberti N, Lisacek F, et al. (2011) pROC: an open-source package for R and S+ to analyze and compare ROC curves. BMC Bioinformatics 12: 77. Available: http://www.pubmedcentral.nih.gov/articlerender.fcgi?artid = 3068975&tool = pmcentrez&rendertype = abstract. Accessed 2013 Aug 7.
21. Stevenson M, Nunes T, Sanchez J, Thornton R, Reiczigel J, et al. (2013) epiR - An R package for the analysis of epidemiological data. Available: http://epicentre.massey.ac.nz.
22. Wickham H (2009) ggplot2: elegant graphics for data analysis.
23. Wickham H (2007) Reshaping Data with the reshape Package. J Stat Softw 21: 1–20. Available: http://www.jstatsoft.org/v21/i12/.
24. Lemon J (2006) Plotrix: a package in the red light district of R. R-News 6: 8–12. Available: http://cran.r-project.org/web/packages/plotrix/citation.html.
25. Siddiqi K, Lambert M-L, Walley J (2003) Clinical diagnosis of smear-negative pulmonary tuberculosis in low-income countries: the current evidence. Lancet Infect Dis 3: 288–296. Available: http://www.ncbi.nlm.nih.gov/pubmed/12726978.
26. Fourie PB, Gatner EMS, Glatthaar E, Kleeberg HH (1980) Follow-up Tuberculosis Prevalence Survey of Transkei. Tubercle 61: 71–79.
27. Buijtels PCAM, van der Sande MAB, de Graaff CS, Parkinson S, Verbrugh HA, et al. (2009) Nontuberculous Mycobacteria, Zambia. Emerg Infect Dis 15: 242–249. Available: http://wwwnc.cdc.gov/eid/article/15/2/08-0006_article.htm. Accessed 2013 Sep 19.
28. Aliyu G, El-Kamary SS, Abimiku A, Brown C, Tracy K, et al. (2013) Prevalence of non-tuberculous mycobacterial infections among tuberculosis suspects in Nigeria. PLoS One 8: e63170. Available: http://www.pubmedcentral.nih.gov/articlerender.fcgi?artid = 3650061&tool = pmcentrez&rendertype = abstract. Accessed 2014 Jan 21.
29. Griffith D, Aksamit T, Brown-Elliot B, Catanzaro A, Daley C, et al. (2006) An Official ATS/IDSA Statement: Diagnosis, Treatment, and Prevention of Nontuberculous Mycobacterial Diseases. Available: http://www.thoracic.org/statements/resources/mtpi/nontuberculous-mycobacterial-diseases.pdf.
30. Ginneken B van, Hogeweg L, Maduskar P, Peters-Bax L, Dawson R, et al. (2012) Performance of inexperienced and experienced observers in detection of active tuberculosis on digital chest radiographs with and without the use of computer-aided diagnosis. at: Annual Meeting of the Radiological Society of North America, 2012.
31. Ministry of Health and Social Welfare (2006) Manual of the National Tuberculosis and Leprosy Programme in Tanzania, 5th Edition.
32. Division of Leprosy Tuberculosis and Lung Disease. Ministry of Public Health and Sanitation Kenya. (2009) Guidelines on management of Leprosy and Tuberculosis.
33. The National Tuberculosis and Leprosy Programme Zambia (2008) TB Manual.
34. Ministry of Health Uganda (2010) Manual of the National Tuberculosis and Leprosy Programme, 2nd Edition.
35. National Department of Health South Africa (2008) National Tuberculosis Management Guidelines.
36. Ministry of Health and Social Services Namibia (2011) National Guidelines for the Management of Tuberculosis, 3rd Edition.
37. Tuberculosis Leprosy and TB/HIV Prevention and Control Programme (2008) Federal Ministry of Health Ethiopia Manual, 4th Edition.
38. Zimbabwe National Tuberculosis Control Programme (2010) National TB Guidelines.
39. WHO (2007) Improving the diagnosis and treatment of smear-negative pulmonary and extrapulmonary tuberculosis among adults and adolescents - Recommendations for HIV-prevalent and resource-constrained settings.

40. Kranzer K, Tomlin K, Golub JE, Shapiro AE, Schaap A, et al. (2013) The benefits to communities and individuals of screening for active tuberculosis disease: a systematic review. Int J Tuberc Lung Dis 17: 432–446.
41. Uplekar M, Creswell J (2013) Programmatic approaches to screening for active tuberculosis. Int J Tuberc Lung Dis 17: 1248–1256. Available: http://www.ingentaconnect.com/content/iuatld/ijtld/2013/00000017/00000010/art00002. Accessed 2013 Dec 9.
42. WHO (2013) Systematic screening for active tuberculosis - Principles and Recommendations.
43. WHO (2013) Workshop to scale up the implementation of collaborative TB/HIV activities in Africa, 10- 11 April, 2013. Maputo, Mozambique: Meeting Report. World Health Organization. Available: http://www.who.int/hiv/pub/meetingreports/maputo_access/en/index.html. Accessed 2013 Nov 24.
44. Zennaro F, Oliveira Gomes JA, Casalino A, Lonardi M, Starc M, et al. (2013) Digital Radiology to Improve the Quality of Care in Countries with Limited Resources: A Feasibility Study from Angola. PLoS One 8: e73939. Available: http://www.pubmedcentral.nih.gov/articlerender.fcgi?artid = 3783475&tool = pmcentrez&rendertype = abstract. Accessed 2013 Nov 23.

10

Discrimination between Weaned and Unweaned Atlantic Cod (*Gadus morhua*) in Capture-Based Aquaculture (CBA) by X-Ray Imaging and Radio-Frequency Metal Detector

Ekrem Misimi*, Svein Martinsen¤, John Reidar Mathiassen, Ulf Erikson

SINTEF Fisheries and Aquaculture, Trondheim, Norway

Abstract

The aim of this study was to investigate the feasibility of two detection methods for use in discrimination and sorting of adult Atlantic cod (about 2 kg) in the small scale capture-based aquaculture (CBA). Presently, there is no established method for discrimination of weaned and unweaned cod in CBA. Generally, 60–70% of the wild-caught cod in the CBA are weaned into commercial dry feed. To increase profitability for the fish farmers, unweaned cod must be separated from the stock, meaning the fish must be sorted into two groups – unweaned and weaned from moist feed. The challenges with handling of large numbers of fish in cages, defined the limits of the applied technology. As a result, a working model was established, focusing on implementing different marking materials added to the fish feed, and different technology for detecting the feed presence in the fish gut. X-ray imaging in two modes (planar and dual energy band) and sensitive radio-frequency metal detection were the detection methods that were chosen for the investigations. Both methods were tested in laboratory conditions using dead fish with marked feed inserted into the gut cavity. In particular, the sensitive radio-frequency metal detection method with carbonyl powder showed very promising results in detection of marked feed. Results show also that Dual energy band X-ray imaging may have potential for prediction of fat content in the feed. Based on the investigations it can be concluded that both X-ray imaging and sensitive radio-frequency metal detector technology have the potential for detecting cod having consumed marked feed. These are all technologies that may be adapted to large scale handling of fish from fish cages. Thus, it may be possible to discriminate between unweaned and weaned cod in a large scale grading situation. Based on the results of this study, a suggestion for evaluation of concept for in-situ sorting system is presented.

Editor: Ronald Thune, Louisiana State University School of Veterinary, United States of America

Funding: This work was funded by Fisheries and Aquaculture Research Fund – FHF through the project "Capture-based Aquaculture". The funders had no role in study design, data collection and analysis, decision to publish, or preparation of the manuscript.

Competing Interests: The authors have declared that no competing interests exist.

* E-mail: ekrem.misimi@sintef.no

¤ Current address: Nekton AS, Smøla, Norway

Introduction

The peak season of the commercial cod fisheries in Norway is from January until April, following the migration of mature cod into the Norwegian fjords [5]. During this period, the market supplies of fresh cod increase up to ten times the average yearly supply, whilst in December the market demand for fresh cod exceeds the supply, due to the use of cod as a raw material in Norwegian and European traditional cuisine. The seasonal dependence and variation of the cod fisheries has triggered strategies such as farming of cod, and conservation of the wild caught cod through capture-based aquaculture (CBA). Products deriving from these activities are more suited in terms of volume and quality for the high-demand market in December. Since the dynamics between fisheries, aquaculture and markets is constantly fluctuating, strong year-groups of wild cod have resulted in increased total catch, from 215.000 tons in 2008 to 340.000 tons in 2011. This increase has resulted in diminishing price levels, from 16 NOK (appr. 2 €) per kg round weight (RW) to 11 NOK (appr. 1.50 €) per kg RW in average. This has made commercial cod farmers unable to cope with the lower prices, as the production costs of farmed cod in Norway, normally exceed 18 NOK (2.50 €) per kg RW. The expected production cost from capture based aquaculture might be lower, given efficient conversion of wild caught cod to formulated feed.

The present CBA of cod, with feeding of wild-caught cod, derives from extended trials in the 1980's [2]. The basic principles of CBA are gentle capture of fish in seine nets and transfer to holding tanks inside fishing vessels. Fish are transferred from the vessels to special flat-bottom cages, specifically developed for storing and resting of cod. Although the operations are performed with caution, the cod can experience physiological changes like gas bladder expansion and severe stress, but the physiological normality is usually established 12 to 24 hours after capture [2].

The captured fish are presented different diets: a) moist feed (frozen herring, mackerel, and capelin); b) semi moist feed

Table 1. Dilution ranges for the metal and glass bead markers used in the investigations/experiments.

Marker weight(%)	Marker weight:20 gr feed sample	Marker weight: 30 gr feed sample
0.1	0.02	0.03
0.5	0.1	0.15
1	0.2	0.3
5	1	1.5
10	2	3

(vacuum soaked commercial fish feed, premix of fishmeal and fish oil); and c) dry feed (commercial fish feed). Captured wild cod traditionally prefer moist feed, and complete weaning (adaption to moist feed) will normally occur shortly after introduction [15]. Moist feed consists of frozen blocks of herring and capelin that slowly thaw and disintegrate inside the cage, with the fish foraging upon the thawed feed. Seen from the cod farmer's point of view, the optimal feed source is commercial dry feed, in terms of nutritionally adequate content, supporting rapid growth, extended storage stability, availability, non-disease carrier and logistics [16]. Fish are reluctant when presented dry feed and the maximum proportion of fully-weaned cod individuals, weaned from moist feed, and varies between 40–70% [16]. Weaned fish achieve satisfying growth, and reportedly increase their weight from 1.5–2 up to 5–6 kg after 5 months. Unweaned fish will not forage on dry feed, resulting in loss of weight and generally poor condition. To achieve viable economy in the cod CBA industry, an efficient method for discriminating unweaned and weaned fish is necessary. Presently, there is no established method for discrimination between weaned and unweaned cod in CBA.

X-ray radiography has been reported as a suitable technique for studying fish feeding, digestion, measuring feed intake and fish growth [14,8,9,10]. In [18], they report use of X-radiography and X-ray dense markers for quantitative determination of gastrointestinal content. [12] used X-ray dense lead glass beads for estimation of individual feed intake of Chinook salmon by X-radiography, while [19] used a similar technique for estimation of feed intake and growth of Atlantic salmon.

The aim of this work was to investigate the required technology platform needed for sorting of wild cod, enabling efficient discrimination between weaned and unweaned cod in CBA. The technological approach involved testing potential methods for in-situ inspection of the gut content after feed intake consisting of commercial dry feed containing markers. Two aspects of the sorting procedure were studied: a) the marking of fish and b) evaluation of detection technology for efficient discrimination. Although the presence of fish feed in fish gut can be possible to detect by use of X-ray images [11], other fish organs such as liver, swim bladder, and gut cavity liquids can disturb the imaging of fish feed. Therefore, marking of fish feed is seen as a potential solution to enhance the detection capability of both X-ray and other detection methods for detection of fish feed.

Two detection technologies that may be suitable for the discrimination between weaned and unweaned cod were evaluated: 1) X-ray imaging in two modes (planar X-ray and dual energy band), with an integrated image analysis, and 2) sensitive radio-frequency metal detection. Five different types of markers were used for discrimination purposes. In addition, the potential of dual energy band X-ray imaging for prediction of fat content in the feed was investigated.

Materials and Methods

Three experiments were conducted, each investigating a separate detection method for the inspection of gut content to facilitate sorting of weaned and unweaned cod. No human participants were used in the study. The fish was delivered by commercial fishery boats that caught wild cod at the coast of Central Norway. From before, they have all necessary permissions to fish, so no specific permission was needed for this study. Fish was delivered to SINTEF SeaLab packed on ice in styrofoam boxes. The wild cod is not an endangered fish species either in Norway or globally.

X-ray Imaging of Fish Fed with Commercial Feed with High Contrast Feed Markers

Fish. Wild Atlantic cod *(Gadus morhua)* (2.1±0.5 kg, n = 20) were caught at the coast of Central Norway. The fish were killed and packed in ice before being shipped to SINTEF Sealab in Trondheim. Their intestinal content was maintained in the body cavity before proceeding with the investigations.

Feed and markers. Fish dry feed [21] was mixed with crude herring oil added as coating for evenly distribution of commercially available markers and to provide a sticky surface of the pellet. The amount of marked feed was 1.0–1.5% of the fish body weight. The markers were chosen so that they were able to provide a good contrast for X-ray image analysis. In addition to metal-based markers shown in Table 1, Ballotini glass beads of 0.6 mm [24] were used at the same dilution ranges (Table 1).

The chosen commercially available markers were added to the fish feed at a dilution range from 0.1% to 10% of feed portion weight (Table 1). The size of each feed portion inserted into the fish was between from 20–30 g of fish feed, corresponding to 1–1.5% of fish round weight. This amount corresponds to a typical meal portion size for a large cod [1,13].

Image acquisition and processing. A line scan X-ray setup [7] was used for acquisition of X-ray images. Prior to the experiment, an image acquisition PC was connected to the Ishida apparatus so that the generated images could be saved directly and online into the PC disk. Line scans were stitched in the X-ray machine, resulting in a sequence of 5–6 images of 90×332 pixels per fish while fish was moving on the conveyer belt. These images were then stitched to a full image (Figure 1a) by implementing a stitching function in Matlab R2011b Image Processing Toolbox [23]. The energy level used for acquisition of X-ray images was 60 kV.

Dual-energy X-ray for Detection of Different Feed Density (Fat Content)

Fish. Wild-caught cod (2.5±0.6 kg, n = 10) were killed, bled and chilled in ice. The fish were transported to the Curato X-Ray

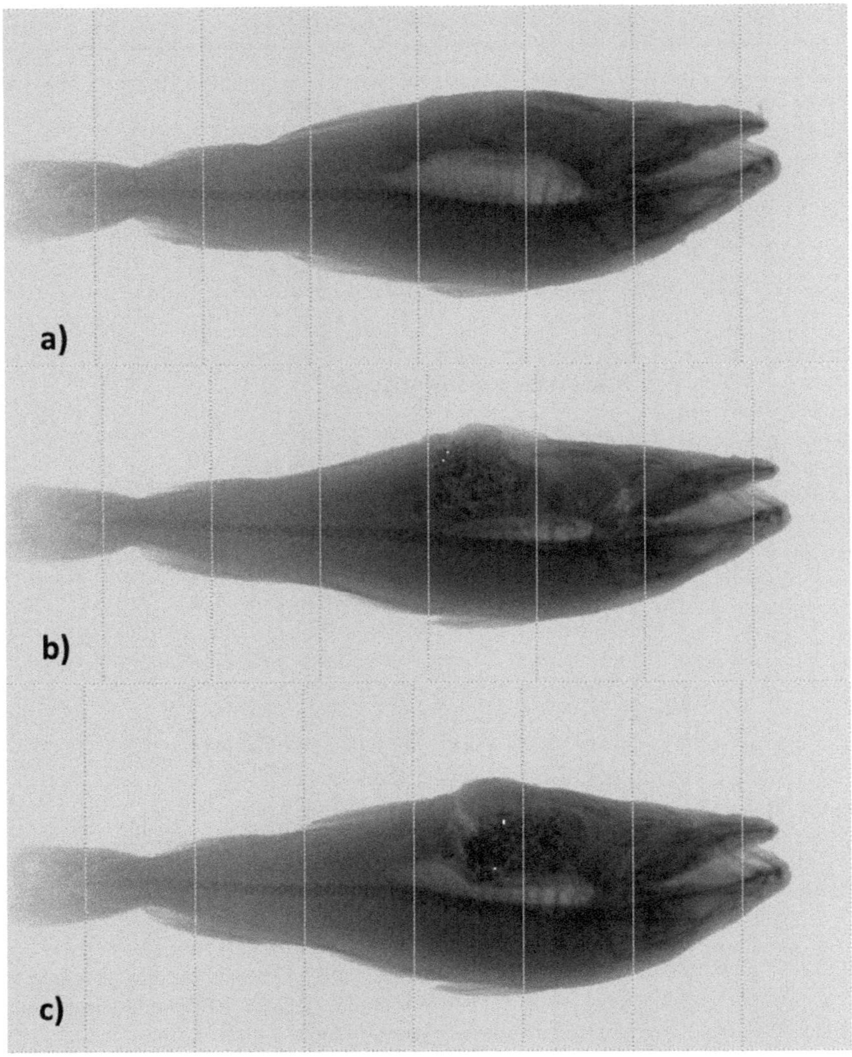

Figure 1. X-ray images of Atlantic cod generated from the Ishida X-ray machine: a) image of a fish without feed, images of a fish with glass beads at b) 0.1% (0.03 g) and c) 10% (3 g) of weight percent of total feed content in gut.

Clinic in Trondheim. Their intestinal content was maintained in the body cavity while the experiments were carried out. To determine the feasibility, of using dual-energy X-ray imaging for discriminating weaned and unweaned cod, a single cod was used for some preliminary experiments.

Feed and markers. Feed samples were weighed and prepared in small plastic bags. Each sample weighed approximately 25 g. The samples were taken from three commercial fish feed diets; Skretting Optiline 2500 (30% fat), Skretting Nutra Parr (22% fat), and BioMar Classic Marine 800 (18% fat). Prior to X-ray imaging, the feed samples were inserted into the fish abdominal cavity through an incision, and the incision was then carefully collated.

Image acquisition and processing. The X-ray images for dual energy X-ray analysis were taken using the commercial medical planar X-ray apparatus [22]. Configuration, setup of parameters, placement and introduction of fish for the imaging system was similar to that described in [20]. To simulate the dual energy X-ray imaging system, fish were imaged with two different X-ray energy levels. A total of 21 planar X-ray images were acquired at both 40 kV (low energy image) and 70 kV (high energy image) (Figure 2). Sets of images of fish without feed, and with NiCr, Steel grit and Cr-Ni alloy markers were generated and saved. The images were transferred then offline into a PC and processed. The Region of Interest (ROI) for dual energy band X-ray image analysis was chosen manually.

These particular voltages were chosen based on the results reported in [20]. Image processing and analysis was done off-line after all images had been acquired. The regions of the images, containing the feed, were segmented from the rest of the fish. Subsequent to this, the regional statistics (consisting on comparing the mean and standard deviation of the image intensity differences between 40 kV and 70 kV images) of the fish regions with feed were compared to those of the same anatomical regions in fish without feed. Features used during the dual energy X-ray image analysis are defined in Table 2, while their mean values are given in Table 3. To test prediction of fat for the fish diets with 18%, 22% and 30% of fat, fat prediction model was developed by using the set of features defined in Table 2 and linear regression. The set of features was extracted from ROI containing fish diets of the abovementioned fat percentages.

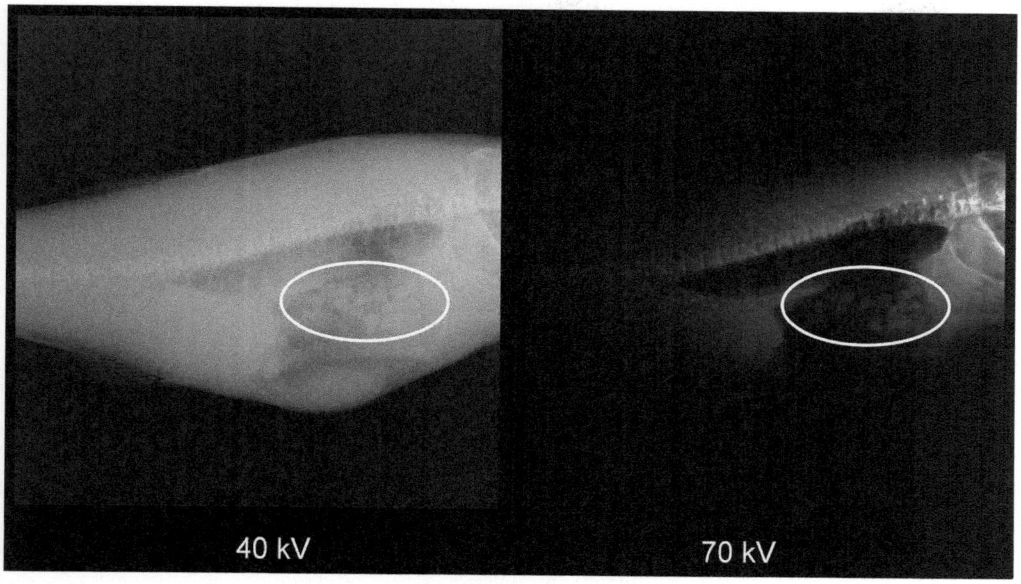

Figure 2. Dual energy X-ray images of Atlantic cod: a) X-ray image at 40 kV, b) X-ray image at 70 kV.

Radio-frequency Metal Detection of Marked Feed in Cod

Fish. Wild-caught cod (2.0±0.8 kg, n = 15) caught at the coast of Central Norway, were killed, packed in ice, and shipped to the ACT Group Lab (Jessheim, Norway). As before, the intestines were kept intact during the experiment.

Feed and markers. Fish feed from [21] was mixed with four different markers (Table 4), and crude herring oil to get a sticky pellet surface and even distributions of marker particles. A dilution series was created to establish the lower detection limit of each marker. The trial feed with markers were packed into small plastic bags in 20 g portions (approximately 1% of fish body weight), equal to a potential daily feed portion, and inserted within the abdominal cavity of the fish. The abdominal cavity was collated by applying plastic strips around the fish body.

Radio-frequency metal detector. The radio-frequency metal detector used for this trial was a CEIA MS21 industrial metal detector [25] supplied by the ACT Group. The detector had a high precision and high sensitivity and was equipped with compensation technology for cancelling external environmental disturbances. The metal detector was arranged over a conveyer belt, approximately 2 m long. The signal strength was given in decibels, and lower detection limit was set to 10 dB (red line in Figure 3). The instrument was calibrated prior to the test by analyzing fish without marked feed and by adjusting the instrument for external disturbance. The metal detector was arranged over a conveyer belt to enable relatively fast and continuous insertion of fish into the detection unit. The sampling/acquisition period per fish was approximately 2 sec, but it can potentially be decreased by optimizing the system setup.

Statistical Analysis

To develop the linear regression model for fat prediction of fish diets inserted in the fish gut cavity, the Minitab [26] statistical software was used. The image features, mean and standard deviation of the X-ray image intensity (Table 2, 3), extracted from dual energy X-ray images, were fed into the Minitab and fat prediction models were generated. The combinations used, in form of multiplication and ratio of features, are motivated from the fundamental principle in dual energy X-ray imaging where the high energy and low energy images are combined in multiplication and division image processing operations [4].

Results and Discussion

X-ray

In Figure 1 and 4 are shown the X-ray images of fish without feed versus fish with feed mixed with glass beads (Figure 1b, 1c) and metal-based markers (Figure 4b, 4c) at the different dilution ranges (Table 1). Figure 1a shows a good visibility of the swim bladder. In Figure 1b and 1c there are also a good visibility of fish feed although its segmentation was not straightforward. The white dots were a result of automatic detection and segmentation of glass

Table 2. Extracted and generated features used for dual energy X-ray image analysis.

$M_{40\,kV}$, $S_{D40\,kV}$	Mean Intensity and standard deviation for ROI image at 40 kV
$M_{70\,kV}$, $S_{D70\,kV}$	Mean Intensity and standard deviation for ROI image at 70 kV
$M_{40/70} = M_{40\,kV}/M_{70\,kV}$	Ratio between mean intensities of the ROI images at 40 kV and 70 kV
$M_{40*70} = M_{40\,kV} * M_{70\,kV}$	Multiplication of mean intensities of the ROI images at 40 kV and 70 kV
$S_{40/70} = S_{40\,kV}/S_{70\,kV}$	Ratio between standard deviation for ROI images at 40 and 70 kV
$S_{40*70} = S_{40\,kV} * S_{70\,kV}$	Multiplication of standard deviation for ROI images at 40 and 70 kV

Table 3. Mean values of the extracted and generated features from the dual energy X-ay 40 kV and 70 kV ROI images of fish diets of the specific fat percentages (18%, 22%, 30%).

Fat(%)	40 kV mean	40 kV std	70 kV mean	70 kV std	40/70 mean	40/70 std	40*70 mean	40*70 std
18(n=6)	2587,65	85,70	37,44	7,11	81,71	25,39	91755,42	35862,59
22(n=6)	2594,17	105,27	40,71	11,06	70,19	17,34	106254,71	32482,88
30(n=6)	2627,30	134,30	45,67	16,72	65,40	21,80	122088,94	49793,78

beads by the Ishida X-ray machine at a certain threshold. It is seen that increase in concentration of glass markers did not result in a better discrimination (Figure 1c).

In Figure 4b and 4c are shown the X-ray images of cod with feed mixed with different concentrations of metal markers. Figure 4b shows a fish with feed containing 0.1% marker (0.03 g), while Figure 4c shows a fish with feed containing 10% marker (3 g). As it is seen in the Figure 4c, the image segmentation of particles was effective at the 10% marker concentration. This is in line with the conclusions of the preliminary study [11], who suggest that the feed could be added particles that absorb X-ray to increase contrast and thereby enable the discrimination of cod weaned to feed.

The advantage of X-ray as a non-invasive method for sorting and discrimination ability at the 10% particle metal concentration (3 g) is shown. Some potential challenges for the methods could be: 1) the need for metal particles to be mixed into the fish feed; 2) to achieve the necessary accuracy, each fish must be singulated prior to imaging. The singulation of fish can be technically solved by use of commercially available singulators. Although prospects of sorting large amounts of fish from a cage containing typically 50.000–100.000 individuals may seem challenging for a concept based on X-ray imaging, there already are commercially available X-ray imaging systems that can cope with harsh environment such as X-ray imaging systems for reservoir studies or pipes provided by InnospeXion [6].

Dual energy X-ray

An example of the visibility of undigested feed [21], with 30% fat, is seen in Figure 2, showing that the feed is visible in both the 40 kV and 70 kV images. Despite the visibility of the feed structure, in the form of cuboid chunks, we conclude that the individual variations in cod thickness, and variations in feed spatial distribution within the gut, makes planar dual-energy X-ray imaging unsuited for the purpose of measuring feed content in the gut. However, the method is promising for measurement of fat percentage in the fish feed diets, assuming the precise extraction of the ROI to be analyzed. Depending on the set of features, the prediction of fat from both linear and multiple linear regression varies from poor $R^2 = 0{,}4476$ (use of only one feature $M_{40*70} = M_{40\ kV} * M_{70\ kV}$) to $R^2 = 0{,}9029$ (use of all generated features) (Table 5). To obtain fat percentage measurements with higher accuracy and throughout the fish gut volume, a dual-energy computed tomography (CT) imaging approach may be convenient, as indicated in previous research [17].

Radio-frequency Metal Detector

The radio-frequency metal detector gave consistent measurements (Table 6). All markers gave detection responses above the detection limit for metal concentrations between 0.1 and 5%. Steel grit marker at 0.1% (0.03 g) concentration provided the strongest signals, while carbonyl iron powder did so at approximately 0.7% (2.1 g) (Figure 3). The steel grit particles were relatively large, with sharp edges and not of uniform shape. The carbonyl-iron powder could be an excellent marker due to its low particle size (a few μm), round particle shape, adaptability to processing in commercial feed mill technology, and benign interaction with the cod digestive system.

Due to efficiency and detection accuracy, radio-frequency metal detectors combined with feed-added carbonyl iron powder at low concentrations seemed like a robust and efficient system for detection of feed in an *in vivo* context. The radio-frequency metal detector could easily be coupled with a conveyer belt or a pipe

Table 4. Particle size of markers used for metal detection.

Marker	Particle size (mm)	Magnetism
Aluminium oxide (AlO2)	0.4–0.6	No
Carbonyl iron (Fe)	0.006–0.009 (powder)	Yes
Steel grit	0.2–0.4	No
Chrome – Nickel alloy (Cr-Ni)	0.6	No

system where fish can be inspected and sorted regardless of positioning and speed.

Use of Fish Feed and Markers

The use of fish feed with added markers (NiCr, AlO_2, Carbonyl Iron, Steel Grit, Ballotini glass beads), as opposed to other marking methods, provided an effective and low-cost method for marking of fish. The general advantage of using this method was that the marked feed could be manufactured in a commercial feed extruder, and the feed could be distributed to all fish in the cohort at once. One potential disadvantage be the variable marking efficiency when feed is unevenly distributed or not accepted by the fish.

Biological Hazards and Fish Welfare

Since we worked with dead fish under laboratory conditions, possible biological hazards and animal welfare issues related to the application of the different markers were not tested in this study.

In practice with live fish, however, it is hardly conceivable that markers such as steel grit, aluminum oxide and Cr-Ni alloys are suitable in fish feed since these compounds are either abrasive, they can have sharp edges, or they can be carcinogen to humans. As such, these compounds might harm the digestive system in fish and their use can therefore result in poor fish welfare. If absorbed in the flesh, they might constitute a hazard to the consumers. Although the abovementioned markers don't have a foreseeable practical use in live fish, we used them for method development as they were commercially available. One of the main hypothesis whether the use of markers would increase the contrast in detection of marked feed to be able to discriminate cod weaned to feed.

On the other hand, results imply that carbonyl iron has an excellent foreseeable practical use in live fish due to the fact that it does not pose biological hazard to live fish. In human beings, single doses of 1–10 g carbonyl iron were tolerated with no evidence of toxicity and only minor gastrointestinal side effects [3].

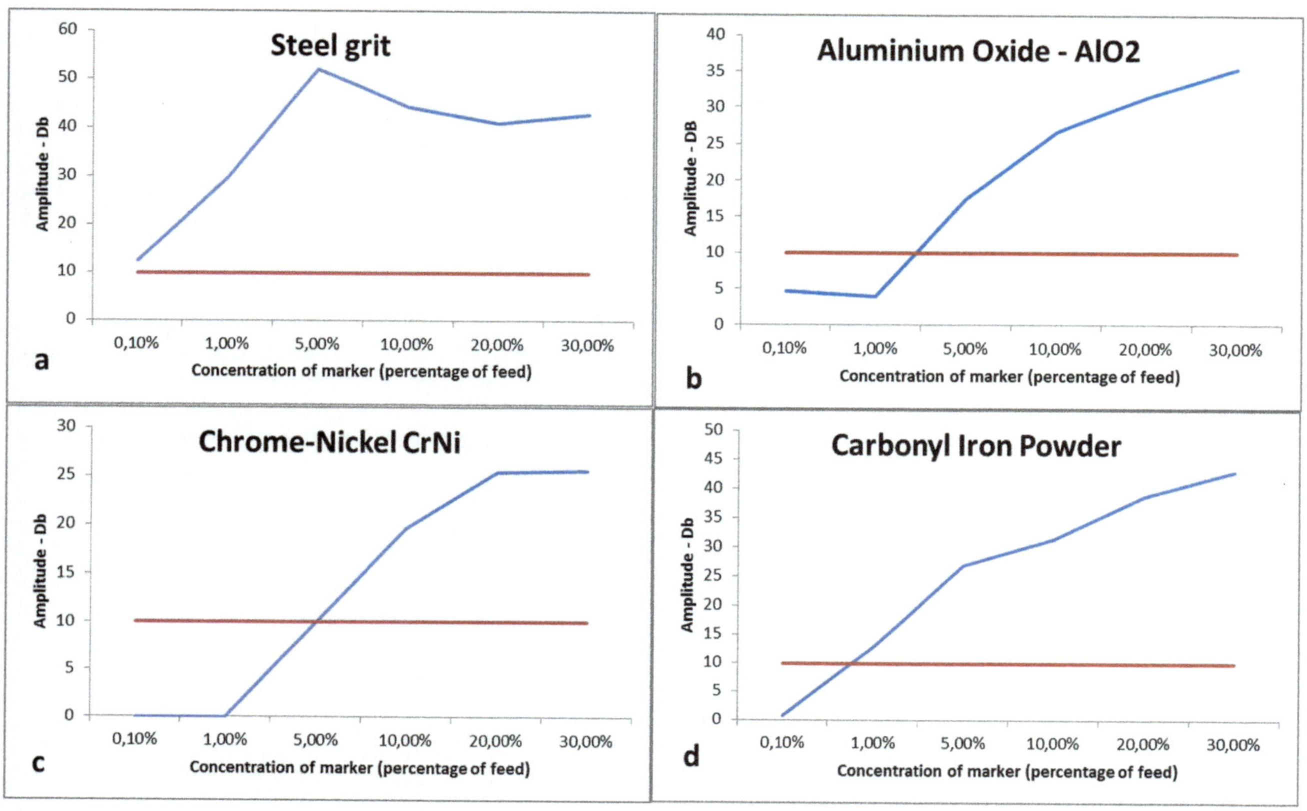

Figure 3. Amplitude of radio frequency metal detector response vs concentration of metal-based markers a) Steel grit, b) Aluminium oxide (AlO_2), c) Chrome-nickel (CrNi), d) Carbonyl iron powder. The red curve is the detection limit at 10 dB.

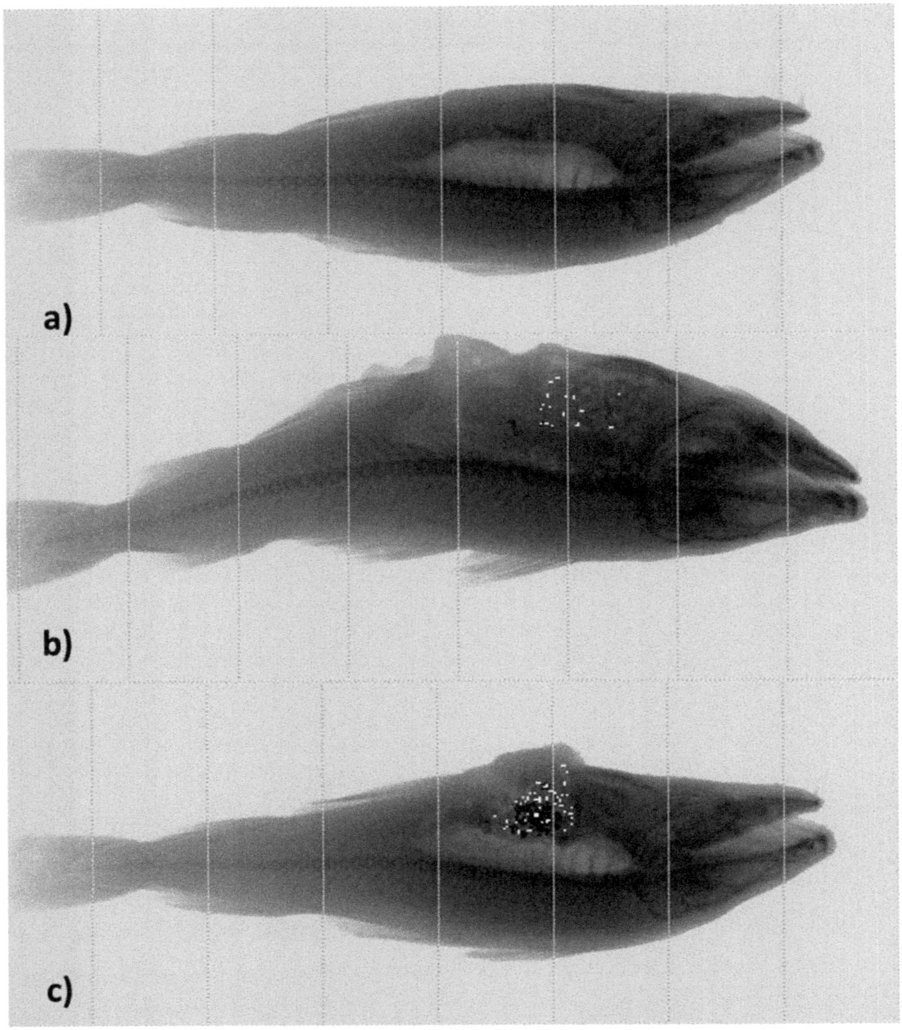

Figure 4. X-ray images of Atlantic cod generated from the Ishida X-ray machine: a) image of fish without feed, b) image of fish with Chrome-Nickel (CrNi) markers at 0.1% (0.03 g) weight percent of total feed content in gut; c) image of fish with Chrome-Nickel (CrNi) markers at 10% (3 g) weight percent of total feed content in gut.

Future work will be concentrated on developing trials with live fish and using carbonyl iron powder as feed marker.

Concept for Implementation of Sorting System

With a detection/discrimination subsystem based on either X-ray imaging or radio frequency metal detection, a suggested concept for implementation of a sorting system for discriminating between weaned and unweaned cod is shown (Figure 5). The discrimination process begins by feeding all the cod with commercial dry feed mixed with a small concentration of carbonyl iron powder. Once the feeding ceases, the cod are pumped from the cage into the sorting system. By mounting a fish pump, detection and sorting unit on a raft, the fish farmer could cut the costs by integrating the discrimination subsystem into the existing pump and sorting system. After drain-off of water, a conveyer belt can be used to transport the fish to the X-ray imaging system or the radio-frequency metal detection unit. Based on the result from the detection unit, with weaned cod being detected by the presence of the metallic carbonyl iron powder in the ingested dry feed, the weaned and unweaned cod can be transported to

Table 5. Prediction of fat of fish diets inserted into fish gut cavity with dual energy band X-ray image features.

Feature set	Prediction model	R^2
$M_{40*70} = M_{40\ kV} * M_{70\ kV}$	Fat(%) = 2,42+0,000196*M_{40*70}	0,4476
All features	Fat(%) = 517+0,00005* 40*70 M −0,203*40 kVmean −0,383 * 40 kV std +0,97* 70 kVmean −15,1 *70 kV std −0,12* 40/70 mean +1,29* 40/70 std +0,00566* 40*70 std	0,9029

Table 6. Response values from the metal detector for different marker types and concentrations (detection limit at 10 dB).

Concentration (%)	AlO_2 (dB)	CrNi (dB)	Steel grit (dB)	Carbonyl Iron powder (dB)
0.10	4.62	0	12.42	0.9
1.00	3.9	0	29.68	**12.84**
5.00	17.52	9.96	52.02	**26.9**
10.00	26.74	19.7	44.22	**31.36**
20.00	31.48	25.34	41	**38.64**
30.00	35.46	25.54	42.78	**42.86**

It is seen that the response value for Carbonyl Iron powder is above the limit for concentrations higher than 1%.

separate cages. From this point on, weaned cod can thus be fed with commercial dry feed, whereas the unweaned cod are fed with the more costly moist feed.

An evaluation of investment costs for the concept solutions based on X-ray, dual energy X-ray and metal detector discrimination methods is reported in [16]. This analysis takes into account the investment need for pumping system, singulation unit, raft, flexible pipes, detection unit, conveyer belts, control software, housing, and costs related to feed production. The cheapest concept solution is the one based on metal detector concept with an estimated cost of 43806 € (361000 NOK), while the concepts based on X-ray are estimated at an approximate cost of 62918 € (518500 NOK).

Conclusions and Future Work

The aim of this work was to investigate the feasibility of X-ray imaging and radio frequency metal detection methods for use in discrimination and sorting of wild cod into two groups – those that are unweaned and those that are weaned from moist feed. Based on the current research, we conclude that both X-ray imaging and radio frequency metal detection were promising methods for discrimination between unweaned and weaned wild cod. In the present investigation, the best results were obtained with the method based on the use of carbonyl iron powder in the commercial dry fish feed combined with the high sensitive radio-frequency metal detector technology. Metal detector based concept was also better when it comes to investment cost,

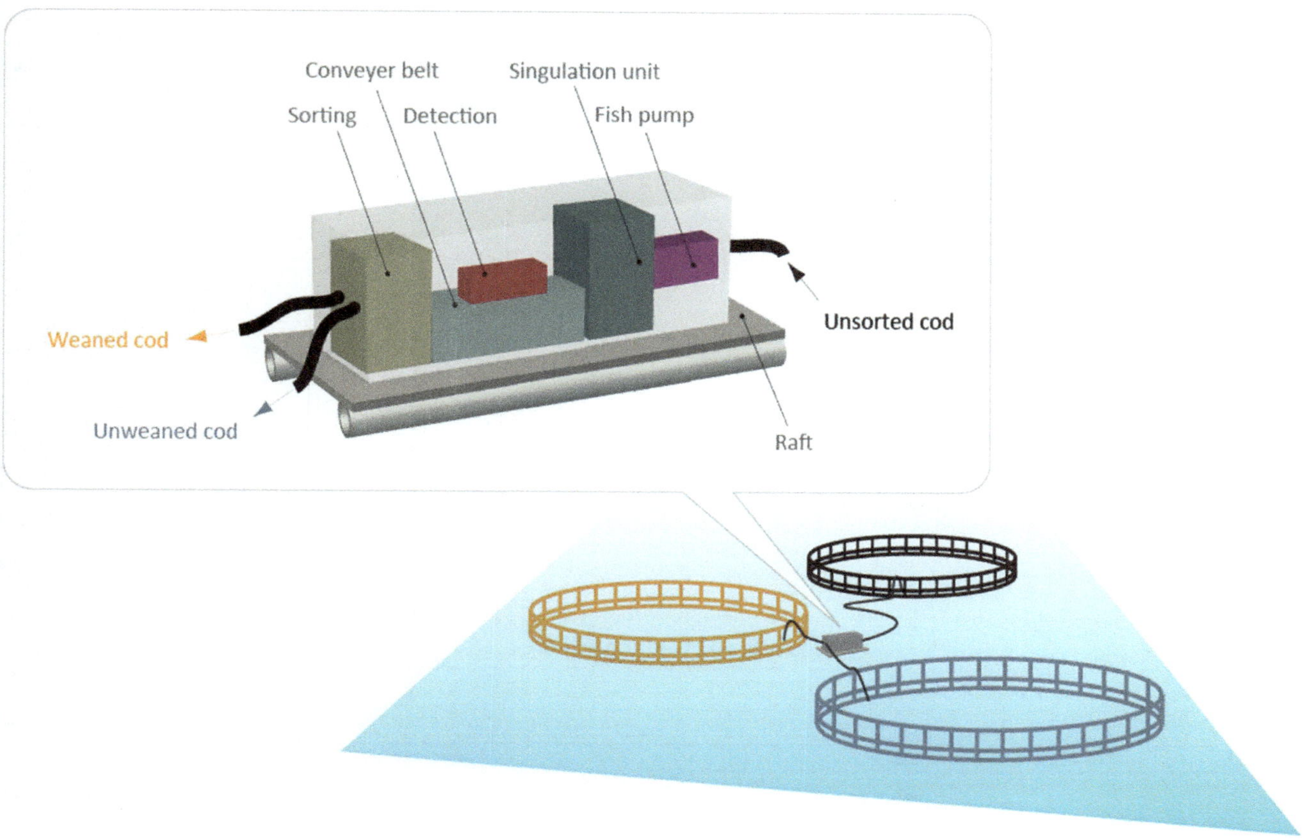

Figure 5. Principle diagram of the concept of sorting system for in situ discrimination of weaned and unweaned Atlantic cod in capture-based aquaculture (CBA) systems.

capacity, accuracy, and use in water. Therefore, as future work we suggest building of a prototype based on metal detector concept, and evaluation of the concept for sorting of live fish in the controlled laboratory conditions. Another important aspect of these trials would be to document the potential biological hazards of carbonyl iron powder to live fish.

Acknowledgments

Dr. Emil Veliyulin is greatly acknowledged for his contribution in preliminary studies that led to the present work. So are Dr. Egis Dauksas for his help in the X-ray investigation experiment, research scientist Andreas Myskja Lien for his work on Figure 5, research scientist Morten Bondø for validation of statistics in Minitab, and Philip Laurence from Ishida Europe for his assistance with the Ishida IX-GA X-ray machine.

Author Contributions

Conceived and designed the experiments: SM EM JRM. Performed the experiments: SM EM. Wrote the paper: EM SM UE JRM. Analyzed the data and images: EM SM JRM. Contributed with fish welfare and biological hazards section: UE.

References

1. Braaten B (1984) Growth of cod in relation to fish size and ration. In: Dahl E, Danielssen D, Moksness E, Solemdal P, editors. The propagation of cod. Institute of Marine Research, Arendal, Norway, 677–710.
2. Dreyer BM, Nøstvold BH, Midling KØ, Hermansen Ø (2008). Capture-based aquaculture of cod. In: Lovatelli A, Holthus PF, editors. *Capture-based aquaculture.* Global overview. FAO Fisheries Technical Paper 508, Rome, 183–198.
3. Gordeuk VR, Brittenham GM, McLaren CE, Hughes MA, Keating LJ (1986) Carbonyl iron therapy for iron deficiency anemia. Blood 67: 745–752.
4. Hamamtsu website: Available http://www.hamamatsu.com/resources/pdf/sys/SFAS0023E06_C10800s.pdf.Accessed 2014 February 20.
5. Hermansen Ø, Isaksen JR, Dreyer B (2012) Challenging spatial and seasonal distribution of fish landings – Experiences from vertically integrated trawlers and delivery obligations in Norway. Marine Policy 36: 206–213.
6. InnospeXion website. Available: http://www.innospexion.dk/index.php/en/pipe-inspection-systems. Accessed 2014 February 20.
7. Ishida Ltd website. Available: http://www.ishida.com/products/ix_g/ix_g_features.html. Accessed 2014 February 20.
8. Jobling M, Christiansen JS, Jørgensen EH, Arnesen AM (1993) The application of X-radiography in feeding and growth studies with fish: a summary of expermients conducted on Arctic charr. Reviews in Fisheries Science 1: 223–237.
9. Jobling M, Arnesen AM, Baardvik BM, Christiansen JS, Jørgensen EH (1995) Monitoring feeding behavior and food intake: methods and applications. Aquaculture Nutrition 1: 131–143.
10. Jobling M, Coves D, Damsgård B, Kristiansen HR, Koskela J, et al. (2001) Techniques for measuring feed intake. In: Houlihan D, Boujard T, Jobling M, editors. Food Intake in Fish. Oxford: Blackwell Science.
11. Martinsen S, Kirkhus T (2009) Codgrade. SINTEF Report Norway : SFH80F094027.
12. Pirhonen J, Schreck CB, Reno PW, Ögüt H (2003) Effect of fasting on feed intake, growth and mortality of chinook salmon, Oncorhynchus tshawytscha, during and induced Aeromonas salmonicida epizootic. Aquaculture 216: 31–38.
13. Refstie S, Førde-Skjærvik O, Rosenlund G, Rørvik KA (2006) Feed intake, growth, and utilization of macronutrients and amino acids by 1- and 2-year old Atlantic cod (*Gadus morhua*) fed standard or bioprocessed soybean meal. Aquaculture 255: 279–291.
14. Santos JD, Jobling M (1991) Factors affecting gastric evacuation in cod, Gadus morhua L., fed single-meals of natural prey. J Fish Biol 38(5): 697–713.
15. Sæther BS, Bjørn PA, Midling KØ, Nilsen R, Jacobsen R, et al. (2009) Fangstbasert Akvakultur, Tilvenning av villtorsk til tørrfôr (Capture-based aquaculture, weaning of wild cod to dry feed). NOFIMA report in Norwegian 4/2009. 25p. http://www.nofima.no/filearchive/Rapport%2004-2009.pdf.
16. Sæther BS, Noble C, Humborstad OB, Martinsen S, Veliyulin E, et al. (2012) Fangstbasert akvakultur: Mellomlagring, oppfôring og foredling av villfanget fisk. NOFIMA report 14/2012.
17. Segtnan VH, Høy M, Sørheim Ø, Kohler A, Lundby F, et al. (2009) Noncontact salt and fat distributional analysis in salted and smoked salmon fillets using X-ray computed tomography and NIR interactance imaging, J Agriculture and Food Chemistry 57: 1705–1710.
18. Talbot C, Higgins PJ (1983) A radiographic method for feeding studies on fish using metallic iron powder as a marker. J Fish Biol 23: 211–220.
19. Toften H, Arnesen AM, Jobling M (2003) Feed intake, growth and ionoregulation in Atlantic salmon (Salmo salar L.) smolts in relation to dietary addition of a feeding stimulant and time of seawater transfer. Aquaculture 217: 647–662.
20. Veliyulin E, Misimi E, Bondø M, Vebenstad PA, Østvik SO (2011) A simple method for weight estimation of whole herring *(Clupea harengus)* using planar X-ray imaging. Journal of Food Science 76: E328–E331.
21. Skretting Optiline website. Available: http://www.skretting.no/internet/SkrettingNorway/webInternet.nsf/wprId/BC7D3F9750A5066DC1257433003E6D02!OpenDocument. Accessed 2013 November 24.
22. SIEMENS Axiom Aristos FDX website. Available: http://www.medwrench.com/?equipment.view/equipmentNo/4418/Siemens/Axiom-Aristos-FX-Plus/. Accessed 2014 February 10.
23. Mathworks website. Available: http://www.mathworks.se/. Accessed 2013 November 24.
24. Potters Industries website. Available: http://www.pottersbeads.com/. Accessed 2014 March 30.
25. Heat and Control website. Available: http://www.heatandcontrol.com/. Accessed 2014 February 20.
26. Minitab website. Available: http://www.minitab.com/en-us/. Accessed 2014 March 30.

Cross-Talk Correction Method for Knee Kinematics in Gait Analysis Using Principal Component Analysis (PCA)

Audrey Baudet[1], Claire Morisset[1,2], Philippe d'Athis[3], Jean-Francis Maillefert[2,4,5], Jean-Marie Casillas[1,2,4,6], Paul Ornetti[2,4,5], Davy Laroche[1,2]*

1 Centre d'Investigation Clinique INSERM 1432, Plateforme d'Investigation Technologique, Dijon University Hospital, Dijon, France, **2** INSERM U1093, Dijon, France, **3** Medical Information department, Dijon University Hospital, Dijon, France, **4** University of Burgundy, Dijon, France, **5** Department of rheumatology, Dijon University Hospital, Dijon, France, **6** Department of physical medicine, Dijon University Hospital, Dijon, France

Abstract

Background: In 3D gait analysis, the knee joint is usually described by the Eulerian way. It consists in breaking down the motion between the articulating bones of the knee into three rotations around three axes: flexion/extension, abduction/adduction and internal/external rotation. However, the definition of these axes is prone to error, such as the "cross-talk" effect, due to difficult positioning of anatomical landmarks. This paper proposes a correction method, principal component analysis (PCA), based on an objective kinematic criterion for standardization, in order to improve knee joint kinematic analysis.

Methods: The method was applied to the 3D gait data of two different groups (twenty healthy subjects and four with knee osteoarthritis). Then, this method was evaluated with respect to three main criteria: (1) the deletion of knee joint angle cross-talk (2) the reduction of variance in the varus/valgus kinematic profile (3) the posture trial varus/valgus deformation matching the X-ray value for patients with knee osteoarthritis. The effect of the correction method was tested statistically on variabilities and cross-talk during gait.

Results: Cross-talk was lower ($p<0.05$) after correction (the correlation between the flexion-extension and varus-valgus kinematic profiles being annihilated). Additionally, the variance in the kinematic profile for knee varus/valgus and knee flexion/extension was found to be lower and higher ($p<0.05$), respectively, after correction for both the left and right side. Moreover, after correction, the posture trial varus/valgus angles were much closer to x-ray grading.

Conclusion: The results show that the PCA correction applied to the knee joint eliminates the cross-talk effect, and does not alter the radiological varus/valgus deformation for patients with knee osteoarthritis. These findings suggest that the proposed correction method produces new rotational axes that better fit true knee motion.

Editor: Alfonso Fasano, University of Toronto, Italy

Funding: The authors have no support or funding to report.

Competing Interests: The authors have declared that no competing interests exist.

* Email: davy.laroche@chu-dijon.fr

Introduction

3D video-based biomechanical models are usually used to evaluate knee motion during gait. It has proved challenging to measure and then to represent this movement [1,2]. 3D knee joint kinematics is commonly expressed using Eulerian or Cardanic description [3]. It requires two coordinate systems (CS), each one associated with an articulating bone of the knee (femur or tibia). Both are defined by positioning reflective markers on the skin on specific bony landmarks [4–8], according to a standard arrangement (marker set). The motion of the distal segment relative to that of the proximal segment, calculated from the coordinates of the markers, is usually reported as three sequential rotations (Euler angles) around three axes: flexion-extension, abduction-adduction and internal-external rotation [9].

Consequently, this technique has to rely on the palpation of external anatomical landmarks, which is an experimental problem [10]. Given the reality of experimental conditions with different examiners and a succession of subjects to examine, this is a serious limitation. Minor changes of marker placements modify the orientation of the coordinate systems and thereafter lead to significant errors in abduction/adduction and internal/external rotation angle curves [11–14]. This error is known as the kinematic "cross-talk" effect [15–18], which particularly affects the kinematics of joints that articulate principally around one major component, e.g. the knee joint [19].

This error leads to overestimation of the ab/adduction and int/external rotation angles [11–13,20–22]. Numerous methods have been proposed to correct this error in the pre-trial phase [23–27] while few methods have investigated correction during the post-trial phase [28,29]. Actually, Woltring proposed to rotate the initial CS until ab/adduction and int/internal rotation are zeroed at the time of maximum knee flexion during gait [29]. In turn, Rivest reduced between-subject variance by minimizing the quadratic variations in the knee abduction/adduction and internal/external rotation angles [28]. However, even though these methods appreciably reduce the cross-talk effect, they may delete existing mechanisms of the pathological knee. Thus, there is still no clear optimal ad hoc method of correcting knee joint motion for purposes of quantitative gait analysis.

The aim of this study is to propose a new method to correct the angles of knee rotation using principal component analysis (PCA) [30]. PCA is a classical statistical method that comes from the mechanical concept of "inertia". It was first formulated thus: "finding lines and planes of closest fit to systems of points in space" [31]. Applied to the knee, it would provide a better representation of knee angles, by transforming the original data of correlated angles into new ones with uncorrelated components.

Materials and Methods

Subjects

Subjects were randomly selected among patients between 50 and 75 years old from two cohorts of healthy (HE) subjects and knee osteoarthritis (OA) patients. The first group of 20 healthy subjects had normal knee function and the second group (4 patients hereafter referred to as OA1 to OA4) had knee OA and symptomatic varus/valgus deformities. The study was conducted in compliance with the principles of Good Clinical Practice and the Declaration of Helsinki and all patients signed an informed consent form. The study protocol was approved by the local ethics committee (CPP Est I, Dijon, France) and was registered under ClinicalTrials.gov Identifier: NCT01884883.

Data collection

Kinematic data were captured using a three-dimensional (3D) Vicon motion analysis system (©VICON Motion Systems Ltd, UK) with eight cameras operating at a sampling rate of 100 Hz, mounted approximately 2.5 m high encircling the 6 m long×3 m wide×2 m tall capture volume. The marker set used for the study was the lower-body Plug-in-Gait provided by Vicon, based on the Newington-Helen Hayes gait model [12,32] (Figure 1.a).

Particularly, the Vicon Plug-in-Gait applies a specific "chord function" in the calculation of the knee joint center (KJC). It estimates the hip joint center (HJC) using four markers on the pelvis and then uses the derived HJC, two other markers (thigh and knee markers) and determined offsets from the subject's measurements to estimate the KJC. The KJC is a point located half a knee width away from the knee marker placed on the lateral epicondyle of the femur. Then, the origin of the knee joint CS is taken as the KJC. The primary Z-axis is taken from the KJC to the hip joint center. The secondary Y-axis is taken parallel to the line from the KJC to the knee marker. For both left and right knees, the Y-axis is directed towards the left of the subject. The X-axis is hence directed forwards from the knee (Figure 1.b).

In each gait protocol, the test session began with a trial to capture static anatomical landmarks for calibration purposes. Then, instructions were given to the participants to walk in a comfortable manner, at a self-selected speed along a 10 m walking path. Each participant performed twenty gait trials. In addition, the four OA patients executed a thirty-second static posture trial in a radiological position in order to compare varus/valgus angles with the measured X-ray angle (see point 3 on 1.5 Statistical evaluation paragraph).

Anatomical varus/valgus angles were assessed on an antero-posterior weight-bearing knee X-ray with a size ratio of 1:1. Knee valgus/varus misalignment was measured accurately in millimeters by an expert rheumatologist using a 0.1 mm graduated magnifying glass, laid directly over the radiograph. In this study, this measurement was considered the gold-standard for assessing valgus/varus misalignment.

Data analysis

Three-dimensional knee joint angular kinematic data were obtained by tracking the trajectories of 14 mm spherical retro-reflective markers. These were mounted over the seven body segments of interest (pelvis, left and right thighs, left and right shanks, left and right foot; for detailed body landmarks see Figure 1).

Coordinate data were filtered using smoothing splines [33]. For missing markers on less than 10 frames, data were interpolated with cubic spline polynomials. Gait cycles containing gaps over 10 frames or more were automatically rejected from the analysis. Temporal events were defined using the position of the heel, toe and sacrum marker [34]. Each stride was time-normalized to 101 points representing equal intervals from 0% to 100% of the gait cycle.

Correction procedure

- Principal Component Analysis

The main goal of PCA is to find a space as close as possible to the observed points [35]. If X is the matrix for n observations by p variables $X = \{x_n\}$, $n \in \{1 \ldots n\}$, the q principal axes $W = \{w_j\}, j \in \{i \ldots q\}$ are orthonormal axes defining such a space. In physics, this means maximizing the inertia of a set of material points around these principal axes.

The vectors $\{w_j\}$ are given by the q dominant eigenvectors (i.e. those with the largest associated eigenvalues λ) of the covariance matrix of the set of observations:

$$C = \frac{1}{n} \times X^T \times X \tag{1}$$

The eigenvalues λ reflect the variance contribution (δ_j) of the j-th principal axis as follows:

$$\delta_j = \frac{\lambda j}{\sum_{i=1}^{n} (\lambda i)} \tag{2}$$

The variables x_n are then linearly transformed into uncorrelated variables for which the covariance matrix is diagonal with elements λ. Finally, it turns out that the q principal components of the observed vector x_n are given by: $x'_n = x_n \times W$.

- PCA calculations

The input data of the PCA analysis were the three angles of the knee joint, i.e. the Euler angles associated with the rotation between the articulating bones of the knee, over the 101 measurements of a gait cycle (n gait cycles for each subject). It was displayed as n (101×3) matrices for each subject:

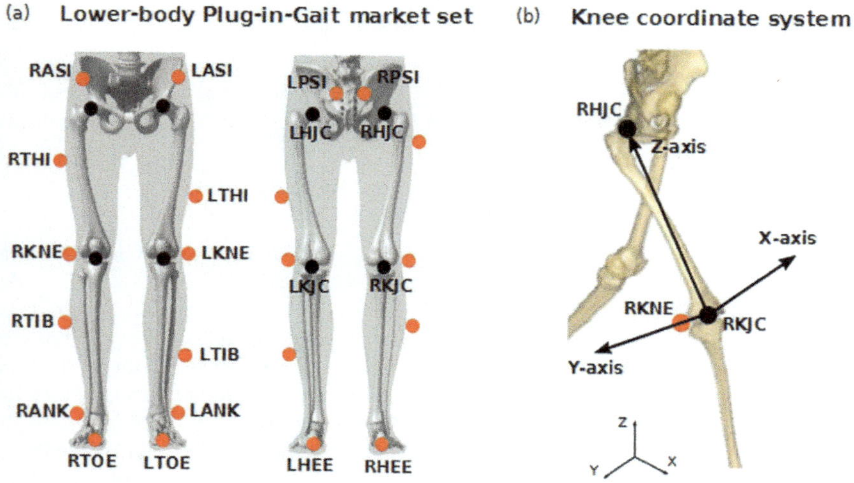

Figure 1. Plug-in-Gait marker set.

$$\underbrace{\begin{pmatrix} \alpha_1 & \beta_1 & \gamma_1 \\ \vdots & \ddots & \vdots \\ \alpha_{101} & \beta_{101} & \gamma_{101} \end{pmatrix}}_{\times n}$$

with α being the motion of flexion/extension, β of ab/adduction and γ of axial rotation.Then, once the matrix of covariance of this set of points has been calculated (see Equation 1), the eigenvalues and the components (a, b, c) of the eigenvectors may be determined in the observational basis:

$$\begin{aligned} w_1 &= (a_1,b_1,c_1) \\ w_2 &= (a_2,b_2,c_2) \\ w_3 &= (a_3,b_3,c_3) \end{aligned} \tag{3}$$

This makes it possible to create the transfer matrix from the observational basis to the principal axes (Equation 4) and to calculate the principal components using the P matrix.

$$P = \begin{bmatrix} a_1 & a_2 & a_3 \\ b_1 & b_2 & b_3 \\ c_1 & c_2 & c_3 \end{bmatrix} \tag{4}$$

Note that the principal axes and the transfer matrix have no physical sense but only a mathematical sense.

- Correction hypothesis

It is hypothesized that each principal component is a corrected anatomical angle.

Therefore, the eigenvectors must be sorted in order to match each principal component to an anatomical angle: the columns of the P matrix are switched depending on the values of the coefficients a_i, b_i, c_i in such a way that the values of the diagonal are maximal.Finally, the corrected angles are determined using the "sorted" P matrix:

$$\begin{pmatrix} \alpha_1 & \beta_1 & \gamma_1 \\ \vdots & \ddots & \vdots \\ \alpha_{101} & \beta_{101} & \gamma_{101} \end{pmatrix} \underset{P\ matrix}{\overset{(PCA)}{\rightarrow}} \begin{pmatrix} \psi_1 & \xi_1 & \rho_1 \\ \vdots & \ddots & \vdots \\ \psi_{101} & \xi_{101} & \rho_{101} \end{pmatrix}$$

with ψ being the corrected flexion/extension angle, ξ the corrected ab/adduction angle and ρ the corrected axial rotation angle.

Statistical evaluation

The method was evaluated on the kinematics of the two groups of subjects to comply with 3 requirements:

(1) The correction must remove cross-talk. In order to quantify the cross-talk, the relationship between the flexion-extension and varus-valgus kinematic profiles was assessed by the correlation between both profiles (r^2), as reported by Schache et al [26].

(2) The variance in the varus/valgus kinematic profile must be minimal. The ab/adductor motion of the knee is physiologically limited, in asymptomatic condition, to approximately 7° due to the restrictions imposed by knee geometry and biomechanical properties [11,18,36]. Thus, an effective correction has to reduce the varus/valgus range of motion (ROM) resulting from cross-talk [23]. To check this, we computed the variance in its kinematic profile (δ^2ab/ad). As a result of this reduction in varus-valgus ROM, the knee flexion-extension ROM has to be increased. To corroborate this, the variance in the flexion-extension kinematic profile (δ^2f/e) was also calculated. Previous studies have used these criteria for a similar purpose [25,28,37,38].

(3) In the case of symptomatic knee OA patients, it is essential for the varus/valgus deformities to remain after correction. The posture trial knee angles (see 1.2 Data collection paragraph) were thus corrected using the transfer matrix P (see 1.4.2 PCA calculations paragraph). We assumed that the varus/valgus angle obtained in the posture trial, after correction, would be close to the x-ray angle because of the similar position for both evaluations. Comparisons were made between the corrected posture angle and the anatomical angle assessed by x-ray.

Statistical analysis

Parameters (variabilities δ^2 and cross-talk r^2) were averaged for all subjects and presented with the standard deviation (SD). Non-parametric tests for paired samples were used to detect whether the correction method had a significant effect: the Wilcoxon test for variabilities and the Friedman test for cross-talk. Comparisons were done for the left and right side separately. Differences were considered significant for $p<0.05$. Statistical analyses were performed using *Statistica 10.0*.

Results

For every subject, 42±19 gait cycles were available, which was sufficient to obtain good reliability of knee joint angles and to overcome intrinsic variability [39].

Figure 2 shows the impact of the cross-talk correction on rotations of the knee. These results are consistent with previous studies [2,12,23.] They demonstrated that the more misaligned the defined CS, the more sensitive to change in flexion/extension the knee varus/valgus became. In contrast, knee axial rotation tended to be offset by approximately 5° but appeared to be less influenced by changes in knee flexion/extension.

The correction method eliminated the presence of knee joint angle cross-talk, as proved by mean r^2 values close to 0 for the left and right side after correction. Cross-talk was significantly lower ($p<0.0001$) than before correction with mean r^2 higher than 0.6 (table 1).

Moreover, the variances in the kinematic profiles for knee varus-valgus (δ^2ab/ad) and knee flexion-extension (δ^2f/e) were found to be significantly ($p<0.05$) lower and higher, respectively, after correction than before correction for both the left and right side (table 1).

To ensure that the PCA did not induce an offset of the abduction/adduction angles, we transferred (see methods) the reorientation of the knee CS during the posture trial in patients with symptomatic OA deformations. Figure 3 shows that the abduction/adduction ROM decreased for subjects OA2, OA3 and OA4. In contrast, OA1 ab/adduction ROM was already small and physiologically acceptable. Interestingly, the X-ray image for OA3 showed varus deformities. However, the initial angles in the frontal plane suggested that the patient had a valgus knee. The PCA correction seemed to have modified this angle to produce a varus knee, as found in previous X-ray images. In order to statically validate the varus/valgus deformation against its X-ray value, we compared the corrected varus/valgus angle during the posture trial with the x-ray angle, obtained in similar positions. As expected, table 2 shows that the varus/valgus angles after correction were much closer to the x-ray grading than before correction.

Discussion

This study aims to propose a new easy-to-apply method using PCA to correct knee kinematics during gait analysis. Particularly, it seems that PCA provided a better representation of the knee angles, reduced the cross-talk effect and did not alter symptomatic deformations for OA patients. To our knowledge, this study is the first to employ this classical statistical tool in order to improve the accuracy of 3D gait kinematic analysis.

Many studies [11–13,20–22] have assessed the influence of errors in aligning the knee flexion/extension axis. All pointed out that misalignment of the CS in the knee joint led to significant errors in abduction/adduction and internal/external rotation angle curves. Several methods for defining the knee joint flexion/extension axis before gait trials have been presented [23–27] while other methods have involved post hoc reorientation of the joint CS to correct axis misalignment. Indeed, data may be corrected by rotating the initial CS until abduction/adduction and internal/external rotation are zeroed at the time of maximum knee flexion during gait [29], or between-subject variance may be reduced by minimizing the quadratic variations in the knee abduction/adduction and internal/external rotation angles [28]. This correction, applied to gait data for a small cohort collected using the same protocol that we used [12,32], was found to appreciably reduce the cross-talk effect. In our study, the corrected joint kinematics gave varus/valgus and axial rotation curves that were similar to those from this method. However, Rivest assumed the flexion/extension angle to be invariant and proposed to minimize ab/adduction and axial rotation angles without reporting these data on the flexion/extension axis [28]. Such a method may delete existing mechanisms of the pathological knee. Since the PCA method uses an objective kinematic criterion for standardization, it is not limited when applied to pathological patients. Besides, the procedure does not have to be implemented during the gait analysis itself and can easily be carried out *a posteriori*, which is useful in the case of large cohorts of patients.

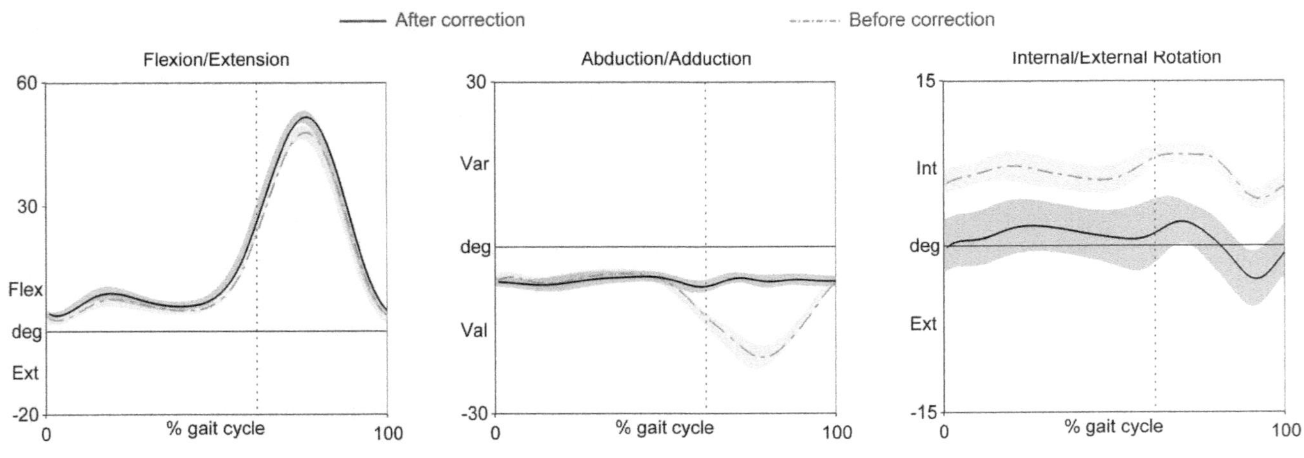

Figure 2. Mean and standard deviation of knee joint rotations during gait for a single typical subject before (grey dash-dotted line and light-grey area) and after correction (black solid line and grey area). Dotted vertical line indicates the mean toe off value for this subject.

Table 1. Mean and S.D. of variability of the flexion/extension axis, the abduction/adduction axis and cross-talk (r^2) between those axes, before (initial) and after (PCA-corrected) correction with PCA method.

Parameter	**Initial**		**PCA-corrected**	
	Mean	**SD**	**Mean**	**SD**
Variability δ^2				
Flex/extension				
Right	16.47	1.82	17.54 *	1.45
Left	16.97	1.30	17.63 *	1.32
Ab/adduction				
Right	3.82	3.15	0.73 *	0.35
Left	3.36	2.07	0.93 *	0.50
Cross-talk (r^2)				
Right	0.71	0.33	0 *	0
Left	0.60	0.39	0 *	0

*: significant difference ($p<0.00625$) between initial and PCA-corrected.

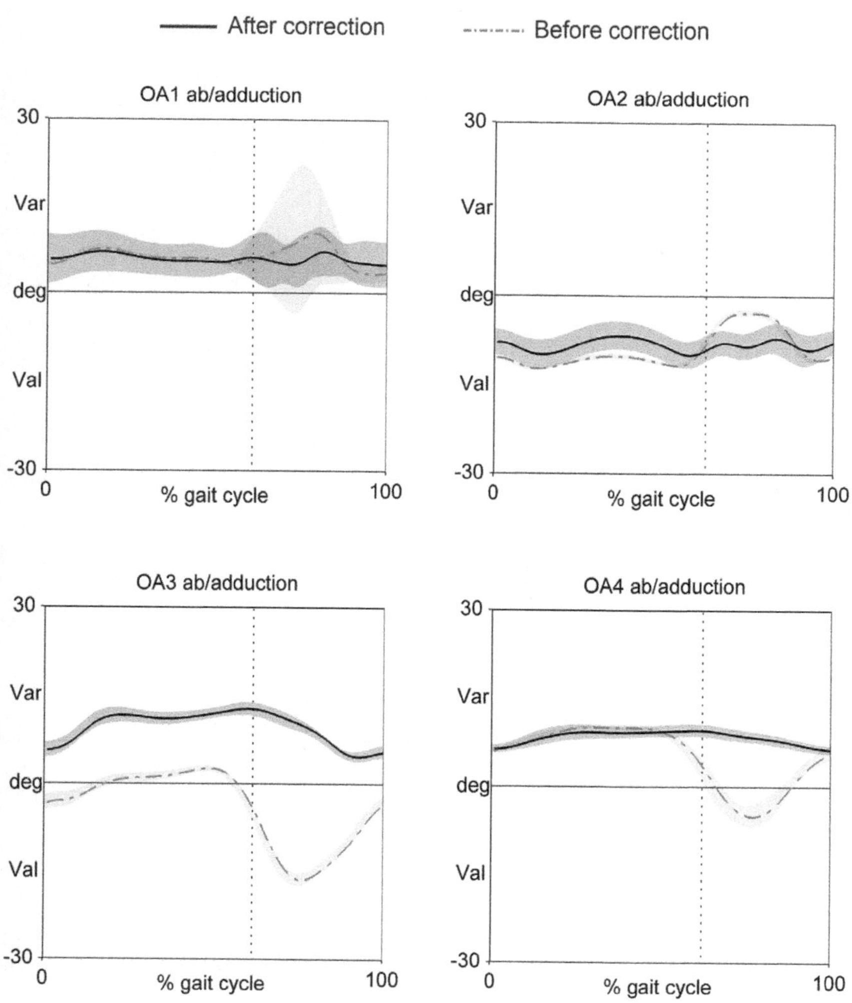

Figure 3. Averaged ab/adduction angle (mean and SD) during gait for each of the four OA patients before (grey dash-dotted line and light-grey area) and after correction (black solid line and grey area). Dotted vertical line indicates mean toe off.

Table 2. Comparison between the x-ray grading and the varus/valgus angle during the posture trial before (b.c.) and after (a.c.) correction.

	Posture trial angle		X-ray grading
	b.c.	a.c.	
OA 1	4.64 °	4.78 °	5.0 °
OA 2	−8.49 °	−4.33 °	−3.6 °
OA 3	−2.71 °	6.20 °	6.0 °
OA 4	−2.26 °	4.03 °	4.3 °

The value of knee varus/valgus ROM of the classical Cardanic angle obtained with the landmark procedure gave data that were out of the range of physiological values for healthy subjects. The errors observed were mainly due to the cross-talk effect, which is assumed to reflect a degree of knee joint flexion-extension axis misalignment [2,12,23]. The PCA corrected the kinematics of the joint by reducing the variance in the space defined by the three principal axes. This method was evaluated with respect to three main criteria: (1) the deletion of knee joint angle cross-talk (2) the reduction of variance in the varus/valgus kinematic profile (3) the postural varus/valgus deformation matching the X-ray value for patients with knee osteoarthritis. Indeed, it has been clearly demonstrated that in a stable knee joint, the physiological ROM of knee varus-valgus is small [11,36]. Furthermore, the kinematic profiles from these studies do not display any obvious evidence of coupling between knee flexion-extension and varus-valgus, unlike that between knee flexion-extension and axial rotation [17,40]. These findings suggest that the presence of cross-talk, measured as the correlation (r^2) between knee flexion-extension and varus-valgus kinematic profiles, is not an expected physiological phenomenon but is rather a reflection of knee flexion-extension axis misalignment. Reduction of knee joint cross-talk using correlation (r^2) and knee varus-valgus variability (δ^2ab/ad) reduction were therefore considered to be valid criteria to evaluate our correction method [25,28,37,38]. This evaluation was strengthened, in the third criterion, by the comparison between corrected angles and x-ray graded angles of symptomatic valgus/varus deformities for patients with knee OA. Finally, the experimental findings are directly in line with the expected findings as the main goal of PCA is to transform original data of correlated variables into new ones with uncorrelated components. However, such corrections applied to the knee joint should have repercussions on adjacent joint kinematics.

Additionally, it should be noted that knee angles are Euler angles associated with rotational motion between the articulating bones of the knee. Therefore, it might be of interest to completely redefine the knee joint CS with respect to the new knee angle curves determined by the PCA correction. This means modifying both femur and tibia CS dynamically during gait and thereafter recalculating lower body kinematics and kinetics. This would make it possible to analyze the repercussions of this correction on "downstream" results: (i) by calculating new hip and ankle angles, as they derive from the rotation matrix between the knee joint CS (i.e. the femur CS) and the hip or ankle CS (i.e. respectively pelvis and tibia CS), and (ii) by determining the new position of the hip joint center (HJC). More accurate methods have been proposed to locate the HJC [41,42]. The combination of such methods and PCA correction should be explored in future studies in order to improve the quality of the results in gait analysis.

Furthermore, some of the variability of lower-body kinematics could be attributed to the operator, and specifically to the operator's ability to identify the external anatomical landmarks. Since the current correction removes the errors introduced by the incorrect positioning of markers on anatomical landmarks, one could easily imagine that it could lead to more reproducible data [43]. In this regard, further investigations should be made in order to analyze the impact of this correction on between-session and between-operator variability.

Conclusion

This paper proposes a post-hoc statistical correction method that is objective, accurate and easy to apply for estimating knee joint kinematics. It is based on the anatomical constraint that the knee articulates principally around one major axis (flexion/extension axis), which allows the use of PCA to retrieve more anatomical knee axes. The findings of this paper, interpreted with an understanding of the knee cross-talk phenomenon, highlight the fact that the correction method produced new rotational axes that correspond more closely to true knee motion.

Acknowledgments

The authors are grateful to P. Bastable for his help in preparing the manuscript.

Author Contributions

Conceived and designed the experiments: CM JFM PO DL. Performed the experiments: AB PO DL. Analyzed the data: AB PA DL. Contributed reagents/materials/analysis tools: CM JMC. Contributed to the writing of the manuscript: AB CM PA JMC PO DL.

References

1. Ball KA, Greiner TM (2008) On the problems of describing joint axis alignment. J Biomech 41: 1599–1603. doi:10.1016/j.jbiomech.2008.02.033.
2. Ramakrishnan HK, Kadaba MP (1991) On the estimation of joint kinematics during gait. J Biomech 24: 969–977.
3. Grood ES, Suntay WJ (1983) A joint coordinate system for the clinical description of three-dimensional motions: application to the knee. J Biomech Eng 105: 136–144.
4. Cappozzo A, Catani F, Della Croce U, Leardini A (1995) Position and orientation in space of bones during movement: anatomical frame definition and determination. Clin Biomech 10: 171–178.
5. Della Croce U, Camomilla V, Leardini A, Cappozzo A (2003) Femoral anatomical frame: assessment of various definitions. Med Eng Phys 25: 425–431. doi:10.1016/S1350-4533(03)00032-8.

6. Donati M, Camomilla V, Vannozzi G, Cappozzo A (2007) Enhanced anatomical calibration in human movement analysis. Gait Posture 26: 179–185. doi:10.1016/j.gaitpost.2007.04.009.
7. Ferrari A, Benedetti MG, Pavan E, Frigo C, Bettinelli D, et al. (2008) Quantitative comparison of five current protocols in gait analysis. Gait Posture 28: 207–216. doi:10.1016/j.gaitpost.2007.11.009.
8. Wu G, Cavanagh PR (1995) ISB recommendations for standardization in the reporting of kinematic data. J Biomech 28: 1257–1261.
9. Tupling SJ, Pierrynowski MR (1987) Use of cardan angles to locate rigid bodies in three-dimensional space. Med Biol Eng Comput 25: 527–532.
10. Szczerbik E, Kalinowska M (2011) The influence of knee marker placement error on evaluation of gait kinematic parameters. Acta Bioeng Biomech Wroc Univ Technol 13: 43–46.
11. Blankevoort L, Huiskes R, de Lange A (1988) The envelope of passive knee joint motion. J Biomech 21: 705–720.
12. Kadaba MP, Ramakrishnan HK, Wootten ME (1990) Measurement of lower extremity kinematics during level walking. J Orthop Res 8: 383–392.
13. Robinson MA, Vanrenterghem J (2012) An evaluation of anatomical and functional knee axis definition in the context of side-cutting. J Biomech 45: 1941–1946. doi:10.1016/j.jbiomech.2012.05.017.
14. Schwartz MH, Trost JP, Wervey RA (2004) Measurement and management of errors in quantitative gait data. Gait Posture 20: 196–203. doi:10.1016/j.gaitpost.2003.09.011.
15. Freeman MAR, Pinskerova V (2005) The movement of the normal tibio-femoral joint. J Biomech 38: 197–208. doi:10.1016/j.jbiomech.2004.02.006.
16. Lafortune MA, Cavanagh PR, Sommer III HJ, Kalenak A (1992) Three-dimensional kinematics of the human knee during walking. J Biomech 25: 347–357. doi:10.1016/0021-9290(92)90254-X.
17. Piazza SJ, Cavanagh PR (2000) Measurement of the screw-home motion of the knee is sensitive to errors in axis alignment. J Biomech 33: 1029–1034.
18. Reinschmidt C, Van Den Bogert AJ, Lundberg A, Nigg BM, Murphy N, et al. (1997) Tibiofemoral and tibiocalcaneal motion during walking: external vs. skeletal markers. Gait Posture 6: 98–109.
19. Ramsey DK, Wretenberg PF (1999) Biomechanics of the knee: methodological considerations in the in vivo kinematic analysis of the tibiofemoral and patellofemoral joint. Clin Biomech 14: 595–611.
20. Chéze L (2000) Comparison of different calculations of three-dimensional joint kinematics from video-based system data. J Biomech 33: 1695–1699.
21. Della Croce U, Cappozzo A, Kerrigan DC (1999) Pelvis and lower limb anatomical landmark calibration precision and its propagation to bone geometry and joint angles. Med Biol Eng Comput 37: 155–161.
22. Most E, Axe J, Rubash H, Li G (2004) Sensitivity of the knee joint kinematics calculation to selection of flexion axes. J Biomech 37: 1743–1748. doi:10.1016/j.jbiomech.2004.01.025.
23. Baker R, Finney L, Orr J (1999) A new approach to determine the hip rotation profile from clinical gait analysis data. Hum Mov Sci 18: 655–667. doi:10.1016/S0167-9457(99)00027-5.
24. Ehrig RM, Taylor WR, Duda GN, Heller MO (2007) A survey of formal methods for determining functional joint axes. J Biomech 40: 2150–2157. doi:10.1016/j.jbiomech.2006.10.026.
25. Marin F, Mannel H, Claes L, Dürselen L (2003) Correction of axis misalignment in the analysis of knee rotations. Hum Mov Sci 22: 285–296. doi:10.1016/S0167-9457(03)00036-8.
26. Schache AG, Baker R, Lamoreux LW (2006) Defining the knee joint flexion–extension axis for purposes of quantitative gait analysis: An evaluation of methods. Gait Posture 24: 100–109. doi:10.1016/j.gaitpost.2005.08.002.
27. Schwartz MH, Rozumalski A (2005) A new method for estimating joint parameters from motion data. J Biomech 38: 107–116. doi:10.1016/j.jbiomech.2004.03.009.
28. Rivest L-P (2005) A correction for axis misalignment in the joint angle curves representing knee movement in gait analysis. J Biomech 38: 1604–1611. doi:10.1016/j.jbiomech.2004.07.031.
29. Woltring HJ (1994) 3-D attitude representation of human joints: a standardization proposal. J Biomech 27: 1399–1414.
30. Jolliffe IT (1986) Principal component analysis. Springer-Verlang. 296 p.
31. Pearson K (1901) On Lines and Planes of Closest Fit to Systems of Points in Space. University College. 572 p.
32. Davis I, Ounpuu S, Tyburski D, Gage J (1991) A gait analysis data collection and reduction technique. Hum Mov Sci 10: 575–587. doi:10.1016/0167-9457(91)90046-z.
33. Woltring HJ (1986) A Fortran package for generalized, cross-validatory spline smoothing and differentiation. Adv Eng Softw 1978: 104–113. doi:10.1016/0141-1195(86)90098-7.
34. Zeni JA, Richards JG, Higginson JS (2008) Two simple methods for determining gait events during treadmill and overground walking using kinematic data. Gait Posture 27: 710–714. doi:10.1016/j.gaitpost.2007.07.007.
35. Hotelling H (1933) Analysis of a complex of statistical variables into principal components. J Educ Psychol 24: 417–441. doi:10.1037/h0071325.
36. Ishii Y, Terajima K, Terashima S, Koga Y (1997) Three-dimensional kinematics of the human knee with intracortical pin fixation. Clin Orthop: 144–150.
37. Charlton IW, Tate P, Smyth P, Roren L (2004) Repeatability of an optimised lower body model. Gait Posture 20: 213–221. doi:10.1016/j.gaitpost.2003.09.004.
38. Noonan KJ, Halliday S, Browne R, O'Brien S, Kayes K, et al. (2003) Interobserver variability of gait analysis in patients with cerebral palsy. J Pediatr Orthop 23: 279–287; discussion 288–291.
39. Laroche D, Duval A, Morisset C, Beis JN, d' Athis P, et al. (2011) Test-retest reliability of 3D kinematic gait variables in hip osteoarthritis patients. Osteoarthr Cartil OARS Osteoarthr Res Soc 19: 194–199. doi:10.1016/j.joca.2010.10.024.
40. Moglo KE, Shirazi-Adl A (2005) Cruciate coupling and screw-home mechanism in passive knee joint during extension–flexion. J Biomech 38: 1075–1083. doi:10.1016/j.jbiomech.2004.05.033.
41. Sangeux M, Pillet H, Skalli W (2014) Which method of hip joint centre localisation should be used in gait analysis? Gait Posture. doi:10.1016/j.gaitpost.2014.01.024.
42. Upadhyaya S, Lee W-S (2013) Survey of Formal Methods of Hip Joint Center Calculation in Human Studies. APCBEE Procedia 7: 27–31. doi:10.1016/j.apcbee.2013.08.007.
43. McGinley JL, Baker R, Wolfe R, Morris ME (2009) The reliability of three-dimensional kinematic gait measurements: A systematic review. Gait Posture 29: 360–369. doi:10.1016/j.gaitpost.2008.09.003.

12

Prediction Equation for Lower Limbs Lean Soft Tissue in Circumpubertal Boys Using Anthropometry and Biological Maturation

João Valente-dos-Santos[1], Manuel J. Coelho-e-Silva[1]*, Aristides M. Machado-Rodrigues[1], Marije T. Elferink-Gemser[2,3], Robert M. Malina[4,5], Édio L. Petroski[6], Cláudia S. Minderico[7], Analiza M. Silva[7], Fátima Baptista[7], Luís B. Sardinha[7]

1 Faculty of Sport Sciences and Physical Education, University of Coimbra, Coimbra, Portugal, **2** Center for Human Movement Sciences, University Medical Center Groningen, University of Groningen, Groningen, The Netherlands, **3** Institute for Studies in Sports and Exercise, HAN University of Applied Sciences, Nijmegen, The Netherlands, **4** Department of Kinesiology and Health Education, University of Texas at Austin, Austin, Texas, United States of America, **5** Department of Kinesiology, Tarleton State University, Stephenville, Texas, United States of America, **6** Research Centre for Kinanthropometry and Human Performance, Federal University of Santa Catarina, Florianópolis, Santa Catarina, Brazil, **7** Exercise and Health Laboratory, CIPER, Faculdade de Motricidade Humana, Universidade de Lisboa, Cruz-Quebrada, Portugal

Abstract

Lean soft tissue (LST), a surrogate of skeletal muscle mass, is largely limited to appendicular body regions. Simple and accurate methods to estimate lower limbs LST are often used in attempts to partition out the influence of body size on performance outputs. The aim of the current study was to develop and cross-validate a new model to predict lower limbs LST in boys aged 10–13 years, using dual-energy X-ray absorptiometry (DXA) as the reference method. Total body and segmental (lower limbs) composition were assessed with a Hologic Explorer-W QDR DXA scanner in a cross-sectional sample of 75 Portuguese boys (144.8±6.4 cm; 40.2±9.0 kg). Skinfolds were measured at the anterior and posterior mid-thigh, and medial calf. Circumferences were measured at the proximal, mid and distal thigh. Leg length was estimated as stature minus sitting height. Current stature expressed as a percentage of attained predicted mature stature (PMS) was used as an estimate of biological maturity status. Backward proportional allometric models were used to identify the model with the best statistical fit: ln (lower limbs LST) $=0.838\times$ ln (body mass) $+0.476\times$ ln (leg length) $-$ $0.135\times$ ln (mid-thigh circumference) $-$ $0.053\times$ ln (anterior mid-thigh skinfold) $-$ $0.098\times$ ln (medial calf skinfold) $-$ $2.680+0.010\times$ (percentage of attained PMS) ($R=0.95$). The obtained equation was cross-validated using the predicted residuals sum of squares statistics (PRESS) method ($R^2_{PRESS}=0.90$). Deming repression analysis between predicted and current lower limbs LST showed a standard error of estimation of 0.52 kg (95% limits of agreement: 0.77 to -1.27 kg). The new model accurately predicts lower limbs LST in circumpubertal boys.

Editor: Amarjit Singh Virdi, Rush University Medical Center, United States of America

Funding: Authors were partially supported by the Portuguese Foundation for Science and Technology (SFRH/BD/64648/2009; PTDC/DTP-DES/1178/2012) and CAPES (BEX0951/10-2). No other current funding sources for this study. The funders had no role in study design, data collection and analysis, decision to publish, or preparation of the manuscript.

Competing Interests: The authors have declared that no competing interests exist.

* Email: mjcesilva@hotmail.com

Introduction

Skeletal muscle mass in the lower extremities is well correlated with a variety of fitness measures in pediatric physiology and health and exercise research [1–6]. Oxygen uptake is probably the most frequently reported physical capacity measurement in children and, for example, is not clear what the pattern of change with age or maturation is once values are dimensionally scaled [7,8]. In heterogeneous samples of boys and men, it has been demonstrated that estimates of lower leg muscle [3] or thigh muscle [6] volume are more relevant allometric scaling denominators for partitioning out the influence of body size on peak oxygen uptake than either body mass or fat-free mass.

Early dissection studies have indicated that the muscles in the lower extremities increase their relative contribution to total muscle mass from about 40% at birth to 55% at maturity [9]. Other studies of regional variation in skeletal muscle were based on radiography and limited largely to the arm and calf [10]. Boys gain about 30% in calf muscle mass width during adolescence [10], but more recent imaging techniques have not yet been used systematically to address this issue in youth.

Multi-scan magnetic resonance imaging (MRI) and computerized axial tomography (CT) are considered the "criterion" methods for evaluating skeletal muscle mass [11]. MRI is not widely available for use in research and clinical practice while CT includes exposure to radiation which limits its application in children and adolescents [12]. Other approaches to estimate skeletal muscle mass, include total-body potassium [13] and bioelectrical impedance [14]. Densitometric techniques rely on specific assumptions concerning the density of fat-free mass (1.1 g/mL) which is assumed to be stable in adults but may vary considerably in children by age, gender, maturity status and perhaps ethnicity [15,16]. The estimated density of fat-free mass increases from 1.0826 to 1.1013 g/mL in boys from 4 to 23 years [17]. Dual-energy X-ray absorptiometry (DXA) is a non-invasive protocol with a minimal radiation dose (1 mSv or 1/100th of the equivalent radiation exposure of a chest x-ray) [18]. The DXA method provides total and lean soft tissue (LST) estimates of the extremities, and a large portion of total-body skeletal muscle is within the fat-free appendicular compartment [19]. DXA-determined appendicular LST has also been validated against criterion methods such as CT [20,21].

Though useful, the availability of DXA in field settings is limited. Estimates of LST based on anthropometry are thus potentially useful, especially among youth. A popular anthropometric method [22] characterizes the lower limb as the sum of six truncated cones based on lengths, circumferences and skinfold thicknesses. The method was originally developed among young adults (with 32 male and 15 female) and has been applied in children and adolescents [4,23,24]. Anthropometric models for appendicular LST (upper and lower limbs combined) in young athletes of both sexes have also been developed and cross-validated [25]. A recent attempt [26] to cross-validate the regression equation of Jones and Pearson [22] in youth (83 girls, 85 boys, 11.0±0.7 years) noted a significantly higher thigh volume with DXA (4.43±1.23 L) than with the anthropometric estimate (4.39±1.22 L). Addition of body mass and the sum of anterior and posterior thigh skinfolds to the model resulted in a new predictive equation ($R^2 = 0.95$). The available research has not systematically considered the potential contribution of biological maturation to inter-individual variability in total and lean soft tissues. Correlations between skeletal age and radiographic widths of upper arm and calf muscle increased from childhood (7–10 years, $r = 0.16$–0.18) to adolescence (11–16 years, $r = 0.51$–0.61) in boys; corresponding correlations in girls, on the other hand, increased with age for arm musculature (7–8 years, $r = 0.27$; 9–14 years, $r = 0.45$) but not for calf musculature (7–8 years, $r = 0.41$; 9–14 years, $r = 0.39$) [27]. The direction of correlations between skeletal age and arm and calf muscle widths in boys across chronological age (CA) groups suggests a need to consider inter-individual differences in maturity status in estimates of lower limbs LST in circumpubertal children. Allowing for the limited data on youth, the present study attempted to develop a non-invasive estimate of lower limbs LST in circumpubertal boys and to cross-validate the new model using DXA measures as the reference.

Materials and Methods

Ethics Statement

The study was approved by the Portuguese Foundation for Science and Technology [PTDC/DTP-DES/1178/2012] and by the scientific board of the Faculty of Human Kinetics at the Technical University of Lisbon. The study was conducted in accordance with the Declaration of Helsinki for human studies by the World Medical Association [28]. All participants, parents or legal guardians were informed about the objectives of the study and provided appropriate informed assent and written informed consent.

Participants

The present study is limited to healthy boys of European ancestry ($n = 75$), 10–13 years of age. Participants were recruited voluntarily from the school population in the Lisbon metropolitan area (Portugal).

Chronological Age and Anthropometry

Chronological age was calculated as the difference between date of birth and date of measurement. Anthropometry was performed by a single experienced observer following standard procedures [29]. Stature and sitting height were measured to the nearest 0.1 cm with a Harpenden stadiometer (model 98.603, Holtain Ltd, Crosswell, UK and Harpenden sitting height table, model 98.607, Holtain Ltd, Crosswell, UK, respectively) and body mass was measured to the nearest 0.1 kg using an electronic scale (Seca, Hamburg, Germany). Leg length was estimated as stature minus sitting height. Circumference at the gluteal furrow (highest possible horizontal circumference), mid-thigh (largest mid-thigh circumference) and distal thigh (minimum circumference above the knee) were measured on the right site of the body. Lengths between each circumference level were also measured to estimate total thigh length. Anterior and posterior mid-thigh and medial calf skinfolds were measured to the nearest mm using a Lange Caliper (Beta Technology, Ann Arbor, MI, USA). Technical errors of measurement were previously reported for the anthropometric dimensions [26] and all were well within the range of several health surveys in the United States and a variety of field surveys [30]. Mid-thigh circumference ($C_{m\text{-}t}$) was corrected for subcutaneous adipose tissue thickness [31]. The corrected mid-thigh circumference ($CC_{m\text{-}t}$) was calculated as $CC_{m\text{-}t} = C_{m\text{-}t} - \pi S$, where S stands for the skinfold measurement, which is assumed to be twice the subcutaneous adipose tissue thickness.

Biological Maturity

Chronological age, stature, and body mass of each boy and midparent stature were used to predict mature (adult) stature using the Khamis–Roche protocol [32]. Parent heights were extracted from national identification cards which included height measured to the nearest centimeter. Measurements were taken by experienced, but not necessarily trained observers. A similar protocol was used in previous studies [33,34]. The median error bound (median absolute deviation) between actual and predicted mature stature (PMS) at 18 years of age is 2.2 cm in boys [32]. Ages at attaining specific percentages of mature stature are related to ages at attaining specific skeletal ages and stages of puberty in boys followed longitudinally from late childhood through adolescence [35]. Percentage of attained PMS (% PMS) is also related to skeletal age in youth football (American) and soccer players of the same age range as the study sample [33,36]. Percentage of attained PMS was expressed as a *z*-score relative to age-specific (half-year intervals) means and standard deviations from the Berkeley Guidance Study [37]; the *z*-score (*z* PMS) was used as the indicator of maturity status for each boy.

Dual energy X-ray absorptiometry

A Hologic Explorer-W, fan-bean densitometer, software QDR for Windows version 12.4 (Hologic, Waltham, MA, USA) was used to perform whole body scans. The procedure also allows measurement of segmental composition: arm, leg and trunk. Daily calibration of the scanner was performed using a phantom spine containing composites of bone, fat and LST. Participants were positioned on the scanner bed according to manufacturer recommendations. A single lab technician positioned the participants and performed the scans according to the manual provided by the manufacturer. The lower limbs on each image were sectioned as follows: all tissue distal to a line drawn through and perpendicular to the axis of the femoral neck and angled with the pelvic brim to the phalange tips. Total lower limb composition was estimated by adding the mass of the left and right legs. Mean variation between measured and reconstructed absolute whole-body mass with DXA software was 0.9%. Based on test-retest in 10 individuals, the coefficients of variation for percent body fat and LST were 1.6% and 0.8%, respectively.

Statistical analyses

Visual inspections of data were made using stem-and-leaf diagram and box-and-whisker plots to examine central tendency, variability, distributions and potential outliers. Subsequently, Gaussian distribution of variables was confirmed with normal Q-Q plots, de-trended normal Q-Q plots and Kolmogorov-Smirnov (*K-S*) test with Lilliefors significance correction. Descriptive statistics were calculated for the total sample (mean, standard deviation and range).

A backward multiple linear regression on ln *y*, based on proportional allometric models [4,38], was used to fit the unknown parameters that best predict lower limb LST determined with DXA. Based on analytical [i.e., Pearson's product moment correlation coefficients ($r_{y,x}$) between lower limbs LST_{DXA} (*y*) with CA, maturity status and body descriptors (*x*)] and biological assumptions, the new model (NM) considered CA, CA^2, % PMS or *z* PMS as exponential terms in addition to body mass, leg length, C_{m-t}, stature × CC_{m-t}^2, anterior and posterior mid-thigh and medial calf skinfolds:

$$\begin{aligned}\ln(\text{lower limbs LST}) = k_1 \times \ln(\text{body mass}) \\ + \ldots k_7 \times \ln(\text{medial calf skinfold}) + a + \quad (1) \\ b_1 \times (CA) + b_2 \times (CA^2) + b_3 \times (\%\ \text{PMS}) + \ln\varepsilon\end{aligned}$$

A tolerance >0.10 and a variance inflation factor <10 was set to avoid collinearity between the explanatory variables [39].

The new model was internally cross-validated by using the predicted residuals sum of squares (PRESS) statistics method [40]. PRESS statistics uses all cases and is considered a statistical jackknife procedure [41]. The technique produces as many models as the number of cases. An independent model is obtained based on *n*-1 data subsets for each participant and this permits the determination of individual residuals. A PRESS residual for a given participant is the difference between the actual response of the left-out case and the predicted response. Prediction of the respective case involves a different prediction equation for a statistical fit that excludes the case [40]. Overall, the PRESS statistic is a function of the sum of squares (SS) of all residuals. The PRESS statistic is always higher than the error (i.e., SS) from MANOVA results. Alternative measures of model adequacy (R^2_{PRESS}) and standard error of estimation (SEE_{PRESS}) were also calculated [40].

Agreement between the reference method (lower limbs LST_{DXA}) and the estimation (lower limbs LST_{NM}) was assessed using Deming regression (i.e., least products regression method which accounts for the error of both *x* and *y* variables) and standard error of estimation ($S_{y \cdot x}$) [42]. Data were then visually inspected by plotting residuals (prediction errors) against predicted values. This plot is similar to the plot suggested by Bland and Altman [43], except that predicted values of lower limbs LST (using the new developed equation) are plotted on the *x*-axis rather than the average of predicted and measures of lower limbs LST [25]. To test for proportional bias, Bland and Altman [43] have recommended plotting error against the average of two the methods. Although they have demonstrated that this is correct when considering the agreement of two existing methods, Hopkins [44] has demonstrated that in criterion/reference validity studies this method will indicate positive proportional bias when no proportional bias exists. This is due to the mathematical relation that occurs when a method is calibrated against a reference using least-squares regression; only vertical error (error in predicting the criterion) is minimized around the regression slope [45]. If errors were associated with the magnitude of the values, heteroscedasticity was examined by calculating the correlation coefficients between the absolute differences and the predicted values of lower limbs LST. Constant error variance (homoscedasticity) can be assumed if the correlations approach zero [46,47]. Correlation coefficients were interpreted as follows: trivial ($r<0.1$), small ($0.1<r<0.3$) moderate ($0.3<r<0.5$), large ($0.5<r<0.7$), very large ($0.7<r<0.9$), nearly perfect ($r>0.9$) and perfect ($r=1$) [48]. Finally, if measurement differences were normally distributed, reliability was assessed on the original scale using the standard error of measurement and 95% limits of agreement [43].

Statistical analyses were performed using IBM SPSS version 19.0 software (SPSS, Inc., IBM Company; NY, USA), GraphPad Prism version 5.03 software (GraphPad Software, Inc.; La Jolla, CA, USA) and MedCalc version 12.2.1 software (MedCalc; Mariakerke, Belgium). Alpha level was set at 0.05.

Results

Descriptive statistics for CA, estimated maturity status and DXA body composition are summarized in Table 1. All variables fitted a normal distribution ($K\text{-}S=0.37$ to 1.18; $p>0.05$). Mean percentage of attained PMS (81.5±2.3%) for the present sample was equivalent of that of the sample on which the physical maturity-prediction protocol was based (81.6±1.2% at 11.0 years) [49]. The means and standard deviations for percent of total body fat_{DXA}, LST_{DXA}, lower limbs fat $percentage_{DXA}$ and lower limbs LST_{DXA} were 26.4 (±8.1%), 29.0 (±4.2 kg), 31.7 (±8.3%) and 10.0 (±1.7 kg), respectively.

Relationships between ln lower limbs LST_{DXA} and the chronovariables [i.e., CA, percent of attained PMS and z-score for age (% attained PMS)] are illustrated in Figure 1 (panels a–c). The relationship between CA and lower limbs LST_{DXA} is linear, while relationships between % PMS and *z* PMS with lower limbs LST_{DXA} are somewhat non-linear. The correlation between CA and lower limbs LST_{DXA} is 0.30, while the corresponding correlations for % PMS and *z* PMS are 0.71 and 0.62, respectively ($p<0.01$).

Anthropometric characteristics for the total sample, results of the Kolmogorov–Smirnov test, and bivariate correlations of anthropometry with CA and estimated maturity status are shown in Table 2. The current sample has a mean stature and mean body mass which approximate, respectively, the 56th and 60th age-specific percentiles for U.S. boys [50]. Correlations between CA and maturity status and anthropometric variables ranged from trivial ($r=0.01$) to very large ($r=0.73$), suggesting the possibility of collinearity occurrence between some exponential terms and body size descriptors.

Table 1. Descriptive statistics ($n = 75$) for chronological age, maturity status and body composition, and results of the Kolmogorov–Smirnov test for checking the normality of the distribution.

	Mean ± SD	Range (min – max)	Kolmogorov–Smirnov	
			Value	p
Chronological age (years)	11.12±0.69	10.27 to 13.08	1.18	0.12
Percentage of PMS (%)	81.5±2.3	77.3 to 90.3	0.70	0.72
z-score for PMS (*z* PMS)	0.04±0.92	−2.07 to 2.40	0.74	0.65
DXA total body				
BMD (g•cm^{-2})	0.84±0.06	0.69 to 0.96	0.37	0.99
BMC (kg)	1.22±0.17	0.86 to 1.66	0.55	0.93
Fat (%)	26.4±8.1	14.0 to 44.6	0.77	0.60
Fat (kg)	11.2±5.8	3.6 to 27.6	1.03	0.24
Lean soft tissue (kg)	29.0±4.2	20.7 to 39.8	0.73	0.66
DXA lower limbs				
BMD (g•cm^{-2})	0.84±0.07	0.68 to 1.04	0.51	0.96
BMC (kg)	0.44±0.08	0.30 to 0.68	0.87	0.43
Fat (%)	31.7±8.3	16.0 to 50.2	0.56	0.92
Fat (kg)	4.9±2.3	1.3 to 10.9	1.16	0.13
Lean soft tissue (kg)	10.0±1.7	6.9 to 13.9	0.74	0.64

Abbreviations: PMS, predicted mature stature; DXA, dual x-ray absorptiometry; BMD, bone mineral density; BMC, Bone mineral content.

The allometric regression model for the prediction of lower limbs LST is given in Table 3. The new model included ln body mass, ln leg length, ln mid-thigh circumference, ln anterior mid-thigh skinfold, ln medial calf skinfold and percent of attained PMS. Its association with lower limbs LST_{DXA} was nearly perfect ($R = 0.95$). The prediction equation was:

$$\begin{aligned}\ln(\text{lower limbs } LST_{DXA}) = {} & 0.838 \times \ln(\text{body mass}) + 0.476 \\ & \times \ln(\text{leg length}) - 0.135 \\ & \times \ln(\text{mid-thigh circumference}) \\ & - 0.053 \times \ln(\text{anterior mid-thigh skinfold}) \\ & - 0.098 \times \ln(\text{medial calf skinfold}) \\ & - 2.680 + 0.010 \times (\%\ \text{PMS})\end{aligned} \quad (2)$$

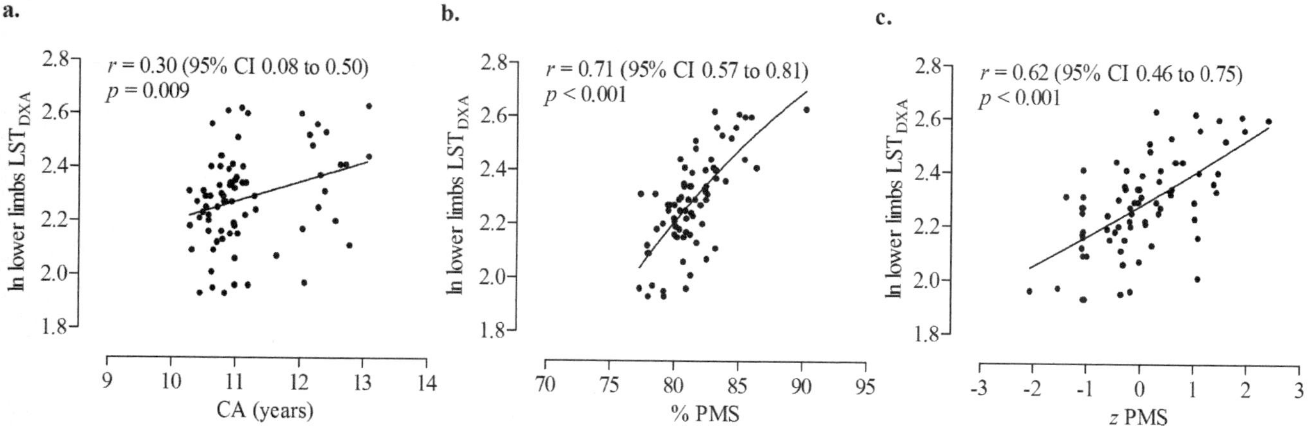

Figure 1. Relationship of the ln transformed lower limbs lean soft tissue (LST_{DXA}) with chronological age (CA, panel a), percentage of predicted mature stature attained at the time of study (% PMS, panel b), and *z*-score for % PMS (*z* PMS, panel c).

Table 2. Descriptive statistics ($n = 75$) for anthropometric variables, results of the Kolmogorov–Smirnov test for checking the normality of the distribution, and bivariate correlations of anthropometry with chronological age and maturity status.

	Mean ± SD	Range (min – max)	Kolmogorov–Smirnov		Correlation					
					CA		% PMS		*z* PMS	
			Value	*p*	*r*	95% CI	*r*	95% CI	*r*	95% CI
Stature (cm)	144.8±6.4	127.9 to 163.5	0.52	0.95	0.36	0.15 to 0.55	0.73	0.60 to 0.82	0.58	0.41 to 0.71
Body mass (kg)	40.2±9.0	24.4 to 66.5	1.17	0.13	0.15	−0.01 to 0.37	0.64	0.48 to 0.76	0.71	0.57 to 0.81
Lengths (cm)										
Leg	69.6±4.2	60.2 to 78.5	0.43	0.99	0.34	0.13 to 0.53	0.63	0.47 to 0.75	0.49	0.30 to 0.65
Thigh	27.8±3.9	17.3 to 36.2	0.58	0.89	0.12	−0.11 to 0.34	0.15	−0.08 to 0.36	0.06	−0.17 to 0.29
Circumferences (cm)										
Proximal thigh	46.8±6.2	36.5 to 66.7	0.97	0.30	0.05	−0.18 to 0.27	0.54	0.35 to 0.68	0.68	0.54 to 0.79
Mid-thigh	41.3±5.4	26.0 to 54.0	0.85	0.47	0.16	−0.08 to 0.37	0.52	0.33 to 0.67	0.54	0.35 to 0.68
Distal thigh	34.3±4.4	27.5 to 47.0	1.19	0.12	0.01	−0.22 to 0.23	0.47	0.27 to 0.63	0.64	0.49 to 0.76
Skinfold thickness (mm)										
Anterior mid-thigh	21±8	7 to 42	0.85	0.47	−0.19	−0.40 to 0.04	0.21	−0.02 to 0.41	0.51	0.32 to 0.66
Posterior mid-thigh	18±8	6 to 37	1.09	0.19	−0.07	−0.30 to 0.16	0.31	0.09 to 0.50	0.53	0.34 to 0.68
Medial calf	14±6	4 to 28	1.11	0.17	−0.04	−0.27 to 0.19	0.41	0.20 to 0.58	0.62	0.46 to 0.74

Abbreviations: CA, Chronological age; PMS, predicted mature stature; *r*, Pearson's product moment correlation coefficient; 95% CI, 95% confidence interval.

Equation (2) (new model) was validated using PRESS statistics (Table 3). The high R^2 (0.90) and low SEE (0.27) emphasize the accuracy of the model.

Deming repression analysis between predicted and measured lower limbs LST showed that the new model had an $R^2 = 0.91$ and a $S_{y \cdot x}$ of 0.52 kg (Figure 2, panel a). The intercept (−0.62, 95% CI −1.40 to 0.17) and slope (1.04, 95% CI 0.96 to 1.11) of the equation did not significantly differ ($p>0.05$) from the identity line (i.e., y-intercept $=0$ when $x=0$ and slope $=1$). Therefore, the possibility of systematic or proportional bias was rejected [51]. The relation between residuals and predicted lower limbs LST values is illustrated in Figure 2 (panel b). No significant mean differences between predicted and measured values and small limits of agreement were found (bias ±1.96 SD = −0.25±1.02 kg, $p>0.05$). The measurement differences (error) relative to predicted lower limbs LST were homoscedastic [46,47], which was confirmed by the correlation ($r=0.09$, $p=0.398$) between the absolute differences and the predicted lower limbs LST values [52].

Discussion

The data detailed total body and segmental (lower limbs) LST in healthy circumpubertal boys in the context of developing and cross-validating a model that included anthropometric dimensions and a non-invasive estimate of maturity status among predictors of lower limbs LST relative to DXA as the reference method. Allometric modeling identified biological maturity status, anterior mid-thigh and medial calf skinfolds, mid-thigh circumference, leg length and body mass among significant predictors of lower limbs LST. The new model showed was valid and non-biased, and accurately predicted lower limbs LST as evident in a nearly perfect correlation between the new model and DXA, an intercept and slope that did not differ from the identity line, small limits of agreement, and errors independent of the magnitude of the values. The equation also had a high R^2_{PRESS} and low SEE_{PRESS}. To our knowledge, this is the first study that obtained and cross-validated an equation to estimate lower limbs LST based on anthropometry and estimated maturity status in circumpubertal boys.

Appendicular skeletal muscle mass can be obtained from DXA [25,53–55] by assuming that all non-bone and non-fat tissue is muscle mass [19]. This assumption is likely to be valid in the legs [56,57] and is most likely to be valid at the regions between the joints such as the mid-thigh and the calf, where the amount of tendons and cartilage is small [20]. Nearly perfect correlations ($r=0.98$–0.99) between appendicular LST assessed by DXA and skeletal muscle mass determined by MRI were noted in a multi-ethnic adolescents and children, consistent with these assumptions [58]. Total body LST of the present sample of boys 11.0±0.5 years was less (29.0±4.2 kg) than that of young boys 13.7±3.0 years (38.1±12.7 kg) [59], reflecting age and body size variation (stature: 144.8±6.4 kg *vs.* 158.1±17.7 cm; body mass: 40.2±9.0 kg *vs.* 50.2±17.4 kg, respectively).

DXA measurements of LST, body fat and bone mineral content were made independently, each with potential measurement error. In the present sample, the difference between whole body DXA mass and scale mass was 0.4 kg (0.9%). Although hydration was not controlled, minimal effects are expected since it has been shown that a subtraction or addition to the Reference Man of 1 kg in extracellular fluid would result in roughly a 0.6% over- or underestimation to total body fat mass using DXA [60]. Errors in the lower limbs LST prediction equation may be attributed in part to the use of skinfolds as predictor variables. The use of skinfold thickness measurements to estimate human body composition is

Table 3. Proportional multiplicative allometric regression model and internal cross-validation for the prediction of DXA-measured lower limbs lean soft tissue*.

Predictors						Model summary			
y	x_i	β Unstandardized	95% CI	Tolerance	VIF	R	SEE	Cross-validation	
								R^2_{PRESS}	SEE_{PRESS}
ln (lower limbs LST_{DXA})	Constant	−2.680	−4.308 to −1.052						
	ln (body mass)	0.838	0.616 to 1.061	0.231	4.332				
	ln (leg length)	0.476	0.067 to 0.884	0.540	1.853				
	ln (mid-thigh circumference)	−0.135	−0.412 to 0.143	0.219	4.568				
	ln (anterior mid-thigh skinfold)	−0.053	−0.129 to 0.024	0.306	3.264				
	ln (medial calf skinfold)	−0.098	−0.176 to 0.020	0.347	2.878				
	% PMS	0.010	−0.002 to 0.021	0.480	2.084				
						0.95	0.07	0.90	0.27

Abbreviations: 95% CI, 95% confidence intervals; VIF, variance inflation factors; LST, lean soft tissue; DXA, dual x-ray absorptiometry; % PMS, percentage of attained predicted mature stature.

*$\ln(\text{lower limbs } LST_{DXA}) = k_1 \times \ln(\text{body mass}) + k_2 \times \ln(\text{leg length}) + k_3 \times \ln(\text{mid-thigh circumference}) + k_4 \times \ln(\text{anterior mid-thigh skinfold}) + k_5 \times \ln(\text{medial calf skinfold}) + a + b \times (\% PMS) + \ln \varepsilon$.

based on two assumptions [61]: the thickness of the subcutaneous adipose tissue reflects a constant proportion of total body fat, and that the sites selected for measurement represent the average thickness of the subcutaneous adipose. Neither assumption, however, has been shown to be consistently generalized [62]. Skinfolds were performed by a single experienced observer following standard procedures [29], in the present study, and intra-observer technical errors of measurement (~0.7 mm) and coefficients of variation (3.7–4.7%) were small [26].

There is no direct measure of leg length [63]. Jones and Pearson [22] measured leg as the length from the ground to the gluteal furrow. In the present study, leg length was estimated as the difference between stature and sitting height. In the DXA protocol, the leg length was defined as the mass of tissue distal to an oblique line passing through the neck of the femur, excluding gluteal muscles.

Leg circumferences were identified as suitable predictor variables. Although the correlation between stature × $CC_{m\text{-}t}^2$ with lower limbs LST_{DXA} was relatively high ($r = 0.72$, $p<0.001$), the interaction term was not a significant predictor of lower limbs LST_{NM}. On the other hand, two studies [25,31] suggested that the square of each corrected muscle girth multiplied by stature is the anthropometric parameter that contributed most to appendicular LST and skeletal muscle mass variance. The discrepancy among results and contribution of corrected muscle circumferences and stature (components of the cylinder's dimensions of the skeletal muscle mass of the human body) may be due to the considerably larger appendicular LST of young athletes [25] and non-obese adults [31] compared to this circumpubertal sample.

The adolescent growth spurt in stature starts, on average, at about 10–11 years of age in boys and reaches peak velocity (age at peak height velocity, PHV) at about 14 years [27]. Predicted time from PHV (erroneously labeled PHV), based on sex-specific anthropometric equations [64], was a significant predictor of total body LST in boys 8–18 years of age [59]. Note, however, predicted years from PHV and in turn age at PHV in boys is dependent on CA at prediction and actual age at PHV in an independent longitudinal sample of boys followed from 8 to 18 years; predicted age at PHV also has a reduced range of variation compared to actual age at PHV [65]. Identical results have been reported for an independent longitudinal sample of girls, highlighting the limitations of the prediction protocol [66]. Given the confounding effect of CA per se on the estimate of maturity timing, it is likely the effect attributed to years from PHV is due largely to CA.

Sexual maturation, based on a five stage scale using the criteria described by Tanner [67], have been considered in studies of skeletal muscle mass in boys 5–17 years [58] and appendicular LST in adolescent athletes 14–17 years [25]. Stages of secondary sex characteristics, though valuable, have limitations analytically. They indicate stage at the time of observation and do not indicate when the stage was entered or how long the individual has been in a stage. Moreover, stages of pubic hair and genital development in boys (or pubic hair and breast stages in girls) are not equivalent [27]. The present study used a non-invasive indicator of maturity status, percentage of predicted mature (adult) stature (% PMS) attained at the time of observation. Results indicated a significant and positive contribution of individual differences in % PMS to the prediction of lower limbs LST.

Although advances in technology permit accurate assessments of segmental tissue mass in vivo, assessments are limited largely to clinical or laboratory settings and are expensive. There is an interest for methods that provide information in a safe, cost-effective and non-invasive manner, and in a non-laboratory setting. The present study offers an equation that compares favorably with those reported in the literature for similar purposes [6,25,26,31,68]. No significant mean differences between measured and predicted lower limbs LST were observed, and the robustness of the model was not compromised by multicollinearity between independent variables. Tolerance (0.22–0.54) and a variance inflation factors (1.85–4.57) were well within the normal ranges (>0.10, <10, respectively) [39]. The adopted method of cross-validation [40] confirmed the effectiveness of the model to predict lower limbs LST with a high internal validity ($R^2_{PRESS} = 0.90$) and low proportional errors of estimation ($SEE_{PRESS} = 0.27$). The PRESS method avoids data-splitting difficulties and provides similar unbiased estimates of future prediction equation performance.

It was deemed important to maintain an appropriate participant-to-variable ratio. In multiple regressions, that ratio was

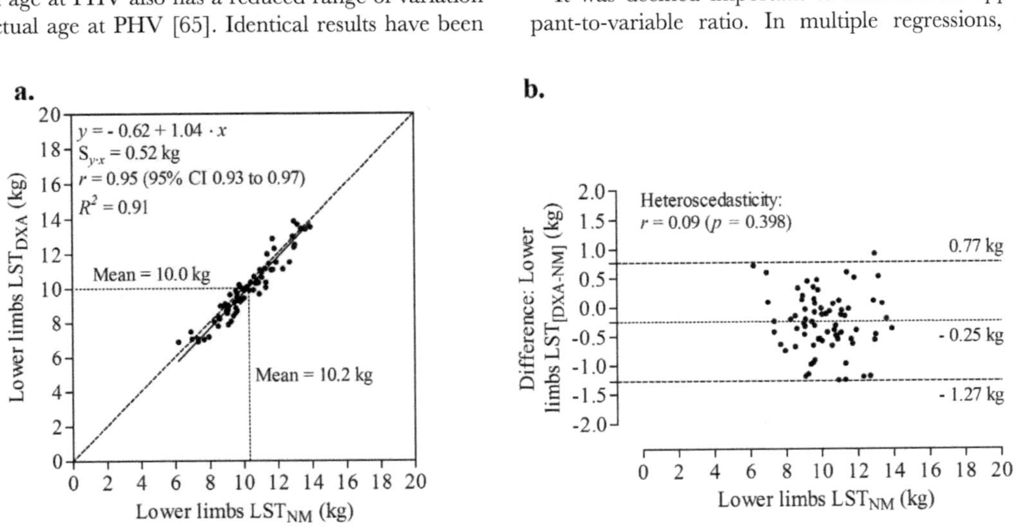

Figure 2. Deming regression analysis between the new anthropometric model (NM) and lower limbs lean soft tissue (LST) measured by dual-energy X-ray absorptiometry (panel a). The reference line from the equation, standard error of estimation ($S_{y \cdot x}$), correlation (r) and coefficient of determination (R^2), are also presented. The right panel (panel b) illustrate the relation between residuals (mean differences between lower limbs LST measured by DXA and predicted by the derived equation) and lower limbs LST_{NM} (heteroscedasticity diagnostic). The dashed lines represent 95% limits of agreement (±1.96 SD).

recommended to be higher than 5:1 and preferably 20:1 [69]. The present ratio was ~13:1. Moreover, it is established that PRESS statistics usually generates less confident estimates of an equation's potential [40]. The least products regression (Deming regression), where random errors in both dependent and independent variables are accommodated in the regression model [42], was used as an alternative to the ordinary least squares method. The new model ($R^2 = 0.91$ and a $S_{y \cdot x}$ of 0.52 kg) did not presented systematic or proportional bias as the equation did not differ significantly from the identity line [51]. Lastly, the measurement differences (error) against the predicted lower limbs LST values were homoscedastic ($r = 0.09$, $p = 0.398$) [46,47], allowing the use of this equation with constant error variance.

Although the current investigation has a number of strengths (e.g., objective measures, analytical procedures), it is not without limitations. First, the method for estimating maturity status was non-invasive, but the prediction equation was based on middle socio-economic class American youth of White/European ancestry in the Fels Longitudinal Study [32]. Validation of the equations in Portuguese youth is needed. Second, the study was limited to a cross-sectional sample of healthy circumpubertal Portuguese boys 10–13 years of age and prediction equations tend to be age and population specific. Additional validation studies are needed to critically validate this model in other samples (e.g., mid- and late-adolescents, youth of other ethnic groups, or specific populations with varying anthropometric characteristics).

Conclusions

In summary, a new model derived from anthropometric variables and maturity status was proposed for assessing lower limbs LST in research dealing with circumpubertal boys. The equation was satisfactorily cross-validated at group and individual basis, ensuring its applicability to similar samples. However, it is important to note that when an equation is applied to groups the associated errors will be always smaller than those for individuals. This equation will allow accurate lower limbs-specific mass information, thus offering a valid alternative to scan participants with technologies such as DXA.

Acknowledgments

The authors gratefully acknowledge the effort of the participants and their parents. The early contribution of Filipe Simões († 2013) in the current project is remembered.

Author Contributions

Conceived and designed the experiments: MJCS JVS MTEG RMM CM LBS. Performed the experiments: ELP CM AMS FB. Analyzed the data: JVS MJCS AMMR MTEG RMM AMS. Contributed reagents/materials/analysis tools: ELP CM AMS FB LBS. Contributed to the writing of the manuscript: JVS MJCS AMMR MTEG RMM ELP CM AMS FB LBS. Intellectual relevant input and critical revision: JVS MJCS AMMR MTEG RMM ELP CM AMS FB LBS. Final approval of the version to be published: JVS MJCS AMMR MTEG RMM ELP CM AMS FB LBS.

References

1. Davies CT, Barnes C, Godfrey S (1972) Body composition and maximal exercise performance in children. Hum Biol 44: 195–214.
2. Docherty D, Gaul CA (1991) Relationship of body size, physique, and composition to physical performance in young boys and girls. Int J Sports Med 12: 525–532.
3. Tolfrey K, Barker A, Thom JM, Morse CI, Narici MV, et al. (2006) Scaling of maximal oxygen uptake by lower leg muscle volume in boys and men. J Appl Physiol 100: 1851–1856.
4. Valente-Dos-Santos J, Sherar L, Coelho-e-Silva MJ, Pereira JR, Vaz V, et al. (2013) Allometric scaling of peak oxygen uptake in male roller hockey players under 17 years old. Appl Physiol Nutr Metab 38: 390–395.
5. Van Praagh E, Fellmann N, Bedu M, Falgairette G, Coudert J (1990) Gender difference in the relationship of anaerobic power output to body composition in children. Pediatr Exerc Sci 2: 336–348.
6. Welsman JR, Armstrong N, Kirby BJ, Winsley RJ, Parsons G, et al. (1997) Exercise performance and magnetic resonance imaging-determined thigh muscle volume in children. Eur J Appl Physiol O 76: 92–97.
7. Armstrong N (2013) Aerobic fitness and physical activity in children. Pediatr Exerc Sci 25: 548–560.
8. Kemper HC, Twisk JW, Van Mechelen W (2013) Changes in aerobic fitness in boys and girls over a period of 25 years: data from the Amsterdam Growth and Health Longitudinal Study revisited and extended. Pediatr Exerc Sci 25: 524–535.
9. Scammon RE (1923) A summary of the anatomy of the infant and child. In: Abt IA, editor. Pediatrics. Philadelphia: Saunders. 257–444.
10. Malina RM (1996) Regional body composition: age, sex, and ethnic variation. In: Roche AF, Heymsfield SB, Lohman TG, editors. Human body composition. Champaign, IL: Human Kinetics. 217–255.
11. Lee SY, Gallagher D (2008) Assessment methods in human body composition. Curr Opin Clin Nutr Metab Care 11: 566–572.
12. Lee RC, Wang ZM, Heymsfield SB (2001) Skeletal muscle mass and aging: regional and whole-body measurement methods. Can J Appl Physiol 26: 102–122.
13. Wang Z, Zhu S, Wang J, Pierson RN, Heymsfield SB (2003) Whole-body skeletal muscle mass: development and validation of total-body potassium prediction models. Am J Clin Nutr 77: 76–82.
14. Salinari S, Bertuzzi A, Mingrone G, Capristo E, Pietrobelli A, et al. (2002) New bioimpedance model accurately predicts lower limb muscle volume: validation by magnetic resonance imaging. Am J Physiol Endocrinol Metab 282: E960–966.
15. Wells JC, Fuller NJ, Dewit O, Fewtrell MS, Elia M, et al. (1999) Four-component model of body composition in children: density and hydration of fat-free mass and comparison with simpler models. Am J Clin Nutr 69: 904–912.
16. Lohman TG (1986) Applicability of body composition techniques and constants for children and youths. Exerc Sport Sci Rev 14: 325–357.
17. Wells JC, Williams JE, Chomtho S, Darch T, Grijalva-Eternod C, et al. (2010) Pediatric reference data for lean tissue properties: density and hydration from age 5 to 20 y. Am J Clin Nutr 91: 610–618.
18. Goran MI (1998) Measurement issues related to studies of childhood obesity: assessment of body composition, body fat distribution, physical activity, and food intake. Pediatrics 101: 505–518.
19. Heymsfield SB, Smith R, Aulet M, Bensen B, Lichtman S, et al. (1990) Appendicular skeletal muscle mass: measurement by dual-photon absorptiometry. Am J Clin Nutr 52: 214–218.
20. Visser M, Fuerst T, Lang T, Salamone L, Harris TB (1999) Validity of fan-beam dual-energy X-ray absorptiometry for measuring fat-free mass and leg muscle mass. Health, aging, and body composition study-dual-energy x-ray absorptiometry and body composition working group. J Appl Physiol 87: 1513–1520.
21. Wang ZM, Visser M, Ma R, Baumgartner RN, Kotler D, et al. (1996) Skeletal muscle mass: evaluation of neutron activation and dual-energy X-ray absorptiometry methods. J Appl Physiol 80: 824–831.
22. Jones PR, Pearson J (1969) Anthropometric determination of leg fat and muscle plus bone volumes in young male and female adults. J Physiol 204: 63–66.
23. Dore E, Bedu M, Franca NM, Van Praagh E (2001) Anaerobic cycling performance characteristics in prepubescent, adolescent and young adult females. Eur J Appl Physiol 84: 476–481.
24. Martin RJ, Dore E, Twisk J, van Praagh E, Hautier CA, et al. (2004) Longitudinal changes of maximal short-term peak power in girls and boys during growth. Med Sci Sport Exer 36: 498–503.
25. Quiterio AL, Carnero EA, Silva AM, Bright BC, Sardinha LB (2009) Anthropometric models to predict appendicular lean soft tissue in adolescent athletes. Med Sci Sport Exer 41: 828–836.
26. Coelho-e-Silva MJ, Malina RM, Simoes F, Valente-Dos-Santos J, Martins RA, et al. (2013) Determination of thigh volume in youth with anthropometry and DXA: Agreement between estimates. Eur J Appl Physiol 13: 527–533.
27. Malina R, Bouchard C, Bar-Or O (2004) Growth, maturation, and physical activity. Champaign, IL: Human Kinetics. 728.
28. World Medical Association (2008) Declaration of Helsinki: ethical principles for medical research involving human subjects. WMJ 54: 122–125.
29. Lohman TG, Roche AF, Martorell R (1988) Anthropometric standardization reference manual. Champaign, IL: Human Kinetics. 177.
30. Malina RM (1995) Anthropometry. In: Maud PJ, Foster C, editors. Physiological assessment of human fitness. Champaign, IL: Human Kinetics. 205–219.
31. Lee RC, Wang Z, Heo M, Ross R, Janssen I, et al. (2000) Total-body skeletal muscle mass: development and cross-validation of anthropometric prediction models. Am J Clin Nutr 72: 796–803.
32. Khamis HJ, Roche AF (1994) Predicting adult stature without using skeletal age: the Khamis-Roche method. Pediatrics 94: 504–507.
33. Malina RM, Coelho-E-Silva MJ, Figueiredo AJ, Carling C, Beunen GP (2012) Interrelationships among invasive and non-invasive indicators of biological maturation in adolescent male soccer players. J Sports Sci 30: 1705–1717.

34. Padez C (2003) Secular trend in stature in the Portuguese population (1904–2000). Ann Hum Biol 30: 262–278.
35. Bielicki T, Koniarek J, Malina RM (1984) Interrelationships among certain measures of growth and maturation rate in boys during adolescence. Ann Hum Biol 11: 201–210.
36. Malina RM, Dompier TP, Powell JW, Barron MJ, Moore MT (2007) Validation of a noninvasive maturity estimate relative to skeletal age in youth football players. Clin J Sport Med 17: 362–368.
37. Bayley N, Pinneau SR (1952) Tables for predicting adult height from skeletal age: revised for use with the Greulich-Pyle hand standards. Journal Pediatr 40: 423–441.
38. Nevill A, Holder R (1994) Modelling maximum oxygen uptake: a case study in non-linear regression model formulation and comparison. J Roy Statistical Society 43: 653–666.
39. Slinker BK, Glantz SA (1985) Multiple regression for physiological data analysis: the problem of multicollinearity. Am J Physiol 249: R1–12.
40. Holiday DB, Ballard JE, McKeown BC (1995) PRESS-related statistics: regression tools for cross-validation and case diagnostics. Med Sci Sport Exer 27: 612–620.
41. Hinkley DV (1977) Jackknifing in unbalanced situations. Technometrics 19: 285–292.
42. Ricker WE (1973) Linear regressions in fishery research. J Fish Res Board Can 30: 409–434.
43. Bland JM, Altman DG (2012) Agreed statistics: measurement method comparison. Anesthesiology 116: 182–185.
44. Hopkins WG (2004) Bias in Bland-Altman but not regression validity analysis. Sportscience 8: 42–46.
45. Evans EM, Rowe DA, Misic MM, Prior BM, Arngrimsson SA (2005) Skinfold prediction equation for athletes developed using a four-component model. Med Sci Sports Exerc 37: 2006–2011.
46. Batterham AM, George KP, Mullineaux DR (1997) Allometric scaling of left ventricular mass by body dimensions in males and females. Med Sci Sport Exer 29: 181–186.
47. Nevill AM, Ramsbottom R, Williams C (1992) Scaling physiological measurements for individuals of different body size. Eur J Appl Physiol O 65: 110–117.
48. Hopkins WG, Marshall SW, Batterham AM, Hanin J (2009) Progressive statistics for studies in sports medicine and exercise science. Med Sci Sport Exer 41: 3–13.
49. Roche AF, Tyleshevski F, Rogers E (1983) Non-invasive measurement of physical maturity in children. Res Q Exerc Sport 54: 364–361.
50. Kuczmarski RJ, Ogden CL, Grummer-Strawn LM, Flegal KM, Mei Z, et al. (2002) 2000 CDC growth charts for the United States: methods and development. Vital Health Stat 11: 1–186.
51. Ludbrook J (2002) Statistical techniques for comparing measurers and methods of measurement: a critical review. Clin Exp Pharmacol Physiol 29: 527–536.
52. Nevill AM, Atkinson G (1997) Assessing agreement between measurements recorded on a ratio scale in sports medicine and sports science. Br J Sports Med 31: 314–318.
53. Ellis KJ (2000) Human body composition: in vivo methods. Physiol Rev 80: 649–680.
54. Kulkarni B, Kuper H, Taylor A, Wells JC, Radhakrishna KV, et al. (2013) Development and validation of anthropometric prediction equations for estimation of lean body mass and appendicular lean soft tissue in Indian men and women. J Appl Physiol 115: 1156–1162.
55. Leahy S, O'Neill C, Sohun R, Jakeman P (2012) A comparison of dual energy X-ray absorptiometry and bioelectrical impedance analysis to measure total and segmental body composition in healthy young adults. Eur J Appl Physiol 112: 589–595.
56. Heymsfield SB, Wang Z, Baumgartner RN, Ross R (1997) Human body composition: advances in models and methods. Annu Rev Nutr 17: 527–558.
57. Snyder WS, Cook MJ, Nasset ES, Karhausen RL, Howells GP, et al. (1975) Report of the Task Group on reference man. ICRP Publication 23. Oxford: Pergamon Press. 40–45.
58. Kim J, Shen W, Gallagher D, Jones A, Wang Z, et al. (2006) Total-body skeletal muscle mass: estimation by dual-energy X-ray absorptiometry in children and adolescents. Am J Clin Nutr 84: 1014–1020.
59. Machado D, Oikawa S, Barbanti V (2013) The multicomponent anthropometric model for assessing body composition in a male pediatric population: a simultaneous prediction of fat mass, bone mineral content, and lean soft tissue. J Obes 2013: e428135.
60. Pietrobelli A, Formica C, Wang Z, Heymsfield SB (1996) Dual-energy X-ray absorptiometry body composition model: review of physical concepts. Am J - Physiol 271: E941–951.
61. Holmes JD, Andrews DM, Durkin JL, Dowling JJ (2005) Predicting in vivo soft tissue masses of the lower extremity using segment anthropometric measures and DXA. J Appl Biomech 21: 371–382.
62. Lukaski HC (1987) Methods for the assessment of human body composition: traditional and new. Am J Clin Nutr 46: 537–556.
63. Martin AD, Carter JE, Hendy KC, Malina RM (1998) Segment lengths. In: Lohman TG, Roche AF, Martorell R, editors. Anthropometric standardization reference manual. Champaign, IL: Human Kinetics. pp. 9–26.
64. Mirwald RL, Baxter-Jones AD, Bailey DA, Beunen GP (2002) An assessment of maturity from anthropometric measurements. Med Sci Sports Exerc 34: 689–694.
65. Malina RM, Kozieł SM (2014) Validation of maturity offset in a longitudinal sample of Polish boys. J Sports Sci 32: 424–437.
66. Malina RM, Kozieł SM (2014) Validation of maturity offset in a longitudinal sample of Polish girls. J Sports Sci. Doi: 10.1080/02640414.2014.889846
67. Tanner JM (1962) Growth at adolescence. Oxford: Blackwell. 325.
68. Fuller NJ, Fewtrell MS, Dewit O, Elia M, Wells JC (2002) Segmental bioelectrical impedance analysis in children aged 8–12 y: The assessment of regional body composition and muscle mass. Int J Obes Relat Metab Disord 26: 692–700.
69. Vincent WJ (2005) Statistics in Kinesiology. Champaign, IL: Human Kinetics. 511.

13

Vitamin D Supplementation Enhances the Fixation of Titanium Implants in Chronic Kidney Disease Mice

Weiqing Liu[1], Shiwen Zhang[1], Dan Zhao[1], Huawei Zou[1], Ningyuan Sun[1], Xing Liang[1], Michel Dard[2], Beate Lanske[3], Quan Yuan[1]*

1 State Key Laboratory of Oral Diseases, West China Hospital of Stomatology, Sichuan University, Chengdu, China, **2** Department of Periodontology and Implant Dentistry, New York University College of Dentistry, New York, United States of America, **3** Department of Oral Medicine, Infection, and Immunity, Harvard School of Dental medicine, Boston, Massachusetts, United States of America

Abstract

Vitamin D (Vit D) deficiency is a common condition in chronic kidney disease (CKD) patients that negatively affects bone regeneration and fracture healing. Previous study has shown that timely healing of titanium implants is impaired in CKD. This study aimed to investigate the effect of Vit D supplementation on implant osseointegration in CKD mice. Uremia was induced by 5/6 nephrectomy in C57BL mice. Eight weeks after the second renal surgery, animals were given 1,25(OH)$_2$D$_3$ three times a week intraperitoneally for four weeks. Experimental titanium implants were inserted into the distal end of femurs two weeks later. Serum measurements confirmed decreased 1,25(OH)$_2$D levels in CKD mice, which could be successfully corrected by Vit D injections. Moreover, the hyperparathyroidism observed in CKD mice was also corrected. X-ray examination and histological sections showed successful osseointegration in these mice. Histomorphometrical analysis revealed that the bone-implant contact (BIC) ratio and bone volume (BV/TV) around the implant were significantly increased in the Vit D-supplementation group. In addition, resistance of the implant, as measured by a push-in method, was significantly improved compared to that in the vehicle group. These results demonstrate that Vit D supplementation is an effective approach to improve the fixation of titanium implants in CKD.

Editor: Emmanuel A. Burdmann, University of Sao Paulo Medical School, Brazil

Funding: This work was supported by grants from the National Natural Science Foundation of China (NSFC 81371173), New Century Excellent Talents in University (NCET-12-0379) and International Team of Implantology (ITI 717_2010) to Q.Y., and the National Institute of Diabetes and Digestive and Kidney Diseases (NIDDK, R01-073944) to B.L. The funders had no role in study design, data collection and analysis, decision to publish, or preparation of the manuscript.

Competing Interests: The authors have declared that no competing interests exist.

* E-mail: yuanquan@scu.edu.cn

Introduction

Chronic kidney disease (CKD) is recognized as a global public health threat. It is a highly prevalent disease with severe complications, such as cardiovascular disease and chronic kidney disease-mineral and bone disorders (CKD-MBD) [1–3]. Screening conducted by nephrologists from all over the world indicates that the incidence of CKD is increasing with ranges of 10.2% to 20% of the population [4–7]. According to a recent cross-sectional survey in China, the prevalence of CKD adults was 10.8%, which means that approximately 119.5 million people are affected by CKD in this rapidly developing country [8].

Declining renal function negatively affects the status of oral health. A recent systematic review showed that poor oral health is a common and often severe side-effect for adults with CKD [9]. Approximately 90% of CKD patients suffer from oral symptom-s,including both hard and soft tissues [10–14]. Studies have demonstrated that CKD profoundly influences bone remolding [15] and the structure of the mandible [16]. Furthermore, cross-sectional radiographic examinations indicate that CKD patients experience much more severe alveolar bone loss [17].

Although dental implants have been widely used in clinical settings, opinions regarding implants for CKD patients vary. Both the oral and nephrological literature suggests that dental implant surgery may be contraindicated in patients with significant renal osteodystrophy [18,19]. However, other investigations into the quantity and quality of the alveolar bone of dialysis patients showed that the residual bone volumes were adequate for implant insertion, suggesting this type of treatment is applicable to CKD patients [20]. Previously, we studied the effect of CKD on osseointegration of titanium implants using a uremic mouse model. Although all implants were able to be successfully integrated, CKD significantly decreased the bone-implant strength at an early stage in healing [21]. Therefore, enhancement of dental implant osseointegration in CKD patients remains a challenge.

Vitamin D deficiency is common in CKD patients [22–26] and this deficiency may negatively affect bone regeneration and fracture healing due to its importance in bone metabolism [27]. Low serum 1,25-dihydroxyvitamin D triggers higher levels of serum PTH [28,29], which in turn promotes high bone turnover, exacerbates osteopenia and finally results in cortical bone loss and pathogenesis of osteoporosis [30–32]. Kelly *et al.* [15] showed that vitamin D insufficiency impairs the osseointegration of Ti6Al4V implants in male Sprague-Dawley rats. Alvim-Pereira F *et al.* [33] observed no association between a vitamin D receptor polymorphism (rs731236, TaqI) and dental implant loss. On the other hand, vitamin D supplementation has demonstrated a significant survival advantage in CKD patients [25], and accelerated cellular events in the process of fracture healing [34]. These findings suggest a potentially beneficial role for vitamin D in promoting implant osseointegration in CKD patients. In this study, we established a CKD mouse model to investigate the effect of vitamin D supplementation on fixation of titanium implants. The results are expected to be a significant contribution to dental implant therapy in CKD patients.

Materials and Methods

Ethics Statement

This study was carried out in strict accordance with the recommendations contained in the Guide for the Care and Use of Laboratory Animals of the National Institutes of Health and the ARRIVE guidelines (http://www.nc3rs.org/ARRIVE). All of the experiments performed were approved by the Subcommittee on Research and Animal Care (SRAC), which serves as the Institutional Animal Care and Use Committee (IACUC) at the Harvard Medical School (protocol number: 03901). All surgery was performed under anesthesia by intraperitoneal injection of a combination of ketamine (100 mg/ml) and xylazine (10 mg/ml), in addition, buprenorphine (0.05 mg/kg) was given for perioperative analgesia to minimize suffering and pain.

Animals

Thirty 9-week-old female C57BL mice (body weight: 22.0+ 2.0 g) were obtained from Charles River Laboratories International Inc. (Wilmington, MA) and randomly assigned to three groups: control(n = 10), CKD(n = 10), and CKD+Vit D(n = 10). The animals were kept under climate-controlled conditions (25°C; 55% humidity; 12 hours of light alternating with 12 hours of darkness) and fed with a standard diet. The workflow is illustrated in Figure 1.

Surgical Procedure to Induce Uremia

CKD is induced in mice by a two-step 5/6 nephrectomy to produce uremia as described previously [21]. Briefly, the first procedure involves electrocautery of the left kidney except for a 2-mm area around the hilum. After 1 week, a total nephrectomy of the right kidney is performed by ligation of the renal hilum and surgical excision. Sham surgery consists of anesthetic administration, flank incision exposing the kidney, and closure of the abdominal wall.

Supplement of Active Vitamin D

The active form of vitamin D [1,25$(OH)_2D_3$], was obtained from Enzo Life Sciences Inc. (Farmingdale, NY) and diluted in saline. Eight weeks after the second kidney surgery, mice in the Vit D-treated group were injected with Vit D (100 ng/kg body weight) 3 times a week until they were sacrificed. Saline was used as a vehicle. The workflow is shown in Fig. S1.

Implant Surgery

Ten weeks after the second surgery (renal ablation), the mice were subjected to implant placement using the method described by Xu *et al.* [35]. Titanium implants with SLA surface (1 mm in diameter and 4 mm in length) were obtained from Institut Straumann AG (Basel, Switzerland). They were cut to the length of 2 mm before insertion. After careful exposure of the distal aspects of the femurs via skin incision and muscle dissection, implant sites were prepared on both sides of the anterior-distal surfaces of the femurs by sequential drilling under cooled sterile saline irrigation with 0.7- and 1.0-mm surgical stainless steel twist drills. Then, the implants were press-fitted into the holes to reach primary stability. After the insertion of the implant, the muscles were carefully sutured with 6-0 silk, which covered the implant and further guaranteed its protection in the biological environment. Then the skin was closed with 5-0 silk.

Serum Biochemical Assays

Two weeks after the insertion of titanium implants, the mice were euthanized by carbon dioxide inhalation. Prior to euthanasia, blood was collected by cheek pouch puncture. Serum biochemistry was performed using commercially available kits: blood urea nitrogen (BUN) (Roche Diagnostics, Indianapolis, IN); 1,25$(OH)_2$D (Immunodiagnostic Systems Ltd., Fountain Hills, AZ); Calcium and Phosphate (Stanbio Laboratory, Boerne, TX). For the assay of serum ALP activity, the serum was diluted 25 times and measured using a SensoLyte *p*NPP Alkaline Phosphatase Assay Kit (AnaSpec Inc., Fremont, CA).

X-ray Examination and Histological Preparation

Two weeks after implant placement, one femur carrying an implant was harvested from each mouse and fixed in 10% buffered formalin for 1 week at 4°C. Specimens were exposed to X-ray (20 kV, 5 seconds), and then dehydrated and embedded in light-curing epoxy resin (TechnoVit 7200VLC, Hereaus Kulzer, Wehrheim, Germany). Embedded specimens were cut perpendicular to the longitudinal axis of the implants at a site 0.5 mm from its apical end. The specimens were then ground to a thickness of about 50 µm with a grinding system (Exakt Apparatebau, Norderstedt, Germany). Sections were stained with Stevenel's blue and Van Gieson's picro fuchsin stain, and observed by light microscopy.

Histomorphometric Measurement

Images of the implant and peri-implant bone tissues were digitized and histomorphometrically analyzed with NIH Image J (National Institutes of Health, USA). Bone-implant contact (BIC) was calculated as the linear percentage of direct bone-to-implant contact to the total surface of the implant. And the bone volume (BV/TV) in the circumferential zone within 100 µm of the implant surface was calculated. The following formulas were used for analysis.

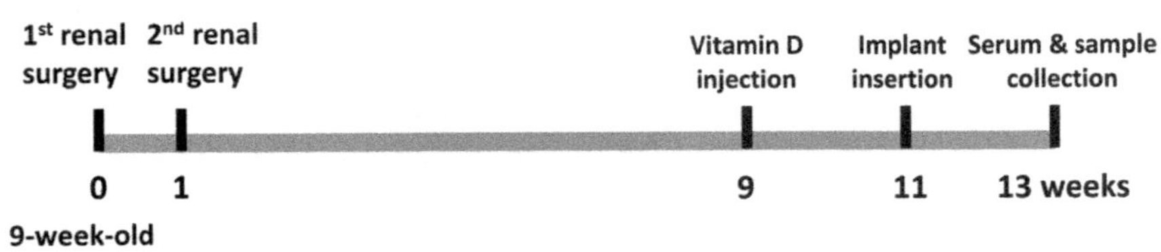

Figure 1. Illustration of the workflow. 1st renal surgery: electrocautery of the left kidney; 2nd renal surgery: a total nephrectomy of the right kidney; Vitamin D injections started at 9th week (100ng/kg body weight, 3 times a week for 4 weeks).

$$Bone-implant\ contact\ (\%) = (sum\ of\ the\ length\ of\ bone\ /\ implant\ contact)/(circumference\ of\ the\ implant) \times 100\%$$

$$Bone\ volume = (bone\ area\ in\ 100\mu m\ zone)/(area\ of\ 100\mu m\ zone) \times 100\%.$$

Implant Biomechanical Push-in Test

The remaining femur from each mouse was harvested and embedded into auto-polymerizing resin with the top surface of the implant level. A test machine (AG-TA electronic universal testing machine, SHIMADZU, Japan) equipped with a pushing rod (diameter = 0.8 mm) was used to load the implant vertically downward at a crosshead speed of 1 mm/min. The push-in value was determined by measuring the peak of the load-displacement curve.

Statistical Analysis

All values were presented as mean ± SD. Statistically significant differences were assessed by ANOVA followed by Tukey's test for multiple comparison, or by independent student *t* test for comparison between two groups. A *p* value of less than 0.05 was considered to be statistically significant.

Results

Animals

As anticipated, all mice tolerated the surgical procedures well and survived the full experimental period. No inflammation or infection at the implant site was observed.

Serum Biochemistry

A significant increase in serum BUN was observed in the CKD (53.87±6.32) and CKD+Vit D (58.45±4.33) groups as compared to that of controls (20.12±3.46) ($p<0.05$), indicating the successful establishment of the uremic mouse model (Figure 2A). Vit D injections did not cause a significant change in the serum BUN level. As shown in Figure 2B, Vit D was significantly decreased in the CKD group (27.51±8.35) ($p<0.05$), while supplementing with Vit D (62.44±26.88) restored it to levels comparable to those in control mice (52.35±16.33). Serum PTH in the CKD group was 3.6-fold that observed in the control group ($p<0.05$). It decreased to the levels comparable to the control upon Vit D treatment (Figure 2C). There was no significant difference in serum calcium (Figure 2D) and phosphate (Figure 2E) levels among the three groups. Serum ALP decreased significantly in the Vit D-treated group as compared to the CKD group ($p<0.05$), although it was still significantly higher than that of control (Figure 2F).

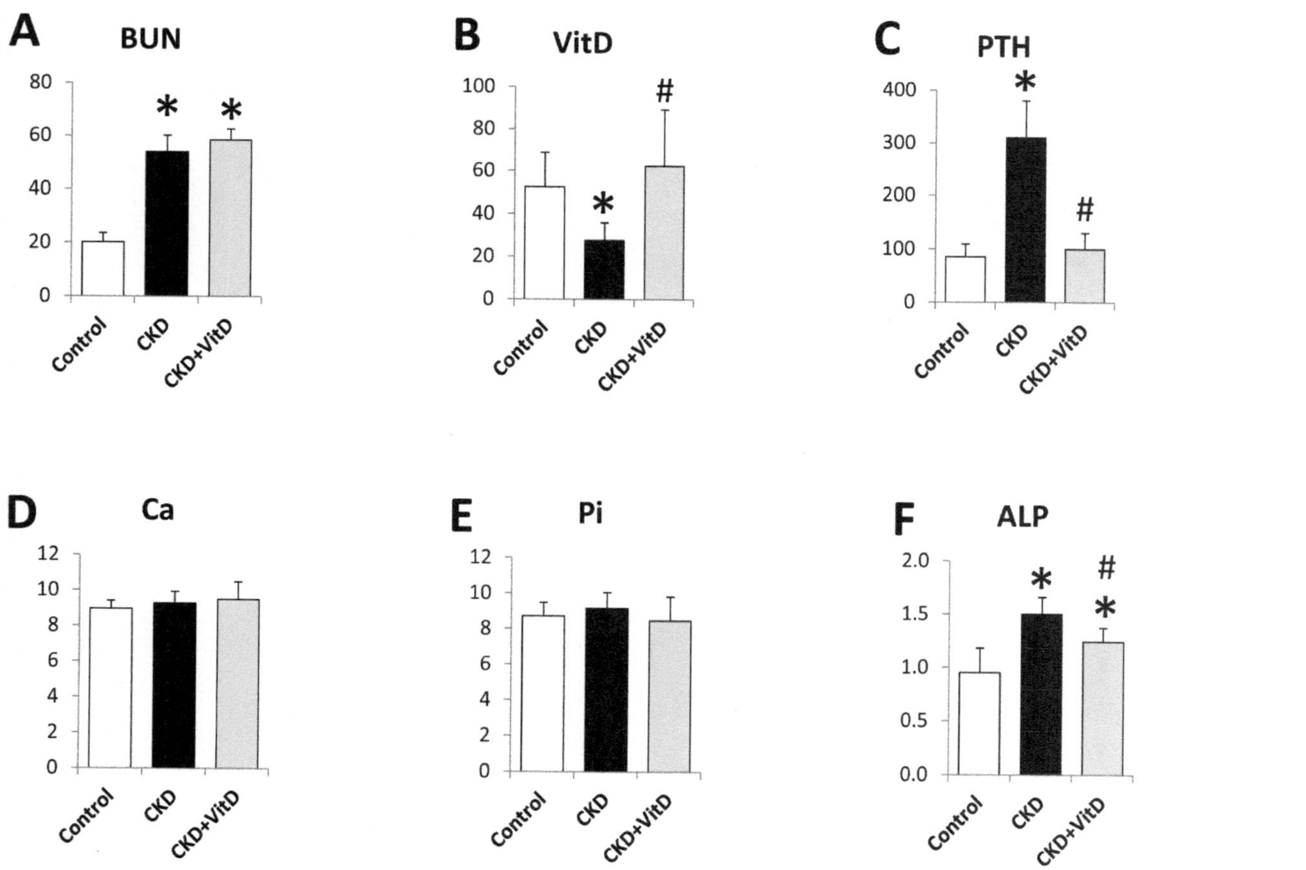

Figure 2. Serum biochemical measurements. (A) Serum BUN; (B) Serum Vitamin D; (C) Serum PTH; (D) Serum calcium; (E) Serum phosphate, and (F) Serum ALP activity. *: $p<0.05$ *vs* Control; #: $p<0.05$ *vs* CKD.

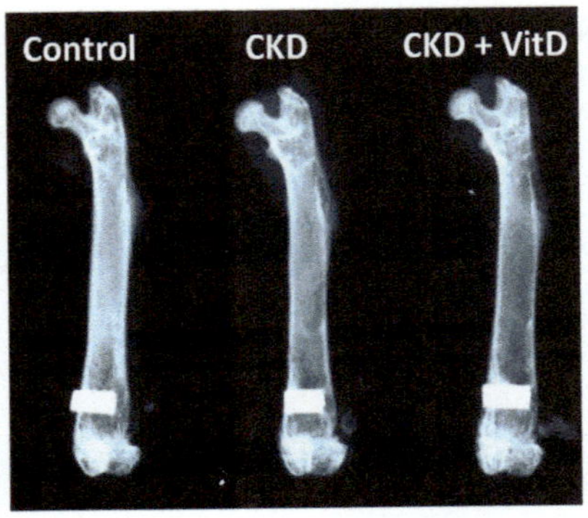

Figure 3. X-ray examination of the femurs after 2-weeks healing. The implants were surrounded with bone without any notable radiotranslucent gap.

X-ray Examination

The *ex vivo* X-ray examination of the femurs showed that the implants were surrounded with bone without any notable radiotranslucent gap, indicating successful osseointegration in all groups (Figure 3).

Histology and Histomorphometry

Examination of histological sections confirmed a direct bone-implant contact in all groups (Figure 4A). Consistent with our previous report [21], the CKD group showed a decrease of bone-implant contact ratio (BIC) when compared to that of control. The contact ratio was successfully restored to the normal level after Vit D treatment. As shown in Figure 4B, the BIC of CKD+VitD group was 75.23±9.92, over 20% higher than that of CKD mice (61.86±10.11) ($p<0.05$). We then calculated the bone volume (BV/TV) in the circumferential zone within 100 μm of the implant surface and were able to observe a 35% increase after Vit D treatment (Figure 4C).

The Resistance of Implant

In the early healing stage (week 2), the resistance of the implant was significantly higher for the Vit D treated group (15.21±4.11) compared to that of the untreated CKD mice (9.86±1.89), indicating an improved strength of bone–implant integration (Figure 5). No significant difference in integration was observed between the control and CKD+VitD groups.

Discussion

Vitamin D is a pleiotropic hormone that plays a critical role in regulating mineral ion metabolism [28]. It is initially biologically inactive and requires sequential hydroxylations in the liver and kidney to produce its active form, 1,25-dihydroxyvitamin D [28].

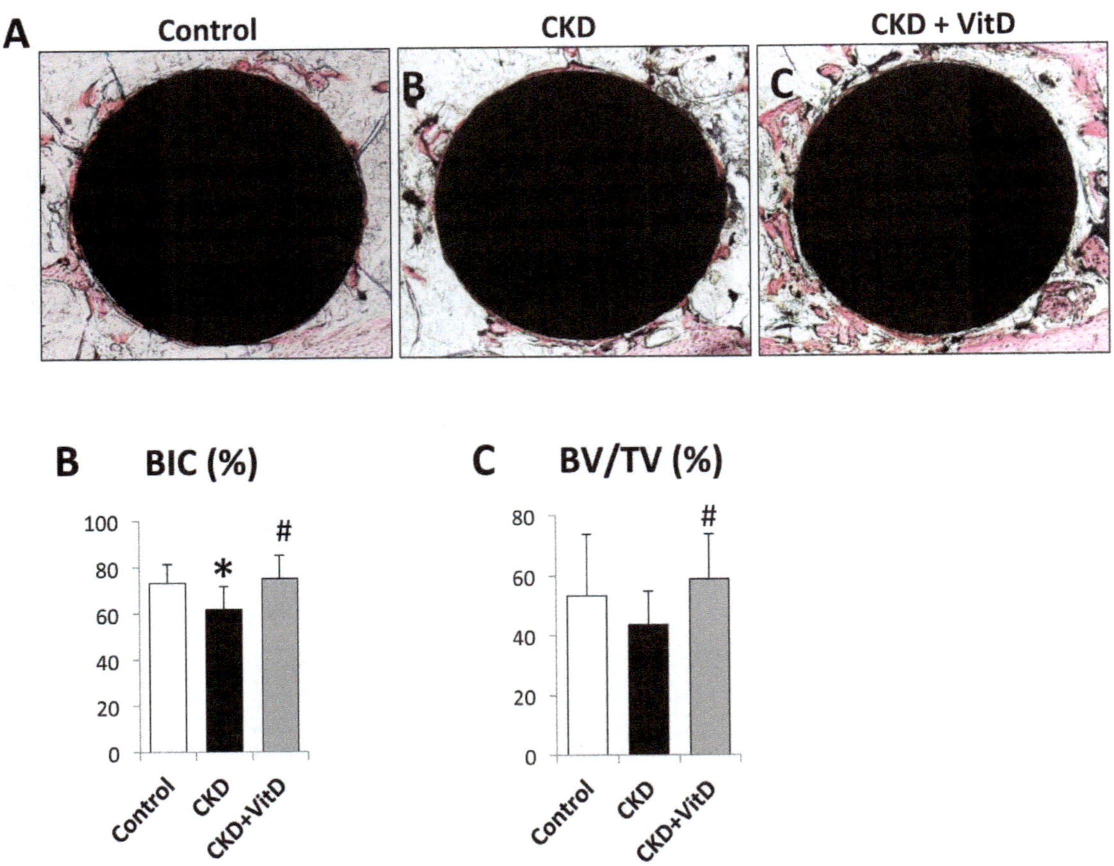

Figure 4. Histological and histomorphometrical analysis of the implants after 2-week healing. (A) Representative images of undecalified sections from all three groups; VitD injection significantly increased (B) Bone-implant contact ratio (BIC, %), and (C) bone volume (BV/TV) in the circumferential zone within 100 μm of the implant surface. *: $p<0.05$ *vs* Control; #: $p<0.05$ *vs* CKD.

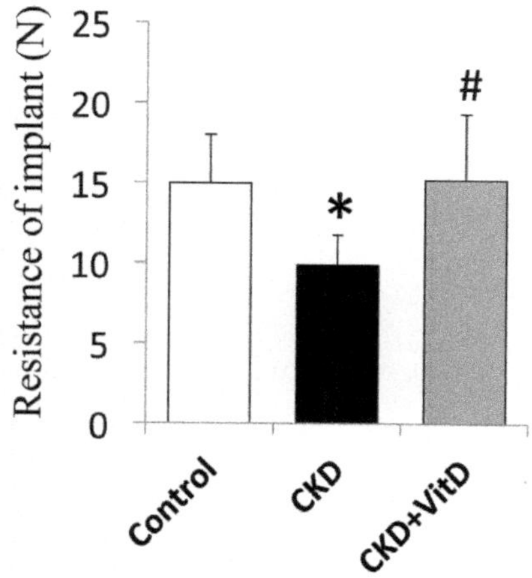

Figure 5. Resistance of push-in tests 2 weeks after implant placement. Vit D supplementation corrected the resistance of implant in CKD. *: $p<0.05$ *vs* control; #: $p<0.05$ *vs* CKD.

Vit D insufficiency is a common medical condition in CKD patients [24], where declining renal function impairs the activity of 1-α hydroxylase (1α-OHase) in kidney, which in turn reduces its ability to convert $25(OH)_2D$ to its activated form, $1,25(OH)_2D$. In this study, we established a uremic mouse model with significantly reduced levels of $1,25(OH)_2D$ using the 5/6 nephrectomy method. These data are consistent with previous studies and similar to the clinical situation in CKD patients [36,37].

Vitamin D deficiency negatively affects bone regeneration, including fracture healing, due to its importance in bone metabolism [27]. Moreover, Kelly *et al.* [15] showed that vitamin D insufficiency decreased the bone-implant contact ratio and the resistance in push-in tests. Recently, Choukroun *et al.* [38] found that Vit D deficiency slows down the process of osseointegration, and also promotes infection in the graft. A genome-wide screening also suggested that Vit D deficiency affects the osseointegration of implants by regulating the circadian rhythm system and the cartilage extracellular matrix [39].

On the other hand, vitamin D supplementation has demonstrated a significant survival advantage in CKD patients [25], including accelerated cellular events in the process of fracture healing [34]. Vitamin D supplementation has been recommended as the primary therapy by the National Kidney Foundation to control secondary hyperparathyroidism and prevent skeletal complications in end stage renal failure patients [40,41]. Two recent studies demonstrated that Vit D supplementation was able to enhance implant fixation in diabetic mellitus rats with Vit D insufficiency [42,43]. Similar results were reported in studies using normal [44] or ovariectomized animals [45,46]. In this study, we successfully corrected the decreased $1,25(OH)_2D$ levels in CKD mice by Vit D injection, and found that both the bone-implant contact (BIC) ratio and the resistance of implant were significantly increased after a 2-week healing period, indicating that Vit D supplementation is an effective approach to improve fixation of titanium implants in CKD.

We also found that Vit D supplementation successfully corrected the increased levels of PTH, a key hormone for bone remodeling. In CKD patients, low serum 1,25-dihydroxyvitamin D triggers higher secretion of PTH [28,29], which precipitates high bone turnover and exacerbates osteopenia and finally results in bone loss [30–32]. A meta-analysis performed by Kandula *et al.* [47] showed that any form of vitamin D (including calcitriol or a vitamin D analog) lowers PTH levels in CKD patients. In this context, we hypothesize that in addition to the direct impact of Vit D on bone healing, the normalization of PTH levels might also contribute to the enhancement of implant fixation. However the direct effect of PTH on osseointegration in CKD needs to be studied further.

It should be noted that this study was performed using a mouse model with the implants placed in the distal end of femurs. Although the rodent model has been widely used for research in implant dentistry[42,45,46], the development and characterization of the femur is different from the jaw bone. A canine or mini pig model might be a better alternative as the implants can be inserted in the jaw bone instead of the femur. However, the establishment of CKD in these large animals is not yet well-established. Clinical trials are expected to confirm whether supplement of Vit D could be a good candidate for clinical approaches to enhance the fixation of titanium implants in CKD patients.

Conclusion

In this study, we found that Vit D supplementation successfully restored serum $1,25(OH)_2D$ levels and corrected the hyperparathyroidism in CKD mice. The bone-implant contact ratio, bone volume around implant and the resistance of the implant were improved at 2 weeks after implantation, indicating that Vit D supplementation is an effective approach to improve the fixation of titanium implants in CKD.

Acknowledgments

We thank Dr. Hans-Peter Weber, Department of Prosthodontics and Operative Dentistry, Tufts University School of Dental Medicine, for the discussion and advice for this study, and Michael Densmore, Department of Oral Medicine, Infection, and Immunity, Harvard School of Dental medicine, for assistance in editing the manuscript.

Author Contributions

Conceived and designed the experiments: QY BL MD. Performed the experiments: WL SZ DZ HZ NS. Analyzed the data: WL XL QY. Contributed reagents/materials/analysis tools: MD BL. Wrote the paper: WL BL QY.

References

1. Moe S, Drueke T, Cunningham J, Goodman W, Martin K, et al. (2006) Definition, evaluation, and classification of renal osteodystrophy: a position statement from Kidney Disease: Improving Global Outcomes (KDIGO). Kidney Int 69: 1945–1953.
2. National Kidney F (2003) K/DOQI clinical practice guidelines for bone metabolism and disease in chronic kidney disease. American journal of kidney diseases : the official journal of the National Kidney Foundation 42: S1–201.
3. Levey AS, Atkins R, Coresh J, Cohen EP, Collins AJ, et al. (2007) Chronic kidney disease as a global public health problem: approaches and initiatives - a position statement from Kidney Disease Improving Global Outcomes. Kidney Int 72: 247–259.
4. Saran R, Hedgeman E, Huseini M, Stack A, Shahinian V (2010) Surveillance of chronic kidney disease around the world: tracking and reining in a global problem. Adv Chronic Kidney Dis 17: 271–281.
5. Kimura G (2007) Predicted prevalence in Japan of chronic kidney disease (CKD). Clinical and experimental nephrology 11: 188–189.
6. Coresh J, Selvin E, Stevens LA, Manzi J, Kusek JW, et al. (2007) Prevalence of chronic kidney disease in the United States. JAMA 298: 2038–2047.
7. Coresh J, Astor BC, Greene T, Eknoyan G, Levey AS (2003) Prevalence of chronic kidney disease and decreased kidney function in the adult US population: Third National Health and Nutrition Examination Survey.

American journal of kidney diseases : the official journal of the National Kidney Foundation 41: 1–12.
8. Zhang L, Wang F, Wang L, Wang W, Liu B, et al. (2012) Prevalence of chronic kidney disease in China: a cross-sectional survey. Lancet 379: 815–822.
9. Ruospo M, Palmer SC, Craig JC, Gentile G, Johnson DW, et al. (2013) Prevalence and severity of oral disease in adults with chronic kidney disease: a systematic review of observational studies. Nephrol Dial Transplant.
10. Jover Cervero A, Bagan JV, Jimenez Soriano Y, Poveda Roda R (2008) Dental management in renal failure: patients on dialysis. Medicina oral, patologia oral y cirugia bucal 13: E419–426.
11. De Rossi SS, Glick M (1996) Dental considerations for the patient with renal disease receiving hemodialysis. Journal of the American Dental Association 127: 211–219.
12. Davidovich E, Schwarz Z, Davidovitch M, Eidelman E, Bimstein E (2005) Oral findings and periodontal status in children, adolescents and young adults suffering from renal failure. Journal of clinical periodontology 32: 1076–1082.
13. Bayraktar G, Kurtulus I, Duraduryan A, Cintan S, Kazancioglu R, et al. (2007) Dental and periodontal findings in hemodialysis patients. Oral Dis 13: 393–397.
14. Davidovich E, Davidovits M, Eidelman E, Schwarz Z, Bimstein E (2005) Pathophysiology, therapy, and oral implications of renal failure in children and adolescents: an update. Pediatric dentistry 27: 98–106.
15. Kelly J, Lin A, Wang CJ, Park S, Nishimura I (2009) Vitamin D and bone physiology: demonstration of vitamin D deficiency in an implant osseointegration rat model. Journal of prosthodontics : official journal of the American College of Prosthodontists 18: 473–478.
16. Lee MM, Chu EY, El-Abbadi MM, Foster BL, Tompkins KA, et al. (2010) Characterization of mandibular bone in a mouse model of chronic kidney disease. Journal of periodontology 81: 300–309.
17. Messier MD, Emde K, Stern L, Radhakrishnan J, Vernocchi L, et al. (2012) Radiographic periodontal bone loss in chronic kidney disease. J Periodontol 83: 602–611.
18. Craig RG, Kotanko P, Kamer AR, Levin NW (2007) Periodontal diseases–a modifiable source of systemic inflammation for the end-stage renal disease patient on haemodialysis therapy? Nephrol Dial Transplant 22: 312–315.
19. Stellingsma C, Vissink A, Meijer HJ, Kuiper C, Raghoebar GM (2004) Implantology and the severely resorbed edentulous mandible. Crit Rev Oral Biol Med 15: 240–248.
20. Dijakiewicz M, Wojtowicz A, Dijakiewicz J, Szycik V, Rutkowski P, et al. (2007) Is implanto-prosthodontic treatment available for haemodialysis patients? Nephrology, dialysis, transplantation : official publication of the European Dialysis and Transplant Association - European Renal Association 22: 2722–2724.
21. Zou H, Zhao X, Sun N, Zhang S, Sato T, et al. (2013) Effect of chronic kidney disease on the healing of titanium implants. Bone 56: 410–415.
22. Ishimura E, Nishizawa Y, Inaba M, Matsumoto N, Emoto M, et al. (1999) Serum levels of 1,25-dihydroxyvitamin D, 24,25-dihydroxyvitamin D, and 25-hydroxyvitamin D in nondialyzed patients with chronic renal failure. Kidney international 55: 1019–1027.
23. Gonzalez EA, Sachdeva A, Oliver DA, Martin KJ (2004) Vitamin D insufficiency and deficiency in chronic kidney disease. A single center observational study. American journal of nephrology 24: 503–510.
24. Rouached M, El Kadiri Boutchich S, Al Rifai AM, Garabedian M, Fournier A (2008) Prevalence of abnormal serum vitamin D, PTH, calcium, and phosphorus in patients with chronic kidney disease: results of the study to evaluate early kidney disease. Kidney international 74: 389–390.
25. Chandra P, Binongo JN, Ziegler TR, Schlanger LE, Wang W, et al. (2008) Cholecalciferol (vitamin D3) therapy and vitamin D insufficiency in patients with chronic kidney disease: a randomized controlled pilot study. Endocrine practice : official journal of the American College of Endocrinology and the American Association of Clinical Endocrinologists 14: 10–17.
26. LaClair RE, Hellman RN, Karp SL, Kraus M, Ofner S, et al. (2005) Prevalence of calcidiol deficiency in CKD: a cross-sectional study across latitudes in the United States. American journal of kidney diseases : the official journal of the National Kidney Foundation 45: 1026–1033.
27. Brinker MR, O'Connor DP, Monla YT, Earthman TP (2007) Metabolic and endocrine abnormalities in patients with nonunions. Journal of orthopaedic trauma 21: 557–570.
28. Lips P (2006) Vitamin D physiology. Progress in biophysics and molecular biology 92: 4–8.
29. Bergwitz C, Juppner H (2010) Regulation of phosphate homeostasis by PTH, vitamin D, and FGF23. Annual review of medicine 61: 91–104.
30. Andress DL (2008) Adynamic bone in patients with chronic kidney disease. Kidney international 73: 1345–1354.
31. Holick MF (2007) Vitamin D deficiency. The New England journal of medicine 357: 266–281.
32. Nickolas TL, Stein E, Cohen A, Thomas V, Staron RB, et al. (2010) Bone mass and microarchitecture in CKD patients with fracture. Journal of the American Society of Nephrology : JASN 21: 1371–1380.
33. Alvim-Pereira F, Montes CC, Thome G, Olandoski M, Trevilatto PC (2008) Analysis of association of clinical aspects and vitamin D receptor gene polymorphism with dental implant loss. Clinical oral implants research 19: 786–795.
34. Jingushi S, Iwaki A, Higuchi O, Azuma Y, Ohta T, et al. (1998) Serum 1alpha,25-dihydroxyvitamin D3 accumulates into the fracture callus during rat femoral fracture healing. Endocrinology 139: 1467–1473.
35. Xu B, Zhang J, Brewer E, Tu Q, Yu L, et al. (2009) Osterix enhances BMSC-associated osseointegration of implants. J Dent Res 88: 1003–1007.
36. Hasegawa H, Nagano N, Urakawa I, Yamazaki Y, Iijima K, et al. (2010) Direct evidence for a causative role of FGF23 in the abnormal renal phosphate handling and vitamin D metabolism in rats with early-stage chronic kidney disease. Kidney international 78: 975–980.
37. Pillar R, MG GL, Rocha LA, Cuppari L, Carvalho AB, et al. (2013) Severe hypovitaminosis D in chronic kidney disease: association with blood pressure and coronary artery calcification. Hypertension research : official journal of the Japanese Society of Hypertension 36: 428–432.
38. Choukroun J, Khoury G, Khoury F, Russe P, Testori T, et al. (2013) Two Neglected Biologic Risk Factors In Bone Grafting And Implantology : High LDL Cholesterol and Low Serum Vitamin D. J Oral Implantol.
39. Mengatto CM, Mussano F, Honda Y, Colwell CS, Nishimura I (2011) Circadian rhythm and cartilage extracellular matrix genes in osseointegration: a genome-wide screening of implant failure by vitamin D deficiency. PloS one 6: e15848.
40. Eknoyan G, Levin A, Levin N (2003) Bone metabolism and disease in chronic kidney disease. American journal of kidney diseases : the official journal of the National Kidney Foundation 42: 1–201.
41. Andress DL (2005) Vitamin D treatment in chronic kidney disease. Seminars in dialysis 18: 315–321.
42. Akhavan A, Noroozi Z, Shafiei AA, Haghighat A, Jahanshahi GR, et al. (2012) The effect of vitamin D supplementation on bone formation around titanium implants in diabetic rats. Dent Res J (Isfahan) 9: 582–587.
43. Wu YY, Yu T, Yang XY, Li F, Ma L, et al. (2013) Vitamin D3 and insulin combined treatment promotes titanium implant osseointegration in diabetes mellitus rats. Bone 52: 1–8.
44. Cho YJ, Heo SJ, Koak JY, Kim SK, Lee SJ, et al. (2011) Promotion of osseointegration of anodized titanium implants with a 1alpha,25-dihydroxyvitamin D3 submicron particle coating. The International journal of oral & maxillofacial implants 26: 1225–1232.
45. Dvorak G, Fugl A, Watzek G, Tangl S, Pokorny P, et al. (2012) Impact of dietary vitamin D on osseointegration in the ovariectomized rat. Clinical oral implants research 23: 1308–1313.
46. Zhou C, Li Y, Wang X, Shui X, Hu J (2012) 1,25Dihydroxy vitamin D(3) improves titanium implant osseointegration in osteoporotic rats. Oral surgery, oral medicine, oral pathology and oral radiology 114: S174–178.
47. Kandula P, Dobre M, Schold JD, Schreiber MJ Jr, Mehrotra R, et al. (2011) Vitamin D supplementation in chronic kidney disease: a systematic review and meta-analysis of observational studies and randomized controlled trials. Clinical journal of the American Society of Nephrology : CJASN 6: 50–62.

Changes in Positive End-Expiratory Pressure Alter the Distribution of Ventilation within the Lung Immediately after Birth in Newborn Rabbits

Marcus J. Kitchen[1], Melissa L. Siew[2]**, Megan J. Wallace[2], Andreas Fouras[4], Robert A. Lewis[5,6], Naoto Yagi[7], Kentaro Uesugi[7], Arjan B. te Pas[3¶], Stuart B. Hooper[2*¶]**

1 School of Physics, Monash Institute of Medical Research, Clayton, Victoria, Australia, 2 The Ritchie Centre, Monash Institute of Medical Research, Clayton, Victoria, Australia, 3 Department of Pediatrics, Leiden University Medical Centre, Leiden, Netherlands, 4 Department of Mechanical and Aerospace Engineering, Monash University, Clayton, Victoria, Australia, 5 Department of Medical Imaging and Radiation Science, Monash University, Clayton, Victoria, Australia, 6 Biomedical Engineering, University of Saskatchewan, Saskatoon, Canada, 7 SPring-8/Japan Synchrotron Radiation Research Institute, Sayo, Hyogo, Japan

Abstract

Current recommendations suggest the use of positive end-expiratory pressures (PEEP) to assist very preterm infants to develop a functional residual capacity (FRC) and establish gas exchange at birth. However, maintaining a consistent PEEP is difficult and so the lungs are exposed to changing distending pressures after birth, which can affect respiratory function. Our aim was to determine how changing PEEP levels alters the distribution of ventilation within the lung. Preterm rabbit pups (28 days gestation) were delivered and mechanically ventilated with one of three strategies, whereby PEEP was changed in sequence; 0-5-10-5-0 cmH_2O, 5-10-0-5-0 cmH_2O or 10-5-0-10-0 cmH_2O. Phase contrast X-ray imaging was used to analyse the distribution of ventilation in the upper left (UL), upper right (UR), lower left (LL) and lower right (LR) quadrants of the lung. Initiating ventilation with 10PEEP resulted in a uniform increase in FRC throughout the lung whereas initiating ventilation with 5PEEP or 0PEEP preferentially aerated the UR than both lower quadrants ($p<0.05$). Consequently, the relative distribution of incoming V_T was preferentially directed into the lower lobes at low PEEP, primarily due to the loss of FRC in those lobes. Following ventilation at 10PEEP, the distribution of air at end-inflation was uniform across all quadrants and remained so regardless of the PEEP level. Uniform distribution of ventilation can be achieved by initiating ventilation with a high PEEP. After the lungs have aerated, small and stepped reductions in PEEP result in more uniform changes in ventilation.

Editor: Edgardo Szyld, Icahn School of Medicine at Mount Sinai, United States of America

Funding: This research was supported by the Australian Research Council (http://www.arc.gov.au), the Australian National Health and Medical Research Council (http://www.nhmrc.gov.au) and the Victorian Government's Operational Infrastructure Support Program (http://www.business.vic.gov.au). The authors acknowledge financial support from the Access to Major Research Facilities Programme (http://www.ansto.gov.au/) which is a component of the International Science Linkages Programme established under the Australian Government's innovation statement, Backing Australia's Ability. The authors also gratefully acknowledge the support provided by the SPring-8 synchrotron facility (http://www.spring8.or.jp) which was granted by the SPring-8 Program Review Committee. Marcus J. Kitchen and Andreas Fouras are the recipients of ARC Australian Research Fellowship and NHMRC Career Development Fellowships respectively. Arjan B. te Pas is recipient of a Veni-grant, The Netherlands Organisation for Health Research and Development (http://www.zonmw.nl/en), part of the Innovational Research Incentives Scheme Veni-Vidi-Vici (project nos. 91612027). The funders had no role in study design, data collection and analysis, decision to publish, or preparation of the manuscript.

Competing Interests: The authors have declared that no competing interests exist.

* E-mail: stuart.hooper@monash.edu

MJK and MLS are joint first authors on this work.

¶ ABtP and SBH are joint senior authors on this work.

Introduction

The lungs of premature newborns are structurally and functionally immature and so have a greater tendency to collapse than the adult lung [1–3]. Specifically, the lung tissue is inelastic and the distal airways lack surfactant [4], which is required to reduce surface tension and promote uniform lung aeration [5,6]. In addition, as their chest walls are highly compliant [7], the premature newborn's ability to oppose lung recoil and maintain functional residual capacity (FRC) is reduced, which may contribute to a lower FRC [8].

Positive end-expiratory pressure (PEEP) and continuous positive airway pressure (CPAP) oppose lung atelectasis by applying an internal distending pressure on the airways, which keeps them aerated at end-expiration [9]. As a result, end-expiratory pressures improve FRC development, gas exchange, lung compliance and reduce lung injury and inflammation [9–11]. However, providing consistent end-expiratory pressure support in the delivery room can be difficult and changing levels often cannot be avoided. Indeed, face mask leak is common [12,13] and assisted ventilation is often interrupted by mask repositioning, suctioning or intubation, which can rapidly decrease lung gas volumes [14]. Little is known about how these pressure changes alter the distribution of ventilation within the immature lung.

In adults with a non-uniform pattern of acute respiratory distress syndrome (ARDS), increasing PEEP levels recruits lung volume preferentially in the apical lobes, which increases compliance to a greater extent in the apical than basal lobes

[15,16]. Similar observations have been made in children with ARDS [17] and a preference for the distribution of air into apical lung regions has also been observed in vertically positioned dead newborn fetal rabbits following consecutive pressure/volume loops applied using air [18]. At birth, as the immature lung lacks surfactant [4] and incompletely clears airway liquid [19], the resulting large regional differences in lung compliance likely contributes to the heterogenous ventilation commonly observed in preterm infants. Thus, it is likely that regional differences in lung compliance, which influence the distribution of ventilation within the lung at FRC, will likely change with different PEEP levels.

We have used phase contrast X-ray imaging [9,18–20] to examine how changing PEEP levels alter the distribution of ventilation within the lung in preterm rabbits ventilated from birth. We hypothesized that air will preferentially enter the apical lobes at low PEEP levels and that once apical regions have aerated, higher PEEP levels mainly affect the distribution of air towards the basal lobes of the lungs.

Methods

Animal Procedures

Experiments were performed in the Biomedical Imaging Centre at the SPring-8 synchrotron in Japan. All experiments were approved by Animal Ethics Committees at SPring-8 in Japan and at the School of Biomedical Science, Monash University. Pregnant near-term New Zealand white rabbits (28 days of gestation; term = 32 days) were initially anaesthetised with propofol (Rapinovet; i.v.; 12 mg/kg bolus), intubated and then maintained by isoflourane inhalation (1.5–4%). Pups were delivered by caesarean section, sedated with pentobarbital (Nembutal; 0.1 mg, i.p.) and intubated with an endotracheal (ET) tube (18G). The ET tube was occluded to prevent spontaneous breathing before ventilation onset. Pups were positioned upright in a pre-warmed (40°C) water-filled, plethysmograph (head out) located in the path of the X-ray beam within the imaging hutch, as previously described [19,21]. The ET tube was connected to the ventilator.

Mechanical Ventilation

Pups were randomised into groups and ventilated with one of three PEEP strategies (Figure 1).

Strategy A: The initial PEEP was set at 0 cmH_2O and was changed to 5, to 10, to 5 and to 0 cmH_2O (0-5-10-5-0PEEP). This strategy was designed to examine the effect of gradually increasing and decreasing PEEP on lung aeration and the distribution of ventilation.

Strategy B: PEEP was initially set at 5 cmH_2O and was then changed to 10, to 0, to 5 and to 0 cmH_2O (5-10-0-5-0PEEP). This strategy was designed to examine the effect of PEEP recruitment (from 5 cmH_2O) on the distribution of ventilation and the ability of 5 cmH_2O of PEEP to re-recruit the lung following a loss of PEEP.

Strategy C: PEEP was initially set at 10 cmH_2O and was then changed to 5, to 0 to 10 and to 0 cmH_2O, (10-5-0-10-0PEEP). This strategy was designed to assess the ability of an initial high PEEP strategy, followed by a normal PEEP level, to aerate the lung and to assess the ability of high PEEP to re-recruit the lung following a loss of PEEP.

Phase contrast X-ray movies, found in the Supporting Information, demonstrate the effect of changing PEEP on lung aeration. Movie S1 shows a representative example of Strategy A, Movie S2 is an example of Strategy B and Movie S3 is an example of Strategy C. Pups were ventilated at each PEEP until FRC and tidal volume (V_T) had reached a plateau; this required ~2–3 minutes. Pups were ventilated using a SAR-830/AP (CWE Inc, Ardmore, Pennsylvania, USA) flow restrictor ventilator, which utilises a pressure-limited system and a variable bias gas flow through the ventilator circuit; in this mode, the pressure wave is triangular in shape. The peak inflation pressure (PIP) was set at 35 cmH_2O and the PEEP was controlled by raising and lowering the expiratory tube outlet in a water-filled PEEP trap; i.e. submerging the tube 5 cm generated a PEEP of 5 cmH_2O. Inspiratory and expiratory times were 1.0 and 1.5 sec, respectively. Changes in

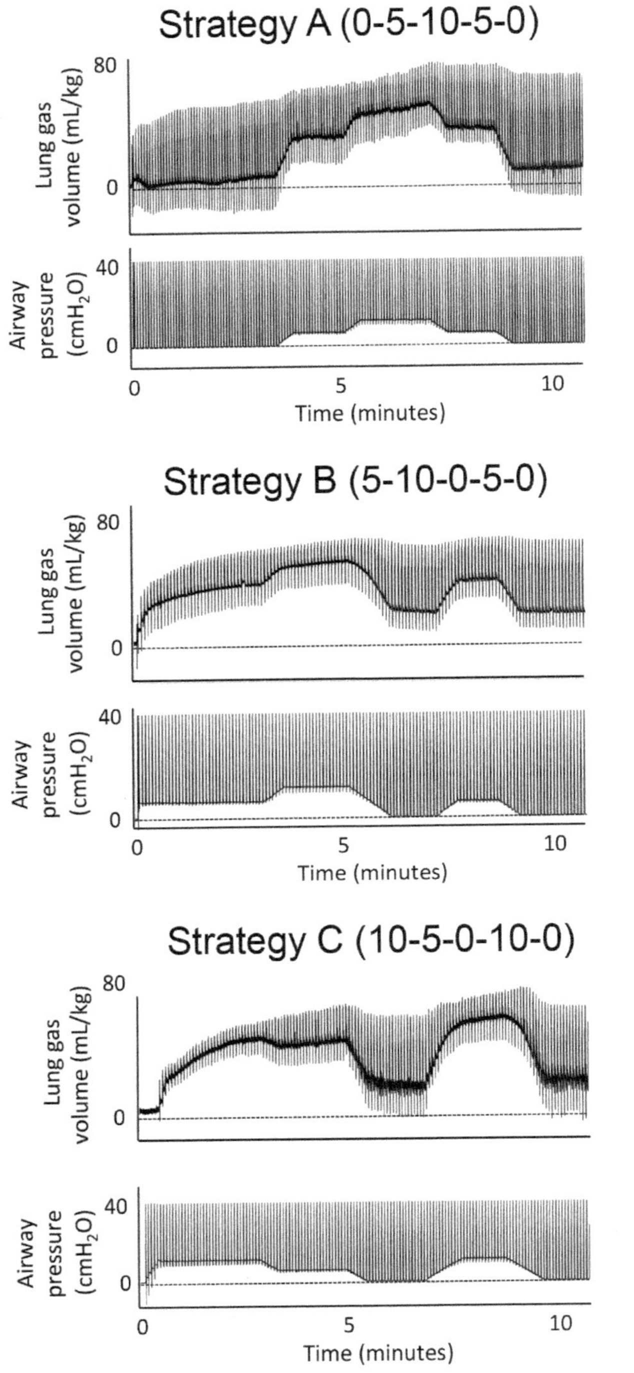

Figure 1. Diagram of ventilation Strategies A, B and C. Plethysmograph and airway pressure recordings of pups that were ventilated from birth using each of the PEEP Strategies A, B or C.

airway pressures were recorded digitally (Powerlab, ADInstruments; Sydney, Australia). At the conclusion of the experiment, pups were euthanized with sodium pentobarbital (Nembutal; 100 mg/kg; i.p.).

Image Acquisition

Phase contrast images were acquired using a monochromatic X-ray beam (24 keV) with the detectors placed 2.0 m downstream from the pups (see [18]). X-rays were converted to visible light and images acquired using an electron multiplying charge-coupled device (EMCCD) camera (Hamamatsu, C9100-02). The effective pixel size was 31.82 μm and the field of view was 32(H) × 32(V) mm^2, which captured the entire pup's chest in a single exposure. Image acquisition was synchronised with ventilation whereby inflation onset triggered the camera to acquire a sequence of six images, 300 ms apart using an exposure time of 80 ms. Three images were acquired during inspiration and three during expiration.

Image Processing and Analysis

The first 4 lung inflations at the onset of lung ventilation and the 4 inflations immediately preceding and following a change in PEEP were used for analysis. Regional lung air volumes were calculated using the image processing technique developed by [18]. This technique utilises differences in X-ray attenuation between air and water to determine changes in gas volume within the image. Despite the images being two-dimensional (2D) projections, this technique enables very small (25 μL) changes in air volumes to be measured without having to reconstruct the three-dimensional (3D) structure using computed tomography [18].

To assess the uniformity of lung aeration, images were partitioned into quadrants using the vertebral column and the 7th rib as landmarks [18]. The four quadrants were labelled upper right (UR), upper left (UL), lower right (LR) and lower left (LL) and are in reference to the image as observed. The position of the regions of interest was held constant within consecutive image by tracking the displacement of the skeleton for each pup using a cross-correlation analysis [18]. Volumetric information extracted from the lung quadrants were used to assess changes in the lung's regional functional residual capacity (FRC), V_T and air volumes at peak inspiratory pressure (V_{PIP}). As the lung volume in each quadrant differs between quadrants and between animals within the same quadrant, lung gas volumes (FRC, V_T and V_{PIP}) were normalised to the maximum lung gas volume obtained in each lung quadrant for each animal within a given imaging sequence. Regional dynamic lung compliance was measured as the change in lung volume in one quadrant divided by the change in airway pressure (PIP-PEEP).

Statistical Analysis

Statistical analysis was performed using Sigmastat (Systat software Inc., USA). Results were presented as mean ± standard error of the mean (SEM) and all data were checked for normality and tested for equal variance. Changes in the distribution of ventilation at FRC, V_T and V_{PIP} were analysed using a 2-way repeated measures ANOVA. Changes in FRC and V_T in response to decreasing or increasing PEEP levels were analysed using a 2-way ANOVA. All statistical tests were followed by a Tukey post hoc test. A $p<0.05$ was considered statistically significant.

Results

Animal data

16 newborn preterm rabbit pups were ventilated from birth and the distribution of air within the lung determined using PC X-ray imaging. 6 pups were ventilated according to PEEP Strategy A, 5 according to PEEP Strategy B and 5 according to PEEP Strategy C. There were no significant differences in mean pup weight between any of the groups ($p>0.05$) and no pups developed a pneumothorax.

Lung air volume distribution between quadrants

Irrespective of the strategy, the lower quadrants had significantly greater maximal lung air volumes (at end inflation) than the upper quadrants ($p<0.05$), which mainly reflects the size differences. The LR and LL quadrants were not significantly different from each other (20.4±1.3 mL/kg vs 17.5±1.7 mL/kg, $p>0.05$) and the UR and UL were also not statistically different from each other (11.7±0.6 mL/kg vs 7.7±0.6 mL/kg, $p>0.05$).

Changes in gas distribution: Strategy A

Air distribution at FRC (Fig 2A). Ventilation with 0PEEP initially resulted in poor aeration of the lung at FRC (<6%) in all quadrants and, although the air volume at FRC gradually increased with time, it was substantially less than with both other strategies by the end of the first ventilation period (Strategy B, Fig 3A and Strategy C, Fig 4A). Furthermore, the relative increase in air volume was unequal and was significantly greater in the UR (28.2±7.3%) than in both LL (13.7±3.0%) and LR (10.3±1.9%) quadrants ($p<0.05$). Subsequent ventilation at 5PEEP, improved aeration in all quadrants but the unequal distribution between quadrants at FRC remained. At 10PEEP, both upper quadrants remained better aerated at FRC than both lower quadrants ($p<0.05$). Following the return to 0PEEP, only the UR quadrant was significantly better aerated than both lower quadrants (UR 42.9±5.3% vs LR 29.1±5.5% and LL 26.1±5.2%, $p<0.05$).

Distribution of incoming V_T (Fig 2B). Following initial lung aeration with 0PEEP, ventilation with 5PEEP and then with 10PEEP did not alter the size of the incoming V_T, which contributed to 20–30% of total lung air volumes at end-inflation (V_{PIP}). However, by the end of the 10PEEP period, the lower quadrants started to receive a significantly ($p<0.05$) greater proportion of this volume than the upper quadrants. With the onset of subsequent 5PEEP ventilation, both lower quadrants persisted in receiving a significantly larger proportion of the incoming V_T than both upper quadrants (~43% vs ~30%; $p<0.05$). This non-uniform distribution of incoming V_T persisted during the subsequent 5PEEP and 0PEEP periods, despite a significant increase in V_T.

Air distribution at end-inflation (V_{PIP}) (Fig 2c). At the initiation of ventilation with 0PEEP, the distribution of air in the lung at V_{PIP} was preferentially directed towards both upper quadrants. By the end of the 0PEEP period, the proportion of air in the upper quadrants at V_{PIP} (range 43–54% of maximal lung gas volume) was significantly greater than the lower quadrants (~33% of maximal lung gas volume; $p<0.05$). During the subsequent 10PEEP ventilation period, when the lung had fully aerated, all quadrants were similarly ventilated at V_{PIP} (>90%, $p>0.05$) and remained so for the rest of the experiment.

Changes in ventilation distribution: Strategy B

Air distribution at FRC (Fig 3A). During ventilation at 5PEEP and then at 10PEEP, the distribution of air in the lungs at FRC was greater in both upper than in both lower quadrants (p<

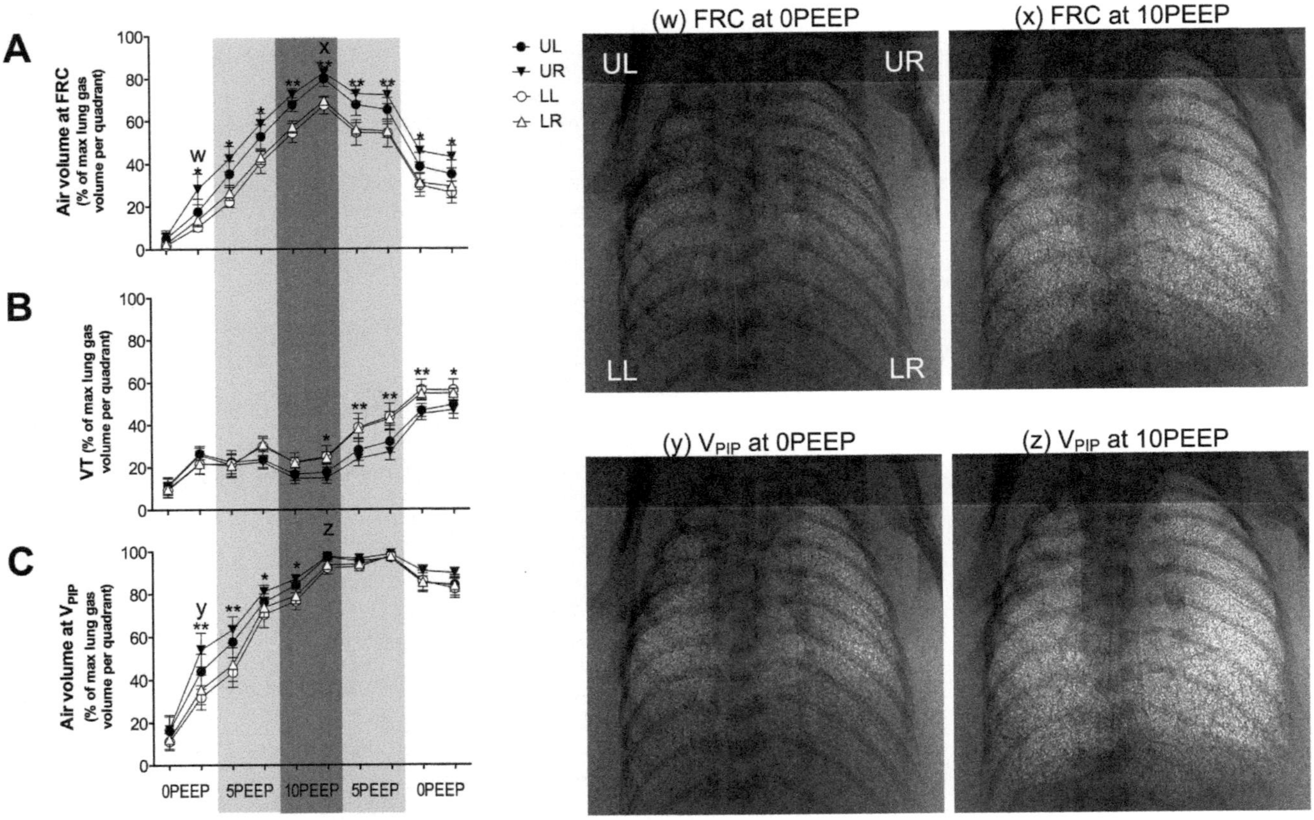

Figure 2. Changes in FRC, V_T and V_{PIP} during ventilation with Strategy A. Distribution of ventilation (A) at functional residual capacity (FRC), (B) of the incoming tidal volume (V_T) and (C) volume at peak inflation pressure (V_{PIP}) in the upper right (open triangles), upper left (closed triangles), lower right (open circles) and lower left (closed circles) regions of the lung during ventilation with Strategy A. Asterisks (*) indicate that UR quadrant is significantly different to the lower quadrants. Double asterisks (**) indicate that the upper quadrants are significantly different to the lower quadrants. Values are significantly different if $p<0.05$. Lower case letters (w-z) correspond to when phase contrast X-ray images of lung aeration at FRC and at V_{PIP} were acquired.

0.05). Reducing PEEP to 0PEEP increased the air volumes in the UR quadrant at FRC and reduced the amount in the LL quadrant (UR 36.3±5.1% and UL 30.6±3.6% vs LL 18.7±3.9% and LR 24.8±5.0%; $p<0.05$). This non-uniform distribution of air in the lungs at FRC persisted during the remainder of the experimental period; relative air volumes in the UR and LL quadrants at FRC remained greater and lower, respectively, than the other quadrants ($p<0.05$).

Distribution of incoming V_T (Fig 3B). Initially at 5PEEP, the distribution of incoming air with each inflation was relatively even across all quadrants, increasing from ~10% to 30% of total volume at end-inspiration. However, following ventilation at 10PEEP, decreasing the PEEP to 0PEEP resulted in a significantly smaller proportion of the V_T entering the UR quadrant ($p<0.05$), compared with the other quadrants, despite the UR quadrant having the highest proportional air volume at FRC. This indicates that some airway closure and gas trapping may have resulted from the sudden reduction in PEEP. Importantly, subsequent ventilation at 5PEEP did not alter this pattern, with the majority of incoming V_T being distributed towards the lower quadrants (~44%; $p<0.05$) rather than upper quadrants (~30%).

Air distribution at V_{PIP} (Fig 3C). During the initial 5PEEP and 10PEEP recruitment periods, the distribution of air in the lung at V_{PIP} predominantly occurred in the upper quadrants, whereas the LL quadrant aerated the least ($p<0.05$). Following ventilation at 10PEEP, all quadrants were similarly aerated at V_{PIP} and subsequent PEEP changes maintained this uniform distribution of air ($p>0.05$).

Changes in ventilation distribution: Strategy C

Air distribution at FRC (Fig 4A). Initiating ventilation with 10PEEP rapidly increased FRC and this air was uniformly distributed across all 4 quadrants of the lung ($p<0.05$). Decreasing the PEEP to 5PEEP, significantly decreased relative air volumes at FRC within the lower quadrants compared with the UR quadrant, which did not change ($p<0.05$). When PEEP was decreased further to 0PEEP, the air volume at FRC in all quadrants rapidly decreased, but the retention of air in the UR quadrant was better than in all other quadrants ($p<0.05$). This pattern of non-uniform air distribution at FRC was abolished by subsequent ventilation with 10PEEP, but returned during the second period of ventilation with 0PEEP.

Distribution of incoming V_T (Fig 4B). Initiating ventilation at birth with 10PEEP resulted in a relatively uniform distribution of the V_T across all quadrants ($p>0.05$). Reducing PEEP to 5PEEP increased V_T in all quadrants, but there was less V_T entering the UR compared to the lower quadrants ($p<0.05$); the UL was not significantly different to any quadrant ($p>0.05$). This non-uniform pattern of incoming V_T distribution was also observed during both 0PEEP ventilation periods but was not observed at the end of the second 10PEEP ventilation period.

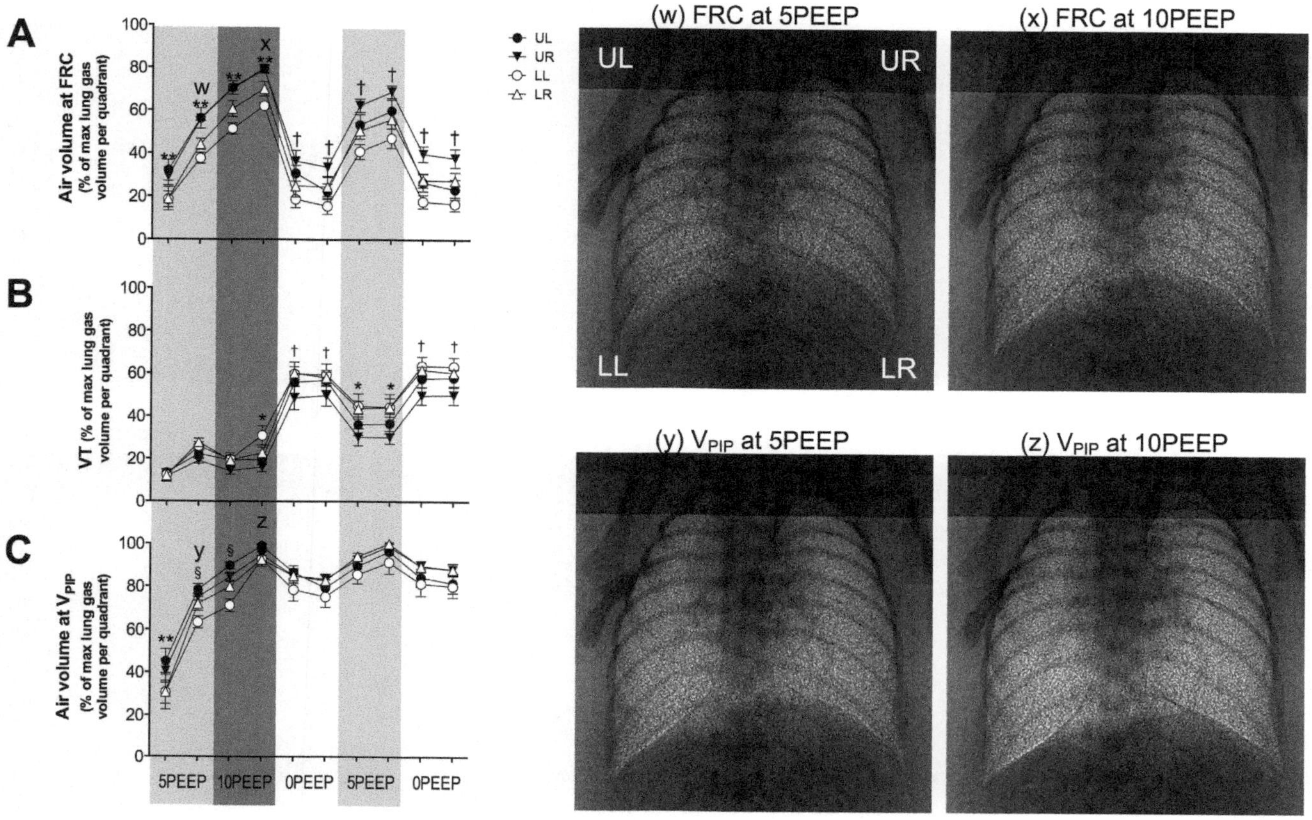

Figure 3. Changes in FRC, V_T and V_{PIP} during ventilation with Strategy B. Distribution of ventilation (A) at functional residual capacity (FRC), (B) of the incoming tidal volume (V_T) and (C) volume at peak inflation pressure (V_{PIP}) in the upper right (open triangles), upper left (closed triangles), lower right (open circles) and lower left (closed circles) regions of the lung during ventilation with Strategy B. Asterisks (*) indicate that UR quadrant is significantly different to the lower quadrants. Double asterisks (**) indicate that the upper quadrants are significantly different to the lower quadrants. Daggers (†) indicate that UR quadrant is significantly different to all other quadrants. Section symbol (§) indicates that the LL quadrant is significantly different to all other quadrants. Values are significantly different if $p<0.05$. Lower case letters (w-z) correspond to when phase contrast X-ray images of lung aeration at FRC and at V_{PIP} were acquired.

During this time, the distribution of V_T was again relatively uniform across all quadrants ($p>0.05$).

Air distribution at V_{PIP} (Fig 4C). Ventilation with 10PEEP rapidly increased lung air volumes at V_{PIP}, which were remarkably uniform across all 4 quadrants. Importantly, this uniform distribution of air between quadrants at V_{PIP} persisted even during both periods of ventilation with 0PEEP, indicating that the initial ventilation with 10PEEP has persisting benefits on the uniformity of ventilation at V_{PIP}.

V_T and FRC changes in response to decreasing PEEP in a ventilated lung

During ventilation strategies A and B, decreasing the PEEP by 5 cmH_2O steps to 0PEEP, (ie from 10 to 5 to 0PEEP during Strategy A or from 5 to 0PEEP during Strategy B) caused a small reduction in FRC and an increase in V_T, with the relative changes in both V_T and FRC being similar in all quadrants (Fig 5). In contrast, a large and continuous decrease in PEEP (ie from 10 to 0PEEP during Strategy C), resulted in changes in V_T and FRC that were not evenly distributed across all quadrants. Indeed, compared to PEEP reductions of only 5cmH_2O, continuous PEEP reductions of 10cmH_2O caused larger reductions in FRC and increases in V_T in both lower quadrants ($p<0.05$; Fig. 5). For instance in the LL quadrant the increase in V_T was markedly greater following the change from 10 to 0PEEP compared with the 10-5-0PEEP change ($42.8\pm3.9\%$ vs $31.1\pm5.5\%$, $p<0.05$, Fig. 6A).

Changes in regional dynamic lung compliance (C_L)

During all PEEP strategies, dynamic lung compliance was higher in the lower than in the upper quadrants, primarily due to size differences between quadrants, and increased with increasing lung aeration. However, this increase was markedly greater in pups that commenced ventilation with PEEP. The gradual time-related increase in dynamic lung compliance for all strategies was associated with both increasing and decreasing PEEP levels (Fig 6). Initiating ventilation with either 5 or 10PEEP resulted in much greater lung compliances, particularly in the lower lobes, irrespective of the PEEP level. Indeed, at the midway point of the experiment, when pups in strategy A were ventilated with 10PEEP and pups in both other strategies were ventilated with 0PEEP, dynamic compliances were markedly higher in all quadrants in pups ventilated with Strategies B and C, compared to Strategy A. Similarly, during the last ventilation phase, when all pups were ventilated with 0PEEP, dynamic lung compliances were higher if ventilation commenced with PEEP, particularly within both lower quadrants.

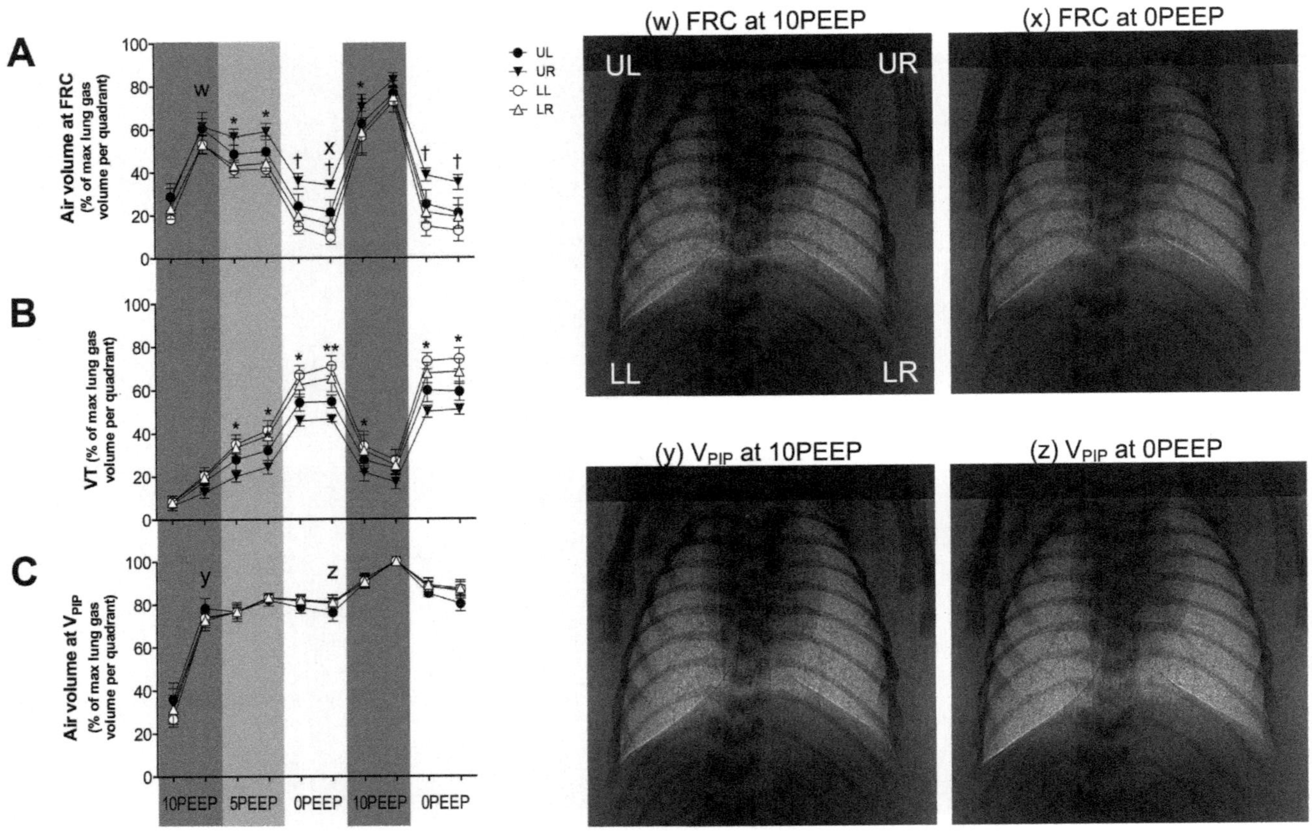

Figure 4. Changes in FRC, V_T and V_{PIP} during ventilation with Strategy C. Distribution of ventilation (A) at functional residual capacity (FRC), (B) of the incoming tidal volume (V_T) and (C) volume at peak inflation pressure (V_{PIP}) in the upper right (open triangles), upper left (closed triangles), lower right (open circles) and lower left (closed circles) regions of the lung during ventilation with Strategy C. Asterisks (*) indicate that UR quadrant is significantly different to the lower quadrants. Double asterisks (**) indicate that the upper quadrants are significantly different to the lower quadrants. Daggers (†) indicate that UR quadrant is different to all other quadrants. Values are significantly different if $p<0.05$. Lower case letters (w-z) correspond to when phase contrast X-ray images of lung aeration at FRC and at V_{PIP} were acquired.

Discussion

Our findings indicate that ventilating preterm rabbits with different and changing PEEP levels markedly effects the distribution of ventilation within the lung and on lung compliance during the immediate newborn period. We have used the quantitative capability [18] and high spatial resolution of phase contrast X-ray imaging to measure the distribution of air in the lung at both FRC and end-inspiration (V_{PIP}) as well as the relative distribution of the incoming V_T with each inflation. We found that, in preterm rabbit pups, changes in PEEP rapidly changed the distribution of air in the lung at FRC and the relative spatial distribution of the incoming V_T. Initiating ventilation at birth with 0PEEP, not only resulted in the lowest air volumes in all quadrants, the relative distribution of air between quadrants was not uniform, resulting in a significantly greater distribution of air towards the upper compared to the lower quadrants at FRC. Importantly, this unequal distribution of air at FRC persisted throughout the experiment even after subsequent ventilation at 5 and 10PEEP. Similarly, although initiating ventilation with 5PEEP increased lung air volumes compared to 0PEEP, the relative distribution of air was again unequal, being significantly greater in the upper compared to the lower quadrants, and persisted throughout the experimental period, even after ventilation with 10PEEP. In contrast, initiating ventilation with 10PEEP resulted in rapid FRC accumulation, which was uniformly distributed across all quadrants at both FRC and V_{PIP}. Although subsequent ventilation with 5PEEP and 0PEEP resulted in the preferential distribution of air into the upper quadrants at FRC, the distribution of air at V_{PIP} remained remarkably uniform across all quadrants. As a result, during ventilation with 5 and 0PEEP in this group, the incoming V_T was preferentially directed into the lower lung quadrants. These data indicate that initiating ventilation at birth with higher PEEP levels has effects on the distribution of ventilation in the lung at both FRC and V_{PIP} that temporarily persist even at different subsequent PEEP levels.

The immature lung is prone to collapse at end-expiration because of its low tissue compliance, high surface tension and a highly compliant chest wall. PEEP or CPAP can prevent atelectasis by acting as an internal "splint" to promote FRC maintenance (see [21–24]. Our results also demonstrate that initiating ventilation with high PEEP levels (i.e. 10PEEP) promoted uniform air distribution at both FRC and V_{PIP} (Fig. 4A) whereas lower PEEPs demonstrated a more non-uniform air distribution, with lower quadrants less ventilated than upper quadrants (Fig. 2A and 3A). It is possible that the momentum of deflating lung tissue during expiration influences the distribution of air in the lung at FRC. As momentum is the product of an object's mass and velocity, the larger mass of lung tissue in the lower quadrants may generate greater momentum during expiration and be more prone to collapse than the upper quadrants, which have a smaller mass. Thus, medium PEEP levels (5PEEP) are able to

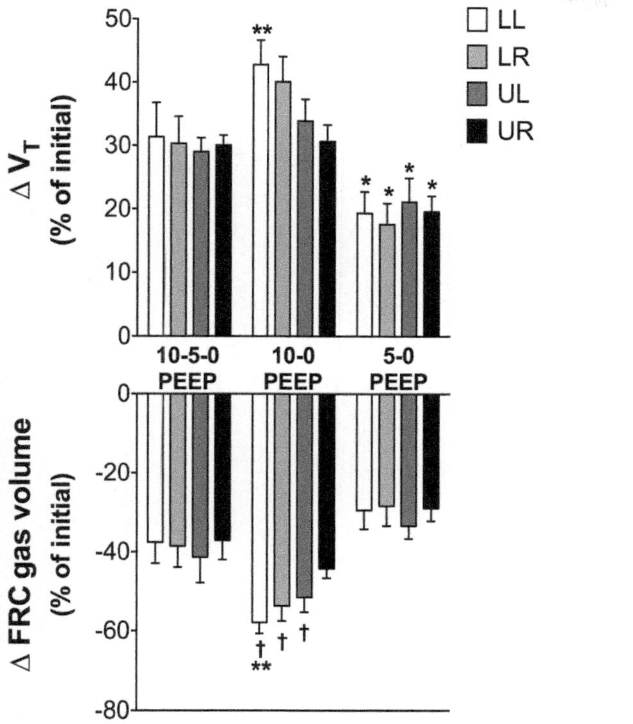

Figure 5. Changes in V_T and FRC during decreasing PEEP. The increase in tidal volume (V_T) and decrease in functional residual capacity (FRC) when positive end-expiratory pressure (PEEP) is decreased in 5 cmH_2O stepwise decrements (10-5-0PEEP), large steps (10-0PEEP) and from a small step (5-0PEEP) in the ventilated lung. Asterisks (*) indicate that values during 5-0PEEP are significantly different to their corresponding quadrant during 10-5-0PEEP and 10-0PEEP. Double asterisks (**) indicate that values during 10-5-0PEEP are significantly different to their corresponding quadrant during 10-0PEEP. Daggers (†) indicate that values during 5-0PEEP are significantly different to their corresponding quadrant during 10-0PEEP. Values are significantly different if $p<0.05$. There was no significant difference between quadrants within any group.

oppose lung collapse in the upper lung quadrants, which have a smaller mass, whereas higher PEEP levels are required to oppose lung collapse in regions with a greater mass. Alternatively, regional differences in chest wall compliance, with the upper chest being less compliant, may account for the regional differences in FRC across the lung.

The persisting effects that the initial PEEP level had on the distribution of air within the lung at FRC during the experiment, despite subsequent changes in PEEP, are difficult to explain. When ventilation was initiated with 0 or 5PEEP, the non-uniform distribution of air at FRC persisted at all PEEP levels throughout the experiment, even during ventilation with 10PEEP. However, when ventilation was initiated with 10PEEP, the distribution of air at FRC was uniform and although the uniformity decreased with decreasing PEEP, it was restored by ventilation with 10PEEP. This indicates that the initial distribution of lung aeration may define the subsequent mechanical behaviour of localised lung regions, with regions that do not initially aerate persisting with lower compliances and lower air volumes at FRC no matter what the subsequent PEEP setting. Further studies are required to determine whether this effect PEEP extends for longer than the duration of this experiment.

In contrast to many studies that investigate the distribution of lung ventilation in supine patients [15–17,25,26], our study imaged newborn rabbit pups positioned upright in a water-filled plethysmograph. It is possible that the upright positioning of the pups during ventilation contributed to the greater distribution of air in the upper compared to the lower quadrants, although we would expect this to have been more apparent if the pups were supine due to the effect of the abdominal contents pushing the diaphragm. In this experiment, the overall influence of gravity on the lung is likely to be minimal as the pups were ventilated whilst suspended in a water-filled plethysmograph. This alleviates the weight of the more vertical lungs regions and the heart on the lower regions thus reducing the dependent/non-dependent lung effect. It also removes the influence of the abdominal contents and the upward displacement of the diaphragm on the lung that would occur if the pup were positioned horizontally. As such, the position of the pup is not expected to significantly influence the distribution of ventilation. As neonates are normally positioned supine or prone, the non-uniform ventilation distributions we observed may exist and be amplified in infants. Ventilation heterogeneity would be expected due to the effects of gravity between non-dependent and dependent lung regions [17,25] and the pressure applied by abdominal contents on the diaphragm, which displaces it into the thorax. Ventilation inhomogeneity has been observed in ventilated infants lying supine, prone and quarter prone, but the authors suggest that ventilation distribution is minimally impacted by gravity [26].

Previous studies have cautioned against the use of high PEEP levels because it can reduce pulmonary blood flow (PBF) [27,28], overexpand alveoli and increase the risk of lung injury [29]. As such, PEEP levels as high as 10 cmH_2O are not recommended for neonates, but in those studies, the newborn lungs were aerated before the high PEEP level was applied. Thus, it is not known whether high PEEP levels during lung aeration at birth cause similar effects. A recent study has shown that an initial sustained inflation of ~1 min (to 35 cmH_2O) induces a greater increase in PBF than conventional ventilation [30]. This indicates that a sustained increase in airway pressure during lung aeration does not have the same negative impact on PBF as it does once the lung has aerated. In our study, none of the rabbit pups developed a pneumothorax, despite appearing maximally aerated at V_{PIP} during ventilation with 10PEEP (see Movies S1–S3, during the period of 10PEEP ventilation). More specifically, when ventilation commenced with 10PEEP, the lungs did not maximally aerate at V_{PIP} during the initial 10PEEP period. This suggests that the lungs were not over-expanded, either globally or in any one region by initiating ventilation with a temporary period of 10PEEP. Furthermore, a short period of ventilation with 10PEEP at birth was found to confer considerable benefit resulting in a remarkably uniform distribution of air across the lung during subsequent ventilation. While there are more familiar methods to promote uniform lung ventilation at birth, such as sustained inflations [23] and prophylactic surfactant [5], initial ventilation with a high PEEP level may be a more practical alternative.

There are many studies demonstrating multiple advantages of PEEP/CPAP on lung aeration and gas exchange in newborns, however, it is difficult to deliver these pressures uninterrupted in the delivery room. Not all positive pressure ventilation devices deliver a set PEEP reliably [31,32] and face mask leak is common [33] and if large (>60%) substantially reduces the effective PEEP level [12]. Our results suggest that if the loss of PEEP is gradual (i.e. 10-5-0PEEP), or if the reduction in PEEP is small (i.e. 5-0PEEP), the changes in V_T and FRC are relatively uniform throughout the lung. (Fig. 5). However, large and continuous reductions in PEEP (i.e. 10-0PEEP) caused large changes in V_T and FRC predominantly within in the lower lung quadrants

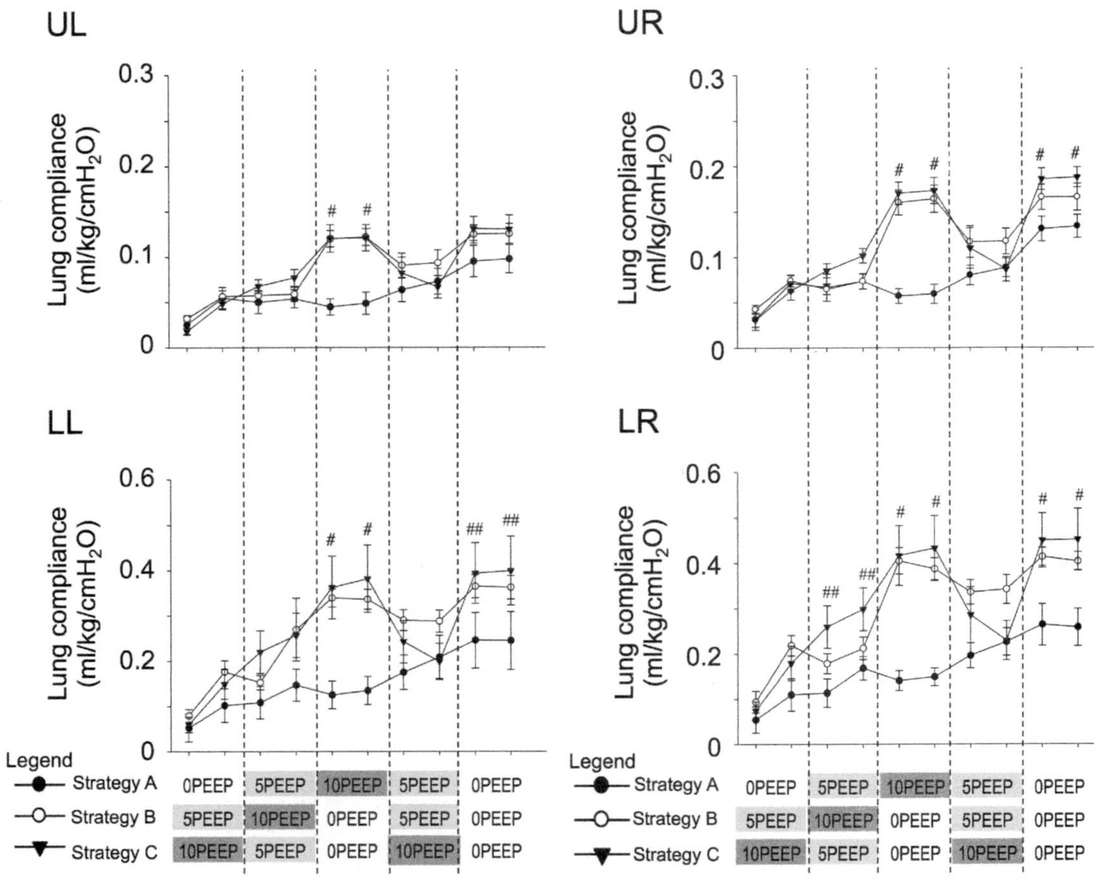

Figure 6. Changes in lung compliance in ventilation strategies A, B and C. Lung compliance of each quadrant (upper left (UL), upper right (UR), lower left (LL) and lower right (LR)) compared between Strategy A (closed circles), Strategy B (open circles) and Strategy C (closed triangles). The x-axis demonstrates the timing and sequence of PEEP change for each strategy. Hashes (#) indicate that Strategy A was significantly different to Strategy B and C. Double hashes (##) indicate that Strategy A was different only to Strategy C. Values are significantly different if $p<0.05$.

(Fig. 5). In the delivery room, respiratory support is often interrupted to reposition the facemask, perform suction, to change mask size, to change the interface for transport and during transfer of the infant to a transportation crib. Previous studies in preterm infants at 7 days of postnatal age have shown that such a rapid reduction in PEEP reduces FRC by as much as 30% within a minute of removing the PEEP [34]. Based on our results, sudden and large losses in PEEP would alter the distribution of ventilation within the lungs, causing marked reductions in FRC and greater V_T changes in the dependent lobes thereby increasing the risk of shear stress injury in these regions. While such interruptions in respiratory support are often necessary, the risks could be minimised by 1) reducing the PEEP gradually and 2) reducing the size of the dependent lung by placing the infant on its side, preferably the left.

It is unclear why the degree of continuous PEEP decrease affected the distribution of air at FRC and the incoming V_T, as the total changes in lung air volumes at 0PEEP were the same between 10-0PEEP and 10-5-0PEEP (data not shown). It is unlikely to be due to the rate of PEEP decrease, because the maximum rate of PEEP decrease was ~1 cmH_2O per inflation, such that a 5 cmH_2O decrease required ~5 inflations and a 10 cmH_2O decrease required ~10 inflations. It is possible that a large continuous decrease in PEEP generates momentum within the lung tissue, particularly in the lower quadrants with larger masses, resulting in larger decreases in FRC with each expiration. However, when the decrease in PEEP was interrupted by a period of ventilation at 5PEEP, the distribution of ventilation between quadrants remained relatively even despite the reduction to 0PEEP, again indicating that previous PEEP history can impact on the distribution of ventilation within the lung.

It is likely that the lower lung quadrants had greater volume changes in response to changes in PEEP because these lung regions are larger and are thus more compliant (Fig. 6). It may appear counter intuitive that dynamic lung compliance in all quadrants gradually increased during ventilation with both an increasing (Strategy A) and decreasing (Strategy B) PEEP strategy. Increasing PEEP and PEEP recruitment strategies are known to increase lung compliance by allowing tidal expansion to occur within a more compliant region of the pressure volume curve [11,35]. However, these pups were premature and surfactant deficient and the initial dynamic compliance measurements are dominated by the presence of airway liquid, which increases airway resistance ~100 fold [20]. Thus, the gradual increase in lung compliance mainly reflects the gradual increase in lung aeration. As such, our findings indicate that the presence of airway liquid is the dominant determinant of dynamic lung compliance during lung aeration. However, following complete lung aeration (usually after ventilation with 10PEEP), increasing PEEP from 0PEEP (Strategies B & C) mostly reduced measures of dynamic lung compliance, whereas decreasing PEEP to 0PEEP increased dynamic lung compliance. Furthermore, during the final 0PEEP ventilation period in all strategies, regional lung compliance, particularly in the lower quadrants, was markedly greater if ventilation had commenced with PEEP (either 5 or 10 cmH_2O) compared with 0PEEP. Although the mechanism is unknown, our study demonstrates that initiating ventilation with PEEP effects subsequent ventilation. These effects were observed for 10 minutes in our experiment but, as lung aeration continues to increase, these affects will likely persist beyond the experimental period.

After the lungs had fully aerated (ie after ventilation with 10PEEP in all strategies), as all pups were ventilated with a set PIP of 35 cmH_2O, the air volumes and the distribution of air at V_{PIP} remained relatively stable at all subsequent PEEP levels. Thus, although V_{PIP} tended to decrease at 0PEEP, the increase and decrease in V_T associated with decreases and increases in PEEP, respectively, mainly resulted from decreases and increases in FRC. This indicates that the effect of PEEP on the pressure-volume (P-V) relationship of the aerating lung immediately after birth is substantially different than it is following complete lung aeration. We found that altering the PEEP level had little or no effect on lung air volumes at V_{PIP}, resulting in a lower V_T when the FRC increased in response to a higher PEEP. How this effects CO_2 clearance is unclear as, although V_T is reduced which would normally increase CO_2 retention, our previous study has shown that V_{PIP} is a primary determinant of CO_2 clearance during lung aeration [36].

At birth, as the lungs make their transition from a liquid-filled to an air-filled organ, changes in PEEP have a marked influence on the distribution of ventilation. Our results demonstrate that when initiating ventilation at birth, the uniformity of ventilation depends on the level of PEEP, with higher PEEPs promoting more uniform ventilation. As such, it is possible that starting infant resuscitation with higher PEEP levels and then gradually reducing the PEEP to currently recommended levels after a few minutes may increase the distribution of ventilation in preterm infants. Furthermore, after the lungs were fully aerated, larger continuous changes in PEEP reduced ventilation within the lower lung quadrants to a greater extent than in the upper lung quadrants. Since providing consistent assisted ventilation at birth is difficult, due to face mask leak or the need to temporarily remove pressure support, it is important to acknowledge that changes in PEEP, even brief, are not without impact on lung volumes and ventilation distribution that can persist. These effects may impair gas exchange or increase the risk of lung damage.

Supporting Information

Movie S1 Phase contrast X-ray movie of a preterm rabbit pup ventilated with Strategy A (0-5-10-5-10PEEP).

Movie S2 Phase contrast X-ray movie of a preterm rabbit pup ventilated with Strategy B (5-10-0-5-0PEEP).

Movie S3 Phase contrast X-ray movie of a preterm rabbit pup ventilated with Strategy C (10-5-0-10-0PEEP).

Author Contributions

Conceived and designed the experiments: ABtP SBH MJK MLS. Performed the experiments: MJK MLS MJW AF RAL NY KU ABtP SBH. Analyzed the data: MJK MLS. Contributed reagents/materials/analysis tools: MJK. Wrote the paper: MJK MLS ABtP SBH MJW AF RAL NY KU.

References

1. Hooper SB, Harding R (2005) Role of aeration in the physiological adaptation of the lung to air-breathing at birth. Current Respiratory Medicine Reviews 1: 185–195.
2. te Pas AB, Davis PG, Kamlin CO, Dawson J, O'Donnell CP, et al. (2008) Spontaneous breathing patterns of very preterm infants treated with continuous positive airway pressure at birth. Pediatric Research 64: 281–285.
3. Mortola JP (1984) Breathing pattern in newborns. J Appl Physiol 56: 1533–1540.
4. Jobe AH, Ikegami M (2000) Lung development and function in preterm infants in the surfactant treatment era. AnnuRevPhysiol 62 825–846.
5. Siew ML, te Pas AB, Wallace MJ, Kitchen MJ, Islam M, et al. (2011) Surfactant increases the uniformity of lung aeration at birth in ventilated preterm rabbits. Pediatr Res 70: 50–55.
6. Enhorning G, Robertson B, Milne E, Wagner R (1975) Radiologic evaluation of the premature newborn rabbit after pharyngeal deposition of surfactant. Am J Obstet Gynecol 121: 475–480.
7. Gerhardt T, Bancalari E (1980) Chestwall compliance in full-term and premature infants. Acta Paediatrica Scandinavica 69: 359–364.
8. Hjalmarson O, Sandberg K (2002) Abnormal lung function in healthy preterm infants. Am J Respir Crit Care Med 165: 83–87.
9. Siew ML, te Pas AB, Wallace MJ, Kitchen MJ, Lewis RA, et al. (2009) Positive end expiratory pressure enhances development of a functional residual capacity in preterm rabbits ventilated from birth. J Appl Physiol 106: 1487–1493.
10. Probyn ME, Hooper SB, Dargaville PA, McCallion N, Crossley K, et al. (2004) Positive end expiratory pressure during resuscitation of premature lambs rapidly improves blood gases without adversely affecting arterial pressure. Pediatric Research 56: 198–204.
11. Nilsson R, Grossmann G, Robertson B (1980) Artificial ventilation of premature newborn rabbits: effects of positive end-expiratory pressure on lung mechanics and lung morphology. Acta Paediatrica Scandinavica 69: 597–602.
12. te Pas AB, Schilleman K, Klein M, Witlox RS, Morley CJ, et al. (2011) Low versus high gas flow rate for respiratory support of infants at birth: a manikin study. Neonatology 99: 266–271.
13. Schilleman K, Schmolzer GM, Kamlin OC, Morley CJ, te Pas AB, et al. (2011) Changing gas flow during neonatal resuscitation: a manikin study. Resuscitation 82: 920–924.
14. Tingay DG, Copnell B, Grant CA, Dargaville PA, Dunster KR, et al. (2010) The effect of endotracheal suction on regional tidal ventilation and end-expiratory lung volume. Intensive Care Med 36: 888–896.
15. Puybasset L, Gusman P, Muller JC, Cluzel P, Coriat P, et al. (2000) Regional distribution of gas and tissue in acute respiratory distress syndrome. III. Consequences for the effects of positive end-expiratory pressure. Intensive Care Medicine 26: 1215–1227.
16. Nieszkowska A, Lu Q, Vieira S, Elman M, Fetita C, et al. (2004) Incidence and regional distribution of lung overinflation during mechanical ventilation with positive end-expiratory pressure. Critical Care Medicine 32: 1496–1503.
17. Wolf GK, Grychtol B, Frerichs I, van Genderingen HR, Zurakowski D, et al. (2007) Regional lung volume changes in children with acute respiratory distress syndrome during a derecruitment maneuver. Crit Care Med 35: 1972–1978.
18. Kitchen MJ, Lewis RA, Morgan MJ, Wallace MJ, Siew MLL, et al. (2008) Dynamic measures of lung air volume using phase contrast X-ray imaging. Phys Med Biol 53: 6065–6077.
19. Hooper SB, Kitchen MJ, Wallace MJ, Yagi N, Uesugi K, et al. (2007) Imaging lung aeration and lung liquid clearance at birth. FASEB J 21: 3329–3337.
20. te Pas AB, Siew M, Wallace MJ, Kitchen MJ, Fouras A, et al. (2009) Effect of sustained inflation length on establishing functional residual capacity at birth in ventilated premature rabbits. Pediatric Research 66: 295–300.
21. Siew ML, Wallace MJ, Kitchen MJ, Lewis RA, Fouras A, et al. (2009) Inspiration regulates the rate and temporal pattern of lung liquid clearance and lung aeration at birth. J Appl Physiol 106: 1888–1895.
22. Dinger J, Topfer A, Schaller P, Schwarze R (2001) Effect of positive end expiratory pressure on functional residual capacity and compliance in surfactant-treated preterm infants. Journal of Perinatal Medicine 29: 137–143.
23. te Pas AB, Siew M, Wallace MJ, Kitchen MJ, Fouras A, et al. (2009) Establishing functional residual capacity at birth: the effect of sustained inflation and positive end expiratory pressure in a preterm rabbit model. Pediatr Res 65: 537–541.
24. Thome U, Topfer A, Schaller P, Pohlandt F (1998) The effect of positive endexpiratory pressure, peak inspiratory pressure, and inspiratory time on functional residual capacity in mechanically ventilated preterm infants. European Journal of Pediatrics 157: 831–837.
25. Frerichs I, Schiffmann H, Oehler R, Dudykevych T, Hahn G, et al. (2003) Distribution of lung ventilation in spontaneously breathing neonates lying in different body positions. Intensive Care Med 29: 787–794.
26. Hough JL, Johnston L, Brauer S, Woodgate P, Schibler A (2013) Effect of body position on ventilation distribution in ventilated preterm infants. Pediatr Crit Care Med 14: 171–177.
27. Polglase GR, Morley CJ, Crossley KJ, Dargaville P, Harding R, et al. (2005) Positive end-expiratory pressure differentially alters pulmonary hemodynamics

and oxygenation in ventilated, very premature lambs. J ApplPhysiol 99: 1453–1461.
28. Schlessel JS, Susskind H, Joel DD, Bossuyt A, Harrold WH, et al. (1989) Effect of PEEP on regional ventilation and perfusion in the mechanically ventilated preterm lamb. JNuclMed 30: 1342–1350.
29. Naik AS, Kallapur SG, Bachurski CJ, Jobe AH, Michna J, et al. (2001) Effects of ventilation with different positive end-expiratory pressures on cytokine expression in the preterm lamb lung. AmJRespirCrit Care Med 164: 494–498.
30. Sobotka KS, Hooper SB, Allison BJ, Pas ABT, Davis PG, et al. (2011) An Initial Sustained Inflation Improves the Respiratory and Cardiovascular Transition at Birth in Preterm Lambs. Pediatric Research 70: 56–60.
31. Dawson JA, Gerber A, Kamlin COF, Davis PG, Morley CJ (2011) Providing PEEP during neonatal resuscitation: Which device is best? Journal of Paediatrics and Child Health 47: 698–703.
32. Morley CJ, Dawson JA, Stewart MJ, Hussain F, Davis PG (2010) The effect of a PEEP valve on a Laerdal neonatal self-inflating resuscitation bag. Journal of Paediatrics and Child Health 46: 51–56.
33. Schmolzer GM, Kamlin OC, O'Donnell CP, Dawson JA, Morley CJ, et al. (2010) Assessment of tidal volume and gas leak during mask ventilation of preterm infants in the delivery room. ArchDisChildFetal Neonatal Ed 95: F393–F397.
34. Vilstrup CT, Bjorklund LJ, Larsson A, Lachmann B, Werner O (1992) Functional residual capacity and ventilation homogeneity in mechanically ventilated small neonates. JApplPhysiol 73: 276–283.
35. Kelly E, Bryan H, Possmayer F, Frndova H, Bryan C (1993) Compliance of the respiratory system in newborn infants pre- and postsurfactant replacement therapy. Pediatric Pulmonology 15: 225–230.
36. Hooper SB, Fouras A, Siew ML, Wallace MJ, Kitchen MJ, et al. (2013) Expired CO2 levels indicate degree of lung aeration at birth. PLoS One 8: e70895.

15

Pilot Quasi-Randomized Controlled Study of Herbal Medicine Hochuekkito as an Adjunct to Conventional Treatment for Progressed Pulmonary *Mycobacterium avium* Complex Disease

Yasunori Enomoto*, Eri Hagiwara, Shigeru Komatsu, Ryuichi Nishihira, Tomohisa Baba, Hideya Kitamura, Akimasa Sekine, Atsuhito Nakazawa, Takashi Ogura

Department of Respiratory Medicine, Kanagawa Cardiovascular and Respiratory Center, Yokohama, Japan

Abstract

Introduction: Hochuekkito, a traditional herbal medicine, is occasionally prescribed in Japan to treat patients with a poor general condition. We aimed to examine whether this medicine was beneficial and tolerable for patients with progressed pulmonary *Mycobacterium avium* complex (MAC) disease.

Methods: This pilot open-label quasi-randomized controlled trial enrolled 18 patients with progressed pulmonary MAC disease who had initiated antimycobacterial treatment over one year ago but were persistently culture-positive or intolerant. All patients continued their baseline treatment regimens with (n = 9) or without (n = 9) oral Hochuekkito for 24 weeks.

Results: Baseline characteristics were generally similar between the groups. Most patients were elderly (median age 70 years), female, had a low body mass index (<20 kg/m^2), and a long-term disease duration (median approximately 8 years). After the 24-week treatment period, no patient achieved sputum conversion. Although the number of colonies in sputum tended to increase in the control group, it generally remained stable in the Hochuekkito group. Radiological disease control was frequently observed in the Hochuekkito group than the control group (8/9 vs. 3/9; p = 0.05). Patients in the Hochuekkito group tended to experience increase in body weight and serum albumin level compared with those in the control group (median body weight change: +0.4 kg vs. −0.8 kg; median albumin change: +0.2 g/dl vs. ±0.0 g/dl). No severe adverse events occurred.

Conclusions: Hochuekkito could be an effective, feasible adjunct to conventional therapy for patients with progressed pulmonary MAC disease. Future study is needed to explore this possibility.

Trial Registration: UMIN Clinical Trials Registry UMIN000009920

Editor: T. Mark Doherty, Glaxo Smith Kline, Denmark

Funding: The authors have no support or funding to report.

Competing Interests: The authors have declared that no competing interests exist.

* Email: yasuyasuyasu29@yahoo.co.jp

Introduction

Mycobacterium avium complex (MAC) is the most common pathogen involved in pulmonary nontuberculous mycobacterium diseases. Recommended treatment regimens offer combinations of drugs including macrolides and others. Patients should ideally be treated for a long period until confirmation of at least 1 year of negative sputum cultures [1]. Majority of patients on macrolide-containing regimens are able to achieve negative sputum cultures within 12 months [2,3]. However, some cases are intractable despite appropriate therapy [4] or due to an intolerance of the recommended therapeutic agents. For those cases, few options are left other than symptom palliation. Although surgery is one of those [1,5], it is difficult to perform it in patients with advanced disease. Alternative and feasible therapeutic agents are awaited.

Hochuekkito (Bu-Zhong-Yi-Qi-Tang in Chinese) is a herbal mixture used in Kampo traditional medicine; it is composed of several plant materials, including *Angelicae radix*, *Astragali radix*, *Atractylodis rhizoma*, *Aurantii nobilis pericarpium*, *Bupleuri radix*, *Cimicifugae rhizoma*, *Ginseng radix*, *Glycyrrhizae radix*, *Zingiberis rhizoma*, and *Zizyphi fructus*. This drug is often used in Japan to treat patients who are in a weakened physical condition, although its pharmacological activity and mechanism of action are not completely understood. Previous studies have demonstrated the immunomodulating effects by increasing serum interferon-γ level [6,7], which is advantageous for killing intracellular pathogens like MAC. On the other hand, Hochuekkito can potentially improve nutritional status and quality of life [8,9]. Actually, beneficial effects of this medicine were reported on some respiratory diseases including chronic lower respiratory tract infection [10] and chronic obstructive pulmonary disease [8]. Therapeutic strategy against chronic wasting disease by immunomodulating activities and/or improving nutritional status would be of a future for progressed MAC disease even without bactericidal effect. In this regard, we conducted a pilot comparative study to evaluate the efficacy and safety of Hochuekkito as an adjunct to conventional treatment in those patients with progressed intractable pulmonary MAC disease.

Methods

Patients

This study was conducted in accordance with good clinical practice and the ethical principles outlined in the Declaration of Helsinki. The protocol was approved by the institutional review board of Kanagawa Cardiovascular and Respiratory Center. All patients provided their written informed consent before registration. The trial was registered under number UMIN000009920 (http://www.umin.ac.jp/). The protocol for this trial and supporting CONSORT checklist are available as supporting information; see Checklist S1 and Protocol S1.

Eligible patients were ≥20 years of age and had been diagnosed with pulmonary MAC disease in accordance with American Thoracic Society/Infectious Diseases Society of America criteria [1] at least 1 year prior to the time of registration. The patients had been treated with antimycobacterial drugs for ≥1 year at our institution but were persistently culture-positive or intolerant and thus met the recommendations for Hochuekkito therapy. Kampo drugs are generally recommended to be used on the basis of the patient's "Sho," which is the special concept in this field and implies the symptoms and/or systemic conditions. Clinicians assess the "Sho," such as Yang (positivity)/Yin (negativity) or Jitsu (fullness)/Kyo (deficiency), and thereafter, choice the most appropriate drug. The recommendation for Hochuekkito therapy included a decline in physical strength, general fatigue, or appetite loss, which are also originated from the concept of "Sho." MAC-positive sputum cultures in solid media within the 3 months prior to registration were confirmed in all patients. Drug susceptibility tests were performed with the broth microdilution method. Macrolides, rifamycins, ethambutol, aminoglycosides, and fluoroquinolones were all regarded as antimycobacterial drugs in this study.

Exclusion criteria included ongoing malignant diseases, interstitial lung diseases or other severe pulmonary diseases, human immunodeficiency virus infection, pregnancy or childbearing potential, and cases in which the antimycobacterial regimen had been changed or who had initiated therapy with herbal drugs (including Hochuekkito) within the 3 months before registration.

Study design and treatment

This was an open-label, single-center, prospective, parallel group, comparative study. The eligible patients were enrolled by each clinician, and sequentially allocated to Hochuekkito or

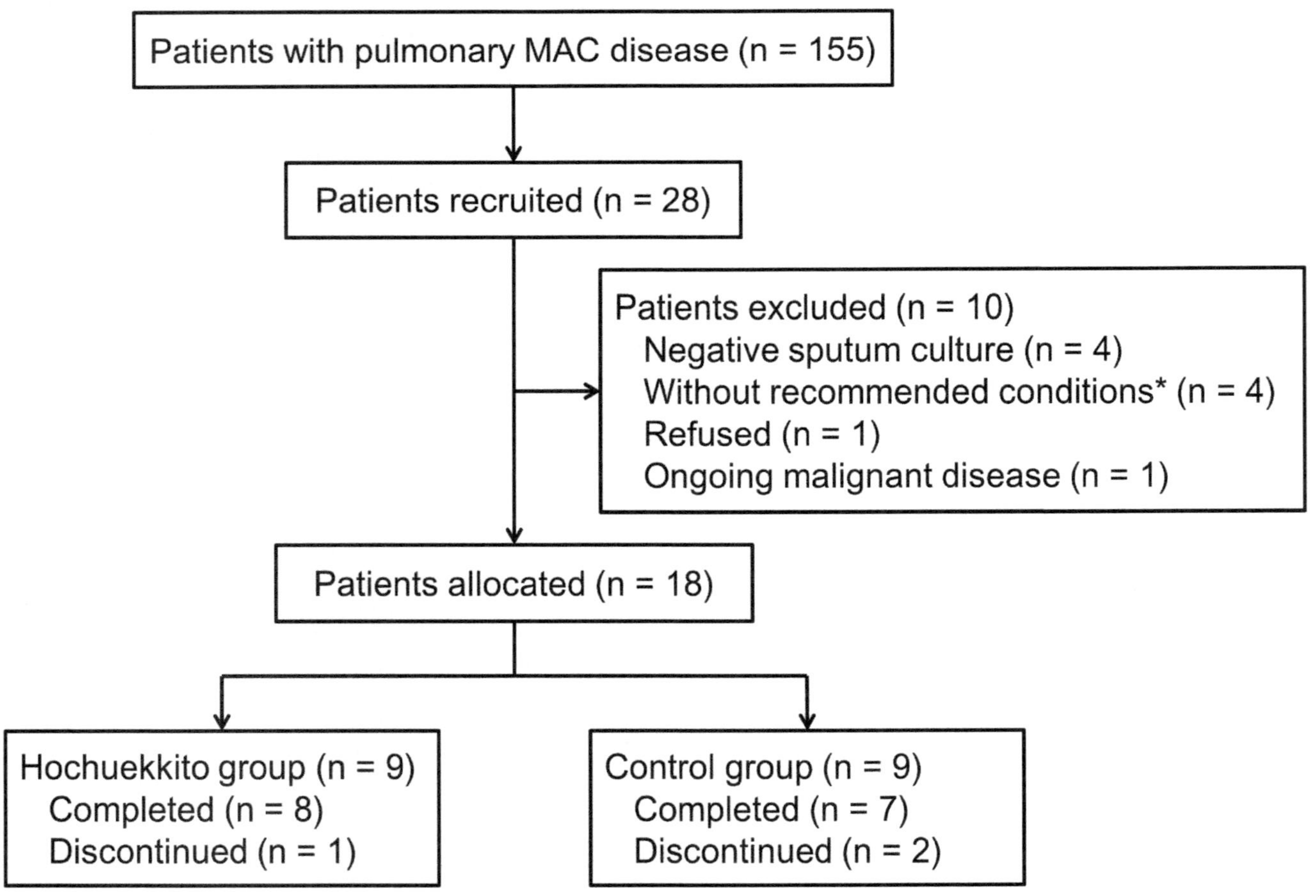

Figure 1. Patient inclusion/exclusion. MAC = *Mycobacterium avium* complex. *Declined physical strength, general fatigue, or appetite loss.

Table 1. Comparison of baseline characteristics in the Hochuekkito and control groups.

	Hochuekkito (n = 9)	Control (n = 9)	p value
Age, years	70 (44, 80)	70 (59, 83)	0.60
Sex, male / female	2/7	2/7	1.00
Smoking status, current and former / never	1/8	4/5	0.29
BMI, kg/m^2	17.6 (16.8, 25.7)	17.4 (15.0, 23.7)	0.40
Disease duration, months	96 (18, 241)	90 (28, 128)	1.00
Number of colonies in sputum culture*	4 (1, 8)	4 (1, 8)	0.50
Extent in chest X-ray, <1/3/1/3–2/3/>2/3	2/2/5	1/2/6	0.81
Cavity in chest X-ray, yes / no	7/2	4/5	0.34
Albumin, g/dl	3.8 (3.5, 4.1)	4.2 (3.6, 4.5)	0.12
CRP, mg/dl	0.62 (0.05, 6.49)	0.19 (0.01, 1.38)	0.20
ESR, mm/hr	60 (9, 100)	35 (11, 49)	0.047
CAT score†	11 (3, 27)	17 (4, 30)	0.43

Data are expressed as the number of patients or median (with observed range: minimum, maximum). All p values are for comparisons between the two groups and were obtained by Fisher's exact test, Pearson's test, or Mann-Whitney U test as appropriate.
BMI = body mass index; CRP = C-reactive protein; ESR = erythrocyte segmentation rate; CAT = chronic obstructive pulmonary disease assessment test.
*Semi-quantitative scoring system: 0 (no colonies), 1 (1–9 colonies), 2 (10–49 colonies), 3 (50–99 colonies), 4 (100–199 colonies), 5 (200–299 colonies), 6 (300–399 colonies), 7 (400–499 colonies), and 8 (≥500 colonies).
†Chronic obstructive pulmonary disease assessment test score ranging from 0 to 40. A higher score means more severe symptoms [11].

control groups in order at the secretariat of our institution. Patients were followed at our institution every 4–8 weeks for up to 24 weeks after allocation. Allocation was stratified by whether patients were currently receiving antimycobacterial medications at the time of registration. All patients continued their preceding treatment regimens at the same dosages over the follow-up period. Those in the Hochuekkito group also received oral Hochuekkito 5.0 g twice daily or 7.5 g three times daily before or after each meal. Daily dosage was determined by each clinician on the basis of patients' physical constitution and/or demands. If a patient had not been prescribed any antimycobacterial drugs at the time of registration, he or she was observed with no medication (control group) or was medicated with Hochuekkito alone (Hochuekkito group).

Efficacy endpoints

The primary endpoint was the sputum conversion rate at 24 weeks after treatment initiation. Sputum culture conversion was defined as confirmation of culture negativity at two consecutive time points (on different days but within a 2-week period). If the patients could not produce sputum, inducement by nebulized hypertonic salt solution was performed. All sputum cultures were grown on solid media, which enables counting the number of colonies. The microbiology technicians were unaware of the treatment assignments throughout the study. The number of MAC colonies in the sputum cultures was also recorded before and after treatment. Because of difficulty counting the exact number of colonies, we used a semi-quantitative scoring system: 0 (no colonies), 1 (1–9 colonies), 2 (10–49 colonies), 3 (50–99 colonies), 4 (100–199 colonies), 5 (200–299 colonies), 6 (300–399 colonies), 7 (400–499 colonies), and 8 (≥500 colonies). Important secondary endpoint was changes in chest X-ray images over the 24-week treatment period. Chest X-ray images were independently reviewed by two experienced clinicians (S. K. and R. N.) who were blinded to the group assignment; they evaluated the disease

Table 2. Comparison of treatment status at the time of registration between patients in the Hochuekkito and control groups.

	Hochuekkito (n = 9)	Control (n = 9)
On medication, yes / no	8/1	8/1
Baseline treatment regimens		
RFP, EB, CAM + others*	3	0
RFP, EB, CAM	3	5
RFP, CAM, LVFX	1	1
RFP, CAM	1	1
EB, CAM	0	1
CAM resistant†, yes / no	4/5	4/5

Data are expressed as number of patients.
RFP = rifampicin (10 mg/kg/day); EB = ethambutol (15 mg/kg/day); CAM = clarithromycin (15–20 mg/kg/day); LVFX = levofloxacin (10 mg/kg/day).
*Aminoglycosides (Kanamycin or Streptomycin: 15 mg/kg two/three times per a week) and/or fluoroquinolones.
†Minimum inhibitory concentration to CAM >32 μg/ml by the broth microdilution method.

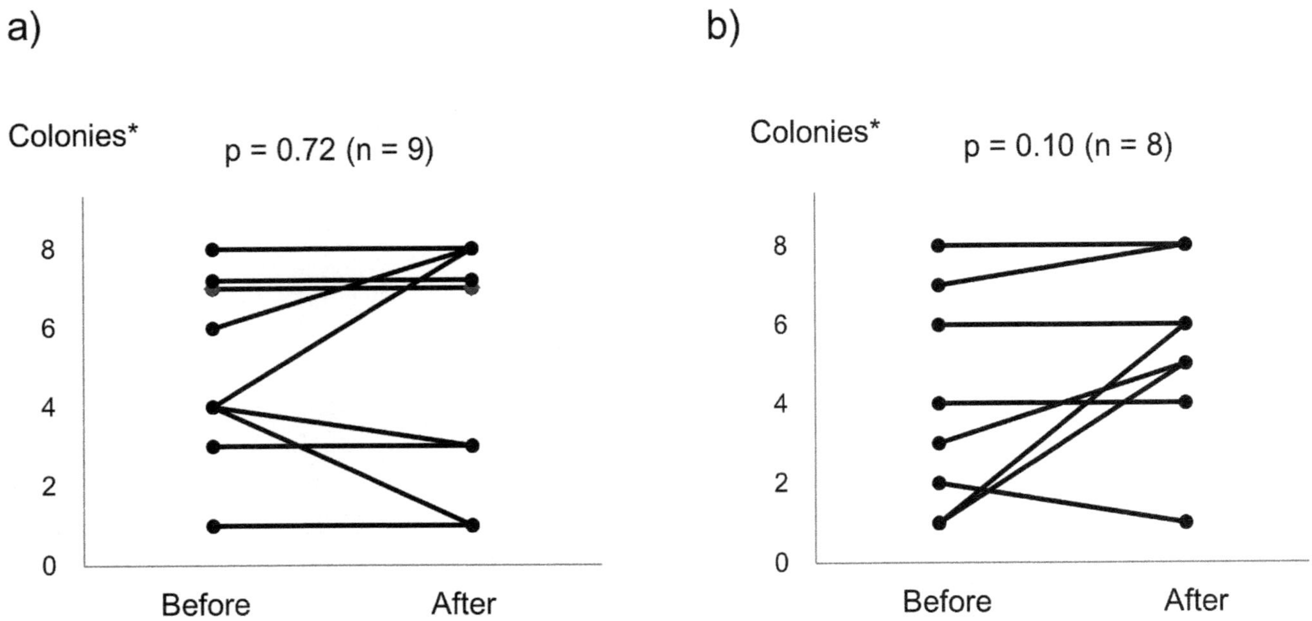

Figure 2. Changes in sputum findings over the 24-week treatment period. The number of MAC colonies in the sputum cultures of patients in the Hochuekkito (a) and control (b) groups. All p values were determined by using Wilcoxon signed-rank test. MAC = *Mycobacterium avium* complex. *Semi-quantitative scoring system: 0 (no colonies), 1 (1–9 colonies), 2 (10–49 colonies), 3 (50–99 colonies), 4 (100–199 colonies), 5 (200–299 colonies), 6 (300–399 colonies), 7 (400–499 colonies), and 8 (≥500 colonies).

extent (<1/3, 1/3–2/3, or >2/3 of the lung area) and the presence/absence of cavities at baseline as well as changes over the 24-week treatment period (improved, stable, or worsened). Disagreements between the two reviewers were resolved by consensus. Additional and exploratory secondary endpoints were changes in chronic obstructive pulmonary disease assessment test (CAT: 0–40) score [11] evaluating patients' symptom, body weight, and three biomarkers over the 24 weeks: serum albumin, C-reactive protein (CRP), and erythrocyte segmentation rate (ESR). In the field of pulmonary MAC disease, evidenced symptom scoring system is not available. Although the validation was not studied, we used CAT score for the substitution.

Safety assessment

Safety was assessed by recording adverse events at least every 8 weeks. These were obtained by clinicians' interview and laboratory results including complete blood counts and the following serum biomarkers: aspartate aminotransferase, alanine aminotransferase, total bilirubin, direct bilirubin, urea nitrogen, creatinine, sodium, and potassium. The severity of each event was determined by the Common Terminology Criteria for Adverse Events v4.0 (CTCAEv4).

Statistical analysis

We assumed negative conversion rates for 5% in the control group and 30% in the Hochuekkito group. With a two-sided alpha level of 0.05, total enrollment of 78 patients was needed to attain power of 80%. Thus, the target sample size was determined as 80. Efficacy and safety were assessed among all allocated patients. Data were expressed as number of patients or as medians with observed ranges. Interobserver agreement with respect to the radiological assessment was determined using kappa statistics (< 0.4: relatively poor; 0.4–0.6: moderate; 0.6–0.8: good; 0.8–1.0: excellent). Group comparisons were performed using Fisher's exact test, Pearson's test, or Mann-Whitney U test as appropriate. Serial changes in the number of colonies in sputum culture were evaluated by Wilcoxon signed-rank test. A p value of <0.05 was considered to be significant. Analyses were performed using SPSS software version 13.0 (SPSS, Inc., Chicago, IL, USA).

Results

Baseline characteristics

Of the 155 patients with pulmonary MAC disease who were diagnosed and followed up at our institution, 28 were recruited for candidates between February and June 2013. Eighteen of these patients were eligible for inclusion and were allocated to the Hochuekkito group (n = 9) or the control group (n = 9) (Figure 1). We were unable to recruit as many patients as expected, and thus decided to end the study with smaller number of patients than the protocol planned. Baseline characteristics are summarized in Table 1, and are mostly similar between the two groups. Most patients were elderly (median age 70 years), female, had a low body mass index <20 kg/m^2, and a long-term disease duration (median approximately 8 years). There were no significant differences in chest X-ray findings between the two groups. Interobserver agreement with respect to the radiological assessment was moderate to excellent (disease extent, $\kappa = 0.45$; presence/absence of cavities, $\kappa = 1.0$). The baseline ESR was significantly higher and the serum albumin level was comparatively lower, in the Hochuekkito group compared with the control group. There were no significant differences in the number of MAC colonies in the sputum cultures and baseline CAT scores between the groups.

Treatment status at the time of registration is summarized in Table 2. Each group included one patient who had not received any antimycobacterial medication at the time of registration. A three-drug regimen consisting of rifampicin, ethambutol, and clarithromycin was most common in both groups. Aminoglycosides and/or fluoroquinolones were frequently added to the

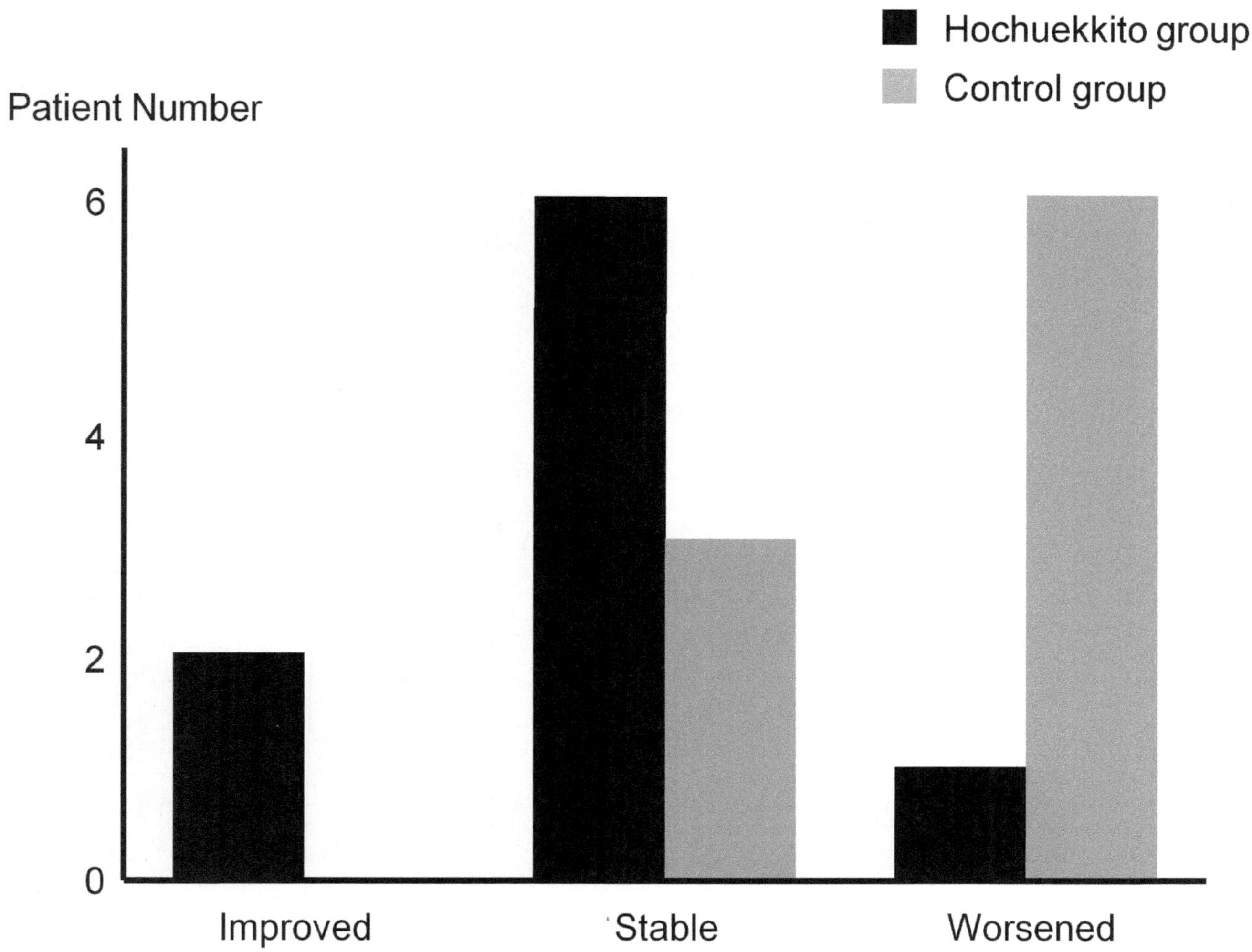

Figure 3. Changes in radiological findings over the 24-week treatment period. Radiological assessment was performed by comparing chest X-ray images before and after treatment.

combination regimen in the Hochuekkito group. However, there was no significant difference in the number of drugs patients had been administered before study initiation [median 4 (range 3–10) in the Hochuekkito group vs. median 4 (range 1–5) in the control group]. Most patients had experienced aminoglycosides administration in past. Drug sensitivity tests identified 8 clarithromycin-resistant MAC cases (more than 32 µg/ml minimum inhibitory concentration) among the entire cohort of patients; these were evenly distributed between the two groups.

Efficacy

After the 24-week treatment period, no patients in either group achieved sputum conversion (95% confidence interval: 0.0–33.6%). The post-treatment sputum of one patient in the control group could not be assessed because of contamination. Changes in the number of colonies in sputum culture are shown in Figure 2. There were no statistically significant changes in either group, although the numbers of colonies were relatively increased in the control group but tended to remain stable in the Hochuekkito group.

There was good interobserver agreement regarding changes in chest X-ray images ($\kappa = 0.72$). Most patients in the Hochuekkito group were categorized as "improved" or "stable" by the radiological assessment, but those in the control group were more frequently categorized as having a "worsened" condition (Figure 3). Disease control (according to the radiological assessment) was greater in the Hochuekkito group compared with the control group (8/9 vs. 3/9; $p = 0.05$). The chest X-ray images of a patient in the Hochuekkito group who was categorized as "improved" is shown in Figure 4. Changes in other secondary and exploratory endpoints over the 24 weeks are summarized in Table 3. CAT score, CRP, and ESR were increased or worsened in most patients of both groups despite the 24-weeks treatment. On the other hand, changes in body weight and serum albumin level seemed to be different. That is, patients in the Hochuekkito group tended to experience increase in body weight and serum albumin level compared with those in the control group (median body weight change: +0.4 kg vs. −0.8 kg; median albumin change: +0.2 g/dl vs. ±0.0 g/dl). Interestingly, patients who achieved improvement in X-ray image all gained weight, whereas most of the patients whose X-ray image was worsened lost weight in both groups.

Safety

None of the patients experienced severe adverse events greater than grade 3. In the Hochuekkito group, two patients developed adverse events. One patient developed pneumonitis (grade 3 on

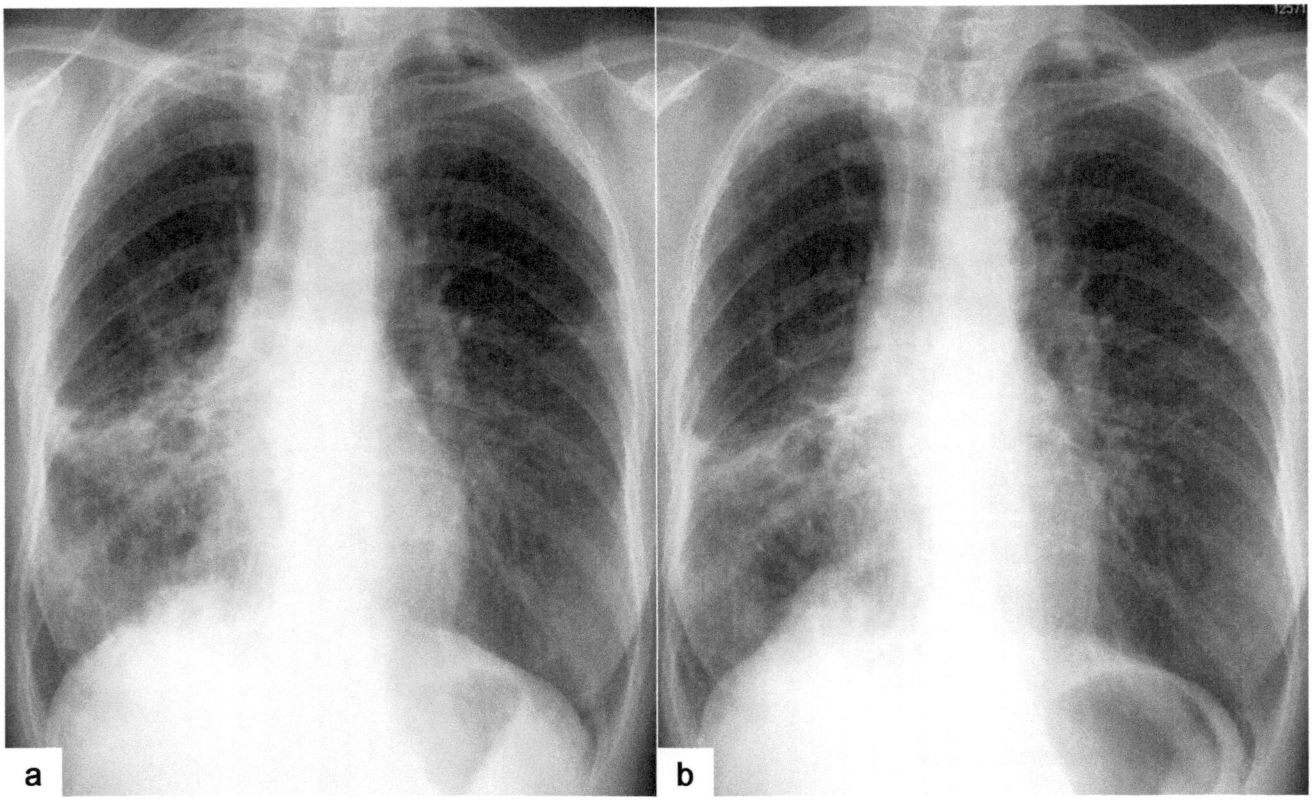

Figure 4. Chest X-ray images of a 61-year-old woman in the Hochuekkito group who achieved radiological improvement. The images shown are before (a) and after 24 weeks of (b) treatment. The consolidation areas in the bilateral lower lesions were decreased after treatment.

day 54), which was improved by discontinuing Hochuekkito and administering intravenous antibiotics (piperacillin/tazobactam). The possibility of Hochuekkito-induced pneumonitis was not excluded. The other patient experienced oral mucositis (grade 2), limb edema (grade 1), diarrhea (grade 1), and a maculopapular rash (grade 1) from day 3 to the end of follow up. Two patients in the control group also experienced adverse events. One developed a lung infection (grade 2 on day 53), which was treated by oral antibiotics (amoxicillin/clavulanate). The other patient developed an optic nerve disorder (grade 2 on day 72) that was induced by ethambutol.

Discussion

Although the sample size was very small, to the best of our knowledge, this is the first prospective comparative study to evaluate the efficacy and safety of Hochuekkito in patients with progressed pulmonary MAC disease. None of the patients in either group achieved sputum conversion despite the 24-week continuation of the baseline treatment with or without Hochuekkito. Nevertheless, we did observe several clinically relevant results and these, in combination with our safety analysis, suggesting that Hochuekkito may be feasible for use because it appears to have several beneficial effects.

It is surprising that 8/9 patients in the Hochuekkito group were able to control the disease progression (assessed by the radiological assessment), particularly because they had more severe status with significantly higher ESR than the control group. This result is partially consistent with the changes in the number of MAC colonies in sputum culture. Most patients in our cohort were elderly, had a low body mass index, and had cavities observed in chest X-ray, all of which have been reportedly poor prognostic factors in pulmonary MAC disease [12]. In addition, about half of the patients in each group had clarithromycin-resistant MAC, which is linked to the low sputum conversion rate [13]. Given the fact that the patients in this study had multiple disadvantages, and that their disease was poorly controlled by the preceding conventional treatment, it is noteworthy that some patients in the Hochuekkito group showed a partial response.

Previous studies have highlighted the immunomodulating effects of Hochuekkito. Some reports have suggested that administration of the drug increases serum interferon-γ levels, which is believed to be related to increased natural killer cell activity [6,7,14,15]. Nakayama et al. reported the possibility of using Hochuekkito for recovering impaired tumor necrosis factor-α production in alveolar macrophages in hyperglycemic mice [16]. They suggested that Hochuekkito may normalize the dysregulated inflammatory response. Interferon-γ and tumor necrosis factor-α play important roles in controlling intracellular infections including MAC diseases [1,17,18]. These mechanisms may thus explain the effectiveness of this drug.

In the present study, interestingly, patients in the Hochuekkito group tended to maintain or gain body weights, and their serum albumin levels tended to remain stable or increased. Although these findings were not based on the statistical evaluation, these imply Hochuekkito may have a favorable impact on nutritional status. In a previous report on patients with moderate-to-severe chronic obstructive pulmonary disease, Hochuekkito was suggested to increase body weight and serum prealbumin levels [8], which

Table 3. Comparison of secondary endpoints between the Hochuekkito and control groups over the 24-week treatment period.

Group/No.	Age/Sex	X-ray	CAT*	BW, kg	ALB, g/dl	CRP, mg/dl	ESR, mm/hr
Hochuekkito							
1	61/F	Improved	+8	+0.9	+0.2	+0.49	+15
2	80/F	Stable	−1	+0.4	−0.5	−0.02	−17
3	44/M	Worsened	+5	−0.7	−0.2	−1.53	+24
4	78/F	Stable	−5	−0.5	+0.3	−0.01	−18
5	63/M	Stable	+3	+2.0	+0.4	+0.20	+9
6	77/F	Stable	+5	±0.0	+0.5	+0.06	+6
7	54/F	Stable	+11	−3.8	−0.5	−0.13	+30
8	70/F	Stable	+3	+1.0	+0.3	+0.71	+18
9	73/F	Improved	−2	+1.4	+0.2	+0.19	+7
Median			+3	+0.4	+0.2	+0.06	+9
Control							
1	73/F	Worsened	+4	±0.0	−0.2	+0.01	+5
2	70/F	Stable	+9	−0.8	±0.0	+0.91	+55
3	70/F	Worsened	−3	+0.8	+0.1	±0.00	+22
4	69/M	Worsened	+7	−2.9	−0.3	+2.37	+44
5	83/M	Worsened	+1	±0.0	−0.5	+4.73	+52
6	67/F	Stable	−1	+0.9	±0.0	−0.01	+1
7	81/F	Worsened	−6	−−2.3	−0.2	−0.15	+10
8	59/F	Stable	+4	−1.5	+0.2	+0.08	+10
9	68/F	Worsened	−1	−3.0	+0.2	+0.02	−3
Median			+1	−0.8	±0.0	+0.02	+10

CAT = chronic obstructive pulmonary disease assessment test; BW = body weight; ALB = albumin; CRP = C-reactive protein; ESR = erythrocyte segmentation rate.
*Chronic obstructive pulmonary disease assessment test score ranging from 0 to 40. A higher score means more severe symptoms [11].

is consistent with our findings. Another herbal drug, Rikkunshito, has been reported to improve anorexia by increasing ghrelin secretion [19,20]. Six of the eight materials present in Rikkunshito (*Atractylodis rhizoma*, *Aurantii nobilis pericarpium*, *Gurantii radix*, *Glycyrrhizae radix*, *Zingiberis rhizoma*, and *Zizyphi fructus*) are common to Hochuekkito. Thus similar effectiveness might be expected. Management of nutritional status is a very important theme in chronic and wasting diseases, including progressed pulmonary MAC. Although it is unclear whether changes in nutritional status are associated with clinical outcome, in fact, all but one (6 of 7) patient who gained body weight in both groups of our study improved their X-ray images or remained stable. Our findings appear to suggest a new therapeutic target for this disease, and Hochuekkito may have particular strengths in this context.

There were several limitations to this study. First, a small number of patients were recruited, which did not provide the study with sufficient statistical power to prove efficacy. Our results should be regarded to be preliminary. Because of the strict criteria for patient entry, it was difficult to recruit additional patients. Second, in open-label study designs, there is a possibility that patients and clinicians may report biased answers, although the majority of our endpoints were considered to be relatively objective. Third, there were several small imbalances at baseline between the treatment groups particularly in terms of the smoking status, preceding treatment regimens, and disease severity. These differences may have influenced several outcomes. To confirm our preliminary findings, further placebo-controlled and large-scale studies are needed.

In conclusion, this pilot study suggests that Hochuekkito could be a feasible and beneficial adjunct to conventional treatment in patients with progressed pulmonary MAC disease, particularly among those for whom no alternative treatments are available. Our results should be confirmed by larger studies in future.

Supporting Information

Protocol S1 Trial protocol.

Checklist S1 CONSORT checklist.

Acknowledgments

The authors would like to thank Enago (www.enago.jp) for the English language review.

Author Contributions

Conceived and designed the experiments: YE EH TO. Performed the experiments: SK RN. Analyzed the data: TB. Wrote the paper: YE EH TO SK RN TB HK AS AN.

References

1. Griffith DE, Aksamit T, Brown-Elliott BA, Catanzaro A, Daley C, et al. (2007) An official ATS/IDSA statement: diagnosis, treatment, and prevention of nontuberculous mycobacterial diseases. Am J Respir Crit Care Med 175: 367–416.
2. Wallace RJ Jr, Brown BA, Griffith DE, Girard WM, Murphy DT (1996) Clarithromycin regimens for pulmonary Mycobacterium avium complex. The first 50 patients. Am J Respir Crit Care Med 153: 1766–1772.
3. Hasegawa N, Nishimura T, Ohtani S, Takeshita K, Fukunaga K, et al. (2009) Therapeutic effects of various initial combinations of chemotherapy including clarithromycin against Mycobacterium avium complex pulmonary disease. Chest 136: 1569–1575.
4. Kobashi Y, Oka M (2008) Long-term observation of pulmonary Mycobacterium avium complex disease treated with chemotherapy– following the guidelines for treatment. Kekkaku 83: 779–784. [Article in Japanese]
5. Corpe RF (1981) Surgical management of pulmonary disease due to Mycobacterium avium-intracellulare. Rev Infect Dis 3: 1064–1067.
6. Kuroiwa A, Liou S, Yan H, Eshita A, Naitoh S, et al. (2004) Effect of a traditional Japanese herbal medicine, hochu-ekki-to (Bu-Zhong-Yi-Qi Tang), on immunity in elderly persons. Int Immunopharmacol 4: 317–324.
7. Matsumoto T, Noguchi M, Hayashi O, Makino K, Yamada H (2010) Hochuekkito, a Kampo (traditional Japanese herbal) Medicine, Enhances Mucosal IgA Antibody Response in Mice Immunized with Antigen-entrapped Biodegradable Microparticles. Evid Based Complement Alternat Med 7: 69–77.
8. Tatsumi K, Shinozuka N, Nakayama K, Sekiya N, Kuriyama T, et al. (2009) Hochuekkito improves systemic inflammation and nutritional status in elderly patients with chronic obstructive pulmonary disease. J Am Geriatr Soc 57: 169–170.
9. Satoh N, Sakai S, Kogure T, Tahara E, Origasa H, et al. (2005) A randomized double blind placebo-controlled clinical trial of Hochuekkito, a traditional herbal medicine, in the treatment of elderly patients with weakness N of one and responder restricted design. Phytomedicine 12: 549–554.
10. Nakayama M, Bando M, Saito T, Yamasawa H, Sugiyama Y, et al. (2011) A case of chronic lower respiratory tract infection in which the traditional herbal medicine Hochuekkito was effective to prevent exacerbation. Nihon Kokyuki Gakkai Zasshi 49: 232–236. (Article in Japanese)
11. Jones PW, Harding G, Berry P, Wiklund I, Chen WH, et al. (2009) Development and first validation of the COPD Assessment Test. Eur Respir J 34: 648–654.
12. Hayashi M, Takayanagi N, Kanauchi T, Miyahara Y, Yanagisawa T, et al. (2012) Prognostic factors of 634 HIV-negative patients with Mycobacterium avium complex lung disease. Am J Respir Crit Care Med 185: 575–583.
13. Kobashi Y, Matsushima T, Oka M (2007) A double-blind randomized study of aminoglycoside infusion with combined therapy for pulmonary Mycobacterium avium complex disease. Respir Med 101: 130–138.
14. Chen R, Moriya J, Luo X, Yamakawa J, Takahashi T, et al. (2009) Hochu-ekki-to combined with interferon-gamma moderately enhances daily activity of chronic fatigue syndrome mice by increasing NK cell activity, but not neuroprotection. Immunopharmacol Immunotoxicol 31: 238–245.
15. Ishimitsu R, Nishimura H, Kawauchi H, Kawakita T, Yoshikai Y (2001) Dichotomous effect of a traditional Japanese medicine, bu-zhong-yi-qi-tang on allergic asthma in mice. Int Immunopharmacol 1: 857–865.
16. Nakayama M, Sugiyama Y, Yamasawa H, Soda M, Mato N, et al. (2012) Effect of hochuekkito on alveolar macrophage inflammatory responses in hyperglycemic mice. Inflammation 35: 1294–1301.
17. Suzuki K, Lee WJ, Hashimoto T, Tanaka E, Murayama T, et al. (1994) Recombinant granulocyte-macrophage colony-stimulating factor (GM-CSF) or tumour necrosis factor-alpha (TNF-alpha) activate human alveolar macrophages to inhibit growth of Mycobacterium avium complex. Clin Exp Immunol 98: 169–173.
18. Winthrop KL, Yamashita S, Beekmann SE, Polgreen PM; Infectious Diseases Society of America Emerging Infections Network (2008) Mycobacterial and other serious infections in patients receiving anti-tumor necrosis factor and other newly approved biologic therapies: case finding through the Emerging Infections Network. Clin Infect Dis 46: 1738–1740.
19. Fujitsuka N, Asakawa A, Amitani H, Hattori T, Inui A (2012) Efficacy of ghrelin in cancer cachexia: clinical trials and a novel treatment by rikkunshito. Crit Rev Oncog 17: 277–284.
20. Takeda H, Muto S, Nakagawa K, Ohnishi S, Asaka M (2012) Rikkunshito and ghrelin secretion. Curr Pharm Des 18: 4827–4838.

16

Bi-Directional X-Ray Phase-Contrast Mammography

Kai Scherer[1]*, Lorenz Birnbacher[1], Michael Chabior[1], Julia Herzen[2], Doris Mayr[3], Susanne Grandl[4], Anikó Sztrókay-Gaul[4], Karin Hellerhoff[4], Fabian Bamberg[4], Franz Pfeiffer[1]

1 Lehrstuhl für Biomedizinische Physik, Physik-Department & Institut für Medizintechnik, Technische Universität München, Garching, Germany, **2** Centre for Materials and Coastal Research, Helmholtz-Zentrum Geesthacht, Geesthacht, Germany, **3** Department of Pathology, Ludwig Maximilian University, Munich, Germany, **4** Department of Clinical Radiology, Ludwig Maximilian University, Munich, Germany

Abstract

Phase-contrast x-ray imaging is a promising improvement of conventional absorption-based mammography for early tumor detection. This potential has been demonstrated recently, utilizing structured gratings to obtain differential phase and dark-field scattering images. However, the inherently anisotropic imaging sensitivity of the proposed mono-directional approach yields only insufficient diagnostic information, and has low diagnostic sensitivity to highly oriented structures. To overcome these limitations, we present a two-directional x-ray phase-contrast mammography approach and demonstrate its advantages by applying it to a freshly dissected, cancerous mastectomy breast specimen. We illustrate that the two-directional scanning procedure overcomes the insufficient diagnostic value of a single scan, and reliably detects tumor structures, independently from their orientation within the breast. Our results indicate the indispensable diagnostic necessity and benefit of a multi-directional approach for x-ray phase-contrast mammography.

Editor: Juri G. Gelovani, Wayne State University, United States of America

Funding: The authors acknowledge financial support through the DFG Cluster of Excellence Munich-Centre for Advanced Photonics (MAP), the DFG Gottfried Wilhelm Leibniz program and the European Research Council (ERC, FP7, StG 240142). This work was carried out with the support of the Karlsruhe Nano Micro Facility (KNMF, www.kit.edu/knmf), a Helmholtz Research Infrastructure at Karlsruhe Institute of Technology (KIT). The funders had no role in study design, data collection and analysis, decision to publish, or preparation of the manuscript.

Competing Interests: The authors have declared that no competing interests exist.

* E-mail: kai.scherer@tum.de

Introduction

Despite the introduction of extensive screening programs in the 80's and a rapid promotion of mammography systems, breast cancer is still the second most common cause of cancer death for women worldwide [1]. The most prevailing difficulties of modern diagnostic mammography are a non-negligible number of false-positive diagnoses, accompanied by redundant medical follow-up (10.7%) and a relatively high rate of undetected tumors (21.9%), most prevalent in the examination of younger women [2]. Especially, dense breast soft-tissue exhibits only minor deviations with respect to attenuation characteristics, resulting in a poor imaging contrast for conventional mammography. Phase-sensitive x-ray imaging methods show the potential to circumvent this problem by utilizing the intrinsically enhanced electron density contrast [3].

Initial mammography studies confirming diagnostic benefits of the superior soft-tissue contrast of phase-sensitive techniques were carried out with synchrotron radiation [4,5]. The introduction of so called Talbot-Lau interferometers in combination with a conventional laboratory x-ray source pushed phase-contrast imaging towards possible clinical applications [6]. In grating-based differential phase-contrast (DPC) imaging, phase stepping enables the simultaneous retrieval of differential phase, dark-field and conventional absorption signal [6–8]. The differential phase signal is obtained by measuring the angular deviations of the transmitted wavefront, which are directly linked to the local gradient of the tissue's phase shift. Recent differential phase-contrast mammography studies conducted with freshly dissected complete breasts showed promising results with respect to clinical relevance and feasibility [9].

However, previous efforts also indicated that a direct translation of radiographic DPC towards conventional mammography is accompanied by two major drawbacks: First, the retrieved local phase gradient is of differential nature, which results in strongly edge-enhanced images with a reduced visual perception of extended structures. One-dimensional integration of the differential data is possible, however requires the implementation of regularization algorithms in order to reduce streak artifacts in direction of the integration (accumulation of statistical errors) affecting the integrated phase [10,11]. Second, since the gratings are only structured along one dimension, DPC imaging sensitivity is highly anisotropic, being only non-zero perpendicular to the grating lines. More precisely, only the component of electron density changes perpendicular to the grating lines can be accessed and contributes to the differential phase-contrast signal. Similarly, tissue-induced small-angle scatter, which determines the dark-field signal, remains undetected if emitted parallel to the grating bars [12]. Consequentially, the risk to overlook oriented, non-uniform structures within the breast such as ducts and tumor branches is high.

In this work, we apply a bi-directional imaging approach, composed of two orthogonal scans, to ensure orientation sensitivity while remaining in a radiographic acquisition mode [13–15]. We investigate the clinical relevance of this method by measuring an invasive ductal carcinoma (IDC) enclosed within the freshly dissected sample. By means of this medically significant tumor which comprises 72.8% of all invasive breast cancer we subsequently prove the necessity of an isotropic detection sensitivity [16]. We evaluate the diagnostic advantages of two-dimensional integrated phase compared to absorption imaging. Furthermore, insights into the tumor morphology are obtained by analysing angular deviations in the scattering signal (directional dark-field imaging) [12,17]. The conclusion of our study is ascertained by a histological verification of our findings.

Materials and Methods

The study was conducted in accordance with the Declaration of Helsinki and was approved by the local ethics committee (Ethikkommission of the Ludwig-Maximilian-University, Munich). Inclusion criteria were indication for surgical removal of a benign or malignant breast tumor after previous core biopsy. Patients had no previous hormonal therapy or chemotherapy. Participants gave written consent before participation after adequate explanation of the study protocol. Indication for breast surgery followed recommendation of the interdisciplinary tumor board of the University of Munich breast center.

The measurements were conducted with a three-grating Talbot-Lau interferometer (Fig. 1), consisting of a conventional x-ray tube, a source grating G_0, a phase grating G_1 (design energy of 27 keV), and an analyser grating G_2 (obtained from Mikroworks GmbH, Germany). A compact layout in the third Talbot order ($\pi/2$-shift) was chosen, with distances $l=106$ cm between G_0 and G_1 and $d=51$ cm between G_1 and G_2, respectively. The corresponding grating periods were $p_0=10$ µm, $p_1=3.24$ µm and $p_2=4.8$ µm. A Varian Paxscan 2550 *D* flat panel with Gadox screen (Gd_2O_2S) and 127×127 mm-pixel size was used as detector. The Nonius FR 591 rotating anode x-ray generator with a molybdenum target was set to 40 kVp/70 mA. The sample was positioned at 2.7 cm directly upstream G_1 in order to optimize the sensitivity of the interferometer [18].

The imaging of the freshly dissected mastectomy specimen was performed in craniocaudal orientation. For reasons of comparability and benchmarking, a digital mammogram (29 kVp, 120 mA, average glandular dose 1.22 mGy) of the specimen within the sample holder was conducted using a Selenia Dimensions scanner from Hologic (Fig. 2a). The sample holder consisted of two 4 mm thin polycarbonate plates bordered in a metal frame to apply a medically reasonable sample compression of 5 cm, while minimizing the reduction of flux by the attenuation.

Firstly, to identify the tumorous region, one image of the complete breast was taken with the interferometer. A total field of view of 12.8×12.8 cm^2 was realized by stitching 4×4 projections. Scans with 9 phase steps and an exposure time of 9 seconds per step (low-statistic) were performed with phase stepping in *x*-direction (Fig. 1). Hence, underlying imaging sensitivity was strongly anisotropic and only components of the signals in *x*-direction detected. Only one flat-field, e.g. projection without the sample in the beam, was taken beforehand. A smooth stitching of the 16 projections was achieved by correcting drift-related offsets within the differential phase. This was done by leveling the overall DPC signal of adjacent projections within the region of joint overlap. The processed and stitched images (Fig. 2) related to absorption (b), differential phase (c) and dark-field (d) were obtained by Fourier analysis [6].

On the basis of the complete DPC breast images (Fig. 2b–d), the position of the tumorous area was determined, by which two-directional differential phase-contrast mammography is showcased in the following: An isotropic DPC imaging sensitivity is realized by combining the two one-dimensional and mutually orthogonal measurements of the IDC with phase stepping in *x* and *y*-direction, respectively. Two high statistic scans were performed with 13 phase steps and an integration-time of 13 seconds per step each, in order to be able to exclude statistical error as the cause of the presented results. The inlays in Figure 2 show the corresponding images of the IDC acquired with phase stepping in *x*-direction. The thereto orthogonal scan in *y*-direction was performed by rotating the sample holder by 90° and then relocating the sample stage to preferably image the same sample volume. For the purpose of demonstrating bi-directional phase-contrast mammography, latter was preferred over the rotation of all three gratings by 90°. Alignment and compression of the breast tissue remain unaltered within the sample holder during the measurement. In the following, images retrieved along one dimension are marked by a subscript "*x*" or "*y*", respectively.

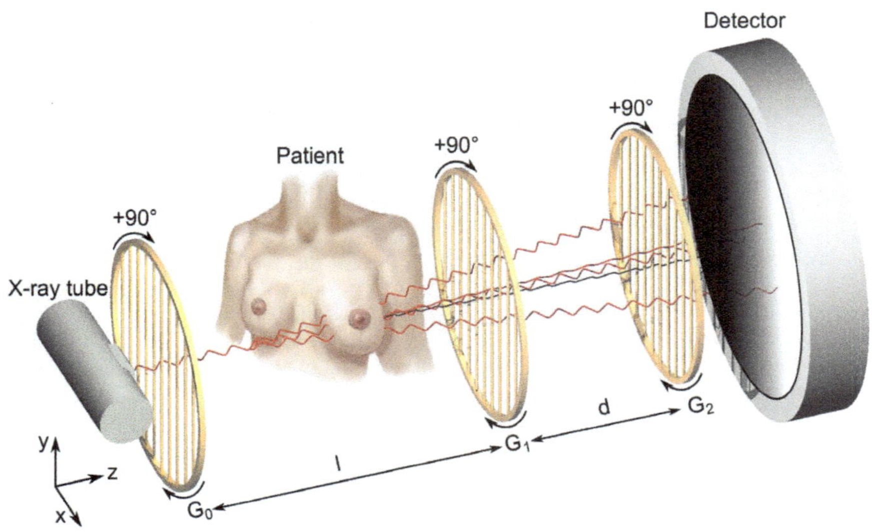

Figure 1. Schematic overview of the bi-directional phase-contrast mammography setup. The setup consists of a conventional x-ray tube, a source grating G_0, a phase grating G_1, an analyser grating G_2 and a flat panel detector. The two-directional, orthogonal scanning approach is indicated by a 90° rotation of the gratings. For practical reasons the rotation of the specimen was preferred.

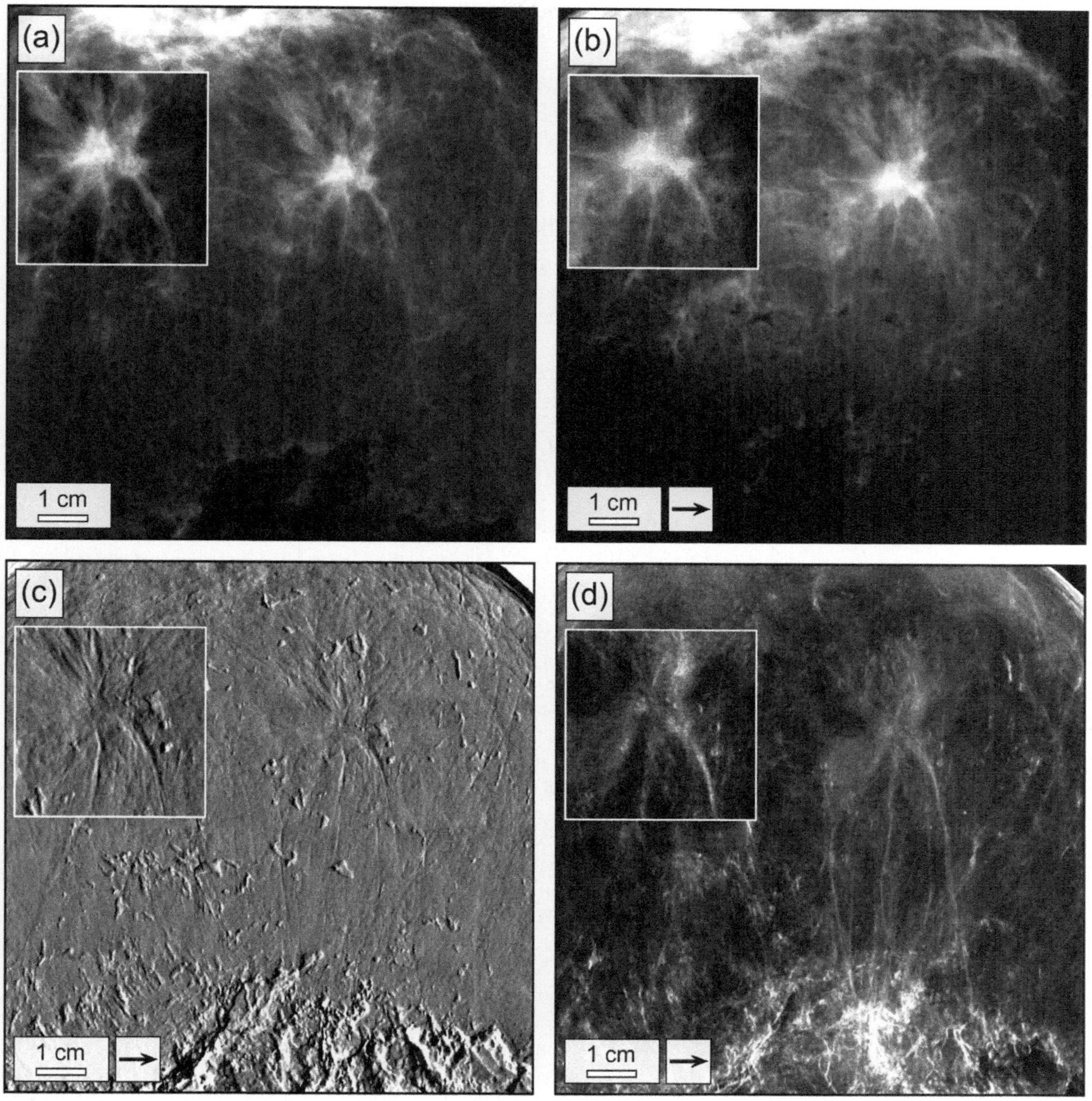

Figure 2. Conventional and grating-based mammograms of a breast specimen with invasive ductal carcinoma. Conventional mammogram (a), grating-based absorption (b), differential phase (c) and dark-field image (d) of the breast specimen. The field of view has a size of 12.8×12.8 cm². Images (b)–(d) were obtained by stitching together 4×4 low-statistic projections. Arrows indicate the direction of scanning. The high-statistic images of the invasive ductal carcinoma are shown as inlays.

Thereafter, the high-statistic set of absorption (A_x, A_y), differential phase ($\partial\phi_x$, $\partial\phi_y$) and dark-field images (D_x, D_y) of the IDC were fused. Firstly, it had to be ensured that the two images of each modality cover precisely the sample section. A possible displacement within the three image sets was reduced by using a least square optimization algorithm, which shifts the two absorption images against each other until the overall discrepancy in intensity between both images is minimized. This is feasible, since the detection of wave attenuation (absorption image) in comparison to wave deviations (differential phase, dark-field image), is independent from the scanning direction. The numerically determined shift (subpixel accuracy) was then used to correct for the displacement within the set of absorption, differential phase and dark-field images.

The fusion of the one-dimensional phase gradients $\partial\phi_x$ and $\partial\phi_y$ was realized via a two-dimensional Fourier transform approach [15]. The two-directional integrated absolute phase Φ is then given by

$$\Phi(x,y)=\mathcal{F}^{-1}\left[\frac{\mathcal{F}[\partial\phi_x(x,y)+i\partial\phi_y(x,y)](k,l)}{2\pi i(k+il)}\right](x,y), \quad (1)$$

where $\mathcal{F}$ is the two-dimensional Fourier transform, x, y the Cartesian and k, l the reciprocal space coordinates. The combined image $\partial\phi_x+i\partial\phi_y$ was mirrored horizontally and vertically to avoid edge discontinuities at the image boundaries, thus providing periodic data in Fourier space [19]. Since the phase integration corresponds to a f^{-1}-filter ($f=\sqrt{k^2+l^2}$) in Fourier space, low frequencies are enhanced compared to high frequencies. The amplification of low frequencies generates a background, that is superimposed on the integrated phase image Φ. The corrected phase image Φ_c is obtained by

$$\Phi_c = \Phi - G(\Phi, \sigma_1), \quad (2)$$

where $G(\Phi, \sigma_1)$ is the integrated phase image Φ, blurred with a Gaussian filter of width σ_1. By intensively blurring (standard deviation of Gaussian kernel of $\sigma_1 = 80$, image size of 384×384 pixels) relevant image contents remain unaffected by the subtraction of the low frequency background.

The noise power spectrum of the input images $A_{x,y}$, $\partial\phi_{x,y}$ and $D_{x,y}$ is approximately inversely proportional to f [20]. Due to integration, the retrieved phase image exhibits a noise power spectrum proportional to f^{-2}. The low amplitude of high frequency noise in the image allows a high frequency boost of Φ_c, in order to pronounce small tumor features and increase image acutance. The sharpened phase image Φ_s (Fig. 3c) is obtained with an unsharp mask operation, given by

$$\Phi_s = \Phi_c + \alpha(\Phi_c - G(\Phi_c, \sigma_2)). \quad (3)$$

To pronounce very fine structures, a slight blur (standard deviation of Gaussian kernel of $\sigma_2 = 5$, image size of 384×384 pixels) was used. The filter strength was set to $\alpha = 3.2$.

The dose-equivalent absorption image is calculated by

$$A(x,y) = e^{\frac{1}{2}(\ln A_X(x,y) + \ln A_Y(x,y))}. \quad (4)$$

To provide comparability to the sharpened phase image Φ_s, the absorption image A was also processed with the unsharp mask filter ($\sigma_2 = 5$). However, in case of the absorption image A, the noise power spectrum is proportional to f^{-1}. This allows sharpening only to a minor extent ($\alpha = 0.5$), until the intrinsic amplification of high frequency noise leads to a degradation of image quality [21]. The sharpened absorption image A_s is shown in Figure 4b.

The mean dark-field image D (Fig. 3f), related to the overall small angle scattering power of the sample, is given by

$$D(x,y) = e^{\frac{1}{2}(\ln D_X(x,y) + \ln D_Y(x,y))}. \quad (5)$$

Moreover, the dark-field images D_x and D_y were utilized to obtain information on the preferred scattering direction of the tissue under investigation. Scattering in x-direction (D_x) is colored red, while scattering in y-direction (D_y) is colored blue. The RGB-composition (Fig. 4c) of the two images, classifies scattering power (brightness) and the preferred scattering direction ranging from *x*-directed (red) over isotropic (purple) to *y*-directed (blue).

The applied radiation dose was measured using the incident air kerma with a Dosimax plus/RQX-detector system. The incident air kerma rate was found to be 2.1 mGy/s at the beam center. For the initial 4×4 low-statistic projections, 9 phase steps with an integration-time of 9 seconds each were taken. In case of the high-statistic projections used for the two-directional proof of principle study the number of steps and integration-time was increased to 13. To calculate the mean glandular dose a Monte-Carlo based conversion factor of 0.389 was chosen, determined by the half-value layer (Al) of 0.8 mm and a sample thickness of 5 cm [22,23]. A mean glandular dose of 66 mSv (total exposure time of 81 seconds, low-statistic) and 138 mSv (total exposure time of 169 seconds, high-statistic) per projection was found. While we acknowledge that these values exceed the dose limits set for clinical mammography, several factors can be addressed to achieve dose-compatible measurements in near future (see discussion).

Results

An overview of the high-statistic differential phase and dark-field images of the IDC, as obtained with the two-directional scanning approach is given in Figure 3. We investigate the dependency between the detection of strongly oriented tumor features and scanning direction, by comparing $\partial\phi_x$ against $\partial\phi_y$ and D_x against D_y, respectively: The tumor branches that are primarily vertically aligned (red framed) are strongly visible in $\partial\phi_x$ (Fig. 3a) and D_x (Fig. 3d). However, the same features cannot be detected in the thereto orthogonal images $\partial\phi_y$ (Fig. 3b) and D_y (Fig. 3e). By contrast the horizontally oriented tumor branch (blue framed), is exclusively detected in $\partial\phi_y$ (Fig. 3b) and D_y (Fig. 3e).

These observations indicate, that tumor branches exhibit a strongly anisotropic contrast for both differential phase and dark-field imaging: Within the tumor branches, electron density variations of the tissue are only minor, resulting in a poor differential phase contrast along the branch. However, compared to the surrounding, healthy tissue, the electron density is differing considerably. Furthermore, scatter caused by the branches and its substructures must be directed mostly perpendicular to the branch orientation.

Hence, the selection of scan direction, and therewith one-dimensional imaging sensitivity, determines to what extent the anisotropic tissue structures like branches, embedded in healthy tissue, can be detected. If scanning is performed parallel to the branch orientation for instance, neither scatter, caused by the branches, is detected, nor sufficient phase-contrast obtained. To secure a full detection of the tumor branches, an isotropic imaging sensitivity is indispensable, as provided by the combination of two orthogonally conducted scans. Comprehensive images, that provide the full range of features (red and blue frames), are obtained by fusing the one-directional differential phase and dark-field images as sharpened, two-directional integrated phase Φ_s (Fig. 3c) and mean dark-field D (Fig. 3f), respectively. Moreover, the sharpened, two-directional integrated phase image Φ_s is free of streak and shadowing artifacts, even though the field of view is exceeded by the sample.

Besides overcoming the limited sensitivity of a one-directional scan, the two-directional approach exhibits further diagnostic advantages, illustrated in a benchmark (Φ_s vs. A_s) and directional dark-field case study (Fig. 4). The sharpened phase image Φ_s (Fig. 4a) enables a diagnostic differentiation of the carcinoma into three locally separated tumor lesions (white frame). Two tumor branches are clearly perceivable, as directly emerging from the single lesions and spreading out to the image borders (arrows). The superior depiction of fine details within the phase image is caused by an enhanced soft-tissue contrast, but also improved local contrast and image acutance gained by image sharpening. By contrast, the same medical details can not be deduced from the dose-equivalent, sharpened absorption image A_s (Fig. 4b): The attenuation-based soft-tissue contrast is insufficient to enable a visual distinction into lesions, but instead displays the tumor mass as pervasive structure (black circle). The tumor branches appear distinctively shortened, since fine branch parts (high frequency features) are blurred within image noise (white circled). To validate

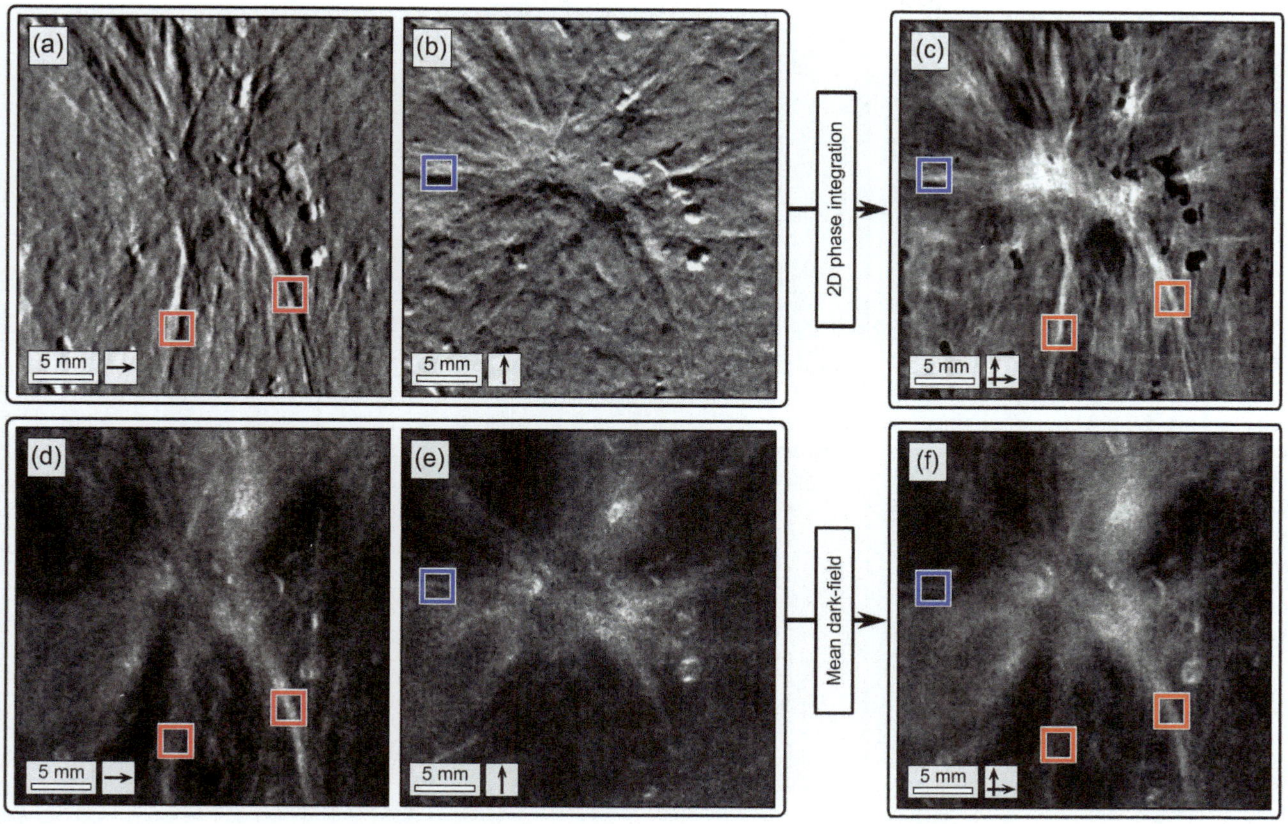

Figure 3. Two-directional, grating-based mammograms of the invasive ductal carcinoma. Two-directional differential phase $\partial\phi_x$ (a), $\partial\phi_y$ (b) and sharpened, two-dimensional integrated phase image Φ_s (c). Dark-field D_x (d), D_y (e) and mean dark-field D image (f). Arrows indicate the direction of scanning. Red and blue boxes indicate tumor branches exclusively perceivable in the images obtained with scanning performed in x- or y-direction, respectively.

the medical relevance of details exclusively perceivable within the phase image and exclude them as being image artifacts, histological evaluations were carried out. The tumorous area was extracted, dissected and stained with Hematoxylin and Eosin (Fig. 4c). We matched the three tumor lesions (white frame) and fine branches (arrows) with respect to size and orientation and confirmed their malignancy. Furthermore, the tumor was classified as apparently trifocal, e.g. containing three locally separated lesions.

We extracted further diagnostic insights on the tumor constitution by examining two spots of the directional dark-field image (Fig. 4d) in more detail. The vertically oriented tumor branch (white diamond) scatters preferably perpendicular to its orientation, identifiable by the red color. This prominent anisotropic scatter can be ascribed to the tissue morphology on the scatter determining length scale, which is in the order of the analyser grating period of $p_2 = 4.8\ \mu m$ [24]. The corresponding histological section of the branch was photographed with a magnification of 200 (Fig. 4e). The magnified image reveals multiple vascular walls (white) and elongated tumor cells (pink) preferably aligned alongside the fibre with diameters in the range of some microns. The elliptically-shaped two dimensional Fourier transform of the image (top right inlay) emphasizes the inherent alignment of the substructure. Since scatter occurs dominantly at edges/tissue-interfaces which are mutually oriented along the fibre, an unilaterally directed scatter is generated.

For a second correlation of directional dark-field with tumor morphology, the top tumor lesion (black diamond) was chosen. Here contributed scatter is uniformly distributed, discernible by the violet color. The corresponding histological section of the branch was photographed with a magnification of 200 (Fig. 4f). The magnified image shows a cluster of tumor cells (violet) surrounded by bunches of elongated cells (pink) and vascular walls (white). By contrast, in this case the morphology seems random, without exhibiting any preferred orientation or distinct alignment of the inherent features. This impression is ascertained by the circular-shaped two-dimensional Fourier transform of the image (top right inlay). Accordingly, scatter in this area is isotropic.

Discussion

In this study, we demonstrated that grating-based mammography faces the problem of a diagnostically limiting imaging sensitivity, if operated with an mono-directional scan only. We identified structures associated with an IDC, that exhibit a strongly anisotropic imaging contrast for both differential phase and dark-field imaging. To provide diagnostic reliability and ensure detection of oriented, tumorous structures, regardless their orientation within the breast, an isotropic imaging sensitivity is indispensable and could be provided by applying a two-directional scanning approach. An isotropic imaging sensitivity is crucial requirement for the successful detection of early stage tumors such as in-situ carcinoma. Here tumor growth is naturally limited to the inner of ducts, resulting in a elongated tumor shape similar to the observed IDC branches [25,26].

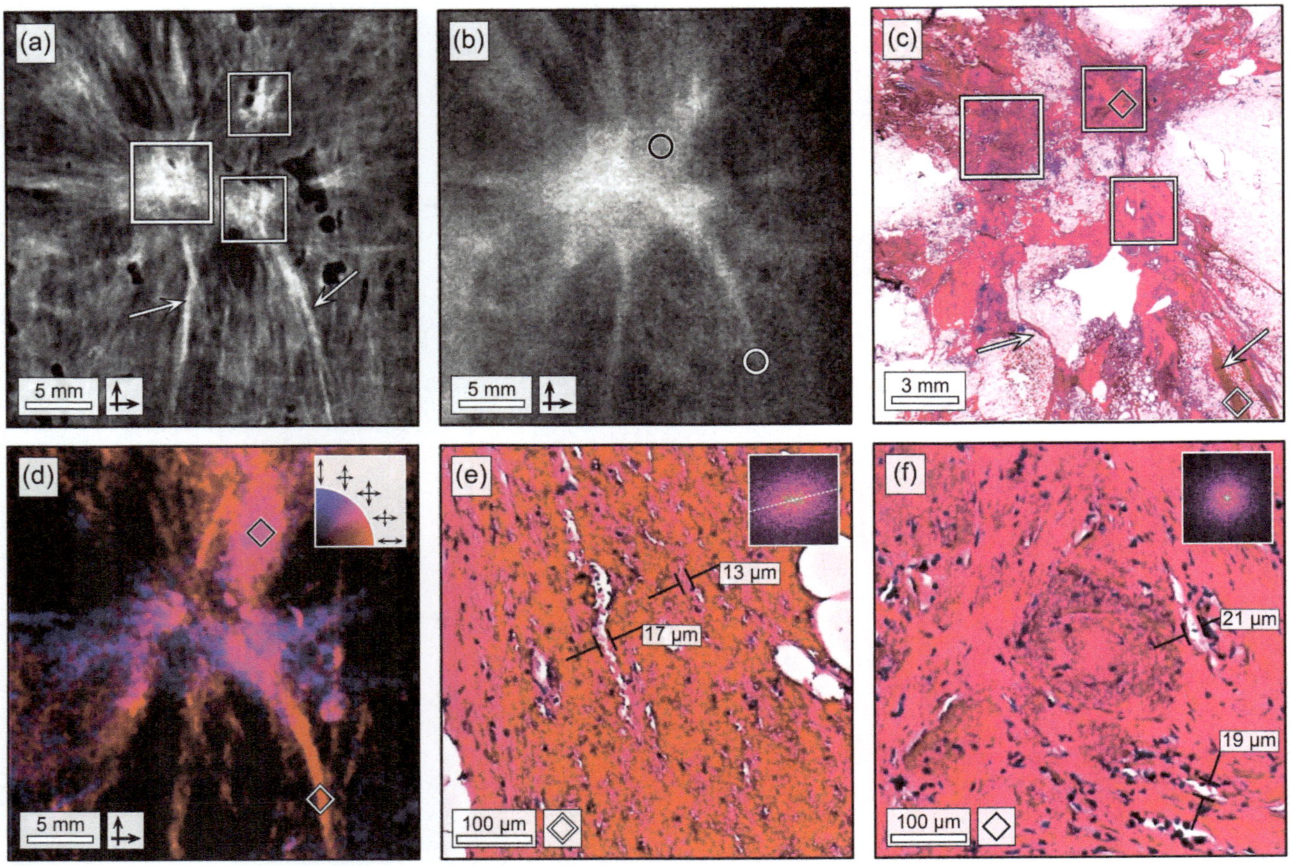

Figure 4. Two-directional, grating-based mammograms of the invasive ductal carcinoma with correlated histopathology. (a) Sharpened, two-dimensional integrated phase image Φ_s of the invasive ductal carcinoma. The frames in (a) and (c) indicate three locally separated tumor lesions (apparently trifocal). Arrows in (a) and (c) indicate fine tumor branches. (b) Sharpened, absorption image A_s of the invasive ductal carcinoma. Circles indicate position of relevant tumor details. (c) Histological slice (Hematoxylin and Eosin stain) of the invasive ductal carcinoma. (d) Directional dark-field image of the invasive ductal carcinoma. Preferred scattering direction is color-coded ranging from x-directed (red) over isotropic (purple) to y-directed (blue). (e) 200x magnified histological image of the tumor branch, as indicated by white diamond in (c) and (d). The 2-dimensional FFT is shown as an inlay. (d) 200x magnified histological image of the tumor lesion, as indicated by black diamond in (c) and (d). The 2-dimensional FFT is shown as an inlay.

We have proven feasibility of the two-directional scanning and phase-integration approach by first localizing the tumor and then subsequently measuring the corresponding enclosed section within the undissected mastectomy specimen.

To exclude statistical errors as cause of the observed anisotropic imaging contrast given by IDC branches, this proof of principle study had to be conducted with high-statistic measurements and thus should neither be considered dose nor time relevantly designed. Stampanoni et al. [9] and Sztrókay et al. [27] already discussed that an acquisition of images within the dose limits required for clinical applications would be possible by optimizing several setup relevant aspects such as design energy, x-ray target material, beam filtration, grating quality, duty-cycle, grating substrate thickness, sample holder and detector efficiency. An increase of currently 13.2% to 49.5% setup fringe visibility by improving beam and grating quality would imply an approximately 14-fold decrease in necessary dose for DPC imaging. Further we expect that an optimization of the detector with respect to the design energy of 27 keV, the replacement of the x-ray target molybdenum with tungsten and the exclusion of polycarbonate plates would double the setup efficiency. These improvements could decrease the current dose of 66 mSv per projection down to 2.4 mSv which is within the dose limits of 2.5 mSv set by the European guidelines for quality assurance in breast cancer screening and diagnosis [28].

We elaborated additional diagnostic advantages accompanied by the two-directional scanning approach which could further motivate the need of acquiring two images: The two-dimensional integration mechanism provides absolute, streak artifact free phase images which proved to facilitate the visual differentiation of medically significant tumor details, yet unseen in the dose equivalent absorption image. The excellent depiction of high frequency features yields the potential to strongly promote the detection of early stage tumors, fine tumor branches and small metastases.

Furthermore, we examined a possible diagnostic application of directional dark-field imaging by characterizing the soft-tissue morphology on the micrometer length scale, far below the actual detector resolution. The morphology of two tumor associated areas could be characterized by their scattering behavior as randomly proliferated and inherently oriented, respectively. This technique may promote the characterization and therewith diagnostic classification of suspicious structures and microcalcifications as linear branching or coarse granular [29,30]. Besides, it might give a hint concerning the neoplastic grading of tumorous tissue by distinguishing between well-differentiated/oriented and fully anaplastic cell domains.

Finally, the 90° rotation of the three gratings could be circumvented by the implementation of two-dimensional structured gratings [13].

Acknowledgments

We would like to thank P. Thibault for providing the least square optimization algorithm, I. Zanette for fruitful discussions and T. Connall for supplying the patient graphic.

Author Contributions

Conceived and designed the experiments: KS LB MC JH FP. Performed the experiments: KS LB. Analyzed the data: KS LB SG KH ASG. Contributed reagents/materials/analysis tools: KS DM SG ASG FB. Wrote the paper: KS MC.

References

1. Siegel R, Naishadham D, Jemal A (2012) Cancer statistics, 2012. CA: A Cancer Journal for Clinicians 62: 1029.
2. Poplack SP, Tosteson AN, Grove MR, Wells WA, Carney PA (2000) Mammography in 53,803 women from the new hampshire mammography network. Radiology 217: 832–840.
3. Keyriläinen J, Bravin A, Fernandez M, Tenhunen M, Virkkunen P, et al. (2010) Phase-contrast x-ray imaging of breast. Acta radiologica 51: 866–884.
4. Takeda T, Momose A, Ueno E, Itai Y (1998) Phase-contrast x-ray CT image of breast tumor. Journal of Synchrotron Radiation 5: 1133–1135.
5. Arfelli F, Bonvicini V, Bravin A, Cantatore G, Castelli E, et al. (2000) Mammography with synchrotron radiation: phase-detection techniques. Radiology 215: 286–293.
6. Pfeiffer F, Weitkamp T, Bunk O, David C (2006) Phase retrieval and differential phase-contrast imaging with low-brilliance x-ray sources. Nature Physics 2: 258–261.
7. Momose A, Kawamoto S, Koyama I, Hamaishi Y, Takai K, et al. (2003) Demonstration of x-ray talbot interferometry. Japanese Journal of Applied Physics 42: L866–L868.
8. Pfeiffer F, Bech M, Bunk O, Kraft P, Eikenberry EF, et al. (2008) Hard-x-ray dark-field imaging using a grating interferometer. Nature Materials 7: 134–137.
9. Stampanoni M, Wang Z, Thring T, David C, Roessl E, et al. (2011) The first analysis and clinical evaluation of native breast tissue using differential phase-contrast mammography. Investigative radiology 46: 801–806.
10. Roessl E, Koehler T, van Stevendaal U, Martens G, Hauser N, et al. (2012) Image fusion algorithm for differential phase contrast imaging. Proc SPIE: 831354.
11. Thring T, Modregger P, Pinzer BR, Wang Z, Stampanoni M (2011) Non-linear regularized phase retrieval for unidirectional x-ray differential phase contrast radiography. Optics express 19: 25545–25558.
12. Jensen TH, Bech M, Bunk O, Donath T, David C, et al. (2010) Directional x-ray dark-field imaging. Physics in Medicine and Biology 55: 3317.
13. Zanette I, Weitkamp T, Donath T, Rutishauser S, David C (2010) Two-dimensional x-ray grating interferometer. Physical Review Letters 105: 248102.
14. Wen H, Bennett EE, Hegedus MM, Rapacchi S (2009) Fourier x-ray scattering radiography yields bone structural information. Radiology 251: 910–918.
15. Kottler C, David C, Pfeiffer F, Bunk O (2007) A two-directional approach for gratingbased differential phase contrastimaging using hard x-rays. Optics Express 15: 1175–1181.
16. Li C, Anderson B, Daling J, Moe R (2003) Trends in incidence rates of invasive lobular and ductal breast carcinoma. JAMA 289: 1421–1424.
17. Jensen TH, Bech M, Zanette I, Weitkamp T, David C, et al. (2010) Directional x-ray dark-field imaging of strongly ordered systems. Physical Review B 82: 214103.
18. Donath T, Chabior M, Pfeiffer F, Bunk O, Reznikova E, et al. (2009) Inverse geometry for gratingbased x-ray phase-contrast imaging. Journal of Applied Physics 106: 054703.
19. Arnison MR, Larkin KG, Sheppard CJR, Smith NI, Cogswell CJ (2004) Linear phase imaging using differential interference contrast microscopy. Journal of Microscopy 214: 712.
20. Cha BK, Kim JY, Kim YJ, Yun S, Cho G, et al. (2012) Design and image-quality performance of high resolution CMOS-based x-ray imaging detectors for digital mammography. Journal of Instrumentation 7: C04020.
21. Polesel A, Ramponi G, Mathews VJ (2000) Image enhancement via adaptive unsharp masking. IEEE Transactions on Image Processing 9: 505–510.
22. Dance DR (1990) Monte carlo calculation of conversion factors for the estimation of mean glandular breast dose. Physics in medicine and biology 35: 1211–1219.
23. Dance DR, Skinner CL, Young KC, Beckett JR, Kotre CJ (2000) Additional factors for the estimation of mean glandular breast dose using the UK mammography dosimetry protocol. Physics in Medicine and Biology 45: 3225.
24. Malecki A, Potdevin G, Pfeiffer F (2012) Quantitative wave-optical numerical analysis of the dark-field signal in grating-based x-ray interferometry. EPL (Europhysics Letters) 99: 48001.
25. Barreau B, Mascarel Id, Feuga C, MacGrogan G, Dilhuydy MH, et al. (2005) Mammography of ductal carcinoma in situ of the breast: Review of 909 cases with radiographicpathologic correlations. European Journal of Radiology 54: 55–61.
26. Menell JH, Morris EA, Dershaw DD, Abramson AF, Brogi E, et al. (2005) Determination of the presence and extent of pure ductal carcinoma in situ by mammography and magnetic resonance imaging. The Breast Journal 11: 382390.
27. Sztrökay A, Diemoz PC, Schlossbauer T, Brun E, Bamberg F, et al. (2012) High-resolution breast tomography at high energy: a feasibility study of phase contrast imaging on a whole breast. Physics in medicine and biology 57: 2931–2942.
28. Perry N, Broeders M, de Wolf C, Trnberg S, Holland R, et al. (2008) European guidelines for quality assurance in breast cancer screening and diagnosis. Annals of oncology: official journal of the European Society for Medical Oncology/ ESMO 19: 614–622.
29. Dinkel HP, Gassel AM, Tschammler A (2000) Is the appearance of microcalcifications on mammography useful in predicting histological grade of malignancy in ductal cancer in situ? The British journal of radiology 73: 938–944.
30. Stomper PC, Connolly JL (1992) Ductal carcinoma in situ of the breast: correlation between mammographic calcification and tumor subtype. AJR American journal of roentgenology 159: 483–485.

Bone Suppression Increases the Visibility of Invasive Pulmonary Aspergillosis in Chest Radiographs

Steven Schalekamp[1]*, Bram van Ginneken[1], Inge A. H. van den Berk[3], Ieneke J. C. Hartmann[4], Miranda M. Snoeren[1], Arlette E. Odink[5], Winnifred van Lankeren[5], Sjoert A. H. Pegge[2], Laura J. Schijf[3], Nico Karssemeijer[1], Cornelia M. Schaefer-Prokop[1,2]

1 Dept. Of Radiology, Radboud University Medical Center, Nijmegen, The Netherlands, **2** Dept. Of Radiology, Meander Medical Center, Amersfoort, The Netherlands, **3** Dept. Of Radiology, Academic Medical Center, Amsterdam, The Netherlands, **4** Dept. Of Radiology, Maasstad Hospital, Rotterdam, The Netherlands, **5** Dept. Of Radiology, Erasmus Medical Center, Rotterdam, The Netherlands

Abstract

Objective: Chest radiographs (CXR) are an important diagnostic tool for the detection of invasive pulmonary aspergillosis (IPA) in critically ill patients, but their diagnostic value is limited by a poor sensitivity. By using advanced image processing, the aim of this study was to increase the value of chest radiographs in the diagnostic work up of neutropenic patients who are suspected of IPA.

Methods: The frontal CXRs of 105 suspected cases of IPA were collected from four institutions. Radiographs could contain single or multiple sites of infection. CT was used as reference standard. Five radiologists and two residents participated in an observer study for the detection of IPA on CXRs with and without bone suppressed images (ClearRead BSI 3.2; Riverain Technologies). The evaluation was performed separately for the right and left lung, resulting in 78 diseased cases (or lungs) and 132 normal cases (or lungs). For each image, observers scored the likelihood of focal infectious lesions being present on a continuous scale (0–100). The area under the receiver operating characteristics curve (AUC) served as the performance measure. Sensitivity and specificity were calculated by considering only the lungs with a suspiciousness score of greater than 50 to be positive.

Results: The average AUC for only CXRs was 0.815. Performance significantly increased, to 0.853, when evaluation was aided with BSI ($p = 0.01$). Sensitivity increased from 49% to 66% with BSI, while specificity decreased from 95% to 90%.

Conclusion: The detection of IPA in CXRs can be improved when their evaluation is aided by bone suppressed images. BSI improved the sensitivity of the CXR examination, outweighing a small loss in specificity.

Editor: Patrick C Y Woo, The University of Hong Kong, Hong Kong

Funding: Riverain Technologies provided a research grant to N. Karssemeijer. The funder had no role in study design, data collection and analysis, decision to publish, or preparation of the manuscript.

Competing Interests: The authors have read the journal's policy and have the following conflicts: Riverain Technologies provided a research grant to N. Karssemeijer. This research is managed by S. Schalekamp. The authors had full access to all of the data in this study and take complete responsibility for the integrity of the data and the accuracy of the data analysis.

* Email: steven.schalekamp@gmail.com

Introduction

Invasive pulmonary aspergillosis (IPA) is a major cause of morbidity and mortality, particularly in patients with hematological malignancies [1–3]. A delay in treatment is associated with substantially increased hospital mortality [4–7]. However, treatment is expensive, and can have serious side effects. From a clinical point of view there is therefore a strong need for prompt recognition and proper onset of treatment to ensure an optimal patient outcome.

Current EORTC/MSG (European Organization for Research and Treatment of Cancer, US Mycoses Study Group) guidelines differentiate three levels of probability for the presence of an invasive fungal infection: proven, probable or possible [8]. While a proven diagnosis requires histological and/or cultural evidence from tissue specimen or positive cultures from body fluids, these criteria are often not met and not applicable at an early stage of infection. This discrepancy between definite diagnostic proof of IPA on one side and the need for treatment as early as possible on the other side has led to different therapeutic strategies ranging from prophylaxis to empirical therapy of persistent neutropenia to pre-emptive approaches of very early, still preclinical disease [9]. In this diagnostic dilemma, imaging still plays an important role. In common with other lung diseases, Computed Tomography (CT) has been proven to be more sensitive than radiography in revealing subtle pathology [10]. As consequence, the imaging criteria of the EORTC/MSG guidelines for the presence of IPA refer to specific CT findings (dense well circumscribed lesions with or without a halo sign, air crescent sign, cavity) and also the guidelines published by the Infectious Diseases Working Party of the German Society of Haematology and Oncology (AGIHO) in

2012 state that in patients with granulocytopenia, high resolution computed tomography (HRCT) should be preferred to chest x-ray for primary diagnosis in high-risk patients [11].

Though CT is currently recommended as the preferred method if there is strong clinical suspicion for an infection, chest x-ray (CXR) remains the first line imaging method because of its immediate availability and lower organizational demands. Chest X-rays are also performed if the clinical suspicion is low and/or clinical symptoms are less obvious or not yet fully developed. Also, guidelines by the American College of Radiology [12] and the Infectious Disease Society of America [13] mention chest radiography as first line method for the work up of a patient with neutropenic fever, but do emphasize the low sensitivity of CXR. Thus, chest radiography is still widely applied despite its known diagnostic limitations, meaning an increased sensitivity for the detection of subtle infiltrations would represent a desirable diagnostic improvement. Early recognition of IPA on CXR would trigger an immediate CT examination of the patient in order to render morphology and accelerate the diagnosis, providing a chance to hasten the onset of treatment.

To improve the detection of IPA on CXR, we tested an advanced image processing solution called bone suppression imaging (BSI). This software solution suppresses bone structures in chest x-rays, which can obscure abnormalities. No special hardware or additional dose for the patient is needed. The processing can be applied to both upright and bedside radiographs using imaging equipment of varying manufacturers.

BSI has been shown to be helpful in the detection of lung nodules and focal pneumonia [14–16]. We believe this means it might also provide an opportunity to improve the detection of IPA. We therefore decided to undertake an observer study to test the effect of BSI on the detection of IPA in neutropenic patients. If BSI would improve detection of IPA, and so possibly avoid delay in treatment, it could result in an optimized use of CXR in immunocompromised patients at risk of developing IPA.

Methods

The selection of study images and study setup were waived by the institutional review board (Commissie Mensgebonden Onderzoek regio Arnhem – Nijmegen; www.cmoregio-a-n.nl; nr. 2011/468). Written informed consent was also waived by the institutional review board.

Image selection

Neutropenic patients with typical signs of invasive pulmonary aspergillosis infection on CT, which had a CXR at a time near the CT scan were selected. Study images were retrospectively retrieved from the image archives of four hospitals (three academic and one non-academic hospital) and anonymized. All images had been obtained for clinical purposes. Patients could have multiple sites of disease per lung, but patients with diffuse lung disease, or large obvious consolidations were excluded. The diagnoses of invasive aspergillus as an underlying disease were taken from the clinical patient charts and included the presence of typical CT findings in all diseased patients. Neutropenic patients with signs of fever with a normal chest radiograph functioned as control subjects. The absence of disease in these control subjects was confirmed by a negative CT after the CXR. Both upright as well as bedside acquisitions were included.

The visibility of disease was retrospectively classified based on the suspiciousness scores assigned by the readers participating in the study. Cases that were assigned an average score above 75 (0 = not suspicious, 100 = very suspicious) were classified as *obvious cases* (Figure 1). Cases with average scores between 50 and 75 were classified as *moderately subtle cases*. Cases with an average score below 50 but higher than 25 were labeled as *subtle cases*. If the average score of a case was below 25 then the case was considered *very subtle*.

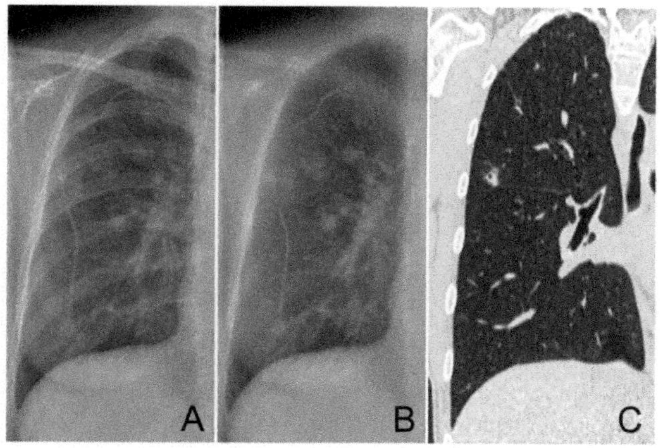

Figure 1. Example of a moderately subtle case of a 35 year old female with multiple focal lesions in the right lung. Without BSI 6 of the 7 observers marked this case with an average suspiciousness score of 63. With BSI all observers marked the case with an average suspiciousness score of 91. Original radiograph (A), bone suppressed image (B), coronal CT slice (C).

Image acquisition

All chest radiographs were obtained with a digital technique using storage phosphor plates (CR, Agfa, Mortsel Belgium), a Selenium drum (Thoravision, Philips, Hamburg Germany) and a flat panel detector DR systems (Siemens, Erlangen, Germany). Bedside images were acquired with the same DR or CR systems. Image processing was applied as recommended by the manufacturers and as used in clinical routine.

Software

Bone suppressed images were generated by ClearRead Bone Suppression 3.2, from Riverain Technologies (Miamisburg, Ohio). This visualization software uses advanced image processing techniques to construct a bone suppressed frontal chest image. Not only bones obscuring the lung fields are being suppressed, but also other skeletal structures superprojecting the lungs such as the claviculae or the scapulae are eliminated. The software product has U.S. Food and Drug Administration (FDA) approval. Since BSI is a post-processing technique, no special hardware is needed and no additional radiation dose is administered to the patient. BSI is applicable to any digital radiographic chest technique, irrespective of whether the images were obtained at the bedside or in the upright position.

After acquisition of the radiograph, data processing is performed automatically in the background. The processed images are made available in the Picture Archiving and Communication System (PACS) system. The bone suppressed images are not designed to replace the original images but rather to serve as supplement to the original frontal chest radiograph. Both the original and bone suppressed image can be visualized side by side or as stack of two images. Both images are equivalent in terms of size and gradation characteristics, with the exception of overlying rib structures.

Table 1. Patient demographics.

	Diseased cases (n = 78)	Normal cases (n = 132)
Age	53.8 (range 16–83)	43.0 (range 8–76)
Male	47 (60%)	87 (66%)
Female	31 (40%)	45 (34%)
Days between CXR and CT (median)	2.6 (2)	3.7 (3)
Bedside	22 (28%)	60 (45%)
Upright	56 (72%)	72 (55%)

Age, gender, average time between the chest radiograph and the CT in days, and projection type are displayed for the diseased and normal cases. n = number.

Observer study

Five radiologists (ranging from 3–17 years of experience) and two radiology residents (3rd and 5th year of residency) read all cases during one sequential reading session. Evaluation was carried out separately for the right and left lung, resulting in 210 images of 105 patients. Radiologists were asked to score the most suspicious lesion per image, if lesions were seen. Images on which the observer did not detect a focal lesion received no score. Scores were given on a scale from 1 to 100. There were no instructions how to use this scoring scale, but the observers were motivated to use the full range of scores of suspicion (1–100). Observers first provided a score for the standard CXR, followed by a second score for the evaluation of the standard radiograph supplemented by the bone suppressed image. Observers were able to add or (re)move marks and adjust their scores. No clinical information, besides the knowledge that it was a neutropenic patient group, was provided to the readers. A training set of 40 lungs was provided in advance, containing pulmonary focal opacities of varying conspicuity to make the observers familiar with the appearance of the processed images.

Statistics

Observer performance was measured using Multi Reader Multi Case (MRMC) receiver operating characteristic (ROC) analysis. ROC analysis calculates the readers' sensitivity as a function of specificity using the assigned ratings per case (suspiciousness scores). The area under the ROC curve (AUC) summarizes the performance of the reader, representing the chance that a positive (diseased) case will be scored with more suspicion than a negative (normal) case. Per reader, each case was assigned the score (1–100) of the most suspicious finding, if present. Differences in observer performance were tested using the Dorfman, Berbaum and Metz method (DBM MRMC package v2.33) which includes case, reader and treatment variance into analysis [17–19]. Non-parametric statistical test was used to generate ROC curves and calculate p-values. Besides ROC analysis, sensitivities and specificities were computed for individual observers considering markings exceeding a confidence score of 50.

Results

Patient demographics

In total 105 patients were selected. In this group there were 78 diseased lungs and 132 normal lungs. The average age of patients with diseased lungs was 53.8 years and average age of patients with normal lungs was 43.0. On average, CT scans were made 2.6 days after the chest radiographs for diseased patients, compared to 3.7 days for patients with normal lungs. Patient characteristics are summarized in Table 1. Radiographs of 128 lungs were obtained upright, and 82 lungs were acquired at the bedside. With respect to the conspicuity of pathology, diseased lungs were classified as being obvious in 17, moderately subtle in 21, subtle in 15, and very subtle in 25 cases (Table 2).

Observer performance: ROC analysis

The average AUC without BSI was 0.815 against 0.853 with BSI ($p = 0.01$). Six of the seven observers improved their performance (Table 3).

ROC analysis for the different subsets of subtlety classification based on reader scores showed that the very subtle cases benefitted the most from BSI. The AUC for very subtle cases increased from 0.579 to 0.659 ($p = 0.02$), AUC for subtle cases increased from 0.809 to 0.856 ($p = 0.07$). For the detection of moderately subtle and obvious cases baseline performance was already very good (AUC = 0.954 and 0.995, respectively) and did not significantly increase with BSI (0.968 and 0.992, $p = 0.26$ and $p = 0.44$, respectively). Examples of cases are illustrated in Figures 1–3.

Table 2. Subtlety categories.

	Bedside	Upright	Total
Obvious	4	13	17
Moderately subtle	8	13	21
Subtle	3	12	15
Very subtle	7	18	25
Total	**22**	**56**	**78**

Number of cases classified into the different subtlety categories.

Table 3. Observer performance.

	AUC		
	Without BSI	*With BSI*	P
All images (n = 210)	0.815	0.853	0.01
Upright images (n = 128)	0.804	0.853	0.02
Bedside images (n = 82)	0.838	0.878	0.15

Average area under the ROC curves (AUC) for all observers. AUCs are displayed for all images and for analysis of the different groups of projection type (bedside and upright).

Analysis of type of projection

The average area under the curve for upright radiographs (n = 128) was 0.804 and significantly increased to 0.853 with BSI (p = 0.02). For bedside images (n = 82) similar improvement was seen with an AUC increasing from 0.838 to 0.878, although the difference did not reach statistical significance (p = 0.15) (Table 3).

Observer performance: Sensitivity and specificity

Overall sensitivity for the detection of IPA was 49 percent without BSI. With the availability of BSI, sensitivity increased to 66%. This resulted, on average, in an additional detection of 13 diseased cases (range 1–38), especially in the more subtle cases (Table 4). Specificity showed a decrease from 95% without BSI to 90% with BSI. On average, 6 normal cases (range 0–13) were marked without BSI, and 14 normal cases (range 2–23) with BSI. Individual sensitivities and specificities are displayed in Table 5. The lower specificity was mainly caused by marking of pseudolesions caused by artifacts of the bone suppression technique (Figure 4).

Discussion

The results of our study indicate a significantly improved detection of focal opacities due to fungal infection, when supported by bone subtracted images. This improvement was especially striking for very subtle lesions, that otherwise would not be reported. With this new processing, the sensitivity for the detection of IPA on chest x-rays could be substantially increased. Although the increase in sensitivity was associated with a small decrease in specificity, ROC analysis indicated a significant improvement in overall performance. These findings are in agreement with previous studies which documented an improved detection performance of nodules or focal pneumonia [14–16]. Our results are noteworthy because they show that BSI is also supportive in a study group of highly variable imaging quality with respect to patient position and inspiration depth.

Whether and to which degree this improved detection performance changes patient management and would prompt earlier treatment can only be hypothesized at this point in time and any quantification is beyond the scope of this publication. Though multiple studies documented the limited sensitivity of CXR for the diagnosis of IPA [20–28], it still remains an important diagnostic procedure in these patients and appears not to necessarily trigger immediate CT imaging as documented by our study group acquired in 4 hospitals: the average time between CXR and CT was about 2.6 days. We do not know whether this delay is due to organizational reasons, a lack of immediate therapeutic consequences (patient was treated anyway) or the fact that a particularly subtle lesions had not been seen during the original readings. We believe that despite its limited sensitivity regarding IPA, or specificity regarding the potential causative organism, CXR has its role in the diagnostic work up of these delicate patients which might not be easily transferrable to CT in all situations. Application of this new processing technique has been shown to improve the detection of focal opacifications in radiographs, which in any case represents the more readily

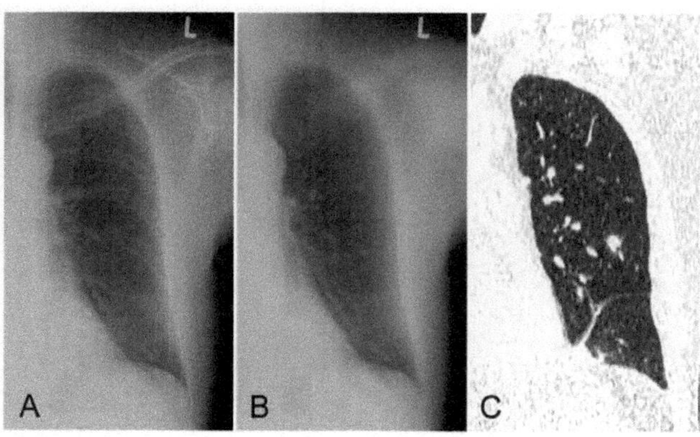

Figure 2. Upright radiograph with a very subtle lesion in the left lower lobe. Without BSI only one observer marked the small lesion. With BSI all 7 observers marked the lesion with an average suspiciousness score of 55. Original radiograph (A), bone suppressed image (B), coronal CT slice (C).

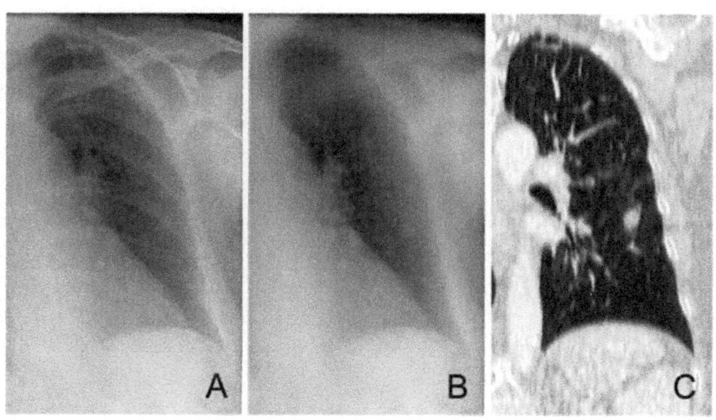

Figure 3. Bedside radiograph of a 58 year old female with neutropenic fever. Without BSI, 3 of the 7 observers called the radiograph suspicious, which increased to 7 observers with BSI. Original radiograph (A), bone suppressed image (B), coronal CT slice (C).

Table 4. Number of, on average, detected cases per subtlety category.

	Without BSI	With BSI
Obvious (n = 17)	16	17
Moderately subtle (n = 21)	15	18
Subtle (n = 15)	6	9
Very subtle (n = 25)	2	8
Total (n = 78)	**39**	**52**

Table 5. Sensitivity and specificity.

	Sensitivity			Specificity		
Observer	**Without BSI (%)**	**With BSI (%)**	**Δ (%)***	**Without BSI (%)**	**With BSI (%)**	**Δ (%)***
Rad 1	44	62	+18	97	91	−6
Rad 2	42	44	+2	98	98	0
Rad 3	62	68	+6	92	87	−5
Rad 4	42	73	+31	97	86	−11
Res 5	15	64	+49	100	91	−9
Res 6	64	69	+5	92	92	0
Rad 7	72	82	+10	90	83	−7
Average	**49**	**66**	**+17**	**95**	**90**	**−5**

Individual sensitivities and specificities for the detection of IPA in chest radiographs without and with BSI, based on marking with a suspiciousness score above 50.
* Δ = difference.

available imaging method.

The ideal situation would be to treat only patients suffering from IPA and to do this without any time delay [29]. In this scenario, imaging plays a crucial role. Current EORTC/MSG guidelines, especially the criteria for CT imaging, are very specific resulting in many non-classifiable cases. A broadening of the radiological criteria by including more non-specific findings would most likely result in an increased sensitivity for the detection of IPA, however, at the expense of a much lower specificity [30]. That way, imaging would be used as a tool to detect any morphological changes rather than revealing findings that indeed are suggestive for IPA.

Widespread nodules with a halo of ground glass in a peribronchovascular distribution have been described as the best discriminator for early IPA [31]. Prematurely obtained CT scans (e.g. immediately after onset of fever and without any radiographic changes) might demonstrate only non-specific findings harboring the risk for false negative interpretation or overdiagnosis, especially if assessed by less experienced radiologists. On the other hand, CT scans obtained in a later stage may provide diagnosis of IPA, but at the price of increased morbidity and mortality for the patient. One can hypothesize that a more sensitive chest radiographic technique may serve as trigger to obtain CT imaging without further delay, thus shortening the time to diagnosis. Meanwhile this CT acquisition, triggered by positive chest radiographic findings, will likely reveal findings indeed suggestive of IPA, consequently increasing its specific diagnostic yield. This hypothesis is supported by the fact that, according to our results, the largest benefit of BSI was seen for the subtle and very subtle cases. With the bone subtracted images, the number of detected very subtle cases quadrupled. Secondly we found a surprisingly long time delay

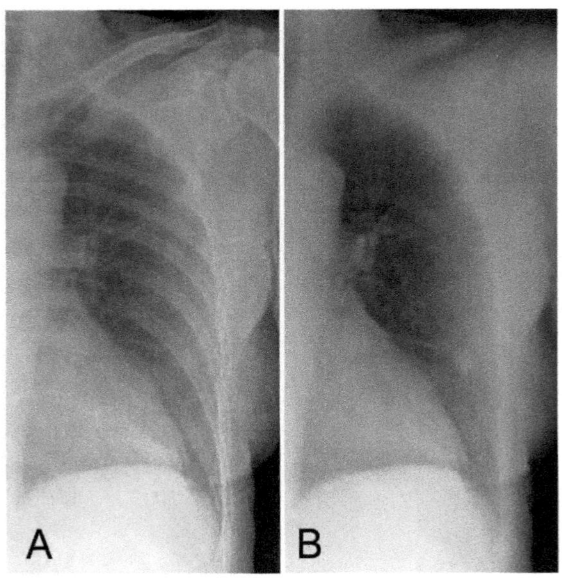

Figure 4. Example of a bedside case that was rated false positive by all 7 observers. Due to an incomplete suppression of the rib crossing of the anterior contour of the 5th rib and the posterior contour of the 8th rib on the BSI, the observers rated the shadow as infectious rounded opacity. Original radiograph (A), bone suppressed image (B).

between radiography and CT of 2.6 days on average for the diseased patients, showing a potential gain in time to diagnosis.

In our study, the baseline performance was higher for bedside images than for the upright images, which was not expected when considering the variable image quality and generally poorer condition of the patients undergoing bedside imaging. The superior baseline performance for the bedside images in our study was likely due to the fact that the group of bedside images contained relatively more obvious cases (group of obvious and *moderately* subtle cases) as compared to the upright group (55% versus 46%). Even so, we found a similar performance increase for both groups with an increase in AUC of 0.49 for upright images and of 0.40 for bedside images which failed to reach significance in the bedside group due to the smaller sample size.

Our study suffers from some limitations. Evaluation was performed separately for the right and left lung to prevent readers from being influenced by the contralateral findings and to be able to assess the performance for various types of lesions independently, with respect to conspicuity. From a clinical point of view this introduced a somewhat artificial component. Although readers did not know the percentage of diseased and normal lungs, they did know that prevalence was enriched which might have lowered their threshold to call opacifications positive. Lastly, the time difference between acquisition of the CXR and the CT does not exclude in this rapidly changing disease that extent and location of lesions differed between the two examinations. All radiographs were carefully evaluated by an experienced chest radiologist and the clinical researcher, confirming the radiographic findings with CT as reference standard. This issue was also considered less important given the fact that readers were asked to score the most obvious lesion per lung and not all lesions.

In conclusion, a new processing technique that digitally subtracts overlying bone structures in chest radiographs significantly improves the detection of fungal infections in chest radiographs. Shortcomings of CXR regarding its low sensitivity for the detection of IPA could be partly eliminated with the use of BSI, since we found an increase in sensitivity of 17%. Despite its inferiority to CT, CXR still represents an important role in the work up of febrile neutropenic patients, serving as a diagnostic screening procedure that is readily available, relatively easy to perform and providing immediate diagnostic information. Prospective studies will have to prove the impact of a substantially improved radiographic technique on the role of radiography in diagnosing IPA more promptly and triggering CT examinations for further morphological analysis.

Author Contributions

Conceived and designed the experiments: SS BG NK CSP. Performed the experiments: SS BG IB IH MS AO WL SP LS NK CSP. Analyzed the data: SS BG NK CSP. Contributed reagents/materials/analysis tools: SS BG IB IH WL NK CSP. Wrote the paper: SS BG IB IH MS AO WL SP LS NK CSP.

References

1. Ninin E, Milpied N, Moreau P, André-Richet B, Morineau N, et al. (2001). Longitudinal study of bacterial, viral, and fungal infections in adult recipients of bone marrow transplants. Clin Infect Dis. 33: 41–47.
2. Upton A, Kirby KA, Carpenter P, Boeckh M, Marr KA. (2007). Invasive aspergillosis following hematopoietic cell transplantation: outcomes and prognostic factors associated with mortality. Clin Infect Dis. 44: 531–540.
3. Pagano L, Caira M, Nosari A, Van Lint MT, Candoni A, et al. (2007). Fungal infections in recipients of hematopoietic stem cell transplants: results of the SEIFEM B-2004 study–Sorveglianza Epidemiologica Infezioni Fungine Nelle Emopatie Maligne. Clin Infect Dis. 45: 1161–1170.
4. von Eiff M, Roos N, Schulten R, Hesse M, Zühlsdorf M, van de Loo J. (1995). Pulmonary aspergillosis: early diagnosis improves survival. Respiration. 62: 341–347.
5. Vandewoude KH, Blot SI, Benoit D, Colardyn F, Vogelaers D. (2004). Invasive aspergillosis in critically ill patients: attributable mortality and excesses in length of ICU stay and ventilator dependence. J Hosp Infect. 56: 269–276.
6. Morrell M, Fraser VJ, Kollef MH. (2005). Delaying the empiric treatment of candida bloodstream infection until positive blood culture results are obtained: a potential risk factor for hospital mortality. Antimicrob Agents Chemother. 49: 3640–3645.
7. Nivoix Y, Velten M, Letscher-Bru V, Moghaddam A, Natarajan-Amé S, et al. (2008). Factors associated with overall and attributable mortality in invasive aspergillosis. Clin Infect Dis. 47: 1176–1184.
8. De Pauw B, Walsh TJ, Donnelly JP, Stevens DA, Edwards JE, et al. (2008). Revised definitions of invasive fungal disease from the European Organization for Research and Treatment of Cancer/Invasive Fungal Infections Cooperative Group and the National Institute of Allergy and Infectious Diseases Mycoses Study Group (EORTC/MSG) Consensus Group. Clin Infect Dis. 46: 1813–1821.
9. Freemantle N, Tharmanathan P, Herbrecht R. (2011). Systematic review and mixed treatment comparison of randomized evidence for empirical, pre-emptive and directed treatment strategies for invasive mould disease. J Antimicrob Chemother. 66 Suppl 1:i25–i35.
10. Heussel CP, Kauczor HU, Heussel GE, Fischer B, Begrich M, et al. (1999). Pneumonia in febrile neutropenic patients and in bone marrow and blood stem-cell transplant recipients: use of high-resolution computed tomography. J Clin Oncol. 17: 796–805.
11. Ruhnke M, Böhme A, Buchheidt D, Cornely O, Donhuijsen K, et al. (2012). Diagnosis of invasive fungal infections in hematology and oncology–guidelines from the Infectious Diseases Working Party in Haematology and Oncology of the German Society for Haematology and Oncology (AGIHO). Ann Oncol. 23: 823–833.
12. Heitkamp DE, Mohammed TLH, Kirsch J, Amorosa JK, Brown K, et al. (2012). ACR appropriateness criteria acute respiratory illness in immunocompromised patients. J Am Coll Radiol. 9: 164–169.
13. O'Grady NP, Barie PS, Bartlett JG, Bleck T, Carroll K, et al. (2008). Guidelines for evaluation of new fever in critically ill adult patients: 2008 update from the American College of Critical Care Medicine and the Infectious Diseases Society of America. Crit Care Med. 36: 1330–1349.
14. Freedman MT, Lo SCB, Seibel JC, Bromley CM. (2011). Lung nodules: improved detection with software that suppresses the rib and clavicle on chest radiographs. Radiology. 260: 265–273.
15. Li F, Engelmann R, Pesce L, Armato SG 3rd, Macmahon H. (2012). Improved detection of focal pneumonia by chest radiography with bone suppression imaging. Eur Radiol. 22: 2729–2735.
16. Schalekamp S, van Ginneken B, Meiss L, Peters-Bax L, Quekel LGBA, et al. (2013). Bone suppressed images improve radiologists' detection performance for pulmonary nodules in chest radiographs. Eur J Radiol. 82: 2399–2405.
17. Dorfman DD, Berbaum KS, Metz CE. (1992). Receiver operating characteristic rating analysis: Generalization to the population of readers and patients with the jackknife method. Invest Radiol. 27: 723–731.
18. Roe CA, Metz CE. (1997). Variance-component modeling in the analysis of receiver operating characteristic index estimates. Acad Radiol. 4: 587–600.
19. Hillis SL, Berbaum KS, Metz CE. (2008). Recent developments in the Dorfman-Berbaum-Metz procedure for multireader ROC study analysis. Acad Radiol. 15: 647–661.
20. Hubbell FA, Greenfield S, Tyler JL, Chetty K, Wyle FA. (1985). The impact of routine admission chest x-ray films on patient care. N Engl J Med. 312: 209–213.
21. Jochelson MS, Altschuler J, Stomper PC. (1986). The yield of chest radiography in febrile and neutropenic patients. Ann Intern Med. 105: 708–709.
22. Feusner J, Cohen R, O'Leary M, Beach B. (1988). Use of routine chest radiography in the evaluation of fever in neutropenic pediatric oncology patients. J Clin Oncol. 6: 1699–1702.
23. Katz JA, Bash R, Rollins N, Cash J, Buchanan GR. (1991). The yield of routine chest radiography in children with cancer hospitalized for fever and neutropenia. Cancer. 68: 940–943.
24. Donowitz GR, Harman C, Pope T, Stewart FM. (1991). The role of the chest roentgenogram in febrile neutropenic patients. Arch Intern Med. 151: 701–704.
25. Korones DN, Hussong MR, Gullace MA. (1997). Routine chest radiography of children with cancer hospitalized for fever and neutropenia: is it really necessary? Cancer. 80: 1160–1164.
26. Oude Nijhuis CSM, Gietema JA, Vellenga E, Daenen SMGJ, De Bont ESJM, et al. (2003). Routine radiography does not have a role in the diagnostic evaluation of ambulatory adult febrile neutropenic cancer patients. Eur J Cancer. 39: 2495–2498.
27. Renoult E, Buteau C, Turgeon N, Moghrabi A, Duval M, et al. (2004). Is routine chest radiography necessary for the initial evaluation of fever in neutropenic children with cancer? Pediatr Blood Cancer. 43: 224–228.
28. Roberts SD, Wells GM, Gandhi NM, York NR, Maron G, et al. (2012). Diagnostic value of routine chest radiography in febrile, neutropenic children for

early detection of pneumonia and mould infections. Support Care Cancer. 20: 2589–2594.

29. Maertens J, Groll AH, Cordonnier C, de la Cámara R, Roilides E, et al. (2011). Treatment and timing in invasive mould disease. J Antimicrob Chemother. 66 Suppl 1:i37–i43.
30. Blot SI, Taccone FS, Van den Abeele AM, Bulpa P, Meersseman W, et al. (2012). A clinical algorithm to diagnose invasive pulmonary aspergillosis in critically ill patients. Am J Respir Crit Care Med. 186: 56–64.
31. Greene RE, Schlamm HT, Oestmann JW, Stark P, Durand C, et al. (2007). Imaging findings in acute invasive pulmonary aspergillosis: clinical significance of the halo sign. Clin Infect Dis. 44: 373–379.

18

Quantitative Assessment of Murine Articular Cartilage and Bone Using X-Ray Phase-Contrast Imaging

Jun Li[1], Huihui Yuan[2], Mingshu Wu[1], Linan Dong[1], Lu Zhang[1], Hongli Shi[1], Shuqian Luo[1]*

1 School of Biomedical Engineering, Capital Medical University, Beijing, China, **2** Department of Rheumatology and Immunology, Capital Medical University, Beijing, China

Abstract

Murine models for rheumatoid arthritis (RA) research can provide important insights for understanding RA pathogenesis and evaluating the efficacy of novel treatments. However, simultaneously imaging both murine articular cartilage and subchondral bone using conventional techniques is challenging because of low spatial resolution and poor soft tissue contrast. X-ray phase-contrast imaging (XPCI) is a new technique that offers high spatial resolution for the visualisation of cartilage and skeletal tissues. The purpose of this study was to utilise XPCI to observe articular cartilage and subchondral bone in a collagen-induced arthritis (CIA) murine model and quantitatively assess changes in the joint microstructure. XPCI was performed on the two treatment groups (the control group and CIA group, n = 9 per group) to monitor the progression of damage to the femur from the knee joint in a longitudinal study (at 0, 4 and 8 weeks after primary injection). For quantitative assessment, morphologic parameters were measured in three-dimensional (3D) images using appropriate image analysis software. Our results showed that the average femoral cartilage volume, surface area and thickness were significantly decreased ($P<0.05$) in the CIA group compared to the control group. Meanwhile, these decreases were accompanied by obvious destruction of the surface of subchondral bone and a loss of trabecular bone in the CIA group. This study confirms that XPCI technology has the ability to qualitatively and quantitatively evaluate microstructural changes in mouse joints. This technique has the potential to become a routine analysis method for accurately monitoring joint damage and comprehensively assessing treatment efficacy.

Editor: Johnny Huard, University of Pittsburgh, United States of America

Funding: This work was supported by the National Natural Science Foundation of China (grant No. 61227802) and by the 7th Framework Program of the European Community (grant No. PIRSES-GA-2009-269124). SL received the funding. The funders had no role in study design, data collection and analysis, decision to publish, or preparation of the manuscript.

Competing Interests: The authors have declared that no competing interests exist.

* Email: shuqian_luo@aliyun.com

Introduction

Rheumatoid arthritis (RA) is characterised by progressive synovial joint inflammation, which results in cartilage erosion and bone destruction [1,2]. Due to the damage to the joints, RA patients suffer from chronic pain, deformity of the joints, and physical disability [3]. Although analysis based on semi-quantitative scoring has contributed to an understanding of RA, detailed structural information on joint damage during RA progression is lacking. To provide sufficient information for the diagnosis and treatment of RA, accurate assessments of the structural changes to joints are needed. Small animal models, which are necessary and complementarity to clinical studies, are well suited for understanding pathogenesis and developing drugs. The collagen-induced arthritis (CIA) mouse model can reliably mimic clinical RA and is an ideal model for morphologic research on joint damage [4].

The current techniques for evaluating joint morphologic changes, such as histologic scoring and biochemical assays, are time consuming, require specimen destruction and cannot provide 3D structural information [5,6]. Magnetic resonance imaging (MRI) and ultrasonography (US), which are non-destructive 3D imaging techniques, are commonly used for the examination of rheumatoid joints in the clinic [7–9]. Unfortunately, these two imaging methods are not feasible to monitor the articular cartilage injury in CIA mouse. At present, the normal spatial resolution of MRI is in the range of 3–5 mm and a few can reach up to 1 mm [10]. High-quality US used for musculoskeletal system even are capable of scanning at spatial resolution of 100 μm [11]. However, compared with the thickness of the cartilage in mice joints, they still are not able to provide adequate spatial resolution for the measurement of thinner joint cartilage in mice. Because the articular cartilage of a normal mouse has an average thickness of 50 μm [12]. So, due to the limitation of spatial resolution, the small lesions in mouse joints are difficult to be detected by MRI and US. In addition, for US, the most important limitation pertains to penetration, that makes it is unable to detect much beyond the bone interface and into the deeper articular structure [10]. In contrast, micro-computed tomography (micro-CT) can provide superb high-resolution at the level of several microns for visualising alterations to the micro-architecture of bone tissue in mice [4,14]. However, biological soft tissues such as articular cartilage are generally undetectable by micro-CT due to low X-ray attenuation [15]. Therefore, the imaging methods described above all have limitations for the visualisation of mouse joints.

X-ray phase-contrast imaging (XPCI) is a novel imaging technique that combines the advantages of high spatial resolution, high phase contrast and 3D non-invasive imaging. It greatly improves the image quality of biological soft tissues. It is well known that X-ray is an electromagnetic radiation. When it propagates through a sample, which may be absorbed, scattered or traverse the sample without interaction. These variations result in changes of the transmitted intensity and the phase shift. This can be described by the complex refractive index $n = 1\text{-}\delta\text{-}i\beta$. The imaginary part β describes the absorption image which is mainly attribute to the X-ray attenuation. Because the variation in X-ray absorption between different biological soft tissues is very small. So, this may lead to low contrast and poor resolution. The real part δ is ascribed to Thorson scattering which is related to the X-ray phase shift. The latter is three orders of magnitude higher than the imaginary part for biological soft tissues. Therefore, the information of X-ray phase shift can be used to achieve an image contrast in sample which do not exhibit significant absorption. Meanwhile, it can provide quite high spatial resolution, even less than 1 μm. Therefore, XPCI is quite suitable for imaging the fine structure to biological soft tissues.

XPCI as a unique method has proven to be a powerful technique for analysing the composition and structure of biological tissues [16,17] and materials [18,19]. To date, this method has been successfully utilised to visualise human articular cartilage [20] and detect damage to mouse articular cartilage [21,22]. Furthermore, a few researchers have applied this technique to assess and quantify changes in the articular cartilage of mice [12]. However, these studies have mostly focused on the destruction of articular cartilage rather than subchondral bone. In reality, these two tissues are intimately related. Anatomically, they are physically connected to one another. Functionally, they play synergistic roles in the conduction of stress [23]. The morphologic changes in one of these tissues inevitably affect the structure and function of the other [24,25]. Thus, simultaneously assessing the destruction of cartilage and bone is crucial for investigating the mechanisms of joint diseases.

The aim of this study was to apply the XPCI technique to the simultaneous visualisation and assessment of articular cartilage erosion and bone loss in a mouse RA model. First, XPCI was used to image the femur of the knee joint in normal and CIA mice. Then, 3D morphologic images of the femoral cartilage, subchondral bone surface and trabecular bone were reconstructed to qualitatively describe the structural changes. In addition, to further enhance the reliability and objectiveness of the results, the morphologic parameters of the articular cartilage and trabecular bone were measured in the 3D images to provide a quantitative assessment.

Materials and Methods

Samples

8-week-old male DBA/1 mice (CIA-susceptible mouse strain, H-2q) were purchased from Beijing HFK Bio-technology Co., Ltd (Beijing, China). All mice were maintained under specific pathogen free conditions and fed standard rodent chow ad libitum. All experimental procedures conformed to the Chinese National Health and Capital Medical University Guidelines and were approved by the Institutional Animal Ethics Committee of the Beijing Military Medical Institution (Permit Number SYXK2007-005).

18 mice were randomly assigned to the two treatment groups: 9 mice for the control group and 9 mice for the RA group. RA was induced by a subcutaneous injection with 100 μL of an emulsion containing 100 μg of bovine type II collagen (CII, Sigma-Aldrich, St Louis, MO) and 100 μg of complete Freund's adjuvant (Sigma-Aldrich, St Louis, MO) at the tail. After 21 days, 100 μl of a booster (100 μg of bovine CII in incomplete Freund's adjuvant) was injected subcutaneously at the tail, but at a different location from the site of first injection. The mice were monitored daily for feeding and signs of pain throughout the experimental period. The mice were killed by cervical vertebra dislocation at 0 week (at the beginning of experimentation) as well as at 4 and 8 weeks after primary immunisation. The fresh femora of the knee joints (left and right) were dissected from the surrounding tissues and immediately fixed in phosphate-buffered formaldehyde (4%, PH 7.0) at 4°C for 24 h.

X-ray phase-contrast imaging

The experiment was conducted at beamline BL13W1 of the Shanghai Synchrotron Radiation Facility (SSRF) in China. A diagram of the experimental setup is shown in Figure 1. The X-ray synchrotron radiation beam line was emitted from a storage ring of electrons with an acceleration voltage of 3.5 GeV and an average beam current of 180 mAn. Subsequently, the beam was monochromatised by a Si(111) double-crystal. The energy range was 8–72 keV, with an energy resolution of $\Delta E/E<5e\text{-}5$. After the monochromatic beam penetrated through the sample, it was detected by a thin(100 μm) $CdWO_4$ cleaved single-crystal scintillator. The projections were recorded by an X-ray sensitive CCD camera. The distance between the sample stage and the CCD camera could be adjusted from 0 to 3 m by moving the CCD.

Because XPCI can provide the quite high contrast for visualization of articular cartilage. In this work, we did not use contrast reagents. Based on our previous experiment, XPCI was carried out using an energy of 14 keV. The distance between sample and the CCD camera was 15 cm. The CCD camera had a resolution of 1768×1768 pixels for a 3.7 μm×3.7 μm area. Seven hundred and twenty projections were recorded (the sample stage was rotated in steps of 180°/720), with an exposure time of 2 seconds for each projection. For the analysis, a volume of interest (VOI) was selected for each sample that extended 4 mm down from the top surface of the cartilage and included cartilage, subchondral bone lamella, and some trabecular bone.

Histological Processing

After the final XPCI scan, the femora of the knee joints were decalcified in 20% EDTA at 4°C for 6 weeks. Subsequently, the specimens were dehydrated using a series of gradient alcohol treatments (immersion in 70%, 80%, 90% alcohol for 3 hours and in 100% alcohol for 4 hours). After dehydration, the samples were embedded in paraffin. For comparison with the 2D images generated by XPCI, the paraffin-embedded samples were sectioned at a thickness of approximately 4 μm. Finally, the sections were stained with Safranin-O using standard protocols.

Image processing

Several factors can influence the quality of projections in the imaging process, such as background noise and ring artifacts. Thus, image preprocessing is crucial prior to analysis. First, We applied the method of image normalisation to remove noise signals from the background. The projection removed background can be written as

$$I = \frac{I_p - I_d}{I_b - I_d} \tag{1}$$

Where, I_p is the projection acquired from XPCI. I_b is the background image and I_d is dark field image.

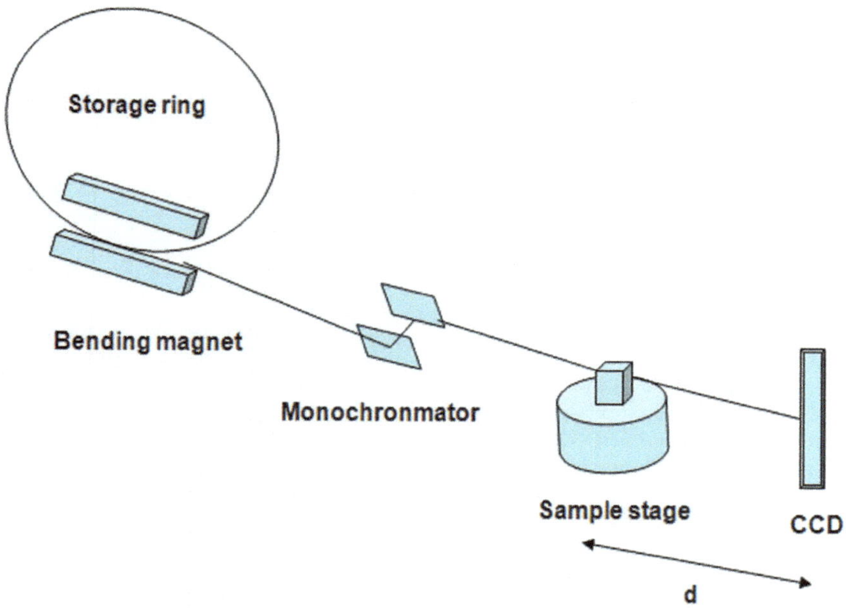

Figure 1. Schematic of the experimental setup of the XPCI system. Femur samples were positioned vertically on the sample stage. During the CT imaging, the sample stage rotated 180° automatically. A CCD camera was used to record the imaging results. In our experiment, the distance between the sample stage and CCD detector was set to 15 cm.

Then, persistent ring artifacts were eliminated by the method of sinogram correction. Actually, the ring artifacts in the reconstructed CT image were due to the vertical stripe artifacts in the sinogram. Therefore, in this method, all operations were performed on the sinogram image instead of the projecton. The first step was to recognise the position of the vertical stripe in the sinogram. And then, a local median filter was executed at this position to depress the vertical stripe. The details of this method were briefly outlined below:

1. Perform the filtering in the sinogram P(β,s). The filtered sinogram P_h(β,s) can be described as:

$$P_h(\beta,\ s) = P(\beta,\ s) \otimes h \tag{2}$$

$$h = \begin{bmatrix} 1 & -2 & 1 \\ \bullet & \bullet & \bullet \\ 1 & -2 & 1 \end{bmatrix} \tag{3}$$

where, h was the filter operator whose size was able to be adjusted according to the noise level. β was the angle of projection, and s was the coordinates of projection. The aim of this step was to enhance the signal of vertical stripe in the sinogram in order to detect the stripe effectively.

2. Calculate the average $\bar{P}$(s) of each row of the filtered sinogram Ph(β,s).

$$\bar{P}(s) = \left| \frac{1}{M} \sum_{i}^{M} P_h(\beta_i, s) \right| \tag{4}$$

Where, M was the total number of projections. After the average, the signal intensity at the position of vertical strip was stronger than others. It would form a peak signal, which was the foundation for the subsequent recognition.

3. Calculate the maximal value $\bar{P}_{max}$ of $\bar{P}$(s). When $0<c\leq 1$, if

$$\bar{P}(s_i) > c\bar{P}_{max}, [\bar{P}(s_i) - \bar{P}(s_{i-1})] \geq 0, \\ [\bar{P}(s_{i+1}) - \bar{P}(s_i)] \leq 0, i = 1.2.\cdots N \tag{5}$$

Coordinates i was detected and regarded as the position of the vertical stripe. Here N was the width of the probe. c was an experimentally determined threshold. Through adjusting the value of c, the ring artifacts of different strength was able to be recognised.

4. After detecting the position of all vertical stripes, the correction was done by using the median filter in the positions of the detected stripes only. By using the above method, we gained the corrected sinogram.

After the above steps, the conventional filtered back projection (FBP) algorithm with a Hamming filter was used to reconstruct CT slices from the 720 projections. The femora were placed in a vertical position during scanning. Therefore, a series of transverse cross-sectional slices was produced. Before and after CT image of removing ring artifacts are shown in Figure 2. We found that the ring artifacts were suppressed effectively, and the quality of image had improved significantly.

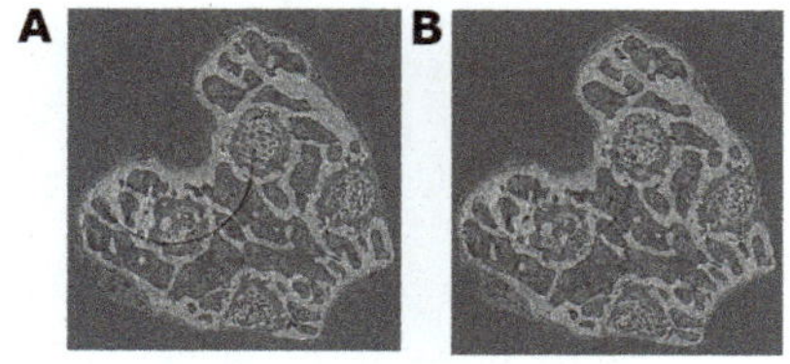

Figure 2. Before and after CT image via image preprocessing. (A) 2D CT image without image preprocessing. (B) 2D CT image after image preprocessing.

Femoral cartilage and subchondral bone are adjacent in the anatomic structure. Thus, for objective analysis of the morphologic changes in these two tissues, it was necessary to separate them from the femur. We applied an image segmentation method based on region growing to separate the cartilage, which was a semi-automatic procedure. It started in manually choosing the seed point in the region of cartilage as well as setting the intensity threshold. Under the control of the intensity threshold, the growing would stop when the cartilage were separated. However, on account of the morphologic disconnection of cartilage, this semi-automatic segmentation approach was not feasible for all the CT slices. To overcome this limitation, the CT slices unsuitable for the above method were loaded in Photoshop software (Adobe, California, USA), and by drawing contour lines to manually extract the femoral cartilage (this part of the work was performed under the guidance of two animal experiment experts). For segmentation of the bone, an appropriate threshold was easy to select. According to a grayscale histogram analysis of the tissues, the valley value in the midpoint of two partially overlapping peaks could be considered as an optimal threshold to separate the bone from the whole femur automatically. After the image segmentation, the 3D morphologies of the entire articular cartilage and subchondral bone were visualised using a surface rendering method. The segmentation methods for the femoral cartilage and bone are shown in Figure 3.

In addition, for quantitative analysis, the 3D data sets of the femoral cartilage and trabecular bone were analysed in Amira software, version 5.2.2 (FEI, Portland, USA) and CTAn software, version 1.8.1.2 (SkyScan, Kontich, Belgium), respectively, to measure the following morphologic parameters: cartilage volume (mm^3), cartilage surface area(mm^2), cartilage average thickness (μm), bone volume to tissue volume ratio (BV/TV, %), bone surface to bone volume ratio (BS/BV, mm^{-1}), trabecular bone thickness (Tb.Th, mm), trabecular bone number (Tb.N, /mm) and trabecular bone space (Tb.Sp, mm).

Statistical analysis

The 3D morphologic parameters of the femoral cartilage and trabecular bone at different time points (0, 4 and 8 weeks after primary injection) were compared using a one-factor repeated generalised linear model with Tukey's test analysis. The data are presented as the mean±standard deviation (SD). P values less than 0.05 were considered statistically significant. Statistical analysis was performed with SPSS, version 17.0(SPSS Inc, Chicago, IL).

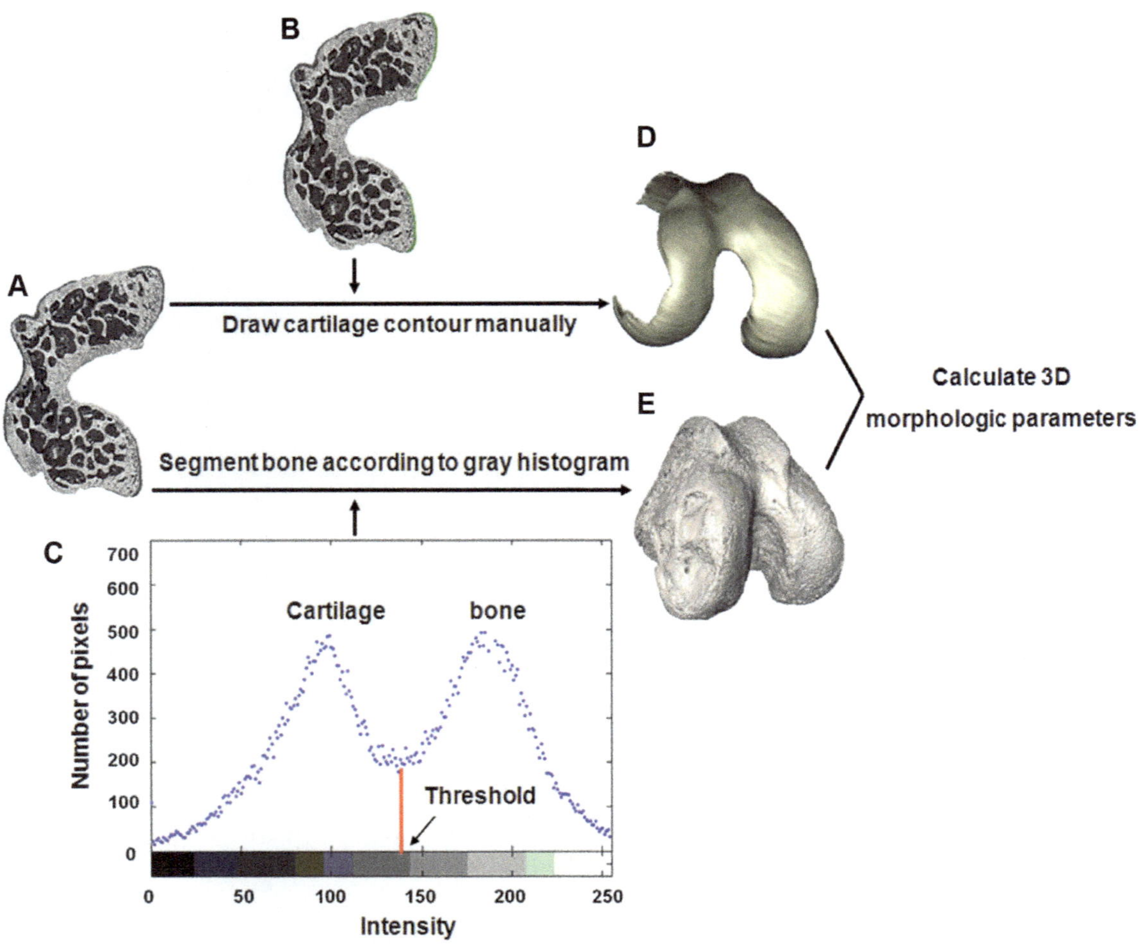

Figure 3. Segmentation methods for quantifying cartilage and bone morphology in the mouse femur. 2D XPCI image of a femoral axial section (A). The method of region growing and manual drawing was used to semi-automatically segment the cartilage, which is indicated in green (B). According to the grayscale histogram (C), an appropriate threshold, indicated by the arrowhead, was selected to separate the bone from the femur. Through the use of the surface rendering method, the 3D morphologies of the femoral cartilage (D) and bone (E) were visualised to calculate the 3D morphologic parameters.

Results

Histological analysis

Representative images of femur sections stained with Safranin-O and the from control and CIA group are shown in Figure 4. At 0 weeks after primary injection, the contour line of the femoral cartilage layer was relatively smooth and the subchondral bone was basically intact. In contrast, at 4 and 8 weeks after primary injection, the thickness of the femoral cartilage was decreased significantly and the contour line was not smooth. Furthermore, part of the subchondral bone surface was obviously eroded. By statistic analysis, the average thickness of femoral cartilage form CIA group at 4 and 8 weeks were respectively low 21% and 34% compared to control group ($P<0.05$).

Morphologic analysis by XPCI

Representative 2D XPCI images are shown in Figure 5. The imaging results clearly show structural changes in the femoral cartilage and subchondral bone in the CIA mice with the RA progression. At 0 weeks after the primary injection, the surface of the subchondral bone was covered with smooth and intact cartilage, and the thickness of the cartilage was uniform. There were no obvious difference between the control and CIA group. At 4 weeks after the primary injection, a portion of the cartilage and bone surface were destroyed, and the cartilage thickness was also decreased significantly compared with the control group. At 8 weeks after the primary injection, femoral structure of normal mouse did not have any significantly change. But, in the CIA group, most of the cartilage was destroyed and had fallen off. Meanwhile, subchondral bone loss was extensive, with more than

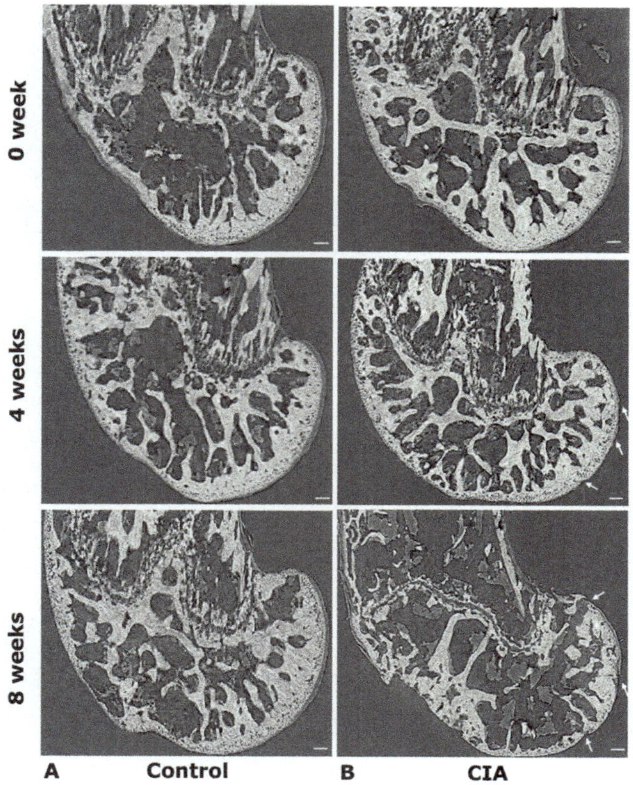

Figure 5. 2D XPCI sagittal images of femora. (A) Femur from a normal mouse at 0, 4 and 8 weeks after the primary injection. (B) Femur from a CIA mouse at 0, 4 and 8 weeks after the primary injection. The red arrowheads indicate the damaged regions in the femora. Scale bars: 100 μm.

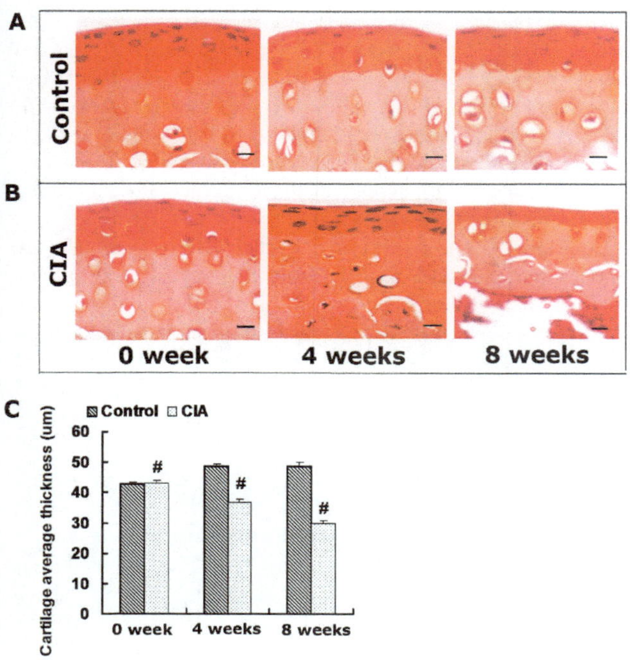

Figure 4. Histological images of femur sections stained with Safranin-O. (A) Femur sections from control group at 0, 4 and 8 weeks after the primary injection. (B) Femur sections from CIA group at 0, 4 and 8 weeks after the primary injection. (C) Average thickness of femoral cartilage assessed by histology. Data are presented as the the mean±SD. 2D CT image before image preprocessing. 2D CT image before image preprocessing. #: $P<0.05$ for differences between the control group and the CIA group. Scale bar: 20 μm.

50% of the surface having been eroded. These imaging results derived from XPCI correlated well with the histological analysis.

The surface rendering method was used to visualise the femur, which provided an intuitive means of identifying 3D architectural anomalies in the femoral cartilage, subchondral bone surface and trabecular bone. Representative 3D images are respectively shown in Figure 6, 7 and 8. At 0 weeks after the primary injection, the structure of femur was basically intact, and no cartilage erosion, subchondral bone lamella denudation or trabecular bone deformities were apparent. As time progressed, we observed that the outer edge of the femoral cartilage, where synovium is densely distributed, was eroded relatively earlier. At later time points, the cartilage damage gradually expanded from the outside to the inside and had an aggravating tendency with the development of the disease. Meanwhile, the subchondral bone was also invaded. Part of the subchondral bone surface was destroyed at 4 weeks, particularly in regions without cartilage coverage, and it had further deteriorated at 8 weeks. At 4 weeks, obvious architectural destruction of the trabecular bone was observed in the form of decreased trabecular bone number and increased trabecular bone separation at 4 weeks. At 8 weeks, there was a progressive increase in the number of bone fragments compared to 4 weeks.

To objectively analyse the structural changes in the articular cartilage and subchondral bone in a quantitative manner, the femoral 3D morphologic parameters of two treatment groups (the control group and CIA group) were measured (Figure 9). At 4 weeks after the primary injection, the femoral cartilage volume, surface area and average thickness in the CIA group were 11%,

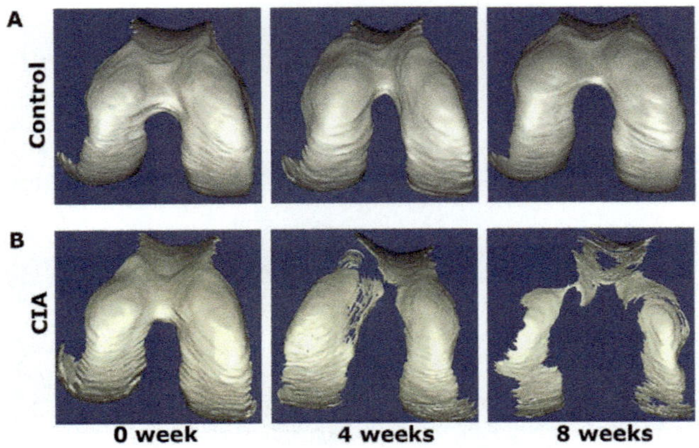

Figure 6. The 3D morphologic images of femoral cartilage. (A) Femoral cartilage from a mouse in control group at 0, 4 and 8 weeks after the primary injection. (B) Femoral cartilage from a mouse in CIA group at 0, 4 and 8 weeks after the primary injection.

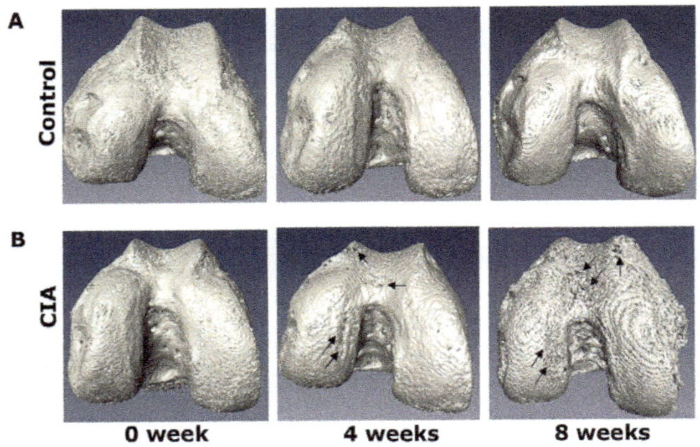

Figure 7. The 3D morphologic images of subchondral bone sufaces. (A) subchondral bone from a mouse in control group at 0, 4 and 8 weeks after the primary injection. (B) subchondral bone from a mouse in CIA group at 0, 4 and 8 weeks after the primary injection. The black arrowheads indicate the damaged regions of the subchondral bone surface.

15% and 12% lower, respectively, than in the control group ($P< 0.05$). In addition, BV/TV, Tb.Th and Tb.N in the CIA group were 6%, 11% and 14% lower, respectively, than in the control group ($P<0.05$), whereas BS/BV and Th.Sp were 10% and 16% higher, respectively ($P<0.05$). At 8 weeks after the primary injection, the cartilage volume, surface area and average thickness in the CIA group were decreased by 32%, 28% and 26%, respectively, compared to the control group ($P<0.05$). Moreover, BV/TV, Tb.Th and Tb.N in the CIA groups were decreased by 28%, 29% and 34%, respectively, corresponding increases of 18% and 43% were measured for BS/BV and Tb.Sp, respectively, compared to the control group ($P<0.05$).

Within the CIA group, the 3D morphologic structure obviously changed in the femora over time. From 0 to 4 weeks, the articular cartilage volume, surface area and average thickness decreased by 7%, 6% and 10% ($P<0.05$), respectively, BV/TV, Tb.Th and Tb.N decreased by 7%, 10% and 9% ($P<0.05$), respectively, and BS/BV and Th.Sp increased by 6% and 7% ($P<0.05$), respectively. At 8 weeks, the femoral cartilage and bone were further eroded compared to the 0 week time point. The cartilage volume, surface area and average thickness were decreased by 20%, 17% and 14%, respectively, and these decreases were accompanied by reductions in BV/TV, Tb.Th and Tb.N by 22%,17% and 26%, respectively ($P<0.05$). Meanwhile, BS/BV and Th.Sp were increased by 15% and 35%, respectively ($P< 0.05$).

Discussion

Although 2D histological analysis is currently regarded as the accepted standard for evaluating the loss of cartilage and bone [6], 3D images obtained from XPCI can provide more structural information for integrated morphologic analysis and precise volumetric assessment. Moreover, histological processing may produce artifacts caused by sample dehydration, embedding and sectionaing in the measurement of morphologic parameters [26]. In contrast, XPCI is a non-invasive imaging method that not only allows for repeated measurements of the same sample but also simplifies the preparative work before imaging to eliminate the possible artifacts and improve the work efficiency.

High-resolution MRI enables 3D non-destructive imaging of cartilage tissue at a resolution of approximately 50 μm [27]. Some studies have used this method to measure the articular cartilage thickness in healthy rats [28] and OA guinea pigs [29]. However, even for high-resolution MRI, according to this level of resolution, quantitative imaging for the accurate measurement of cartilage thickness and volume in a RA mouse is still limited, because the knee joint cartilage of a RA mouse has an average thickness of 30–60 μm. Moreover, the intrinsically poor contrast between cartilage and joint fluid makes it difficult to distinguish them by MRI [13], which may make it difficult to interpret pathological changes.

Compared with routine micro-CT, micro-CT arthrography improves the deficiency of X-ray insensitivity to soft tissues, making it possible to observe morphologic changes in the articular cartilage of mice [26]. However, this technique relies on the use of X-ray absorbing contrast agents that could lead to a risk of comorbidity, such as joint infection or allergic reaction. In addition, another limitation is that micro-CT arthrography, at best, provides functional rather than truly structural information because of differential binding of contrast agents to healthy versus diseased cartilage [21].

Importantly, RA is a condition that affects both articular cartilage and subchondral bone. Elucidating the pathology of these

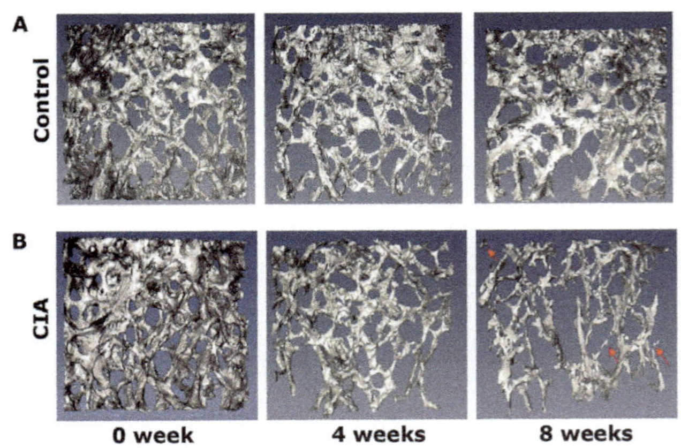

Figure 8. The 3D morphologic images of Trabecular bone. (A) Trabecular bone from a mouse in control group at 0, 4 and 8 weeks after the primary injection. (B) Trabecular bone from a mouse in CIA group at 0, 4 and 8 weeks after the primary injection. The red arrowheads indicate fragments of trabecular bone.

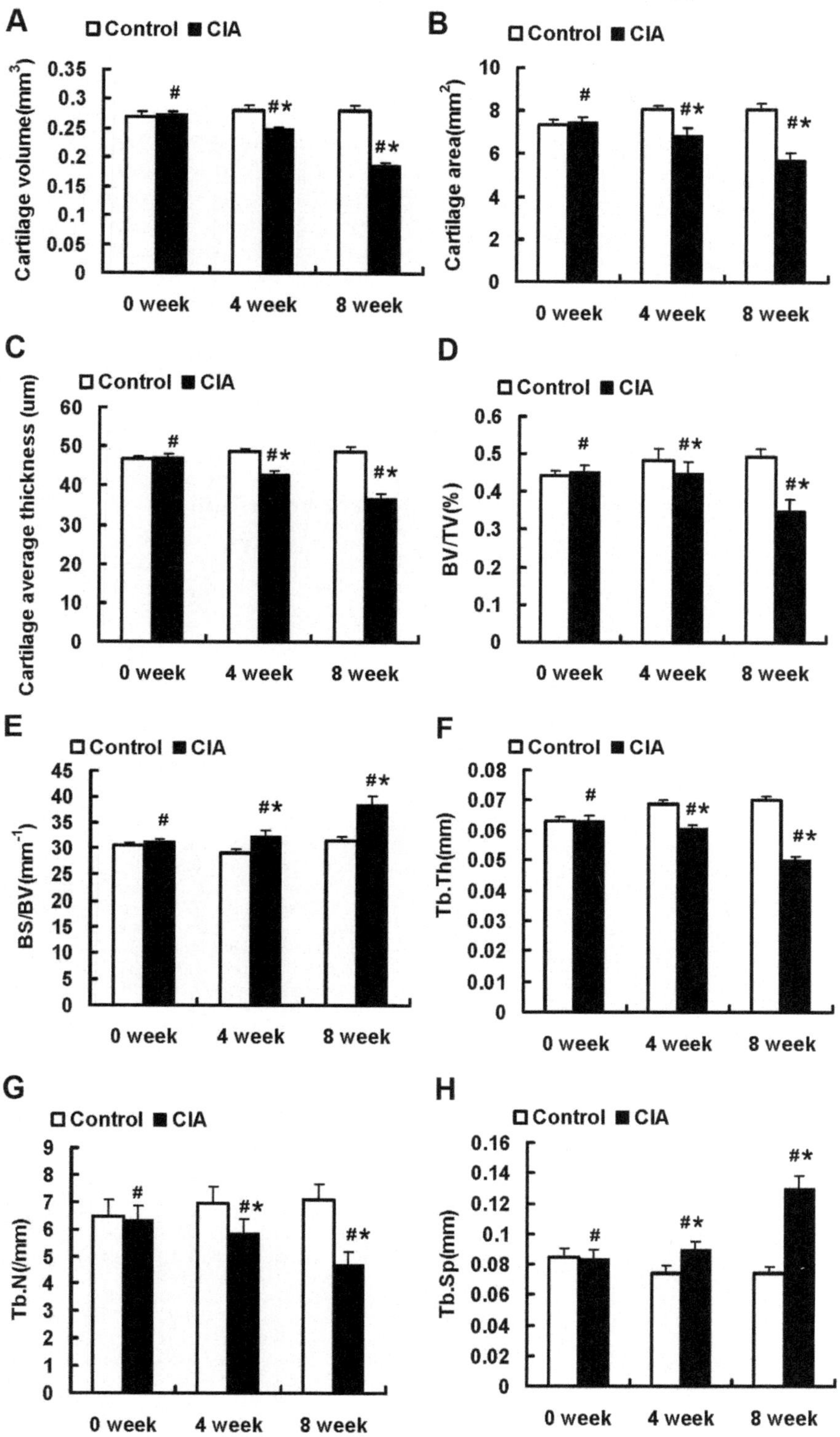

Figure 9. Evaluation of femoral morphology changes between control and CIA groups. (A) Cartilage volume. (B) Cartilage surface area. (C) Average cartilage thickness. (D) Bone volume to tissue volume ratio (BV/TV). (E) Bone surface to bone volume ratio (BS/BV). (F) Trabecular bone thickness (Tb.Th). (G) Trabecular bone number (Tb.N). (H) Trabecular bone space (Tb.Sp). Data are presented as the mean±SD. *: $P<0.05$ for differences between the control group and the CIA group; #: $P<0.05$ for differences within the CIA group.

two tissues is important for the comprehensive diagnosis and treatment of RA. The optimal simultaneous imaging of cartilage and bone is not possible with current MRI and CT systems. In contrast, XPCI can provide high resolution, an order of magnitude higher than MRI, and distinguish the border between cartilage and other tissues without the need for contrast agents [30]. This technique presents opportunities to realise repetitive and accurate measurements of cartilage and bone tissues.

Thereby, we adopted XPCI to study progressive joint damage in a mouse RA model.

The CII induced murine RA model has excellent repeatability, sensitivity and reliability. Furthermore, it specifically demonstrates progression of human RA in a timely manner [31]. The use of CII as an exogenous alloantigen stimulates an autoimmune response and induces pannus formation [32]. The articular cartilage is a barrier covering the surface of the subchondral bone, and it is attacked first by destructive enzymes and inflammatory mediators. Following damage of the articular cartilage, the exposed subchondral bone is eroded. When the structure of the articular cartilage is badly destroyed, the pressure and friction on the subchondral bone are increased [33,34]. This interplay between biochemical and mechanical factors causes a vicious cycle of cartilage damage and bone loss. In our study, the measurements made by XPCI definitively showed morphologic changes in the joint, including obvious decreases in cartilage thickness, area, volume, BV/TV, Tb.Th and Tb.N, as well as corresponding increases in BS/BV and Tb.Sp.

Conclusions

XPCI technology has ability to qualitatively and quantitatively evaluate changes in the joints of RA mice. Moreover, the analysis of 3D morphologic parameters by XPCI here revealed important pathologic features during RA progression. This technique can potentially provide new insights to improve the understanding of RA pathogenesis and be extended to the development of new therapeutic strategies. We believe that with instrumentation and methodological developments, this advanced imaging method has the potential to be applied broadly for the comprehensive and accurate evaluation of joint diseases.

Acknowledgments

Authors thank Tiqiao Xiao, Guohao Du, Yanan Fu and other staffs from beamline BL13W1 of Shanghai Synchrotron Radiation Facility (SSRF) for their guidance and assistance.

Author Contributions

Conceived and designed the experiments: JL SL. Performed the experiments: JL MW LD LZ. Analyzed the data: JL SL HS. Contributed reagents/materials/analysis tools: HY JL. Wrote the paper: JL.

References

1. Alamanos Y, Voulgari PV, Drosos AA (2008) Incidence and prevalence of psoriatic arthritis: a systematic review. J Rheumatol 35:1354–1358.
2. Carmona L, Cross M, Williams B, Lassere M, March L (2010) Rheumatoid arthritis. Best Pract Res Clin Rheumatol 24:733–745.
3. Smolen JS, Alletaha D, Redlich K (2012) The pathogenesis of rheumatoid arthritis: new insights from old clinical data? Nat Rev Rheumatol 8:234–243.
4. Dusad A, Duryee MJ, Shaw AT, Klassen LW, Anderson DR, et al. (2014) Induction of bone loss in DBA/1J mice immunized with citrullinated autologous mouse type II collagen in the absence of adjuvant. Immunol Res 58:51–60.
5. Roemhildt ML, Coughlin KM, Peura GD, Fleming BC, Beynnon BD (2006) Material properties of articular cartilage in the rabbit tibial plateau. J Biomech 39:233–237.
6. Glasson SS, Chambers MG, Little CB (2010) The OARSI histopathology initiative: recommendations for histological assessments of osteoarthritis in the mouse. Osteoarthritis Cartilage 18:17–23.
7. Roemer FW, van Holsbeeck M, Genant HK (2005) Musculoskeletal ultrasound in rheumatology: a radiologic perspective. Arthritis and Rheumatism 53: 491–493.
8. Peterfy CG, Olech E, DiCarlo JC, Merrill JT, Countryman PJ, et al. (2013) Monitoring cartilage loss in the hands and wrists in rheumatoid arthritis with magnetic resonance imaging in a multi-center clinical trial: IMPRESS (NCT00425932). Arthritis Res Ther 15: 44–54.
9. Perry D, Stewart N, Benton N, Robinson E, Yeoman S, et al. (2005) Detection of erosions in the rheumatoid hand; a comparative study of multidetector computerized tomography versus magnetic resonance scanning. J Rheumatol 32:256–267.
10. Ley-Zaporozhan J, Ley S, Eberhardt R, Kauczor HU, Heussel CP (2010) Visualization of morphological parenchymal changes in emphysema: comparison of different MRI sequences to 3D-HRCT. Eur J Radiol 73: 43–49.
11. Smith J, Finnoff JT (2009) Diagnostic and interventional musculoskeletal ultrasound: part 1. Fundamentals PM R 1:64–75.
12. Ruan MZ, Dawson B, Jiang MM, Gannon F, Heggeness M, et al. (2013) Quantitative imaging of murine osteoarthritic cartilage by phase-contrast micro-computed tomography. Arthritis and Rheumatism 65:388–396
13. Fran WR, Michel DC, Siegfried T, Ali G (2011) Advances in imaging of Osteoarthritis and Cartilage. Radiology 260:332–354.
14. Piscaer TM, van Osch GJ, Verhaar JA, Weinans H (2008) Imaging of experimental osteoarthritis in small animal models. Biorheology 45:355–364.
15. Bech M, Jensen TH, Feidenhans R, Bunk O, David C, et al. (2009) Soft tissue phase-contrast tomography with an x-ray tube source. Phys Med Biol 54:2747–2753.
16. Pinzer BR, Cacquevel M, Modregger P, McDonald SA, Bensadoun JC, et al. (2012) Imaging brain amyloid deposition using grating-based differential phase contrast tomography. Neuroimage 4:1336–1346.
17. Grandl S, Willner M, Herzen J, Mayr D, Auweter SD, et al. (2013) Evaluation of phase-contrast CT of breast tissue at conventional X-ray sources-presentation of selected findings. Z Med Phys 23:212–221.
18. Dai C, Guo H, Lu J, Shi J, Wei J, et al. (2011) Osteogenic evaluation of calcium/magnesium-doped mesoporous silica scaffold with incorporation of rhBMP-2 by synchrotron radiation-based μCT. Biomaterials 33:8506–8517.
19. Yang F, Wang J, Hou J, Guo H, Liu C (2013) Bone regeneration using cell-mediated responsive degradable PEG-based scaffolds incorporating with rhBMP-2. Biomaterials 5:1514–1528.
20. Stutman D, Beck TJ, Carrino JA, Bingham CO (2011) Talbot phase-contrast x-ray imaging for the small joints of the hand. Phys Med Biol 17:5697–5720.
21. Marenzana M, Hagen CK, Das Neves Borges P, Endrizzi M, Szafraniec MB, et al. (2012) Visualization of small lesions in rat cartilage by means of laboratory-base x-ray phase contrast imaging. Phys Med Biol 24:8171–8184.
22. Lee YS, Heo EA, Jun HY, Kang SH, Kim HS, et al. (2010) Articular cartilage imaging by the use of phase-contrast tomography in a collagen-induced arthritis mouse model. Acad Radiol 17:244–250.
23. Imhof H, Sulzbacher I, Grampp S, Czerny C, Youssefzadeh S, et al. (2000) Subchondral bone and cartilage disease: a rediscovered functional unit. Invest Radiol 35:581–588.
24. Blair-Levy JM, Watts CE, Fiorentino NM, Dimitriadis EK, Marini JC, et al. (2008) A type I collagen defect leads to rapidly progressive osteoarthritis in a mouse model. Arthritis Rheum 58:1096–1106.
25. Mrosek EH, Lahm A, Erggelet C, Uhl M, Kurz H, et al. (2006) Subchondral bone trauma causes cartilage matrix degeneration: an immunohistochemical analysis in a canine model. Osteoarthritis Cartilage 14:171–178.
26. Kotwal N, Li J, Sandy J, Plaas A, Sumner DR (2012) Initial application of EPIC-μCT to assess mouse articular cartilage morphology and composition: effects of aging and treadmill running. Osteoarthritis and Cartilage 20:887–895.
27. Goebel JC, Pinzano A, Grenier D, Perrier AL, Henrionnet C, et al. (2010) New trends in MRI of cartilage: Advances and limitations in small animal studies. Biomed Mater Eng 2010;20:189–194.
28. Rengle A, Armenean M, Bolbos R, Goebel JC, Pinzano-Watrin A, et al. (2009) A dedicated two-channel phased array receiver coil for high resolution MRI of the rat knee cartilage at 7 T, IEEE Trans Biomed Eng 2891–2897.
29. Bolbos R, Benoit CH, Langlois JB, Chomel A, Chereul E, et al. (2008) Measurement of knee cartilage thickness using MRI: a reproducibility study in a meniscectomized guinea pig model of osteoarthritis. NMR Biomed 366–375.
30. Li J, Zhong Z, Connor D, Mollenhauer J, Muehleman C (2009) Phase-sensitive X-ray imaging of synovial joints. Osteoarthritis Cartilage 17:1193–1196.
31. Brand DD, Latham KA, Rosloniec EF (2007) Collagen-induced arthritis. Nat Protoc 2:1269–1275.
32. Hegen M, Keith JC Jr, Collins M, Nickerson-Nutter CL (2008) Utility of animal models for identification of potential therapeutics for rheumatoid arthritis. Ann Rheum Dis 67:1505–1515.
33. Rieppo J, Toyras J, Nieminen MT, Kovanen V, Hyttinen MM, et al. (2003) Structure-function relationships in enzymatically modified articular cartilage. Cells Tissues Organs 175:121–132.
34. LeRoux MA, Arokoski J, Vail TP, Guilak F, Hyttinen MM, et al. (2000) Simultaneous changes in the mechanical properties, quantitative collagen organization, and proteoglycan concentration of articular cartilage following canine meniscectomy. J Orthop Res 18:383–392.

19

A Novel Weighted Total Difference Based Image Reconstruction Algorithm for Few-View Computed Tomography

Wei Yu[1,3], **Li Zeng**[1,2]*

1 Key Laboratory of Optoelectronic Technology and System of the Education Ministry of China, Chongqing University, Chongqing, China, **2** College of Mathematics and Statistics, Chongqing University, Chongqing, China, **3** Engineering Research Center of Industrial Computed Tomography Nondestructive Testing of the Education Ministry of China, Chongqing University, Chongqing, China

Abstract

In practical applications of computed tomography (CT) imaging, due to the risk of high radiation dose imposed on the patients, it is desired that high quality CT images can be accurately reconstructed from limited projection data. While with limited projections, the images reconstructed often suffer severe artifacts and the edges of the objects are blurred. In recent years, the compressed sensing based reconstruction algorithm has attracted major attention for CT reconstruction from a limited number of projections. In this paper, to eliminate the streak artifacts and preserve the edge structure information of the object, we present a novel iterative reconstruction algorithm based on weighted total difference (WTD) minimization, and demonstrate the superior performance of this algorithm. The WTD measure enforces both the sparsity and the directional continuity in the gradient domain, while the conventional total difference (TD) measure simply enforces the gradient sparsity horizontally and vertically. To solve our WTD-based few-view CT reconstruction model, we use the soft-threshold filtering approach. Numerical experiments are performed to validate the efficiency and the feasibility of our algorithm. For a typical slice of FORBILD head phantom, using 40 projections in the experiments, our algorithm outperforms the TD-based algorithm with more than 60% gains in terms of the root-mean-square error (RMSE), normalized root mean square distance (NRMSD) and normalized mean absolute distance (NMAD) measures and with more than 10% gains in terms of the peak signal-to-noise ratio (PSNR) measure. While for the experiments of noisy projections, our algorithm outperforms the TD-based algorithm with more than 15% gains in terms of the RMSE, NRMSD and NMAD measures and with more than 4% gains in terms of the PSNR measure. The experimental results indicate that our algorithm achieves better performance in terms of suppressing streak artifacts and preserving the edge structure information of the object.

Editor: Christof Markus Aegerter, University of Zurich, Switzerland

Funding: This work is supported by the National Natural Science Foundation of China under grant (61271313) (http://www.nsfc.gov.cn), National Instrumentation Program of China (2013YQ030629) (http://www.most.gov.cn), and Chongqing science and technology research plan project (cstc2012gg-yyjs70016) (http://www.ctin.ac.cn/). The funders had no role in study design, data collection and analysis, decision to publish, or preparation of the manuscript.

Competing Interests: The authors have declared that no competing interests exist.

* Email: drlizeng@cqu.edu.cn

Introduction

As an extremely valuable diagnostic tool, computed tomography (CT) has been widely used in medical area. With this powerful tool, many valuable internal features can be extract without cutting the object [1,2]. However, during clinical exams, excessive X-ray radiation exposure may increase the lifetime cancer risk [3,4]. Thus, it has great significance to use shorter time of radiation exposure and lower patient radiation dose to reconstruct numerically accurate tomographic images. To reduce radiation dose, few-view CT has been an important CT imaging modality. In this scanning data situation, tomographic image is reconstructed from the projection data collected by sparse angular sampling [5–9]. For few-view CT, due to the projection data obtained is not theoretically sufficient for exact reconstruction of tomographic images, conspicuous streak artifacts are present in reconstructed images by conventional analytic algorithms such as filtered back-projection [5,10–12]. In this paper, we mainly focus the iterative reconstruction algorithm for few-view CT.

Since the development of the large computational capacities in graphical processing unit and the ongoing efforts towards lower doses have made in CT, iterative reconstruction has become a hot topic for all major vendors of clinical CT systems in the past years [13–17]. The algebraic reconstruction technique and simultaneous algebraic reconstruction technique (SART) are two classical reconstruction algorithms for CT image reconstruction [18,19]. Since the projection data are incomplete, using the two algorithms, obvious artifacts and noise are present in reconstructed images. With the development of compressed sensing theory [20–22], compressed sensing based iterative reconstruction algorithm has drawn much attention in the medical imaging and other tomographic imaging modalities. By adopting the compressed sensing based iterative reconstruction algorithm, the image can be reconstructed from rather limited projection data [23]. In mathematics, actually, CT image reconstruction with few-view projection data is taken as an ill-posed inverse problem. To solve this problem, regularization method is usually adopted, and corresponding unconstrained optimization problem can be formulated [24]. In the unconstrained optimization problem, the objective function usually contains two terms. The first term is data fidelity term which constraints the data consistency between measured projection data and model data. The second term is regularization term which is designed according to the priori information of the image.

In the CT reconstruction field, it is likely that images are not sparse themselves, but image coefficients in some transform domains show sparsity. In image gradient transform, the L1 norm of the image gradient magnitudes (also known as total variation (TV) of image) are approximately sparse. If D_h and D_v represent the horizontal and vertical gradient operators respectively, then TV regularization term can be expressed as $\mathrm{TV}(\mathbf{u}) = \sum_i \sqrt{(D_h\mathbf{u})_i^2 + (D_v\mathbf{u})_i^2}$. This regularization term which was originally proposed for image denoising [25], has been extended in the field of few-view CT image reconstruction [5]. Subsequently, many other related reconstruction algorithms have been developed [6–8,23,26].

In 1996, Li and Santosa suggested that total difference (TD) which was defined as $\mathbf{TD(u)} = \|D_h\mathbf{u}\|_1 + \|D_v\mathbf{u}\|_1$, was a reliable and computationally efficient approximation to the TV in image restoration [27]. In 2010, by constructing a pseudo-inverse of the discrete TD, a TD minimization algorithm with soft-threshold filtering (TDM-STF) was developed for few-view CT. It can improve the convergence and efficiency of TV based minimization methods [28]. In the TDM-STF algorithm, TD is taken as the regularization term. Later, the TDM-STF algorithm was applied to a multisource x-ray interior imaging system [29]. In their work, they accelerated the convergence speed of TDM-STF by incorporating a fast iterative shrinkage thresholding algorithm [30]. It shows that when obtaining the same image quality, the TDM-STF may need less iterations and total computational cost for practical application. However, the TD seeks the gradient sparsity horizontally and vertically, but fails to enforce the gradient continuity. Thus, the TD is prone to recovering an image of sharp horizontal and vertical edges. To overcome this shortcoming of TD, a new measure (called weighted total difference (WTD) measure hereafter) was utilized by Shu and Ahuja for compressive sampling [31]. In their work, they proposed a hybrid compressive sampling method for recovering a piecewise smooth image from limited measurements. Since the WTD measure exploits the continuity and sparsity simultaneously in the partial gradient domain, all possible sharper edges of the image can be recovered from limited measurements. In [31], WTD measure was taken as the regularization term. Note that model investigated in [31] is different from the model for CT reconstruction since WTD combines two complementary sampling systems for image recovery. In this work, we consider incorporating WTD measure into the model for CT reconstruction due to the good property of WTD.

With the aim to eliminate the undesired streak artifacts and preserve the edge structure information of the object, in this paper, we propose a novel reconstruction algorithm based on WTD minimization for few-view CT. The proposed reconstruction model combines the CT imaging model and the WTD measure. In the proposed reconstruction model, the WTD measure is taken as the regularization term. The differences between the WTD in current study and in the study [31] lie in the application fields and the corresponding problems need to solve. To solve our model effectively, the soft-threshold filtering (STF) method and a fast iterative shrinkage thresholding algorithm are employed to accelerate the converging speed of our algorithm. For simplicity, in the following sections, we referred to our algorithm as WTDM-STF.

The rest of the paper is organized as follows. In section Method, we illustrate the CT imaging model and describe the WTDM-STF reconstruction algorithm for few-view CT, together with an efficient iterative scheme. Moreover, the data acquisitions and performance evaluations are also outlined in this section. In the following section, numerical results and discussion are presented and conclusions are given in final section.

Methods

CT imaging model

The model of fan beam CT imaging can be approximated as following discrete linear system [19]:

$$\mathbf{Au} = \mathbf{g}, \tag{1}$$

where $\mathbf{g} = [g_1, g_2, \ldots, g_M]^T \in R^M$ is the measured projection data which can be represented by a vector of size M, M is the number of the transmission rays, g_i is the ray-sum measured with the ith ray, $\mathbf{u} = [u_1, u_2, \ldots, u_N]^T \in R^N$ denotes the image to be reconstructed which can be represented by a vector of size N, N is the number of image pixels. $\mathbf{A} = (a_{i,j}) \in R^M \times R^N$ is the system matrix which represents forward projection. The system matrix weight $a_{i,j}$ represents the contribution of the jth pixel to the ith ray-sum. In our experiments, the system matrix weights $a_{i,j}$ are computed by calculating the intersection length of the ith ray through the jth pixel. Given the projection data acquired from the detector, the aim for image reconstruction is to solve the Eq. (1) for $\mathbf{u}$ from the measured data $\mathbf{g}$. As for few-view CT problem, the number of the measured projection data M is much smaller than the number of image pixels N, then, the Eq. (1) is underdetermined. Therefore,

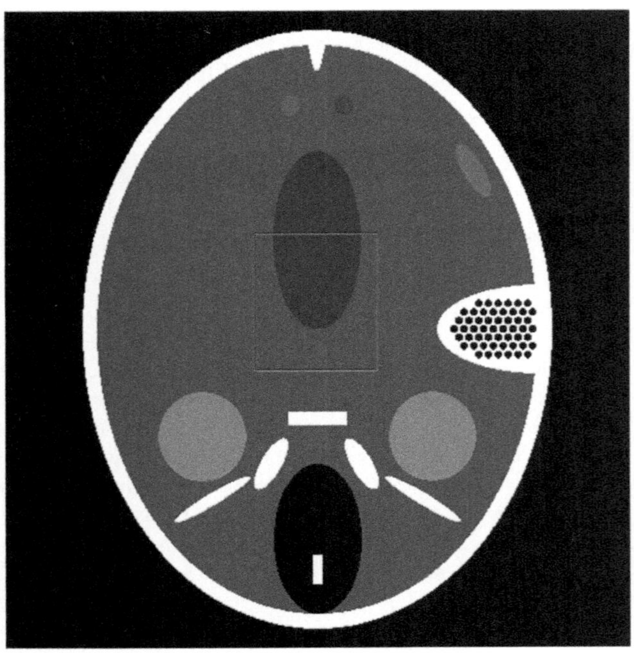

Figure 1. A typical slice of the FORBILD head phantom.

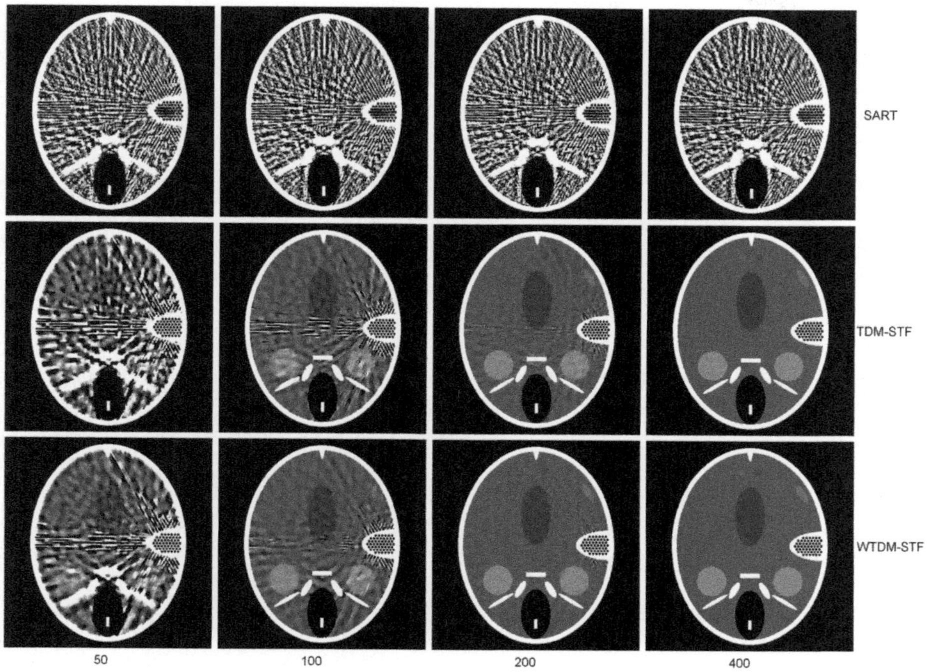

Figure 2. Images reconstructed by SART (first row), TDM-STF (second row) and WTDM-STF (third row) algorithms after 50, 100, 200, 400 iterations using noise-free projections, respectively. The gray scale window is set to [1.03, 1.08].

how to reconstruct approximately accurate CT image is important for practical applications.

The WTDM-STF algorithm

Inspired by the wok in [31], the WTD measure not only enforces the gradient sparsity horizontally and vertically, but also enforces the gradient continuity. By the WTD measure, the sharp and clear edges can be better preserved than TD. The WTD of image **u** is defined as follows

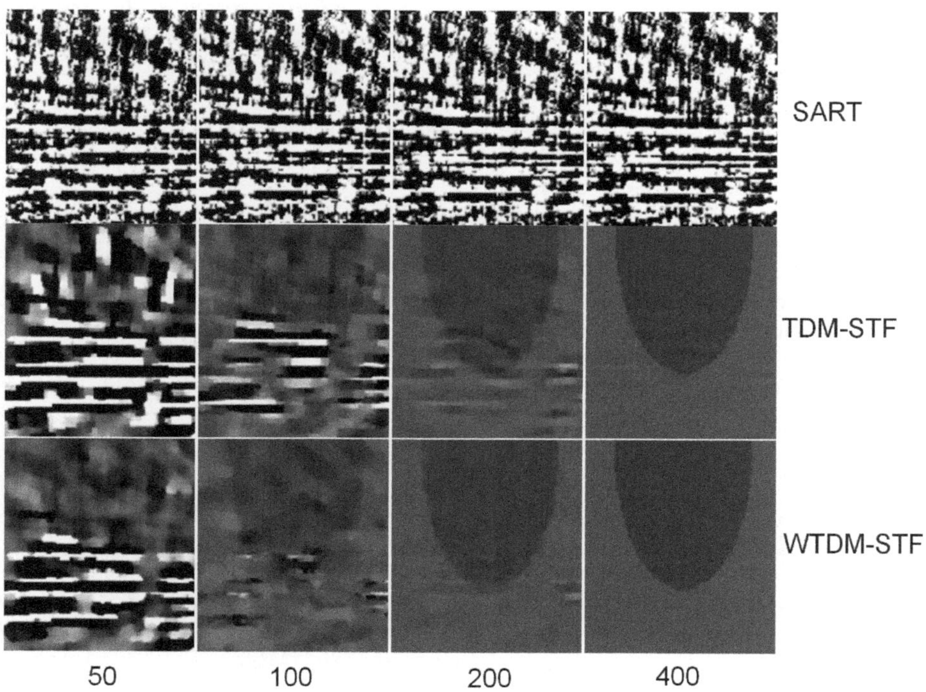

Figure 3. Zoom-in views of images reconstructed by SART (first row), TDM-STF (second row) and WTDM-STF (third row) algorithms after 50, 100, 200, 400 iterations, respectively. The gray scale window is set to [1.03, 1.08].

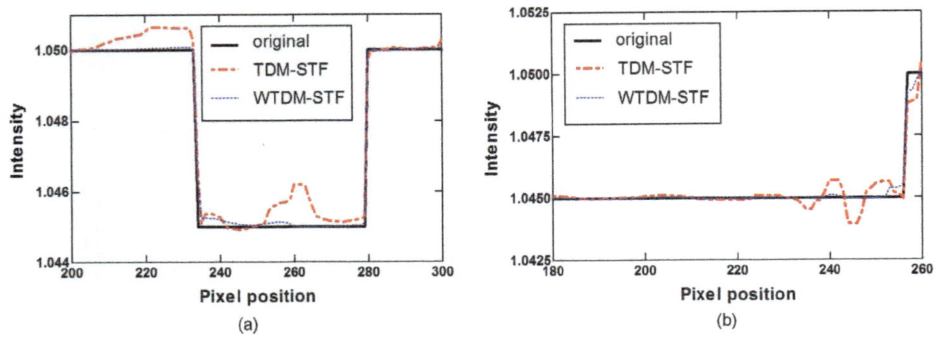

Figure 4. 1D profiles of the images reconstructed by different algorithms using noise-free projections. (a) Horizontal profiles (240th row, 200th column to the 300th column); (b) Vertical profiles (258th column, 180th row to the 260th row).

$$\begin{aligned}\mathbf{WTD(u)} &= \|D_h\mathbf{u}\|_1 + \|D_v\mathbf{u}\|_1 + \alpha(\|D_{hv}\mathbf{u}\|_1 + \|D_{vh}\mathbf{u}\|_1) \\ &= \sum_i \sum_j |D_h u_{i,j}| + |D_v u_{i,j}| + \alpha(|D_{hv} u_{i,j}| + |D_{vh} u_{i,j}|)\end{aligned} \quad (2)$$

Where D_h, D_v, D_{hv} and D_{vh} are respectively horizontal, vertical and two diagonal partial gradients operators, i.e., $D_h u_{i,j} = u_{i+1,j} - u_{i,j}$, $D_v u_{i,j} = u_{i,j+1} - u_{i,j}$, $D_{hv} u_{i,j} = u_{i+1,j+1} - u_{i,j}$, $D_{vh} u_{i,j} = u_{i,j+1} - u_{i+1,j}$. The first two terms measure the gradient sparsity; the last two terms measure the gradient continuity, and the parameter α plays a crucial role in balancing the gradient sparsity and the gradient continuity. In this work, we combine the WTD (see also in Eq. (2)) and CT imaging model (see also in Eq. (1)) to formulate a novel reconstruction model for few-view CT. Using **WTD(u)** as the regularization term, the developed image reconstruction model can be expressed as

$$\begin{aligned}&\min_{\mathbf{u}} \|\mathbf{Au} - \mathbf{g}\|_2^2 + 2\omega \cdot \sum_i \sum_j |u_{i+1,j} - u_{i,j}| + |u_{i,j+1} - u_{i,j}| \\ &+ \alpha(|u_{i+1,j+1} - u_{i,j}| + |u_{i,j+1} - u_{i+1,j}|),\end{aligned} \quad (3)$$

From the model above, the TD-based image reconstruction model [28] is one special case of model (3), which is equivalent to the model (3) when α equals to zero. In our work, we fix the parameter α equals to 1.0, which equally penalizes the gradient sparsity and the gradient continuity. The difference between TD-based image reconstruction model and our model lies in the original TD-based regularization just enforces the sparsity horizontally and vertically in the gradient domain, while the sparsity diagonally and the directional continuity of gradients are not considered. Therefore, the sharp and clear edges in the CT image can be well preserved along more directions by our reconstruction algorithm.

To solve the above model in (3), there are many ways, such as soft-threshold filtering (STF) method [32,33] and Split Bregman method [34]. The STF method, whose convergence and efficiency have been theoretically proven, has already been applied for CT reconstruction in [28,29]. Similar to [29], in this work, we solve our reconstruction model in the soft-threshold filtering framework. After the soft-threshold filtration, we need to construct a pseudo-inverse of the WTD. The detailed iterative steps of our WTDM-STF algorithm can be summarized as the following:

(1) Initialization:

$n = 0$, $\mathbf{u}^{(n)} = 0$, $\mathbf{u}_{\text{temp}} = 0$, $t_n = 1$, $\alpha = 1.0$.

(2) The data constraint step. Update $\mathbf{u}^{(n)}$ using the SART formula:

$$\tilde{u}_j^{n+1} = u_j^n - \gamma^n \frac{1}{\sum_{i=1}^{M} a_{i,j}} \sum_{i=1}^{M} \frac{a_{i,j}}{\sum_{j=1}^{N} a_{i,j}} (g_i - \mathbf{A}_i \mathbf{u}^n),\ j = 1, 2, \ldots, N.$$

where γ^n is a relax parameter.

(3) Soft-threshold filtering step, the pseudo-inverse of $u_{i,j}^{(n+1)}$ is constructed similar to reference [28],

$$\begin{aligned}u_{i,j}^{(n+1)} = \frac{1}{4 + 4\cdot\alpha}&(q(\omega, \tilde{u}_{i,j}^{(n+1)}, \tilde{u}_{i+1,j}^{(n+1)}) + q(\omega, \tilde{u}_{i,j}^{(n+1)}, \tilde{u}_{i,j+1}^{(n+1)}) + q(\omega, \tilde{u}_{i,j}^{(n+1)}, \\ &\tilde{u}_{i,j-1}^{(n+1)}) + q(\omega, \tilde{u}_{i,j}^{(n+1)}, \tilde{u}_{i-1,j}^{(n+1)}) + \alpha\cdot((q(\omega, \tilde{u}_{i,j}^{(n+1)}, \tilde{u}_{i+1,j+1}^{(n+1)}) + q(\omega, \tilde{u}_{i,j}^{(n+1)}, \\ &\tilde{u}_{i+1,j-1}^{(n+1)}) + q(\omega, \tilde{u}_{i,j}^{(n+1)}, \tilde{u}_{i-1,j-1}^{(n+1)}) + q(\omega, \tilde{u}_{i,j}^{(n+1)}, \tilde{u}_{i-1,j+1}^{(n+1)})),\end{aligned}$$

where

Table 1. Evaluations of the results reconstructed by different algorithms (with 400 iterations from noise-free projections for a typical slice of the FORBILD head phantom).

	RMSE	PSNR	NRMSD	NMAD
SART	0.0843	21.9048	34.4883	0.0618
TDM-STF	0.000266	71.9376	0.1087	0.000155
WTDM-STF	0.000102	80.2738	0.0416	0.000037

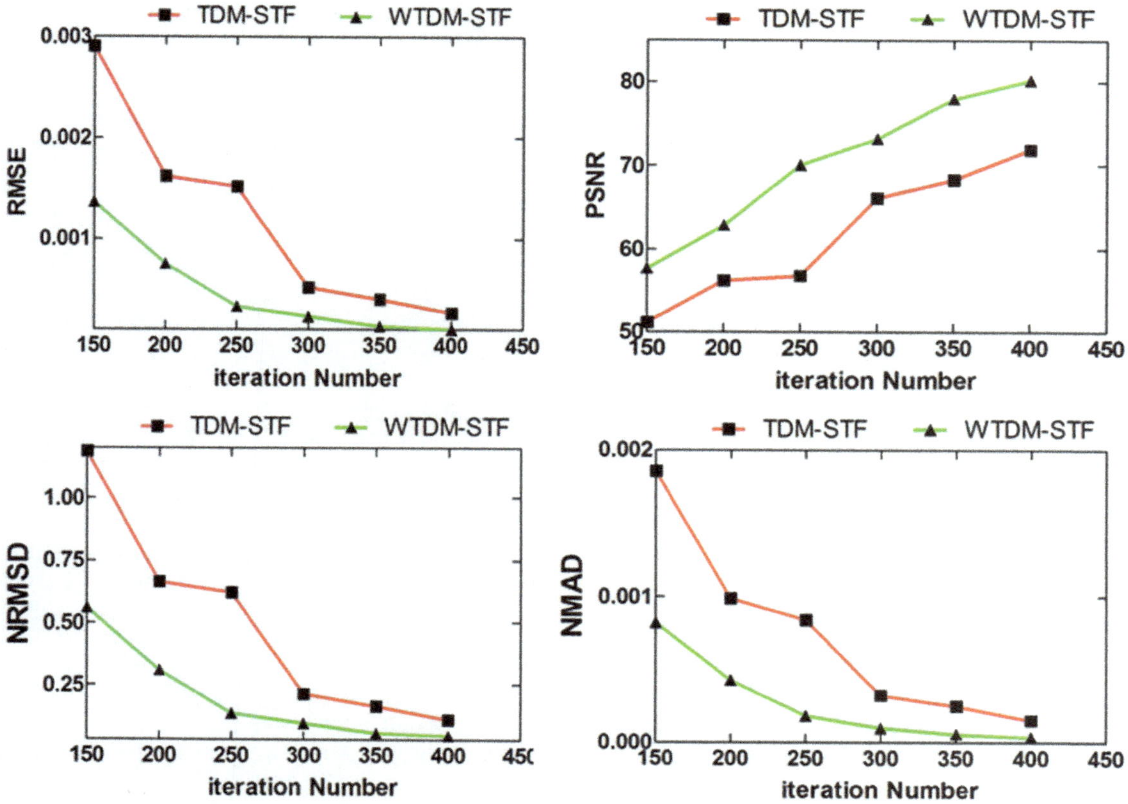

Figure 5. Different performance evaluations as a function of iteration numbers on the reconstructions by TDM-STF and WTDM-STF.

$$q(\omega,y,z)=\begin{cases}(y+z)/2, \text{ if } |\text{y-z}|<\omega\\ y-\omega/2, \text{ if y-z}\geq\omega\\ y+\omega/2, \text{ if y-z}\leq-\omega.\end{cases}$$

the threshold $\omega=\max_i |r_i|$, $\mathbf{r}=\mathbf{A}^*(\mathbf{g}-\mathbf{Au})$ [33].

(4) Acceleration technique:

$$\mathbf{h}=\mathbf{u}^{(n)};$$

$$t_{n+1}=\frac{1+\sqrt{1+4t_n^2}}{2};$$

$$\mathbf{u}^{(n+1)}=\mathbf{h}+\left(\frac{t_n-1}{t_{n+1}}\right)(\mathbf{h}-\mathbf{u}_{\text{temp}});$$

$$\mathbf{u}_{temp}=\mathbf{h};$$

(5) Initialize next loop:

$$n=n+1,\ \mathbf{u}^{(n)}=\mathbf{u}^{(n-1)};$$

Return to step (2) until the stopping criteria is satisfied.

From the iterative reconstruction algorithm mentioned above, each main loop of WTDM-STF algorithm is divided into three steps. These three steps are performed in the manner of alternating iteration in each of main loop. The first step is the data constraint step, which utilizes SART formula to reduce the data discrepancy between original projection data and the forward projection of the reconstructed image. The second step is the soft-threshold filtering step, which is adopted to reduce the WTD of the image. In the third step, an acceleration technique is employed to accelerate the converging speed of the WTDM-STF algorithm. From the Soft-threshold filtering step mentioned above, it is found that the pseudo-inverse of $u_{i,j}^{(n+1)}$ not only related to the results of soft-threshold filtration function $q(\omega,y,z)$, but also related to the parameter α. The parameter α here determines the weight of the contribution of four diagonal pixels to the center pixel. By this process, the directional continuity of gradients can be effectively enforced. Thus, the edge structure information of the object can be effectively preserved and the streak artifacts can be significantly reduced.

Data acquisitions

To demonstrate the validity of our WTDM-STF algorithm, we implemented it on a PC (2.67 GHz Intel Core i5 CPU, 4.0 G memory, Windows 7 operating system) coded in Microsoft Visual C++2008. We tested the reconstruction algorithms for few-view CT using a typical slice of low-contrast FORBILD head phantom with matrix size 512×512 [35] shown in Figure 1. Since the high-frequency and high-contrast fine inner ear structures caused severe artifacts overlapping with the low-contrast structures, more projections were used to reconstruct low-contrast structures well. In our experiments, the projection data is generated at 40 view angles specified by:

$$\theta_i = \begin{cases} 9^\circ \times (i-1) & 1 \leq i \leq 20 \\ 9^\circ \times (i-0.5) & 20 < i \leq 40 \end{cases} \quad (4)$$

Though sparse, the angles cover 360° about the object. We chose a circular scanning locus of radius 51.1 cm and fan-beam geometry. The object was fixed, the X-ray source and the detector rotated around the rotation axis synchronously. The distance between source and rotation axis was set to 293.1 cm. The pixel size of the reconstructed image was 0.1×0.1 cm^2. The equi-distance virtual detector array we used had 1025 elements, each of which had an aperture 0.05 cm. The noise-free projection data are generated by applying the system matrix to the typical slice of the FORBILD head phantom. For the noisy case, the noisy projection data are generated by adding Gaussian noise to the noise-free projection data generated previously. The standard deviation of the Gaussian noise is 0.05% of the maximum value of the projection data and the average value is zero.

Performance evaluations

To evaluate the performance of the WTDM-STF for few-view CT image reconstruction, the following four metrics were utilized: (1) root-mean-square error (RMSE); (2) peak signal-to-noise ratio (PSNR); (3) normalized root mean square distance (NRMSD) [36]; (4) normalized mean absolute distance (NMAD) [36]:

$$RMSE = \sqrt{\frac{1}{Q}\sum_{m=1}^{Q}(u(m) - u_{true}(m))^2} \quad (5)$$

$$PSNR = 10\log_{10}\left(\frac{MAX^2(u_{true})}{\frac{1}{Q}\sum_{m=1}^{Q}(u(m)-u_{true}(m))^2}\right) \quad (6)$$

$$\text{NRMSD} = \sqrt{\frac{\sum_{m=1}^{Q}(u(m)-u_{true}(m))^2}{\sum_{m=1}^{Q}(\bar{u}_{true}-u_{true}(m))^2}} \quad (7)$$

$$\text{NMAD} = \frac{\sum_{m=1}^{Q}|u(m)-u_{true}(m)|}{\sum_{m=1}^{Q}|u_{true}(m)|} \quad (8)$$

where u denotes the image reconstructed, u_{true} denotes the original phantom image, $MAX(u_{true})$ denotes the maximum density value of the original phantom image, $|x|$ denotes the absolute value of x, $\bar{u}_{true}$ denotes the average of the densities in the interest of region (ROI) wherein m indexes the pixels in the ROI. Q is the number of pixels in the ROI. Both the values of NRMSD and NMAD are close to 0 if the reconstruction is approximately equal to original phantom image. The NRMSD and NMAD measures emphasize different aspects of image quality. A large difference in a few places causes the value of NRMSD to be large. Note that the value of NRMSD is 1.0 if the reconstruction is a uniformly dense image with the correct average density. As opposed to NRMSD, NMAD emphasizes the importance of a lot of small errors rather than of a few large errors. Note that the value of NMAD is 1.0 if the reconstruction is a uniformly dense image with zero density.

Statistical Analysis

Statistical analysis is performed using a user-friendly statistical software (MedCalc [37], Ostend, Belgium). To assess the performance evaluations of image quality (RMSE, PSNR, NRMSD, NMAD) presented in (5)–(8), the tests of statistical significance are performed using 500 slices of the FORBILD head phantom. First, we perform the F-test. If the associated (two-sided) P-value is less than the conventional 0.05, the null hypothesis is rejected and the conclusion is that the two variances do indeed differ significantly. If the P-value is low ($P<0.05$), the variances of the two samples cannot be assumed to be equal and it should be considered to use the t-test with a correction for unequal variances (Welch's t test, [38]). The variables are expressed as Mean ± SD (standard deviations). For Welch's t test, when the P-value is less than the conventional 0.05, the null hypothesis is rejected and the conclusion is that the two means do indeed differ significantly.

Results and Discussion

In order to verify the superiority of our WTDM-STF algorithm, we made the comparison with the following two algorithms: (1) the classical SART algorithm and (2) the acceleration version of TDM-STF algorithm [28], respectively. For all the above reconstruction algorithms, the stopping criterion was defined as reaching the maximum iteration number 400. In all the experiments, we set the relax parameter $\gamma^n = 0.1$ in the SART iteration formula. For all iterative reconstruction algorithms, the initial image was $\mathbf{u}^{(n)} = 0$.

Figure 2 shows the images reconstructed by different algorithms using 40 noise-free projections. The images from up to bottom are reconstructed by SART, TDM-STF and WTDM-STF, respectively. The images from left to right are reconstructed with 50, 100, 200, 400 iterations respectively. The gray scale window is set to [1.03, 1.08]. It can be found that the images reconstructed by SART have severe streak artifacts due to the few-view projection data. While the artifacts can be better suppressed by TDM-STF and WTDM-STF after certain iterations. In the earlier iterations (such as 50 and 100 iterations), the reconstructed images are distorted nearby the high-contrast fine inner ear structures. With the increase of the iteration numbers, the streak artifacts are effectively reduced by WTDM-STF and TDM-STF. As can be seen from the first column of Figure 2, the WTDM-STF has more advantage of reducing the streak artifacts than TDM-STF. From the following two columns of Figure 2, we also come to the conclusion that the streak artifacts can be suppressed more effectively by WTDM-STF than TDM-STF. From the last column of Figure 2, it shows that when the iteration number is big enough, the reconstruction results have similar quality of vision. However, since the WTD measure enforces the gradient sparsity and the

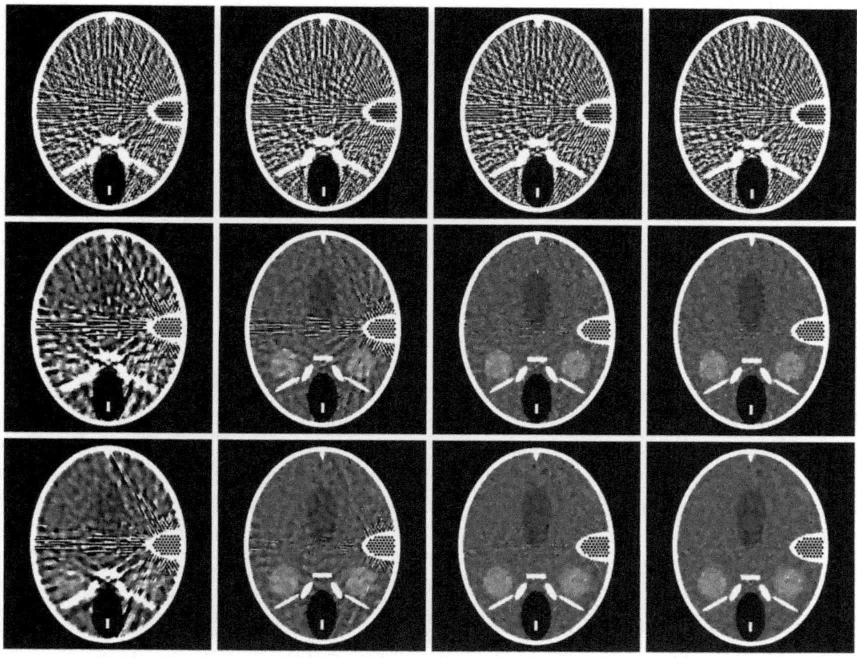

Figure 6. Images reconstructed by SART (first row), TDM-STF (second row) and WTDM-STF (third row) algorithms after 50, 100, 200, 400 iterations using noisy projections, respectively. The gray scale window is set to [1.03, 1.08].

gradient continuity, the streak artifacts can be better suppressed by WTDM-STF than TDM-STF.

To further demonstrate the superiority of our algorithm, the zoom-in views of the images reconstructed corresponding to the selected region in Figure 1 are shown in Figure 3. It illustrates that the images reconstructed by WTDM-STF have superior image quality for different iterations. And the streak artifacts are significantly reduced by WTDM-STF and TDM-STF with the increase of iterations. Moreover, it shows that the edges are more accurate and better preserved by WTDM-STF in term of maintaining the structure information of ROI.

To visualize the difference between WTDM-STF and TDM-STF, Figure 4 displays the horizontal and vertical profiles of the images reconstructed by WTDM-STF and TDM-STF. Figure 4(a) shows the horizontal profiles across the 240th row from the 200th column to the 300th column. Figure 4(b) shows the vertical profiles across the 258th column from the 180th row to the 260th row. It can be seen that the profiles of WTDM-STF match well with that from the typical slice of original phantom. The results indicate that the gains than from the WTDM-STF are more noticeable compared with those from the TDM-STF.

In addition to visual inspection of the results, Table 1 lists the RMSE, PSNR, NRMSD and NMAD measures of the images (as shown in Figure 3) reconstructed by SART, TDM-STF and WTDM-STF with 400 iterations. The quantitative results from both the TDM-STF and WTDM-STF exhibited better results than that from the SART algorithm in terms of the four measures. As can be observed from the Table 1, the WTDM-STF outperforms the TDM-STF with more than 60% gains in terms of the RMSE, NRMSD and NMAD measures and with more than 10% gains in terms of the PSNR measure. In Table 1, the WTDM-STF shows better performance since the artifacts near the edge of the object affect the accuracy of the image reconstructed. Considering the gradient sparsity and gradient continuity simultaneously in WTDM-STF, the reconstruction is more closer to typical slice of original phantom image, where the edge structure information of the object has been better preserved. In the experiments, it finds that the more the iterations, the better the image quality. Thus, to clearly demonstrate the superiority of WTDM-STF, the reconstructions after 150 iterations are considered. Figure 5 shows different performance evaluations as a function of iteration numbers on the reconstructions. It can be observed that the WTDM-STF consistently outperforms TDM-STF in these profiles.

In the practical applications, the projection data usually contains measurement noise. Then, we repeated the aforemen-

Table 2. Evaluations of the results reconstructed by different algorithms (with 400 iterations from noisy projections for a typical slice of the FORBILD head phantom).

	RMSE	PSNR	NRMSD	NMAD
SART	0.0858	21.7519	35.1011	0.0630
TDM-STF	0.0030	50.7433	1.2467	0.0019
WTDM-STF	0.0024	52.8677	0.9762	0.0016

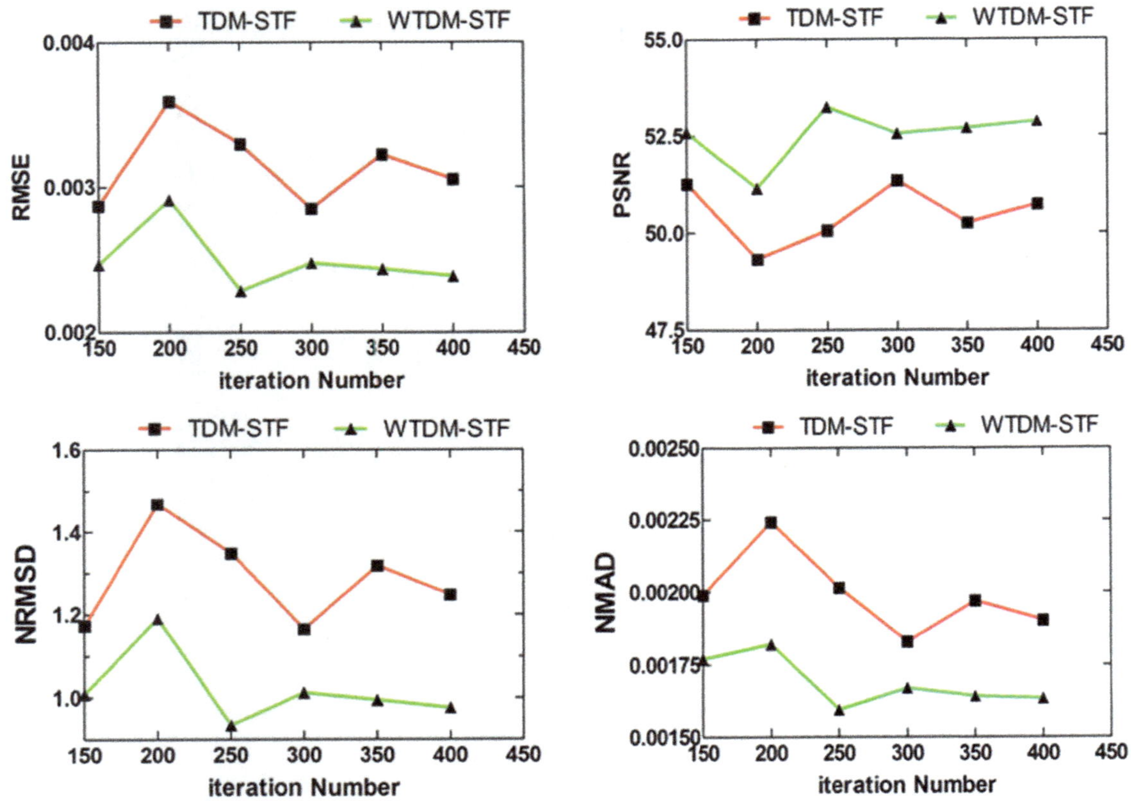

Figure 7. Different performance evaluations as a function of iteration numbers on the reconstructions by TDM-STF and WTDM-STF from noisy projection data.

tioned experiments. Figure 6 gives the reconstructed images from noisy projection data. It can be found that the SART suffers severe streak artifacts. Compared with TDM-STF and SART, WTDM-STF causes fewer artifacts and the edges are better kept. Table 2 lists the same quantitative evaluations as in Table 1 but from noisy cases with 400 iterations. From Table 2, it shows that the results by our algorithm have better performance which are consistent with the results presented in Table 1. As can be observed from the Table 2, the WTDM-STF outperforms the TDM-STF with more than 15% gains in terms of the RMSE, NRMSD and NMAD measures and with more than 4% gains in terms of the PSNR measure. The good performance of WTDM-STF is attributed to the WTD measure which can better suppress noise and preserve the edge of the object. Figure 7 also shows different performance evaluations curves as Figure 5. It can be observed that, for noisy case, the WTDM-STF slightly outperforms TDM-STF in terms of these performance evaluations. Therefore, the WTDM-STF is a more robust algorithm for few-view CT.

To further support the conclusion statements and assess the performance evaluations of image quality presented in Tables 1 and 2, we performed the tests of statistical significance using 500 slices of the FORBILD head phantom. For the experiments mentioned above, we perform the F-test first. Since the P-values are low ($P<0.05$), the variances of the these samples cannot be assumed to be equal. Thus, we perform the Welch's t test. The statistical analysis results of performance evaluations of image quality between different algorithms with 100 iterations for 500 reconstruction images are summarized in Tables 3 and 4, respectively. The variables are expressed as Mean ± SD. From Table 3, there are obvious statistical differences in the values of RMSE, PSNR, NRMSD, NMAD between any two algorithms ($P<0.0001$). And the values of RMSE, NRMSD, NMAD by

Table 3. Summary of Welch's t test analysis results of performance evaluations of image quality between different algorithms (with 100 iterations from noise-free projections for 500 slices of the FORBILD head phantom).

				P-value		
Item	**SART (A)**	**TDM-STF (B)**	**WTDM-STF (C)**	**A vs. B**	**A vs. C**	**B vs. C**
RMSE	0.03849±0.01882	0.002728±0.002386	0.002208±0.001087	<0.0001	<0.0001	<0.0001
PSNR	34.5921±5.3182	57.8400±4.2862	58.8675±3.0864	<0.0001	<0.0001	<0.0001
NRMSD	0.06671±0.02806	0.004786±0.003732	0.003935±0.001619	<0.0001	<0.0001	<0.0001
NMAD	0.03223±0.01181	0.001692±0.001054	0.001284±0.0006269	<0.0001	<0.0001	<0.0001

Table 4. Summary of Welch's t test analysis results of performance evaluations of image quality between different algorithms (with 100 iterations from noisy projections for 500 slices of the FORBILD head phantom).

				P-value		
Item	**SART(A)**	**TDM-STF(B)**	**WTDM-STF(C)**	**A vs. B**	**A vs. C**	**B vs. C**
RMSE	0.03983±0.01872	0.004180±0.002491	0.003789±0.001351	<0.0001	<0.0001	0.0021
PSNR	34.2103±5.1016	53.7299±4.1429	54.1347±3.4225	<0.0001	<0.0001	0.0925
NRMSD	0.06913±0.02764	0.007311±0.003742	0.006676±0.001774	<0.0001	<0.0001	0.0006
NMAD	0.03487±0.01112	0.003098±0.001014	0.002659±0.0005893	<0.0001	<0.0001	<0.0001

WTDM-STF are significantly lower than that of TDM-STF and SART. The value of PSNR by WTDM-STF is higher than that of TDM-STF and SART. From Table 4, the values of RMSE, PSNR, NRMSD, NMAD of WTDM-STF and TDM-STF had significant statistical difference from that of SART ($P<0.0001$). It shows that both WTDM-STF and TDM-STF have better performance than SART. There are significant statistical differences between WTDM-STF and TDM-STF in RMSE ($P=0.0021<0.05$), NRMSD ($P=0.0006<0.05$), NMAD ($P<0.0001$). The values of RMSE, NRMSD, NMAD show that WTDM-STF has better performance than TDM-STF. There is no obvious statistical difference in the PSNR value between WTDM-STF and TDM-STF ($P=0.0925>0.05$).

For the experiments implemented mentioned above on a PC (2.67 GHz Intel Core i5 CPU), the average computation time per iteration of WTDM-STF, TDM-STF and SART are 2.01 s, 1.97 s and 0.95 s respectively. The average computation time of WTDM-STF, TDM-STF are longer than SART, which are due to the extra time that takes by soft-threshold filtering step. And there is small difference between the average computation time of WTDM-STF and TDM-STF. However, the parallel technique such as GPU implementation can be adopted to speed up these algorithms.

Conclusion

To solve the problem in few-view CT image reconstruction, we present a novel iterative reconstruction algorithm based on weighted total difference minimization with soft-threshold filtering (WTDM-STF). In this algorithm, the weighted total difference (WTD) is taken as our regularization term to constrain the gradient sparsity and the gradient continuity for image reconstruction in space domain. Compared with TDM-STF algorithm in which the total difference (TD) acts as the regularization term, our WTDM-STF algorithm is more effective for few-view CT. It is inferred from the experiments that from limited projection data, our WTDM-STF algorithm shows more advantages than other algorithms in terms of image quality and convergence speed. The streak artifacts can be better suppressed and more accurate images can be generated by our WTDM-STF algorithm for few-view CT. And more edge structure information of the object can be preserved compared with the traditional ones. While for limited-angle CT, that is the projections are collected in a limited angular range less than π, our algorithm may need to be improved since the artifacts caused by this case are more complicated than that of few-view CT. As limited-angle CT is also an important CT imaging modality for reducing the patient radiation dose, we will investigate the method for this case in the future work. For this work, while the few-view reconstruction problem was investigate only in fan-beam CT, the WTDM-STF algorithm can be extended to cone-beam CT straightforward.

Acknowledgments

We would like to thank associate professor Baodong Liu (Institute of High Energy Physics, Chinese Academy of Sciences, China) for providing us with many valuable discussions on the subject.

Author Contributions

Conceived and designed the experiments: WY LZ. Performed the experiments: WY. Analyzed the data: WY LZ. Contributed reagents/materials/analysis tools: WY LZ. Contributed to the writing of the manuscript: WY LZ.

References

1. Takx RAP, de Jong PA, Leiner T, Oudkerk M, de Koning HJ, et al. (2014) Automated Coronary Artery Calcification Scoring in Non-Gated Chest CT: Agreement and Reliability. Plos One 9.
2. Kambara K, Shimizu K, Makita H, Hasegawa M, Nagai K, et al. (2014) Effect of Lung Volume on Airway Luminal Area Assessed by Computed Tomography in Chronic Obstructive Pulmonary Disease. Plos One 9.
3. Vandeghinste B, Vandenberghe S, Vanhove C, Staelens S, Van Holen R (2013) Low-Dose Micro-CT Imaging for Vascular Segmentation and Analysis Using Sparse-View Acquisitions. Plos One 8.
4. Frush DP, Donnelly LF, Rosen NS (2003) Computed tomography and radiation risks: What pediatric health care providers should know. Pediatrics 112: 951–957.
5. Sidky EY, Kao CM, Pan XC (2006) Accurate image reconstruction from few-views and limited-angle data in divergent-beam CT. Journal of X-Ray Science and Technology 14: 119–139.
6. Ritschl L, Bergner F, Fleischmann C, Kachelriess M (2011) Improved total variation-based CT image reconstruction applied to clinical data. Physics in Medicine and Biology 56: 1545–1561.
7. Han X, Bian JG, Ritman EL, Sidky EY, Pan XC (2012) Optimization-based reconstruction of sparse images from few-view projections. Physics in Medicine and Biology 57.
8. Lu Y, Zhao J, Wang G (2012) Few-view image reconstruction with dual dictionaries. Physics in Medicine and Biology 57: 173–189.
9. Han XA, Bian JG, Eaker DR, Kline TL, Sidky EY, et al. (2011) Algorithm-Enabled Low-Dose Micro-CT Imaging. IEEE Transactions on Medical Imaging 30: 606–620.
10. Bian JG, Siewerdsen JH, Han XA, Sidky EY, Prince JL, et al. (2010) Evaluation of sparse-view reconstruction from flat-panel-detector cone-beam CT. Physics in Medicine and Biology 55: 6575–6599.
11. Jin SO, Kim JG, Lee SY, Kwon OK (2012) Bone-induced streak artifact suppression in sparse-view CT image reconstruction. Biomedical Engineering Online 11.
12. Pan XC, Sidky EY, Vannier M (2009) Why do commercial CT scanners still employ traditional, filtered back-projection for image reconstruction? Inverse Problems 25: 123009.
13. Beister M, Kolditz D, Kalender WA (2012) Iterative reconstruction methods in X-ray CT. Physica Medica-European Journal of Medical Physics 28: 94–108.

14. Bajpai M, Gupta P, Munshi P, Titarenko V, Withers PJ (2013) A Graphical Processing Unit–Based Parallel Implementation of Multiplicative Algebraic Reconstruction Technique Algorithm for Limited View Tomography. Research in Nondestructive Evaluation 24: 211–222.
15. Karonis NT, Duffin KL, Ordonez CE, Erdelyi B, Uram TD, et al. (2013) Distributed and hardware accelerated computing for clinical medical imaging using proton computed tomography (pCT). Journal of Parallel and Distributed Computing 73: 1605–1612.
16. Flores LA, Vidal V, Mayo P, Rodenas F, Verdu G (2014) Parallel CT image reconstruction based on GPUs. Radiation Physics and Chemistry 95: 247–250.
17. Zhao X, Hu JJ, Yang T (2013) GPU based iterative cone-beam CT reconstruction using empty space skipping technique. Journal of X-Ray Science and Technology 21: 53–69.
18. Andersen AH, Kak AC (1984) Simultaneous algebraic reconstruction technique (SART): A superior implementation of the ART algorithm, Ultrasonic Imaging 6: 81–94.
19. A.C. Kak, M. Slaney, Principles of Computerized Tomographic Imaging, IEEE Press, New York, 1988.
20. Candes EJ, Romberg J, Tao T (2006) Robust uncertainty principles: exact signal reconstruction from highly incomplete frequency information. IEEE Transactions on Information Theory 52: 489–509.
21. Candès EJ, Romberg JK, Tao T (2006) Stable signal recovery from incomplete and inaccurate measurements. Communications on Pure and Applied Mathematics 59: 1207–1223.
22. Donoho DL (2006) Compressed sensing. IEEE Transactions on Information Theory 52: 1289–1306.
23. Chen GH, Tang J, Leng SH (2008) Prior image constrained compressed sensing (PICCS): A method to accurately reconstruct dynamic CT images from highly undersampled projection data sets. Medical Physics 35: 660–663.
24. Wright SJ, Nowak RD, Figueiredo MAT (2009) Sparse Reconstruction by Separable Approximation. IEEE Transactions on Signal Processing 57: 2479–2493.
25. Rudin LI, Osher S, Fatemi E (1992) Nonlinear total variation based noise removal algorithms. Physica D: Nonlinear Phenomena 60: 259–268.
26. Chang M, Li L, Chen ZQ, Xiao YS, Zhang L, et al. (2013) A few-view reweighted sparsity hunting (FRESH) method for CT image reconstruction. Journal of X-Ray Science and Technology 21: 161–176.
27. Li YY, Santosa F (1996) A computational algorithm for minimizing total variation in image restoration. IEEE Transactions on Image Processing 5: 987–995.
28. Yu HY, Wang G (2010) A soft-threshold filtering approach for reconstruction from a limited number of projections. Physics in Medicine and Biology 55: 3905–3916.
29. Liu BD, Wang G, Ritman EL, Cao GH, Lu JP, et al. (2011) Image reconstruction from limited angle projections collected by multisource interior x-ray imaging systems. Physics in Medicine and Biology 56: 6337–6357.
30. Beck A, Teboulle M (2009) A Fast Iterative Shrinkage-Thresholding Algorithm for Linear Inverse Problems. Siam Journal on Imaging Sciences 2: 183–202.
31. Shu XB, Ahuja N (2010) Hybrid Compressive Sampling via a New Total Variation TVL1. In: Daniilidis K, Maragos P, Paragios N, editors. Computer Vision - Eccv 2010, Pt Vi. Berlin: Springer-Verlag Berlin. 393–404.
32. Daubechies I, Defrise M, De Mol C (2004) An iterative thresholding algorithm for linear inverse problems with a sparsity constraint. Communications on Pure and Applied Mathematics 57: 1413–1457.
33. Daubechies I, Fornasier M, Loris I (2008) Accelerated Projected Gradient Method for Linear Inverse Problems with Sparsity Constraints. Journal of Fourier Analysis and Applications 14: 764–792.
34. Goldstein T, Osher S (2009) The Split Bregman Method for L1-Regularized Problems. Siam Journal on Imaging Sciences 2: 323–343.
35. Head Phantom website. Available: http://www.imp.uni-erlangen.de/forbild/deutsch/results/head/head.html. Accessed 2014 Jan 10.
36. Herman G (2009) Fundamentals of computerized tomography: image reconstruction from projections. Springer Verlag.
37. MedCalc Statistical Software website. Available: http://www.medcalc.org. Accessed 2014 Aug 19.
38. Armitage P, Berry G, Matthews JNS (2002) Statistical methods in medical research. 4th ed. Oxford, England: Blackwell Science.

20

X-Ray Phase-Contrast Tomography of Renal Ischemia-Reperfusion Damage

Astrid Velroyen[1], Martin Bech[1,2], Irene Zanette[1], Jolanda Schwarz[1], Alexander Rack[3], Christiane Tympner[4], Tanja Herrler[5], Claudia Staab-Weijnitz[6,7], Margarita Braunagel[6], Maximilian Reiser[6], Fabian Bamberg[6,8], Franz Pfeiffer[1], Mike Notohamiprodjo[6,8]*

1 Chair of Biomedical Physics, Department of Physics (E17), Munich, Bavaria, Germany, **2** Medical Radiation Physics, Lund University, Lund, Sweden, **3** European Synchrotron Radiation Facility, Grenoble, France, **4** Institute of Pathology, Ludwig-Maximilians-University Munich, Munich, Germany, **5** Department of General, Trauma, Hand, and Plastic Surgery, Ludwig-Maximilians-University Hospital Munich, Munich, Germany, **6** Institute for Clinical Radiology, University Hospitals Munich, Munich, Germany, **7** Comprehensive Pneumology Center, University Hospital, Ludwig-Maximilians-University and Helmholtz Zentrum Munich, Munich, Germany, **8** Department of Radiology, University Hospital Tuebingen, Tuebingen, Germany

Abstract

Purpose: The aim of the study was to investigate microstructural changes occurring in unilateral renal ischemia-reperfusion injury in a murine animal model using synchrotron radiation.

Material and Methods: The effects of renal ischemia-reperfusion were investigated in a murine animal model of unilateral ischemia. Kidney samples were harvested on day 18. Grating-Based Phase-Contrast Imaging (GB-PCI) of the paraffin-embedded kidney samples was performed at a Synchrotron Radiation Facility (beam energy of 19 keV). To obtain phase information, a two-grating Talbot interferometer was used applying the phase stepping technique. The imaging system provided an effective pixel size of 7.5 μm. The resulting attenuation and differential phase projections were tomographically reconstructed using filtered back-projection. Semi-automated segmentation and volumetry and correlation to histopathology were performed.

Results: GB-PCI provided good discrimination of the cortex, outer and inner medulla in non-ischemic control kidneys. Post-ischemic kidneys showed a reduced compartmental differentiation, particularly of the outer stripe of the outer medulla, which could not be differentiated from the inner stripe. Compared to the contralateral kidney, after ischemia a volume loss was detected, while the inner medulla mainly retained its volume (ratio 0.94). Post-ischemic kidneys exhibited severe tissue damage as evidenced by tubular atrophy and dilatation, moderate inflammatory infiltration, loss of brush borders and tubular protein cylinders.

Conclusion: In conclusion GB-PCI with synchrotron radiation allows for non-destructive microstructural assessment of parenchymal kidney disease and vessel architecture. If translation to lab-based approaches generates sufficient density resolution, and with a time-optimized image analysis protocol, GB-PCI may ultimately serve as a non-invasive, non-enhanced alternative for imaging of pathological changes of the kidney.

Editor: Mauricio Sendeski, Charité Universitätsmedizin Berlin, Germany

Funding: The authors acknowledge financial support through the DFG Cluster of Excellence Munich-Centre for Advanced Photonics (MAP, Grant no. DFG EXC-158), the DFG Gottfried Wilhelm Leibniz program and the European Research Council (ERC, FP7, StG 240142). This work was carried out with the support of the Karlsruhe Nano Micro Facility (KNMF, www.kit.edu/knmf), a Helmholtz Research Infrastructure at Karlsruhe Institute of Technology (KIT, www.kit.edu). A. Velroyen acknowledges the TUM Graduate School. The funders had no role in study design, data collection and analysis, decision to publish, or preparation of the manuscript.

Competing Interests: The authors have declared that no competing interests exist.

* Email: mike.notohamiprodjo@uni-tuebingen.de

Introduction

Renal ischemia-reperfusion (I/R) accounts for the majority of acute kidney injury cases [1], which often progress to chronic kidney disease [2]. Its consequences such as cortical and tubular necrosis are commonly encountered after renal transplantation [3] and form a potential basis for development of renal fibrosis, which is the final path of most renal diseases [4].

Clinically ill patients present with a decrease of renal function, i.e. glomerular filtration, however, there are no established laboratory tests for a reliable diagnosis of ischemia-reperfusion damage, so that renal biopsy remains the diagnostic standard of reference with all its risks and potential complications [5].

Morphological imaging modalities such as ultrasonography, computed tomography and magnetic resonance imaging are not ideally suited for detection of renal parenchymal disease, as early changes rather affect the ultrastructure and function than gross morphology [6]. Functional techniques such as perfusion and diffusion weighted MR imaging may reveal microstructural and functional changes [7–9], but spatial resolution is low [10], acquisition is not standardized and analysis is heavily influenced by the post-processing method [11].

X-ray phase-contrast imaging (PCI) and dark-field imaging (DFI) techniques, which exploit the refraction and small-angle scattering of x-rays in the investigated tissue in addition to their absorption, provide a novel contrast and complementary information [12–14] and thus may form a potential modality for non-enhanced, non-invasive kidney imaging [15]. The majority of PCI-studies on biological tissue have been performed at synchrotron radiation sources [16] which provide monochromatic x-rays with high flux and are used in combination with high-resolution imaging systems. PCI of the kidney without the use of a contrast agent has so far only been performed using crystal-based phase imaging techniques [15,17–19]. These studies already demonstrate the innovative potential of this technique to depict the smallest anatomical structures and detect parenchymal renal disease such as glomerulosclerosis in hamster kidneys [15]. However, both the applied crystal-interferometer technique [17] as well as the analyzer-crystal based diffraction enhanced imaging (DEI) require a monochromatic, highly collimated x-ray beam. Consequently, their transfer from highly brilliant synchrotron sources to conventional x-ray sources suffers from long exposure times [20] and does not allow for the clinically widely used cone-beam geometry, thus rendering a transfer to a clinical setting difficult. Grating-based (GB) Talbot interferometry [21,22] was successfully implemented in laboratory-based settings using conventional polychromatic x-ray sources by introduction of a third grating [13]. In synchrotron studies, it has proven excellent soft-tissue contrast and high-resolution volumetric data of various biomedical samples [23,24]. Several studies on biomedical samples conducted at polychromatic x-ray sources have shown improved imaging of parenchymal lung disease [25], breast lesions [26,27], cartilage [28], and atherosclerotic plaques [29] at good density resolution and reasonable spatial resolution.

The aim of this study was to investigate microstructural changes occurring in parenchymal renal disease, e.g. acute unilateral ischemic kidney injury in a murine animal model, using GB-PCI at a synchrotron radiation source. We hypothesize that GB-PCI allows depiction of volumetric and microstructural changes as well as vessel imaging without the use of contrast media.

Materials and Methods

Animals

Two male Balb/C nude (nu/nu) mice, aged 10–12 weeks and weighing 21–24 g, purchased from Charles River Laboratories (Sulzfeld, Germany) were included in this study. Animals were fed a standard diet and allowed free access to water. All animal experiments were conducted in accordance with institutional guidelines and were approved by the Administrative Panel on Laboratory Animal Care (AZ 55.2-1-54-2532-19-11, Government of Upper Bavaria, Germany).

Renal Ischemia-Reperfusion Injury Model

Mice were anesthetized by intraperitoneal injection of a combination of 0.05 mg/kg fentanyl, 0.5 mg/kg medetomidine (Pfizer, Berlin, Germany), and 5 mg/kg midazolam (Ratiopharm, Ulm, Germany) and placed on a heated surgical pad to keep the body temperature constant. The right kidney was exposed through median abdominal incision, and mice were subjected to ischemia by clamping the renal pedicle with a nontraumatic microaneurysm clamp (Braun, Melsungen, Germany), which was removed after 45 min. The incision was closed with a 5–0 suture (Ethicon, Livingston, Scotland, UK) and surgical staples (Hugo Sachs GmbH, March, Germany). Postoperatively, anesthesia was antagonized by subcutaneous injection of a combination of 2.5 mg/kg atipamezole (Pfizer), 0.5 mg/kg flumazenil (Delta Select, Pfullingen, Germany), and 1.2 mg/kg naloxone (Inresa, Bartenheim, France). Mice were sacrificed by combined cervical dislocation and exsanguination. Tissue specimens of the ischemic right and the contralateral nonischemic kidney were collected on day 18 for histological analysis and embedded in paraffin according to standard protocols.

GB-PCI Setup and Image Acquisition

GB-PCI of the paraffin-embedded kidney samples was performed at beam line ID19 of the European Synchrotron Radiation Facility (ESRF), Grenoble, France. To extract the phase information of the x-ray beam passing through the sample, a two-grating Talbot interferometer was used [30], which was operated at a photon energy of 19 keV with an inter-grating distance corresponding to the 11th fractional Talbot order to assure high sensitivity. The periods and heights of the π-shifting silicon phase grating G1 and the gold analyzer grating G2 were $p_1 = 4.78$ µm, $h_1 = 21$ µm, and $p_2 = 2.4$ µm, $h_2 = 100$ µm, respectively. For x-ray detection the standard system at ID19, consisting of a Gadox scintillator coupled via lenses to a charge-coupled device camera, was used, providing an effective pixel size of 7.5 µm. A photograph of the setup is shown in **Figure 1**.

For image acquisition, the samples, embedded in paraffin blocks, were placed in an Eppendorf vial (Sigma Aldrich, St. Louis, USA). In order to ensure complete wetting of the paraffin surface and avoid trapping of air bubbles that cause image artifacts, a non-polar fluid, i.e. oil, was used to fill up the vial. To avoid phase-wrapping artifacts, the sample container was additionally placed into a box-shaped water basin. Tomographies of all four samples were acquired using the phase stepping procedure (as described

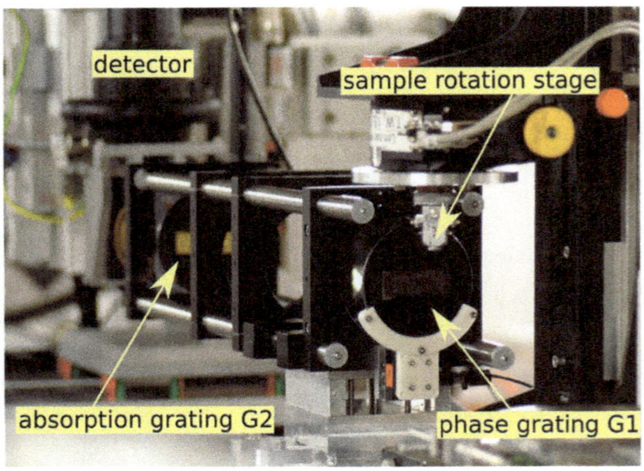

Figure 1. Photograph of the Interferometer Setup at Beamline ID19, ESRF, Grenoble, France. Monochromatic, coherent X-rays travel through the sample and introduce distortions in the interference pattern created by the phase grating. Those are evaluated by a lateral movement of the phase grating located behind the sample. Photograph adapted from I. Zanette, *Interférometrie X à réseaux pour l'imagerie et l'analyse de front d'ondes au synchrotron*, PhD thesis, University of Grenoble, 2011.

earlier [21]) with 4 phase steps per projection and an exposure time of 5 seconds per step. Accounting for their difference in size, 701 projections were taken of the control kidneys, whereas only 501 projections of the clamped kidneys were acquired, each over 360 degrees.

Post-Processing

The raw projection data was processed according to the standard phase stepping Fourier processing [12,21]. The resulting attenuation, differential phase and dark-field projections were tomographically reconstructed using standard filtered back-projection, with a Ram-Lak (for attenuation and dark field) and a Hilbert filter (for phase data). To obtain quantitative volumetric data, the three-dimensional tomograms were segmented using the commercial software VGStudio MAX 2.0 (Volume Graphics, Heidelberg, Germany). Because the expenditure of time for this procedure is about 40 to 50 hours per dataset, the segmentation was only performed exemplarily on the dataset of one contralateral control and one I/R kidney. On the I/R dataset rough regions of interest were defined manually beforehand, in which the more precise segmentation was then performed by a combination of region growing, thresholding and manual segmentation. In the control kidney dataset the borders between the compartments appeared clearly defined, so that segmentation was mainly performed using thresholding, region-growing algorithms and occasional manual segmentation. The juxtacortical outer stripe of the outer medulla could not be distinguished from the cortex in the control kidney and not from the inner stripe in the I/R dataset.

Histology

The specimens were stained with hematoxylin-eosin stain, iron stain, and Periodic acid-Schiff reaction for protein for conventional histopathologic evaluation. The slides were examined by an experienced uropathologist (C.T., with 7 years pathology experience). Histology was evaluated with respect to increased cellularity, disturbance of cellular polarity, failure of differentiation from the base to the surface, irregularity in the size of cells, variations of shape, protein cylinders and loss of brush borders and infiltration of leukocytes. A radiologist (M.N., with 7 years urogenital radiology experience), a physicist (A.V.), and the above-mentioned pathologist assessed the correlation between the PCI and histopathology findings in consensus.

Statistical Analysis

Statistical analysis was performed with IBM SPSS Software 20 (IBM, Armonk, New York, USA). The gray values were extracted from the respective three-dimensional segmentations of the phase-contrast volumes of each dataset. A low quantity represents low electron density and vice versa. Due to the enormous data size (> 100 million data points), statistical analysis was performed using the "random sampling" function, randomly selecting 10 000 datapoints from each kidney compartment. Significant differences between the gray values of the compartments were assessed with paired t-tests. Significance was assumed at $p<0.05$.

Results

Kidney Morphology

A qualitative overview of exemplary slices of the contralateral non-ischemic control kidney and the I/R kidney on day 18 in all three different contrast modalities (phase contrast, dark-field, attenuation) is provided in **Figure 2**. Phase-contrast images of the contralateral kidney (**Figure 2a**) allowed to differentiate the functional compartments of the kidney. Inner medulla, inner stripe of the outer medulla and cortex were clearly distinguishable by decreasing gray values. The outer stripe of the medulla showed gray values similar to the cortex. Also, an abundance of tubular structures and blood vessels was visible. In dark-field contrast images of control kidneys (**Figure 2b**) scattering at tubule-to-tissue interfaces was detected. The conventional absorption-based images (**Figure 2c**) exhibited a considerably lower contrast and relatively higher noise than the phase-contrast images. Phase-contrast images of I/R kidneys (**Figure 2d**) showed considerably less variation in gray values between the different compartments. Also, the tissue appeared hypotrophic and the number of visible tubular structures was markedly reduced. The outer stripe of the outer medulla showed a dramatic change in gray values after ischemia-reperfusion injury and could not be distinguished from the inner stripe. Correspondingly, in dark-field images the number of scattering structures was reduced in injured kidneys (**Figure 2e**). In the absorption-based images no additional information could be obtained (**Figure 2f**).

Quantitative Analysis

For a quantitative comparison, semi-automated segmentation and volumetry of a control and an I/R kidney was performed (**Table 1**). In the control kidneys, the different kidney compartments showed a distinct and substantial contrast ($p<0.01$) (**Figure 3**), whereas in I/R kidneys there was no significant difference between gray values of the inner and the stripes of the outer medulla. Histogram analysis of gray values exhibited in agreement with the visual appearance a wider range of gray values in the control kidney as compared to the I/R kidney (**Figure 4a**). In the control kidney three significantly different peaks corresponding to the cortex and outer stripe of the outer medulla, inner stripe of the outer medulla and the inner medulla could be identified (**Figure 4b**). In contrast, the histogram of gray values of the I/R kidney consisted of one merged peak with considerably overlapping sub-volumes (**Figure 4c**). Ischemia-reperfusion induced an overall organ-shrinkage by more than 50% compared to the contralateral kidney. The decrease in volume was clearly dominated by the cortex and outer medulla whereas the inner medulla remained a relatively constant volume with a ratio of 0.94.

Vessel Imaging

GB-PCI allowed for visualization and segmentation of the renal vasculature without the use of a contrast agent. The high contrast and spatial resolution allowed to track vessel ramification from the renal hilus to the cortical branches and back to the medulla. 3D-Rendering techniques facilitated to visualize the vasculature on a single image (**Figure 5**). In I/R kidneys a dramatic reduction of vascular structures compared to the contralateral kidney could be observed and quantified (ratio 0.18).

Correlation to Histology

Generally no signs of gross necrosis were found in the cortex or the tubules of the I/R kidneys. The inner and outer medulla and its stripes as well as the cortex of the healthy kidney could be distinguished by their different morphological structure of nephron and the cellularity, similarly to the phase-contrast image (**Figure 6**). No protein cylinders were detected in the tubules of the control kidneys.

In good agreement with the findings from the phase-contrast dataset, I/R kidneys exhibited severe tissue damage prominent in the juxtamedullary nephron (**Figure 7**). The proximal tubules showed consecutive atrophy with small lumen, cellular damage and denudation of the basement membrane with segmental

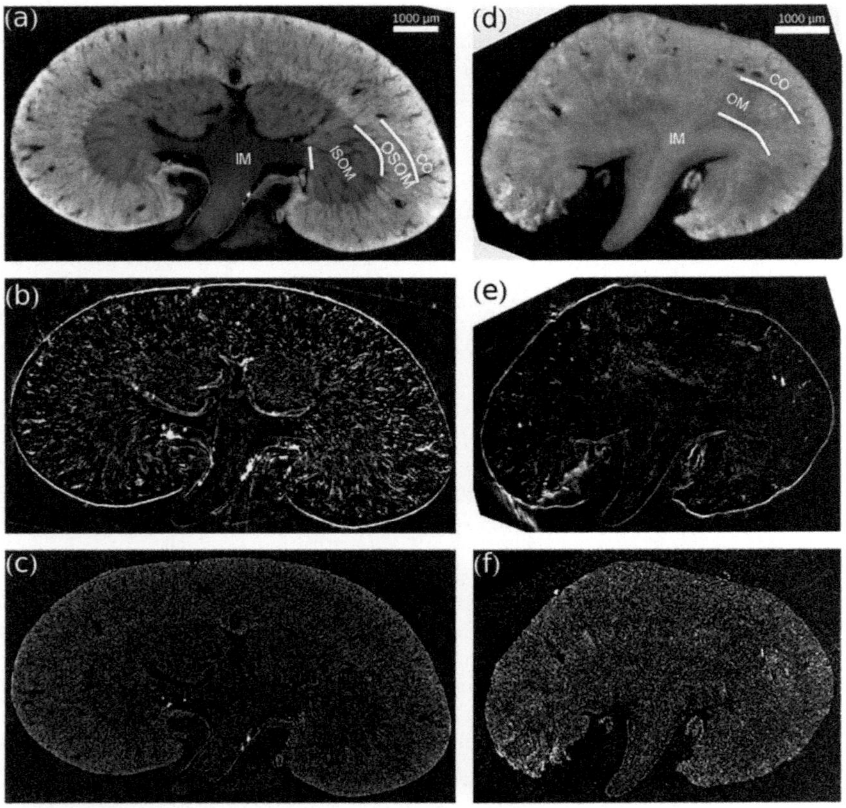

Figure 2. Contralateral Control Kidney and Ischemic Kidney in three Different Contrast Modalities. (a), (d) Phase contrast. (b), (e) Dark-field contrast. (c), (f) Attenuation contrast. All images are scaled individually for best visual appearance. (a) Phase-contrast images of the contralateral kidney allow to differentiate the functional compartments of the kidney. (d) Phase-contrast images of I/R kidneys show considerably less variation in gray value between the different compartments. Stripes of the outer medulla cannot be distinguished. The number of visible tubular structure or voids is highly reduced. In dark-field contrast, (b) control kidneys show scattering at interfaces, which is reduced in (e) I/R kidneys. Conventional absorption-based images show considerably lower contrast and relatively higher noise in both (c) control and (f) ischemic kidney. CO – cortex; OM – outer medulla; OSOM – outer stripe outer medulla; ISOM – inner stripe outer medulla; IM – inner medulla.

shedding of both necrotic and viable epithelial cells into the tubular lumen. Focal tubules were dilated and lined with a flattened epithelium. In periodic acid-Schiff (PAS) stain, the brush border of proximal tubules was thinned or absent. Hyaline, granular casts were seen in the distal portions of the nephron and particularly prominent in the collecting ducts with focal calcification. The edematous interstitium was enlarged with a fibrillary appearance and a minimal interstitial infiltrate with lymphocytes and clustered iron macrophages could be documented. The glomeruli differed segmentally in volume with widening of Bowman's space refers to shrinkage of the glomerular capillary tuft accompanied by an apparent decrease in the number of normal glomerular lobules and by apparent loss of mesangial matrix and cells.

Discussion

By performing volumetric and histogram analysis of the functional kidney compartments after ischemia-reperfusion damage, we demonstrate quantitative non-invasive assessment of pathophysiological processes with GB-PCI. Day 18 after unilateral clamping was chosen as an appropriate time point to assess the effects of acute kidney injury, when advanced remodeling and repair processes are highly active [31]. We chose Balb/C nu/nu mice, because the nude mice variant is more susceptible to renal ischemia-reperfusion injury than their wild-type counterparts [31]. This is in line with recent studies on the pathophysiological role of B-cells and the protective effects of regulatory T-cells in ischemia-reperfusion injury. GB-PCI can be translated from synchrotron to more accessible experimental laboratory based conditions [12]. Other studies performed at lab-based GB-PCI-settings confirmed an increase in soft-tissue contrast and a gain of complementary information for example in arteries [29] and human breast tissue [26] despite the lower density- and spatial resolution compared to synchrotron experiments. We anticipate a similar benefit for imaging of renal tissue. The feasibility of in-vivo studies with GB-PCI on small animals with acceptable radiation dose has been shown [32] for projection-based imaging at a dedicated phase-contrast and dark-field small-animal scanner. A study on dose-compatible small-animal CT imaging is ongoing. Translation to a clinical setting is still dependent on further technological developments, such as larger gratings to cover a larger field of view. Optimization of the technique in terms of acquisition time and radiation dose, for example with alternative phase extraction methods such as fourier-based single-shot imaging [33–35] or iterative reconstruction algorithms [35] is ongoing research.

Diagnostic Impact of GB-PCI

MR-Imaging studies investigating acute kidney injury observed indirect changes such as alteration of the cortical and medullary T2-relaxation-time or reduced perfusion [36–39]. A MR-tech-

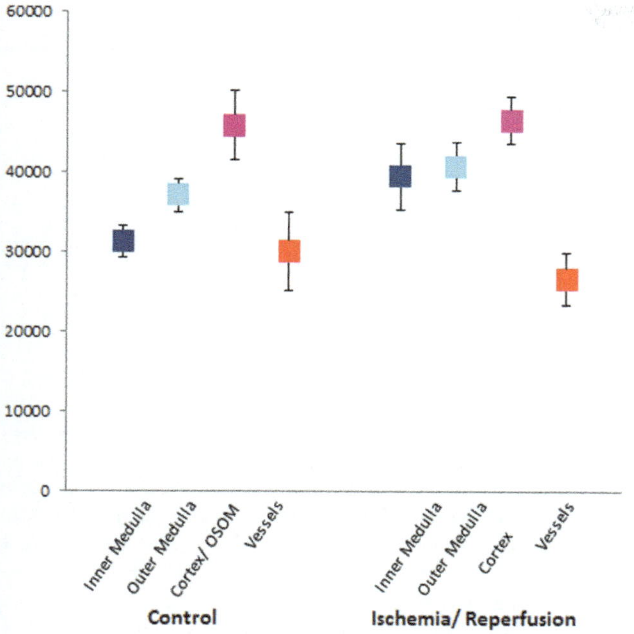

Figure 3. Mean Gray Values of Kidney Compartments. Mean value and standard deviations of phase gray values of the respective compartment. Note that OSOM and cortex were assessed together in healthy kidneys and OSOM and ISOM together in I/R kidneys. OSOM – outer stripe outer medulla ISOM – inner stripe outer medulla.

nique quantifying tissue anisotropy as an indirect measure of tubular integrity is Tensor Imaging, commonly based on diffusion (DTI) [7,40–42] or as described recently on susceptibility (STI) [43]. However MRI techniques are limited in spatial resolution due to the magnetic field (in the latter reference to 55 μm). Also above mentioned MR-techniques only indirectly depict pathophysiologic changes, while GB-PCI directly assesses morphological changes of the medulla, albeit *ex vivo*. STI also still suffers from limitations that have to be overcome before translation to in-vivo scenarios, i.e. long acquisition times and necessary sample rotation relative to the magnetic field, because datasets acquired for at least 6 different orientations are necessary.

This proof-of-principle experiment clearly demonstrates the applicability of GB-PCI in renal research and pathology: Highly resolved GB-PCI using synchrotron radiation can be used to three-dimensionally examine structural changes caused by parenchymal renal disease on the level of a few micrometers facilitating volumetry. Histological sectioning only provides two-dimensional information with inevitable destruction of the sample.

After acute kidney injury we observed a significantly decreased discrimination of the different functional compartments in GB-PCI, which are presumably related to pathophysiologic changes. Usually the pathway of tubular atrophy conceptualized from morphological studies of diseased kidneys involves simplification of epithelial structure progressing to autophagy and apoptosis accompanied by marked thickening of tubule basement membranes [44]. Furthermore failed re-differentiation of the epithelial cells leads these abnormal tubules to develop thick basement membranes, autophagy and apoptosis [44]. Paracrine signaling gives rise to inflammation and finally fibrosis [2]. This evolving tubulointerstitial remodeling process may increase the average electron density particularly of the medullary compartments, and thus cause the blending-in of measured gray values, which was particularly evident for the inner and outer stripe of the outer medulla.

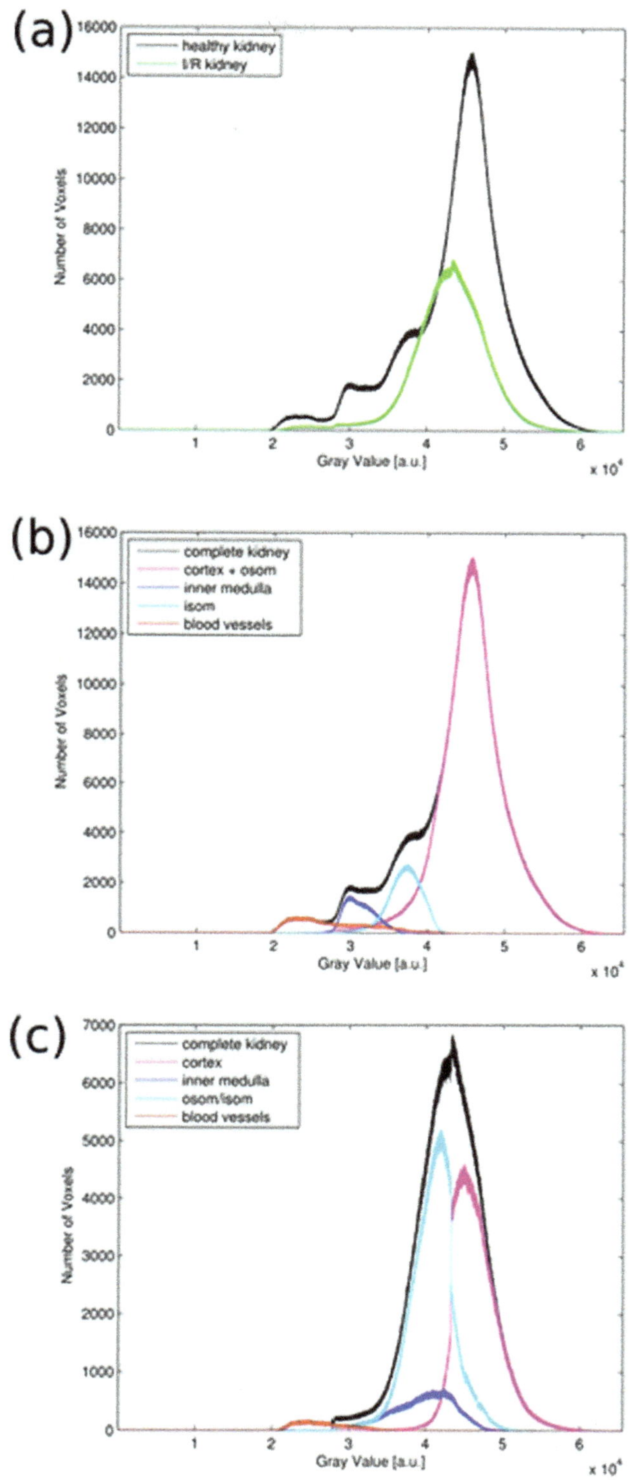

Figure 4. Volumetry of Healthy and I/R Kidney. Gray values are proportional to electron densities. (a) Histogram for both complete kidney volumes in comparison. (b) Histogram of healthy kidney and the contributions of the different compartments. (c) Histogram of post-ischemic kidney and the contributions of the different compartments. OSOM – outer stripe outer medulla; IS – inner stripe.

Interestingly, we could observe significant shrinkage of the cortex and the outer medulla. The latter forms the critical zone in ischemic injury [45–48]. Our visual and volumetric data directly

Table 1. Volumetric data from three-dimensional segmentation of the functional compartments of the kidneys.

	Volume ischemic kidney [mm^3]	Volume contralateral kidney [mm^3]	Ratio ischemic/contralateral
total	27.96	61.14	0.46
inner medulla	2.62	2.76	0.95
Cortex/outer medulla	24.90	56.96	0.49
blood vessels	0.44	2.42	0.18

The voxel size is equal to $4.22 \cdot 10^{-7}$ mm^3.

correspond to the current pathophysiological knowledge of acute kidney injury. The earliest pathophysiological description of acute kidney injury were made by Reinhard in 1850 [49], who noted that the kidneys of patients dying from "the acute Bright's disease" had a hyperemic medulla with a pale cortex. Many investigators have demonstrated the concept of a decreased medullary blood flow as a consequence of medullary congestion [45–48]. Furthermore upregulation of pro-inflammatory molecules and leukocyte infiltration are most commonly observed in the outer medulla [45]. While the volume of the medulla is usually preserved, cortical atrophy follows the obstruction of the collecting ducts as described above [50,51] We must acknowledge that in control specimen the discrimination of the outer stripe of the outer medulla from the cortex and in I/R kidney discrimination of the inner stripe of the outer stripe an inner stripe was not possible by means of gray values. The density resolution, i.e. the ability to differentiate between differences in electron density in the different tissues, can be in principle improved by the use of grating-structures with finer bars, i.e. smaller periods.

Further studies may explore the impact of the dark-field contrast, in which signal strength is determined by small-angle scattering of x-rays at microstructures that can lie on a scale below the spatial resolution of the imaging system [52,53] thus revealing structural information that is inaccessible for transmission and phase-contrast images [32]. We have observed decreased scattering at tubular interfaces in injured kidneys, similar to what can be seen in pulmonary emphysema [25,54] [55]. The scattering may theoretically serve as a quantifiable indirect injury marker. The absorption cross-section was inferior to phase-contrast imaging in depicting the morphological changes.

These morphological findings can be generally observed on histopathological slices, which provide abundant information on a microstructural level. However, this technique is destructive and provides only two-dimensional information on single slices. In contrast, the GB-PCI provides valuable volumetric information while maintaining an intact sample.

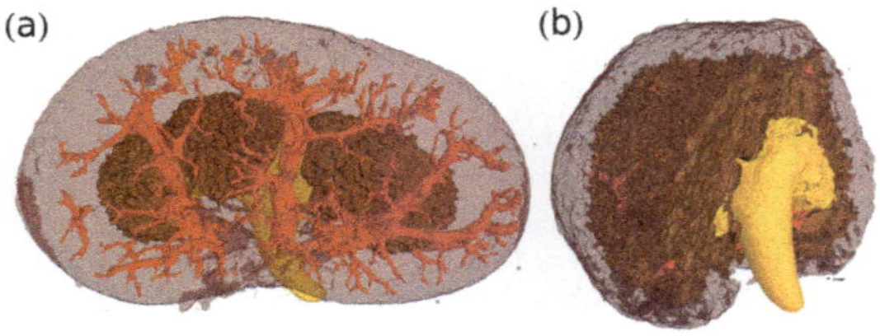

Figure 5. Three-Dimensional Renderings of the Renal Vasculature. (a) Healthy and (b) post-ischemic kidney from the segmented phase-contrast tomographies. The injured kidney shows a dramatic reduction of the vasculature.

Furthermore GB-PCI allows for non-enhanced 3D-imaging of the renal vessels by using semi-automated segmentation of the vessel data. This is of particular interest, as many patients who would undergo renal imaging suffer from chronic kidney disease and are thus at high risk for either contrast induced nephropathy or nephrogenic systemic fibrosis. The observed differences in soft-tissue contrast were obtained without the use of any contrast agent. One must acknowledge that gray-value based differentiation between arteries and veins is not possible, but only by visual selection. The applicability of contrast agents in phase-sensitive x-ray imaging is still under investigation. Besides iodinated contrast agents, the main focus is currently on contrast media with x-ray scattering properties for dark-field imaging such as microbubbles, which can be also administered in patients with renal insufficiency [56].

Challenges and Limitations

One challenge to overcome is the optimization of automatic segmentation of the kidney compartments, as this is a potential error source. The outer stripe of the outer medulla could be identified in the healthy kidney by means of the different tissue texture but not gray value and was virtually not distinguishable from the inner stripe in the I/R kidney. So quantitative comparison of the cortex and the outer medulla could not reliably performed in this study. While the other functional compartments could be readily discriminated in the healthy kidney, the segmentation of the I/R kidney dataset was more prone to errors. Here the compartments could not be separated by thresholding and region growing only, so that additional manual segmentation

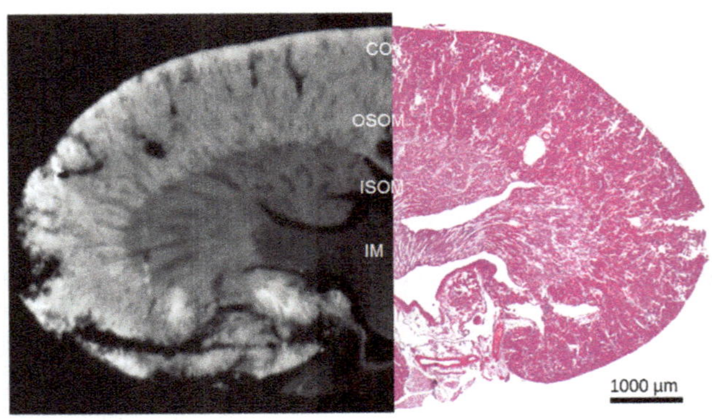

Figure 6. Comparison of a HE-Stained Histological Slice of Control Kidney. Phase contrast images provide similar morphological information as a HE-stained slice. The different functional compartments (IM, ISOM, OSOM/CO) can be readily differentiated. CO – cortex; OSOM – outer stripe outer medulla; ISOM – inner stripe outer medulla; IM – inner medulla.

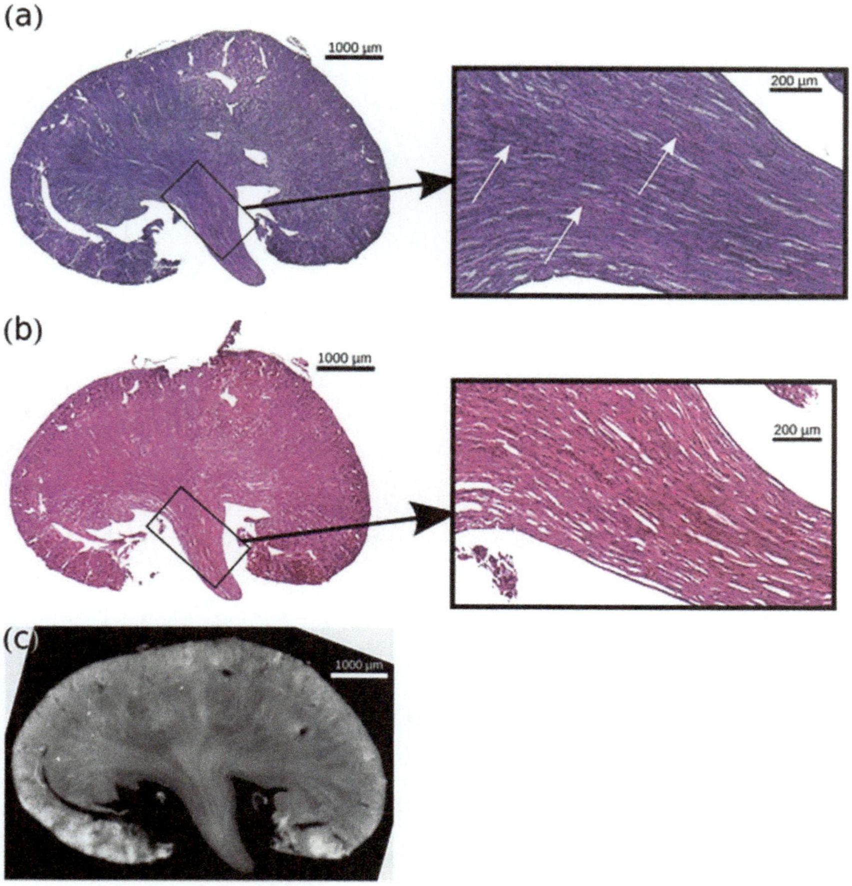

Figure 7. Comparison of Histological Slices of Clamped Kidney. (a) PAS histological slice of the clamped kidney. (b) HE-stained histological slice of the clamped kidney, with a similar slice of the phase-contrast volume (c). For both histology slices a respective zoom view of the inner medulla is given. Scarring and beginning tubular atrophy as well proteinaceous casts could be detected correlating with increasing medullary density in PCI.

had to be performed, introducing a potential human source for segmentation errors. For a more objective segmentation, the area of image processing and machine learning provides a wide variety of adaptive dedicated algorithms [57,58].

Another potential source of error is the influence of formalin fixation on soft-tissue signal characteristics in phase-contrast imaging. This has only been examined for brain tissue [16] and is currently under investigation for other tissue types [19]. Security regulations at the synchrotron radiation facility did not allow for the measurement of fresh kidney samples. Thus the gray values displayed in this work are proportional to the respective electron density of the formalin fixated sample. We do not present absolute numbers of electron density or their respective conversion to phase-contrast Hounsfield units, because the values measured here may not exactly represent the values for fresh or *in-vivo* tissue because of potential effects of the fixation process.

In general, GB-PCI is still associated with high radiation doses and the presented study has not been optimized in this regard. However, alternative acquisition and post-processing techniques as well as dedicated iterative reconstruction algorithms [35] are currently being developed to reduce the necessary radiation dose [59,60]. Furthermore, the facilitated access to laboratory-based setups with polychromatic x-ray sources and a larger – however still limited - field of view, in contrast to synchrotron radiation facilities, allows for studies with an increased number of samples and larger sample sizes. It remains to be determined if similar image quality can be achieved in a potential human in-vivo setting at acceptable radiation doses.

Another limitation to this study is that the assessment of volumetric data is subject to particular biases. First of all, the imaged kidney samples were cut in half after excision to allow for proper formalin fixation. This was performed similarly for both kidneys, so that the deduced ratios are still valid, however the absolute values would have to be doubled. Actually, our findings were in line with a previous study investigating kidney volume with ultrasound. Here a mean volume of 0.1 cm^3 was determined for wt/wt mice [61]. Another study investigated kidney volume of CD1-mice. Here a mean volume of 0.2 cm^3 was determined [62]. If doubled, the volume of our control kidney would result in 0,12 cm^3. Secondly, the contralateral kidney served as internal control. After unilateral renal ischemia the contralateral kidney may undergo a certain hypertrophy [39], so that the observed volumetric shift may also be partly due to this process.

Conclusions

GB-PCI with synchrotron radiation allows for noninvasive and non-destructive assessment of parenchymal kidney disease on the microstructural level and vessel architecture in three dimensions and thus serves well as a volumetric alternative to histological slicing. Since GB-PCI using conventional polychromatic x-ray tube sources has been proven successful, the value of laboratory-based GB-PCI on the investigation of parenchymal renal disease of murine and human kidney samples has to be assessed in further studies. If the density resolution achieved with polychromatic sources is sufficient to differentiate between diseased and healthy tissue, GB-PCI may serve ultimately as a non-invasive, non-contrast media enhanced method to study pathological changes of the kidney and become an alternative to current imaging methods.

Author Contributions

Conceived and designed the experiments: MN AV M. Bech FP FB MFR. Performed the experiments: AV JS IZ AR TH. Analyzed the data: MN AV JS M. Bech CT M. Braunagel. Contributed reagents/materials/analysis tools: CSW CT. Wrote the paper: AV MN FP MFR CSW FB M. Bech M. Braunagel.

References

1. Hoste EA, Kellum JA (2007) Incidence, classification, and outcomes of acute kidney injury. Contrib Nephrol 156: 32–38.
2. Venkatachalam MA, Griffin KA, Lan R, Geng H, Saikumar P, et al. (2010) Acute kidney injury: a springboard for progression in chronic kidney disease. Am J Physiol Renal Physiol 298: F1078–1094.
3. Yalavarthy R, Edelstein CL, Teitelbaum I (2007) Acute renal failure and chronic kidney disease following liver transplantation. Hemodial Int 11 Suppl 3: S7–12.
4. Singh P, Ricksten SE, Bragadottir G, Redfors B, Nordquist L (2013) Renal oxygenation and haemodynamics in acute kidney injury and chronic kidney disease. Clin Exp Pharmacol Physiol 40: 138–147.
5. Sidebotham D (2012) Novel biomarkers for cardiac surgery-associated acute kidney injury: a skeptical assessment of their role. J Extra Corpor Technol 44: 235–240.
6. Notohamiprodjo M, Reiser MF, Sourbron SP (2010) Diffusion and perfusion of the kidney. Eur J Radiol 76: 337–347.
7. Notohamiprodjo M, Dietrich O, Horger W, Horng A, Helck AD, et al. (2010) Diffusion tensor imaging (DTI) of the kidney at 3 tesla-feasibility, protocol evaluation and comparison to 1.5 Tesla. Invest Radiol 45: 245–254.
8. Notohamiprodjo M, Pedersen M, Glaser C, Helck AD, Lodemann KP, et al. (2011) Comparison of Gd-DTPA and Gd-BOPTA for studying renal perfusion and filtration. J Magn Reson Imaging 34: 595–607.
9. Kang SK, Huang WC, Wong S, Zhang JL, Stifelman MD, et al. (2013) Dynamic contrast-enhanced magnetic resonance imaging measurement of renal function in patients undergoing partial nephrectomy: preliminary experience. Invest Radiol 48: 687–692.
10. Rossi C, Sharma P, Pazahr S, Alkadhi H, Nanz D, et al. (2013) Blood oxygen level-dependent magnetic resonance imaging of the kidneys: influence of spatial resolution on the apparent R2* transverse relaxation rate of renal tissue. Invest Radiol 48: 671–677.
11. Braunagel M, Graser A, Reiser M, Notohamiprodjo M (2013) The role of functional imaging in the era of targeted therapy of renal cell carcinoma. World J Urol.
12. Pfeiffer F, Bech M, Bunk O, Kraft P, Eikenberry EF, et al. (2008) Hard-X-ray dark-field imaging using a grating interferometer. Nat Mater 7: 134–137.
13. Pfeiffer F, Kottler C, Bunk O, David C (2007) Hard x-ray phase tomography with low-brilliance sources. Phys Rev Lett 98: 108105.
14. Donath T, Pfeiffer F, Bunk O, Grunzweig C, Hempel E, et al. (2010) Toward clinical X-ray phase-contrast CT: demonstration of enhanced soft-tissue contrast in human specimen. Invest Radiol 45: 445–452.
15. Wu J, Takeda T, Lwin TT, Momose A, Sunaguchi N, et al. (2009) Imaging renal structures by X-ray phase-contrast microtomography. Kidney Int 75: 945–951.
16. Schulz G, Waschkies C, Pfeiffer F, Zanette I, Weitkamp T, et al. (2012) Multimodal imaging of human cerebellum - merging X-ray phase microtomography, magnetic resonance microscopy and histology. Sci Rep 2: 826.
17. Momose A (2003) Phase-sensitive imaging and phase tomography using X-ray interferometers. Opt Express 11: 2303–2314.
18. Gang L, Zhihua C, Ziyu W, Ando M, Lin P, et al. (2005) Image quality dependence on thickness of sliced rat kidney taken by a simplest DEI construction. Nuclear Instruments and Methods in Physics Research Section A, , 548: 200–206.
19. Shirai R, Kunii T, Yoneyama A, Ooizumi T, Maruyama H, et al. (2014) Enhanced renal image contrast by ethanol fixation in phase-contrast X-ray computed tomography. J Synchrotron Radiat 21: 795–800.
20. Nesch I, Fogarty DP, Tzvetkov T, Reinhart B, Walus AC, et al. (2009) The design and application of an in-laboratory diffraction-enhanced x-ray imaging instrument. Rev Sci Instrum 80: 093702.
21. Weitkamp T, Diaz A, David C, Pfeiffer F, Stampanoni M, et al. (2005) X-ray phase imaging with a grating interferometer. Opt Express 13: 6296–6304.
22. Momose A, Yashiro W, Maikusa H, Takeda Y (2009) High-speed X-ray phase imaging and X-ray phase tomography with Talbot interferometer and white synchrotron radiation. Opt Express 17: 12540–12545.
23. Noel PB, Herzen J, Fingerle AA, Willner M, Stockmar MK, et al. (2013) Evaluation of the potential of phase-contrast computed tomography for improved visualization of cancerous human liver tissue. Z Med Phys 23: 204–211.
24. Hetterich H, Fill S, Herzen J, Willner M, Zanette I, et al. (2013) Grating-based X-ray phase-contrast tomography of atherosclerotic plaque at high photon energies. Z Med Phys 23: 194–203.
25. Yaroshenko A, Meinel FG, Bech M, Tapfer A, Velroyen A, et al. (2013) Pulmonary Emphysema Diagnosis with a Preclinical Small-Animal X-ray Dark-Field Scatter-Contrast Scanner. Radiology 269: 427–433.
26. Sztrokay A, Herzen J, Auweter SD, Liebhardt S, Mayr D, et al. (2013) Assessment of grating-based X-ray phase-contrast CT for differentiation of invasive ductal carcinoma and ductal carcinoma in situ in an experimental ex vivo set-up. Eur Radiol 23: 381–387.
27. Hauser N, Wang Z, Kubik-Huch RA, Trippel M, Singer G, et al. (2013) A Study on Mastectomy Samples to Evaluate Breast Imaging Quality and Potential Clinical Relevance of Differential Phase Contrast Mammography. Invest Radiol.
28. Tanaka J, Nagashima M, Kido K, Hoshino Y, Kiyohara J, et al. (2013) Cadaveric and in vivo human joint imaging based on differential phase contrast by X-ray Talbot-Lau interferometry. Z Med Phys 23: 222–227.
29. Saam T, Herzen J, Hetterich H, Fill S, Willner M, et al. (2013) Translation of Atherosclerotic Plaque Phase-Contrast CT Imaging from Synchrotron Radiation to a Conventional Lab-Based X-Ray Source. PLoS One 8: e73513.
30. Weitkamp T, Zanette I, David C, Baruchel J, Bech M, et al. (2010) Recent developments in X-ray Talbot interferometry at ESRF-ID19. Proceedings of SPIE 7804.
31. Herrler T, Wang H, Tischer A, Schupp N, Lehner S, et al. (2013) Decompression of inflammatory edema along with endothelial cell therapy expedites regeneration after renal ischemia-reperfusion injury. Cell Transplant 22: 2091–2103.
32. Bech M, Tapfer A, Velroyen A, Yaroshenko A, Pauwels B, et al. (2013) In-vivo dark-field and phase-contrast x-ray imaging. Sci Rep 3: 3209.
33. Bennett EE, Kopace R, Stein AF, Wen H (2010) A grating-based single-shot x-ray phase contrast and diffraction method for in vivo imaging. Med Phys 37: 6047–6054.
34. Takeda M, Hidek I, Seiji K (1982) Fourier-transform method of fringe-pattern analysis for computer-based topography and interferometry. Journal of the Optical Society of America 72: 156–160.
35. Hahn D, Thibault P, Fehringer A, Bech M, Noel PB, et al. (2013) Bone artifact reduction in differential phase-contrast CT. Fully3D: 416.
36. Herrler T, Wang H, Tischer A, Bartenstein P, Jauch KW, et al. (2012) 99mTc-MAG3 scintigraphy for the longitudinal follow-up of kidney function in a mouse model of renal ischemia-reperfusion injury. EJNMMI Res 2: 2.
37. Hueper K, Gutberlet M, Rong S, Hartung D, Mengel M, et al. (2013) Acute Kidney Injury: Arterial Spin Labeling to Monitor Renal Perfusion Impairment in Mice-Comparison with Histopathologic Results and Renal Function. Radiology.
38. Hueper K, Rong S, Gutberlet M, Hartung D, Mengel M, et al. (2013) T2 relaxation time and apparent diffusion coefficient for noninvasive assessment of renal pathology after acute kidney injury in mice: comparison with histopathology. Invest Radiol 48: 834–842.
39. Zimmer F, Zollner FG, Hoeger S, Klotz S, Tsagogiorgas C, et al. (2013) Quantitative renal perfusion measurements in a rat model of acute kidney injury at 3T: testing inter- and intramethodical significance of ASL and DCE-MRI. PLoS One 8: e53849.
40. Lanzman RS, Ljimani A, Pentang G, Zgoura P, Zenginli H, et al. (2013) Kidney transplant: functional assessment with diffusion-tensor MR imaging at 3T. Radiology 266: 218–225.
41. Hueper K, Gutberlet M, Rodt T, Gwinner W, Lehner F, et al. (2011) Diffusion tensor imaging and tractography for assessment of renal allograft dysfunction-initial results. Eur Radiol 21: 2427–2433.
42. Hueper K, Hartung D, Gutberlet M, Gueler F, Sann H, et al. (2012) Magnetic resonance diffusion tensor imaging for evaluation of histopathological changes in a rat model of diabetic nephropathy. Invest Radiol 47: 430–437.
43. Xie L, Dibb R, Cofer GP, Li W, Nicholls PJ, et al. (2014) Susceptibility tensor imaging of the kidney and its microstructural underpinnings. Magn Reson Med.
44. Kaissling B, Lehir M, Kriz W (2013) Renal epithelial injury and fibrosis. Biochim Biophys Acta 1832: 931–939.
45. De Greef KE, Ysebaert DK, Persy V, Vercauteren SR, De Broe ME (2003) ICAM-1 expression and leukocyte accumulation in inner stripe of outer medulla in early phase of ischemic compared to HgCl2-induced ARF. Kidney Int 63: 1697–1707.
46. Mason J, Torhorst J, Welsch J (1984) Role of the medullary perfusion defect in the pathogenesis of ischemic renal failure. Kidney Int 26: 283–293.
47. Mason J, Welsch J, Torhorst J (1987) The contribution of vascular obstruction to the functional defect that follows renal ischemia. Kidney Int 31: 65–71.

48. Karlberg L, Kallskog O, Nygren K, Wolgast M (1982) Erythrocyte and albumin distribution in the kidney following warm ischemia. A study in rats. Scand J Urol Nephrol 16: 173–177.
49. Reinhard B (1850) Zur Kenntnis der Brithschen Krankheit. Charité Ann 1: 185.
50. Hellberg PO, Bayati A, Kallskog O, Wolgast M (1990) Red cell trapping after ischemia and long-term kidney damage. Influence of hematocrit. Kidney Int 37: 1240–1247.
51. Bayati A, Christofferson R, Kallskog O, Wolgast M (1990) Mechanism of erythrocyte trapping in ischaemic acute renal failure. Acta Physiol Scand 138: 13–23.
52. Bech M, Bunk O, Donath T, Feidenhans'l R, David C, et al. (2010) Quantitative x-ray dark-field computed tomography. Phys Med Biol 55: 5529–5539.
53. Chen GH, Bevins N, Zambelli J, Qi Z (2010) Small-angle scattering computed tomography (SAS-CT) using a Talbot-Lau interferometerand a rotating anode x-ray tube:theory and experiments. Opt Express 18: 12960–12970.
54. Meinel FG, Schwab F, Schleede S, Bech M, Herzen J, et al. (2013) Diagnosing and mapping pulmonary emphysema on X-ray projection images: incremental value of grating-based X-ray dark-field imaging. PLoS One 8: e59526.
55. Schleede S, Meinel FG, Bech M, Herzen J, Achterhold K, et al. (2012) Emphysema diagnosis using X-ray dark-field imaging at a laser-driven compact synchrotron light source. Proc Natl Acad Sci U S A 109: 17880–17885.
56. Velroyen A, Bech M, Malecki A, Tapfer A, Yaroshenko A, et al. (2013) Microbubbles as a scattering contrast agent for grating-based x-ray dark-field imaging. Phys Med Biol 58: N37–46.
57. Chen X, Summers RM, Cho M, Bagci U, Yao J (2012) An automatic method for renal cortex segmentation on CT images: evaluation on kidney donors. Acad Radiol 19: 562–570.
58. Nordsletten DA, Blackett S, Bentley MD, Ritman EL, Smith NP (2006) Structural morphology of renal vasculature. Am J Physiol Heart Circ Physiol 291: H296–309.
59. Diemoz PC, Coan P, Zanette I, Bravin A, Lang S, et al. (2011) A simplified approach for computed tomography with an X-ray grating interferometer. Opt Express 19: 1691–1698.
60. Zanette I, Bech M, Rack A, Le Duc G, Tafforeau P, et al. (2012) Trimodal low-dose X-ray tomography. Proc Natl Acad Sci U S A 109: 10199–10204.
61. Pollard R, Yunis R, Kultz D, Martin P, Griffey S, et al. (2006) Ultrasound detection and characterization of polycystic kidney disease in a mouse model. Comp Med 56: 215–221.
62. Wallace DP, Hou YP, Huang ZL, Nivens E, Savinkova L, et al. (2008) Tracking kidney volume in mice with polycystic kidney disease by magnetic resonance imaging. Kidney Int 73: 778–781.

High Fidelity System Modeling for High Quality Image Reconstruction in Clinical CT

Synho Do[1]*, William Clem Karl[2], Sarabjeet Singh[1], Mannudeep Kalra[1], Tom Brady[1], Ellie Shin[1], Homer Pien[1]

1 Department of Radiology, Massachusetts General Hospital and Harvard Medical School, Boston, Massachusetts, United States of America, **2** Department of Electrical and Computer Engineering, Boston University, Boston, Massachusetts, United States of America

Abstract

Today, while many researchers focus on the improvement of the regularization term in IR algorithms, they pay less concern to the improvement of the fidelity term. In this paper, we hypothesize that improving the fidelity term will further improve IR image quality in low-dose scanning, which typically causes more noise. The purpose of this paper is to systematically test and examine the role of high-fidelity system models using raw data in the performance of iterative image reconstruction approach minimizing energy functional. We first isolated the fidelity term and analyzed the importance of using focal spot area modeling, flying focal spot location modeling, and active detector area modeling as opposed to just flying focal spot motion. We then compared images using different permutations of all three factors. Next, we tested the ability of the fidelity terms to retain signals upon application of the regularization term with all three factors. We then compared the differences between images generated by the proposed method and Filtered-Back-Projection. Lastly, we compared images of low-dose in vivo data using Filtered-Back-Projection, Iterative Reconstruction in Image Space, and the proposed method using raw data. The initial comparison of difference maps of images constructed showed that the focal spot area model and the active detector area model also have significant impacts on the quality of images produced. Upon application of the regularization term, images generated using all three factors were able to substantially decrease model mismatch error, artifacts, and noise. When the images generated by the proposed method were tested, conspicuity greatly increased, noise standard deviation decreased by 90% in homogeneous regions, and resolution also greatly improved. In conclusion, the improvement of the fidelity term to model clinical scanners is essential to generating higher quality images in low-dose imaging.

Editor: Arrate Muñoz-Barrutia, University of Navarra, Spain

Funding: The authors have no funding or support to report.

Competing Interests: The authors have declared that no competing interests exist.

* Email: sdo@mgh.harvard.edu

Introduction

Computed tomography (CT) is one of the most commonly used diagnostic imaging modalities in modern medicine. CT enables rapid, non-invasive image acquisition at high resolutions. However, CT also exposes the patient to radiation [1,2]. CT dosage can be decreased by lowering either the voltage or the flux. Lowering the voltage implies that the emitted photons are less energetic, reducing their ability to penetrate through the body. Lowering the flux reduces the number of photons emitted, further degrading the signal-to-noise ratio of the acquired data. Therefore, the consequence of low-dose CT imaging is that the resulting images are considerably noisier than images acquired with todays clinical doses [3].

The drive towards lower dose CT imaging (while maintaining the diagnostic quality of CT) has been an area of focus for the entire CT community [4–9]. Numerous approaches to dose reduction have been implemented in commercial systems including the use of filters [10–12], collimators [13], dose modulation [14,15], prospective triggering [6], patient-specific protocols [16,17], and more [12,18]. One additional component to the current repertoire of low-dose CT scanning techniques is the use of new image reconstruction techniques.

Through recent studies, iterative reconstruction (IR) algorithms have been shown to be more robust than FBP algorithms in regards to the presence of noise and artifacts [8,19–25]. Numerous researchers have discussed different aspects of formulations [26–31] and optimization approaches [32–36]. However, we have found that having a high fidelity model of the imaging system is also a critical factor in the reconstruction of high quality images; this is an aspect of iterative reconstruction algorithms which has often been either neglected or substantially simplified [37,38].

A critical component of tomographic IR algorithms is the accuracy of the forward system model. In positron emission tomography (PET), the forward system model consists of a geometric projection matrix and a sinogram blurring matrix, which can be either measured or simulated [39,40]. It is shown that the combined model improves resolution and contrast-to-noise ratio in PET imaging [41]. It is also possible to reuse the

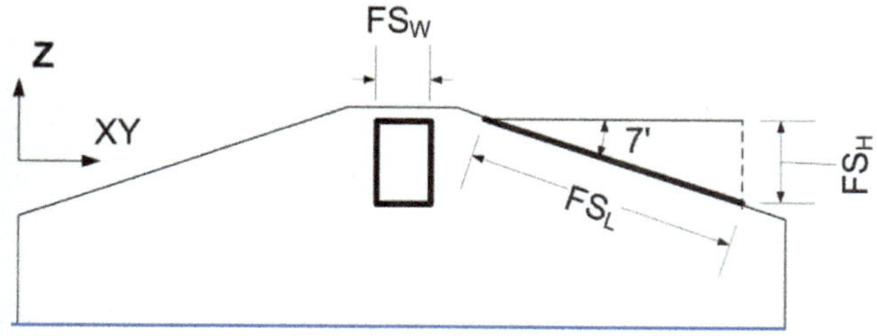

Figure 1. Focal spot area diagram: The length (*FSL*), width (*FSW*), and height ($FSH = FSL \times sin(7)$) of the focal spot area (rectangular shape) are denoted in the diagram.

stored system matrix to improve computation time because the PET scanner is stationary, making it relatively easy to factorize the system model based on symmetric geometry. A similar method is applied to single photon emission computed tomography (SPECT) for the estimation of the depth-dependent component of the point spread function (PSF) [42]. However, it is a challenging task to derive an explicit system matrix in clinical CT for the following reasons: i) each scan has a different scan length and pitch based on the scanning protocol, and ii) it is very hard to find symmetries in cone beam helical CT scans because the source-detector set has a functional misalignment (i.e., a quarter of a detector offset [43]) and view-by-view deflections of the X-ray source spot (i.e., flying focal spot (FFS) [44]).

In this paper, we show the systematic implementation of accurate system modeling for an IRT in clinical CT. A similar approach for PET [45] was derived from an analytical formula for calculating error propagation in a reconstructed image from the system matrix. In addition, in the cone-beam CT, the beam divergence and the rotation of the X-ray source and detector unit give space-variant effect on image. Since we do not use a system matrix as in PET, we integrate all the functional misalignment and fabrication limitations with on-the-fly calculation method so that the space-invariant nature is embedded in the forward model. Therefore, when we run image reconstruction algorithm, we set up on/off parameters for each modular model. That is one of major differences of our results compared to the previous 2D or phantom simulation works.

Also, there are algorithms (ASIR, IRIS, iDose, VEO, etc.) implemented in clinical scanners by vendors, but the technical description and detailed methods are not available to the research community. In this paper, we systematically demonstrate the necessity of implementing focal spot area, flying focal spot, and detector area in the forward system model to generate higher quality images. We also compare our raw-data-domain IRT with a mathematical formulation of image domain iteration called Iterative Reconstruction in Image Space (IRIS). The purpose of this paper is to examine the role of high-fidelity system models in the performance of the iterative image reconstruction approach minimizing energy functional. This paper is organized as follows. In section 2, we mathematically describe iterative image reconstruction and the components of proposed system models. In section 3, we present some initial results on phantom and in vivo data. In section 4, we summarize our findings and conclusions.

Methods

In this section, we describe the mathematical formulation of IRT and a detailed forward system modeling method. The forward system modeling method can be decomposed into a series of components to increase modeling accuracy. We structure a three-component model that incorporates the most important elements of the system model. Each component can be replaced by a specific scanner parameter or vendor-specific model. The accuracy of this system model is critical in the improvement of image quality of a reconstructed image.

On-the-fly System Modeling and Reconstruction Formulation for Clinical Scanner

We assume a transmission CT system with a field of x-ray attenuation coefficients x and projection operator H as modeled by:

$$y = Hx + \eta \qquad (1)$$

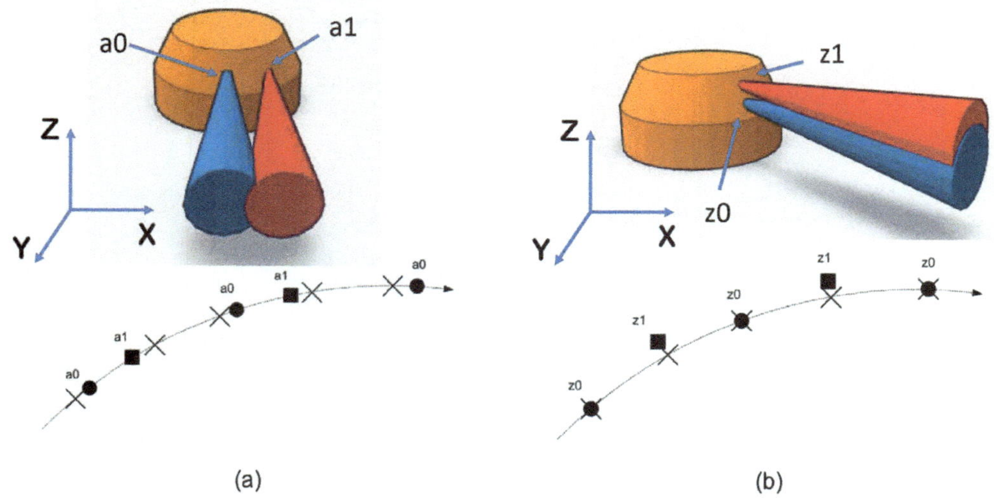

Figure 2. Flying Focal Spot (*FFS*) modeling: (a) $\alpha - FFS$ model shows deflected *FFSs* to the angular direction and (b) $z - FFS$ model shows z-directional deflections.

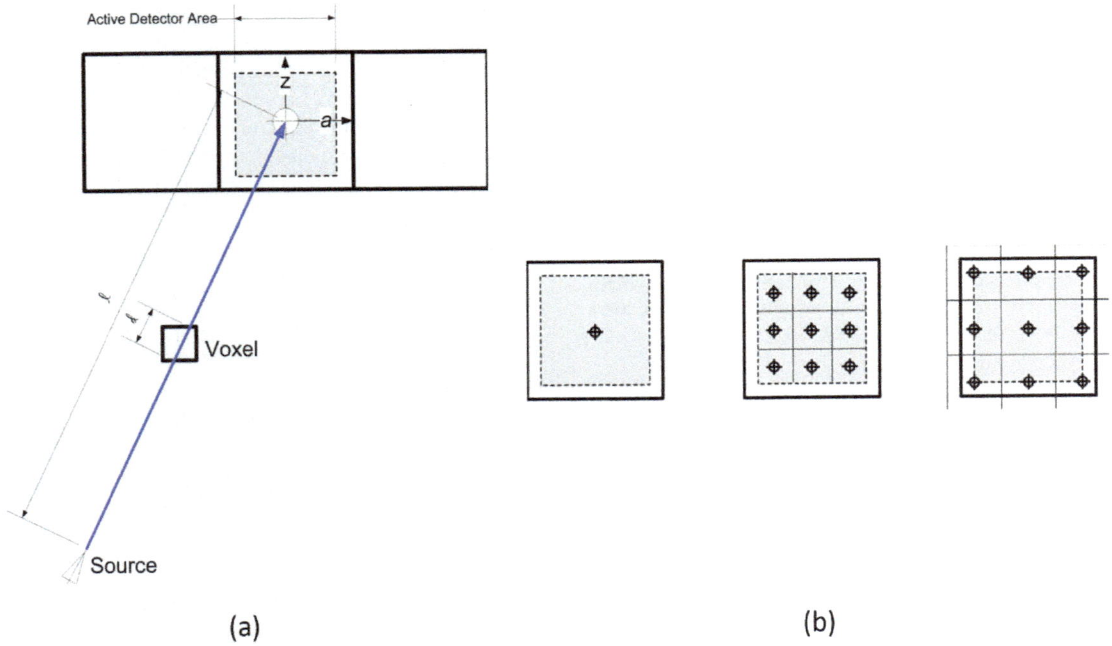

Figure 3. Diagram of active area of detector element: (a) Siddon-type ray-based projector calculates the ratio of intersections of the ray (i.e., d/l), (b) Gray area is the active region of single detector element, Left: single element model, middle: multiple elements by limiting active area of detector, right: multiple elements by assigning rays to the boundary of active area of detector element.

where y denotes the projection sinogram, and η denotes noise. We formulate our reconstruction problem by the following equation:

$$\hat{x}=\underset{x}{\operatorname{argmin}}\, E_d(y,x)+\alpha E(x) \tag{2}$$

where $E_d(y,x)$ is the data fidelity term between image x and sinogram y via the projection process. The second term $E(x)$ is the prior, or regularization term, and α is the weighting term. We formulate the fidelity term as:

$$E_d(y,x)=\|y-Hx\|_2^2 \tag{3}$$

where H is the system matrix, or projection process. One example of the regularization term $E(x)$ is the L_p norm:

$$E(x)=\|Lx\|_p^p=(\|Lx\|_p)^p=((|Lx_1|^p+|Lx_2|^p+\cdots+|Lx_n|^p)^{\frac{1}{p}})^p \tag{4}$$

When $L=\nabla$ and $p=1$, $E(x)$ becomes a Total Variation (TV) regularizer, which is commonly used to suppress noise and preserve edges in the image [46,47]. From a modeling perspective, we make the assumption that H, the system matrix, can be decomposed into a series of component models:

$$H=A_{det}A_{fs}P_{geom} \tag{5}$$

The models include a geometric projector (P_{geom}), a focal spot model (A_{fs}), and an active detector response function (A_{det}). By decomposing a system matrix H into sub-components, the implementation of complex clinical scanner modeling becomes more feasible. This approach also increases the usability of a single developed code across multiple CT systems, as opposed to requiring entirely different projectors for each system.

In this paper, we used the least-squares (LS) solution without the regularization term and TV solution in Equation (2) and (4) for comparison. The lagged diffusivity fixed-point method [46,48], where we iteratively approximated the cost by a weighted quadratic cost and then solved the resulting linear normal equations using pre-conditioned conjugated gradient (CG) iterations, is used to minimize the energy functional in Equation (2) [49].

Focal Spot Area Modeling

A focal spot is the region where electrons transfer their energy to target atoms in order to generate X-rays. In many cases, the focal spot is approximated as a point model, but in reality, the focal spot consists of a finite area (i.e., 0.3 mm to 0.8 mm) [50]. Furthermore, the size of this area changes with scanner settings (kVp or mA), an important consideration in regards to image reconstruction of low dose scans. Figure 1 illustrates the focal spot area with the length (FS_L), width (FS_W), and height ($FS_H=FS_L\times sin(7)$) of the area in the diagram. This sub-module should be included for accurate forward system modeling.

Flying Focal Spot (FFS) Modeling

The detector elements form an equiangular concentric cylindrical structure with 32 rows and 672 channels (i.e., 1st generation Dual Source CT, Siemens, Definition) with FFS models as shown in Figure 2. We assume the active area of all detector elements (i.e., $32\times 672=21504$) is identical for all elements according to manufacturer specifications. In Siddon-type ray-based projectors, a single ray sum is calculated for a single detector element by using the ratio of intersections of the ray with equally spaced parallel lines [51]. For our IR technique, we calculate a bundle of rays to simulate the virtual ray, which shapes the volume from the focal spot area to the active detector area. The ratio of the active

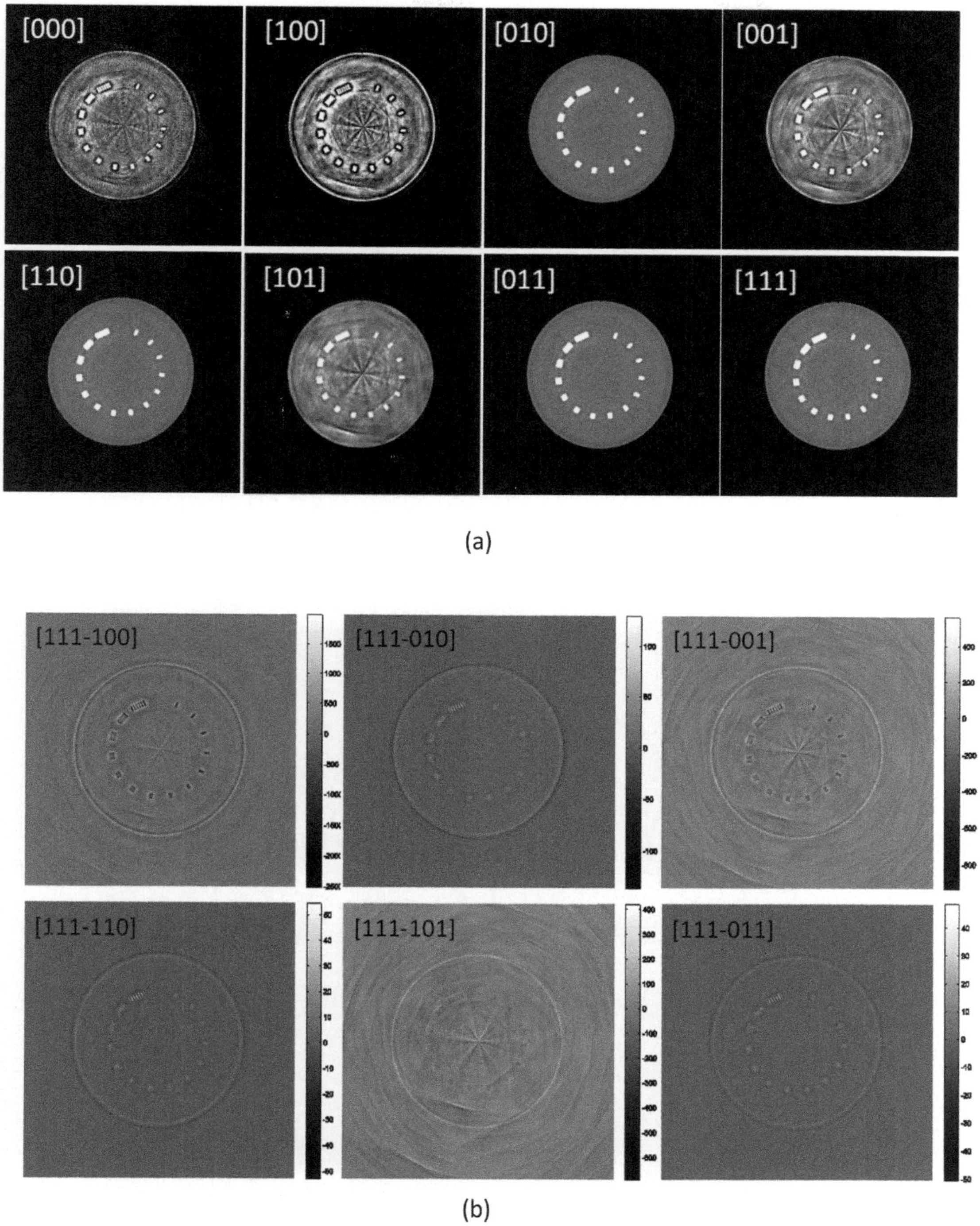

Figure 4. Modular system model effects: (a) Images are displayed in $[-1000,500]$ **HU and (b) difference maps are displayed in dynamic contrast range.** $[FS,FFS,DM]$: *FS*: Focal Spot model, *FFS*: Flying Focal Spot model, and *DM*: Detector model.

detector area to physical spacing between detector elements was provided to us by the scanner manufacturer as 85% in the angular direction and 80% in the z-direction as shown in Figure 3. These ratios can be changed for different systems.

The Siddon projector calculates only the weighted sums of the portion of the ray that intersects through each voxel without considering and compensating for the neighboring voxels, generating aliasing artifacts [52]. Multiple rays in the volume beam can be used to compensate for this aliasing effect at the expense of over-sampling the image grid [53]. We have additionally implemented a version of the Siddon projector which does not require recursion [54], thus making it amendable to parallel implementations [55].

Figure 3-(b) shows how we divide active sub-elements to compute ray-sums. In Figure 3-(b), a single element model, as well as a multiple element model that strictly limits the active area of the detector (i.e., middle sub-figure), is depicted. We have noticed, however, that applications with reconstructions on voxel

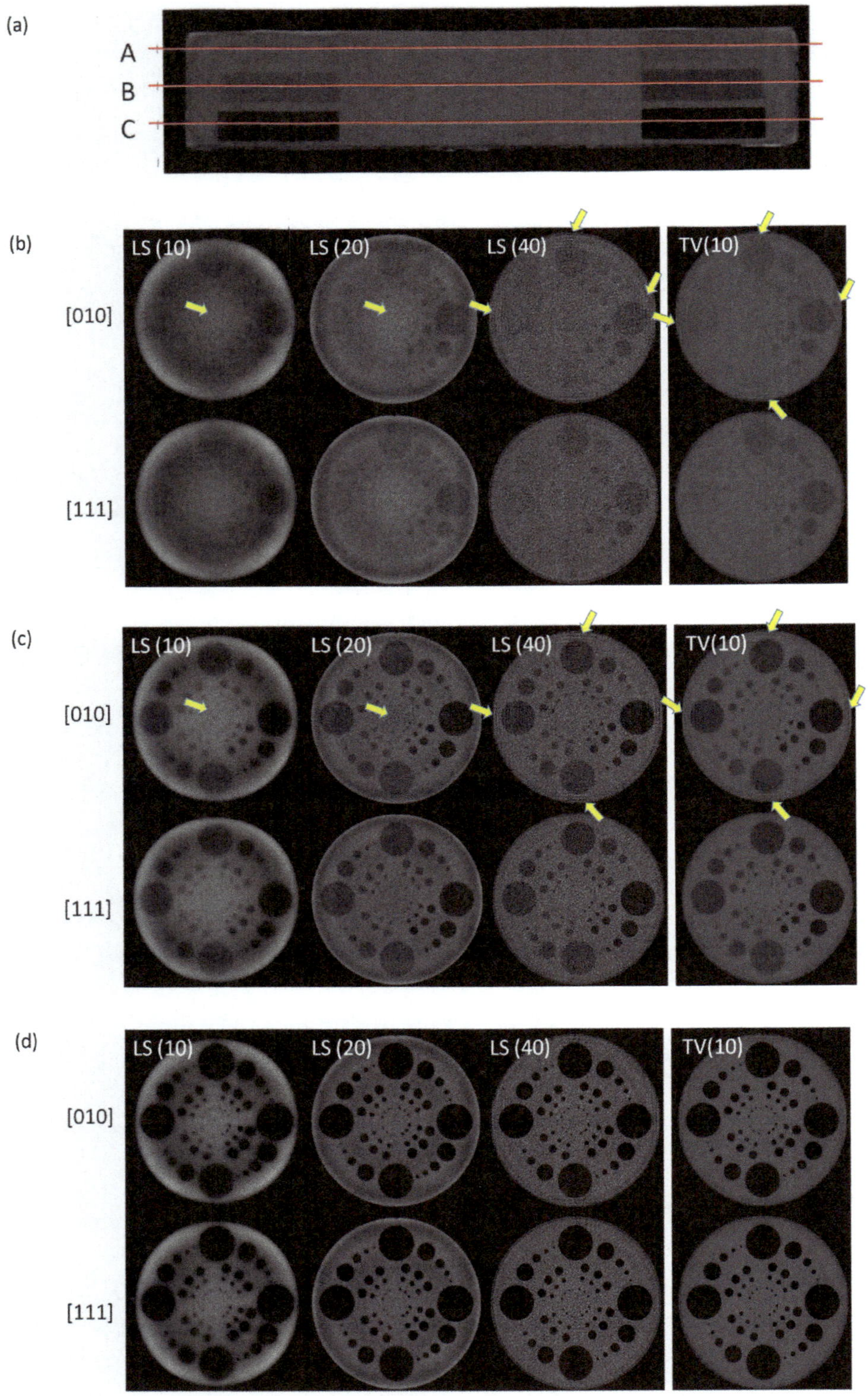

Figure 5. A modeling effect comparison on LS and TV images: (a) Coronal view of soft contrast section of phantom, (b), (c), and (d) show axial views of line A, B, and C respectively. The FFS only model (so called Siddon Model, (0,1,0)) shows circular line artifacts in LS and TV as well. In contrast, the proposed model ((1,1,1)) shows high quality image even in LS without regularization term and significant noise suppression effect on TV.

sizes that are finer than the detector size itself requires a greater over-sampling of the detector. In this case, not only does the computational demand increase, but the gap between the active areas of two adjacent detectors begin to introduce artifacts. As such, we have implemented the active area model depicted in the right sub-figure of Figure 3-(b), where the rays intersect the major boundary points, leading to a higher quality reconstruction.

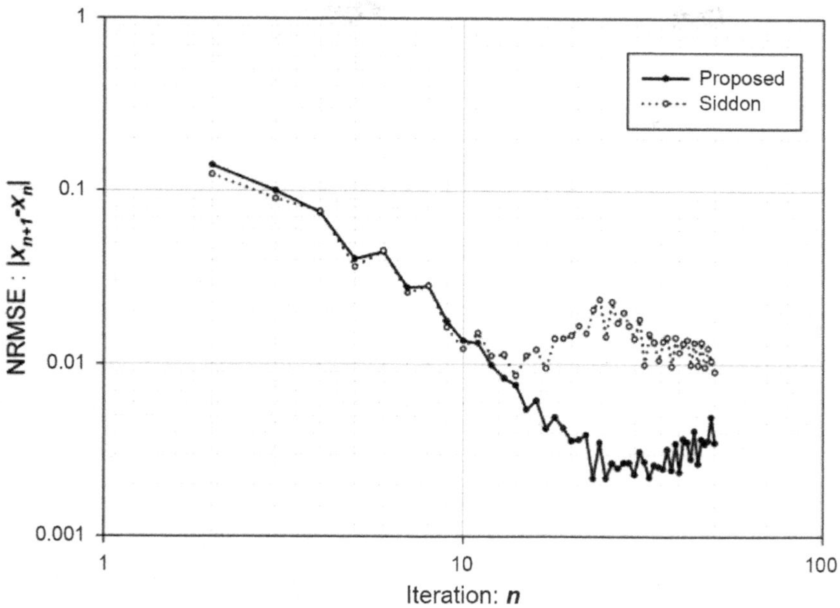

Figure 6. Consecutive error plot of Siddon (0,1,0) **and the proposed method** (1,1,1)**.** The NRMSEs of two consecutive images are calculated and displayed in log-log plot. The proposed method exhibits smaller consecutive errors after 15 iterations compared to Siddon method and reaches smaller modeling error.

Results

We show two experimental results in this section. For the phantom study, we focus on the comparison between the effects of each model on the LS images with a cone beam phantom (QRM, Moehrendorf, Germany) with respect to conspicuity improvement, noise statistics, and resolution. In an in vivo study, we show clinical evidence that supports the proposed approach with subjective assessment. The proposed method is compared with conventional FBP and image domain IR (IRIS) algorithms in a low dose scan. In this case, we used the same raw data for image reconstructions.

Phantom Study

A cone beam phantom with a spatial resolution section with 14 circularly aligned line-patterns varying from 4 to 30 lp/cm was scanned on a dual source 64-slice multi-detector row CT (Definition, Siemens Healthcare, Forchheim, Germany) using the following parameters: detector collimation $=0.6mm$, table speed $=3.8mm$ per gantry rotation, gantry rotation $=330msec$, tube current $=515mA$, and tube voltage $=120kV$.

In the following sections we demonstrate the impact of our various system modules. We will use the following notation: the triplet (FS,FFS,DM) to denote with a 1 or 0, whether the focal spot model, flying focal spot model, and detector model, respectively, are turned on $(=1)$ or off $(=0)$. Thus, for example, $(FS,FFS,DM)=(0,1,0)$ indicates that the flying focal spot model is turned on, while the other two system models are turned off.

Figure 4 shows the LS solutions reconstructed using all permutations of (FS,FFS,DM). Additionally, the differences between these permutations and the case in which all models are turned on $((FS,FFS,DM)=(1,1,1))$ are shown. All reconstructed images are shown with a windowing level of $[-1000,500]$, and difference images are shown with the full dynamic range of each difference so that patterns of artifacts are visible. The model without FFS generates the stellar shape artifact from the center of the rotation and it causes major deterioration of image quality. Therefore, FFS modeling is one of the most important components of clinical system modeling. The image quality evaluations in analytic reconstruction methods are shown in papers [44,56]. In analytic reconstruction methods, the locations of X-ray source and detector elements are the only models that can be implemented in the algorithm, so it is easy to overlook the importance of FS and DM.

In Figure 4, we can visually compare image qualities of Siddon-type model with FFS (0,1,0) and the proposed method (1,1,1) including focal spot and detector models to acquire a more accurate system model and to remove Moire patterns. There are only small differences between the two models, especially around the edges of the image, but eventually these will cause a significant change in the final image (i.e., TV regularization), especially in low dose scans. To suppress noise in low dose imaging, we frequently use regularization terms in Equation (2) with which we suppress noise by keeping the structure components of the image. When there are small model discrepancies related to the fidelity term in Equation (3), the mismatches can be concealed by noise and may cause resolution degradation and eventually poor contrast.

To compare artifact propagation, we compare the LS and TV images with a soft contrast section of the phantom. The three cross-sections of the soft contrast region are displayed in Figure 5-(a). Figure 5-(b), (c), and (d) show the axial views of line A, B, and C respectively. The top images are from Siddon-type model with $FFS(0,1,0)$ and the bottom images are from the proposed method (1,1,1). By the number of iteration (i.e., LS: 10,20, and 40 iteration, TV: 10 iteration), we can observe circular line artifacts on LS and TV, as well as on the Siddon-type model. It is especially more obvious in a very low contrast case (Figure 5-(b)). However, the images reconstructed by the proposed method show high quality images without any artifacts in both LS and TV. As expected, the TV images show significant noise suppression.

To observe the effects of iterations, we simulated a Siddon-type projector with proper FFS model (0,1,0) without FS and DM, and a complete model (1,1,1) including all modular models in Section 2. Both methods used the same optimization algorithm

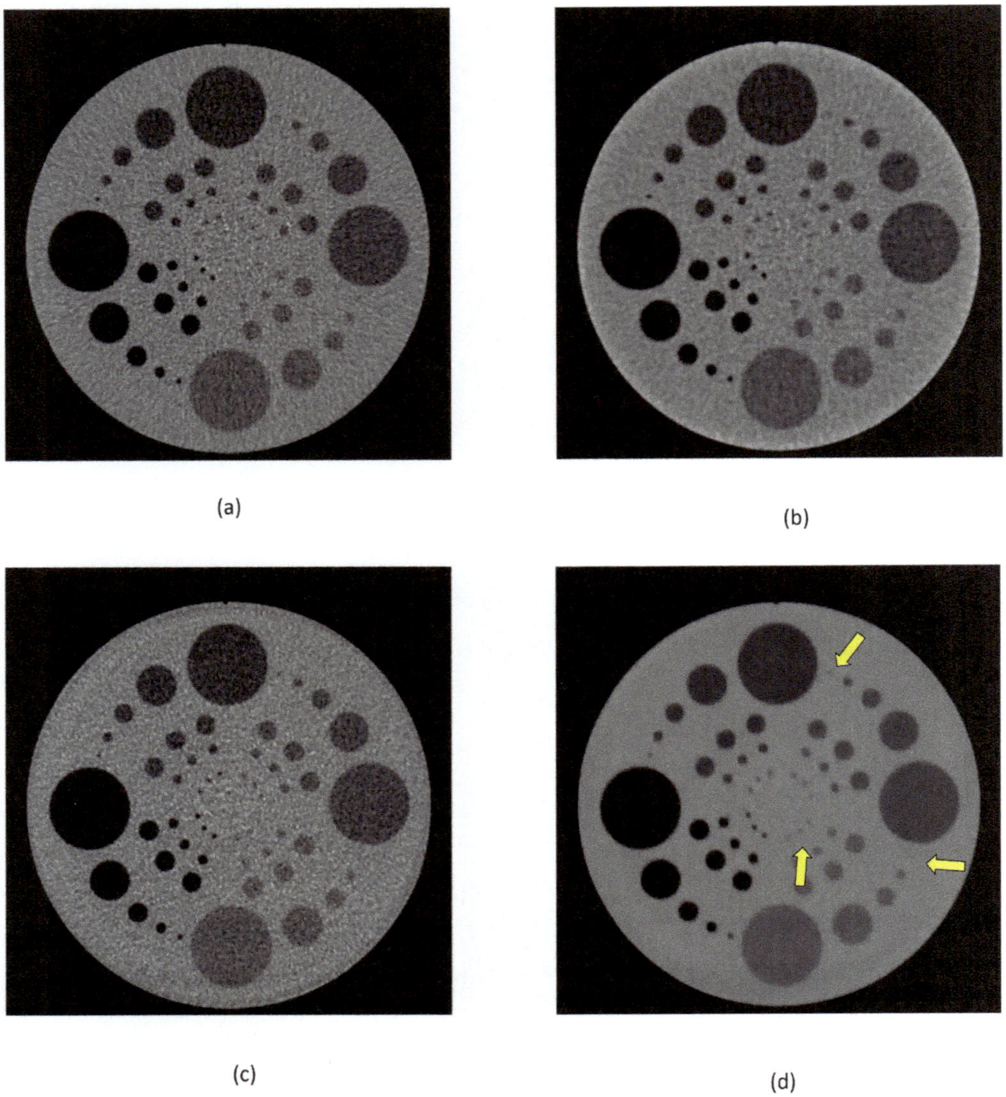

Figure 7. Soft contrast and conspicuity comparison for (a) FBP with sharp kernel filtering, (b) FBP with soft kernel filtering, (c) Least-Squares solution after 30-iteration, and (d) Total Variation (TV) image after 10-iteration with (c) initialization $[-200,300]$.

and code (C++ and Open MPI) to reconstruct images and consecutively calculate the NRMSE (Normalized Root Mean Square Error):

$$\varepsilon=\sqrt{\frac{\sum(\|X_n-X_{n+1}\|^2)}{\sum(\|X_{n+1}\|^2)}} \tag{6}$$

where X_n is the $n-th$ iteration result of LS-solution with L elements.

Figure 6 compares the consecutive errors with iteration for Siddon (0,1,0) and the proposed method (1,1,1) in the log-log scale. The Siddon-type projector shows similar updates to the proposed method until iteration-15, where it plateaus and then fluctuates. The resulting image from the Siddon projector does not provide the best image even though it reaches the solution of Equation (3). In contrast, the NRMSEs for our proposed method become smaller even after 15-iterations because the modeling error decreases with increasing iterations. However, the high frequency and noise components of the 30 iterations become dominant in the system modeling.

Note that the proposed method exhibits significant modeling error reduction in terms of visual evaluation and NRMSE taking into account the nonlinear scaling of log-log plot.

Conspicuity Improvements. In Figure 7, we display a contrast resolution section of QRM phantoms scanned in the clinical system. We show four groups of circles with different attenuation coefficients in Hounsfield Units (HU) $(-60,-90,-120,$ and -200 HU) in tissue equivalent background (35 HU) at $120kVp$. Each group consists of 14 circular inserts with different diameters (2,4,8,16, and $32mm$). We used the same raw data for the comparison of four different reconstruction methods: Figure 7-(a) FBP with sharp kernel filtering, (b) FBP with soft kernel filtering, (c) Least-Squares (LS) solution after 30-iterations, and (d) Total Variation (TV) image after 10-iterations with (c) initialization.

We found that it is difficult to detect low contrast circles (for example, $2mm$ circles in -60 and -90 HU groups) visually as shown in Figure 7-(a), (b), and (c). Notice that there is no improvement of conspicuity in small circles with low contrast even

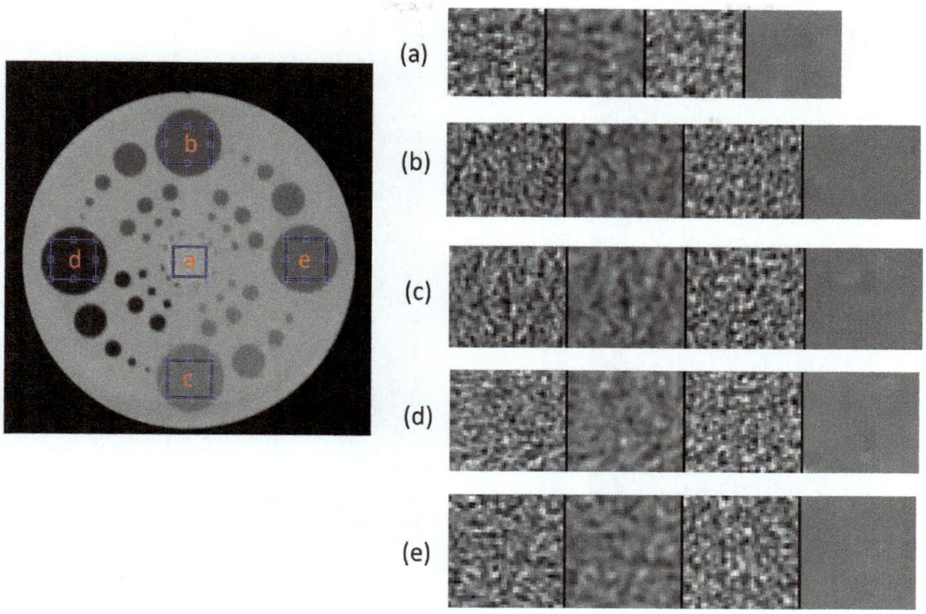

Figure 8. Noise patches comparison for the four images in Figure 8. Each sampled region is concatenated with dividing columns (zeros) and displayed in dynamic contrast window to show noticeable differences. From left to right, FBP with sharp kernel filtering, FBP with soft kernel filtering, IRT (LS), and IRT (TV).

with the smoothing kernel, Figure 7-(b). Basically, it suppresses high frequency noise components on the image without keeping small and low contrast information, which is key to the evaluation of low contrast tissues and lesions in most soft tissues such as the brain, liver, spleen, and lymph nodes, given subtle or low differences in HU values between organs and several of these legions (i.e., neoplasms and infarcts).

However, we can easily identify $2mm$ circles in -60 and -90 HU groups from Figure 7-(d). The TV image can be initialized on FBP image and can replace the LS solution.

Noise Statistics. Figure 8 compares noise patches from five noise regions for each image in Figure 7: one from each tissue equivalent region at the center of the Phantom and four $32mm$ circles from different HU groups ($-60, -90, -120$, and -200 HU). Each sampled region is concatenated with dividing columns (zeros) and displayed in a dynamic contrast window to show noticeable differences. The FBP with sharp kernel filtering and LS solutions show similar noise patterns. As shown in Table 1, a smoother and lower spatial frequency kernel FBP with soft kernel filtering has lower noise compared to that of a sharper and higher spatial frequency kernel FBP (sharp kernel). However, TV shows a strong noise suppression capability and retains visibility of small and low-contrast circular objects that are, in our opinion, from accurate system modeling.

The image reconstruction formulation in Equation (2) emphasizes that the energy functional aggregates a fidelity term and a regularization term. When the system model is not accurate enough to model details of the system, the TV-regularization (Equation (4)) of the energy functional (Equation (2)) smears or even loses the signal components associated with lower HU rather

Table 1. Shows the measurements of noise mean (m) and standard deviation (σ) for each patch from four difference reconstruction images.

		FBP(sharp kernel)	FBP(soft kernel)	IRT(LS)	IRT (TV)
Patch a	m	35.41	35.67	43.09	40.82
	σ	28.39	17.78	26.60	2.31
Patch b	m	−83.25	−84.19	−78.41	−78.92
	σ	21.81	13.14	22.35	2.04
Patch c	m	−26.99	−27.02	−24.23	−24.58
	σ	20.25	12.09	23.11	2.05
Patch d	m	−163.35	−164.98	−163.40	−163.64
	σ	19.07	11.66	21.90	2.29
Patch e	m	−54.57	−54.60	−51.37	−52.48
	σ	21.04	12.40	21.60	1.28

FBP (soft kernel) has smaller standard deviation than FBP (sharp kernel) and IRT (LS) but the IRT (TV) shows the smallest noise standard deviation.

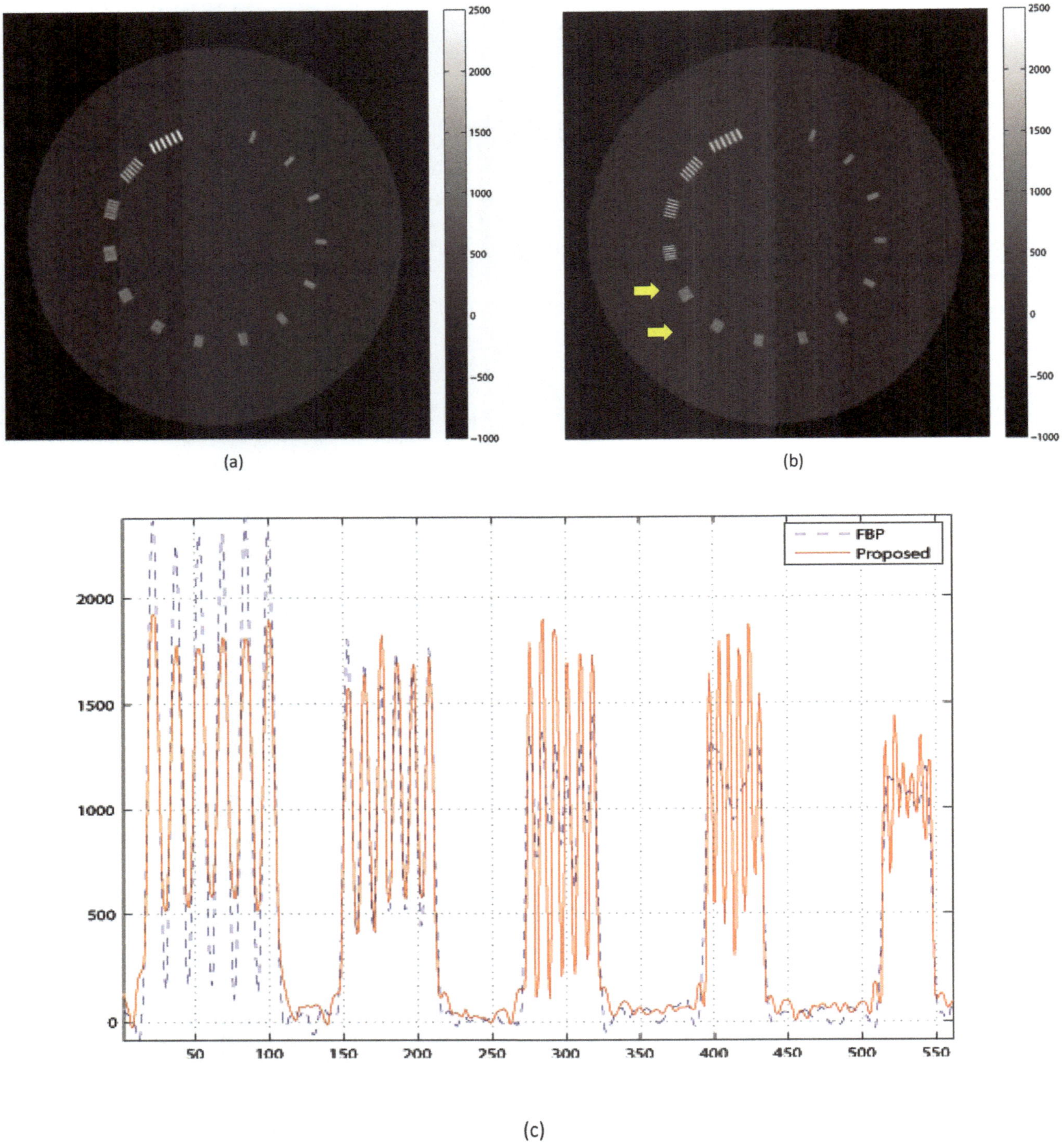

Figure 9. Spatial resolution bar pattern comparison: (a) FBP (sharp kernel) and (b) TV with high fidelity term image with proposed model (111) are displayed in [800, 2300] HU. (a) shows clear separations of 4, 6, and 8 lp/cm and (b) presents improved resolution showing 10 and 12 lp/cm bar patterns. (c) compares profiles of spatial resolution inserts.

than noise when enforcing the smoothness constraint (i.e., L_1-norm) as in Equation (4). This can even occur to greater signal components in low dose CT data, when the system model is inaccurate and iteration proceeds to suppress amplified noise.

On the other hand, the accurate system model sustains small signal components in the fidelity term so that it eventually reveals hidden signal components under the noise components.

Resolution. The reconstruction parameters of FBP and the proposed IRT method (1,1,1) are set to be the same as slice-thickness (0.6mm).

The spatial resolution bar patterns are displayed in Figure 9 with a [800,2300] contrast window. FBP (sharp kernel) and FBP (soft kernel) had similar resolutions, so only the better FBP (sharp kernel) is displayed in Figure 9-(a) and compared to the TV with

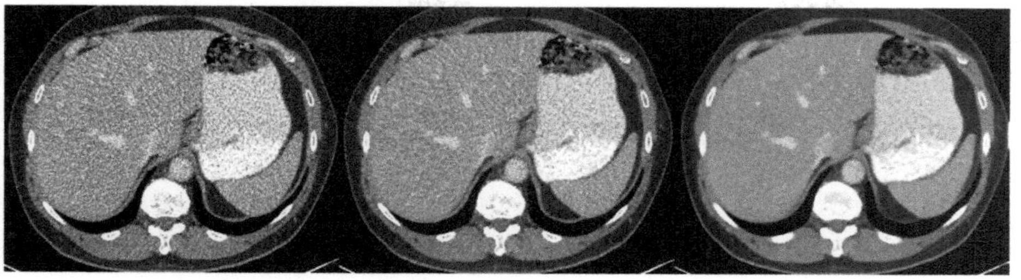

(a)

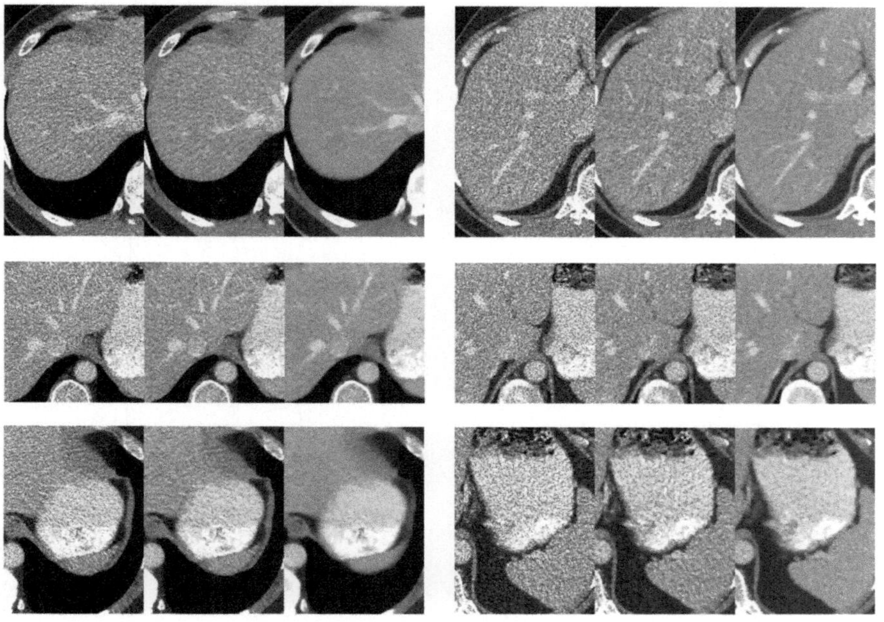

(b)

Figure 10. Comparison of reconstruction methods on half-dose images: (a) Reconstructed images, with (L) FBP, (M) IRIS, and (R) TV with advanced system modeling, (b) Zoomed images from different slices; each sub-figure shows (L) FBP, (M) IRIS, and (R) TV with advanced system modeling. Display in [5,155] **HU.**

advanced model in Figure 9-(b). Note that the arrows in Figure 9-(b) indicate 10 and 12 lp/cm inserts, which points to clear improvement of spatial resolution on the TV with advanced modeling image.

In vivo study

In the in vivo study, we only show clinical evidences of the proposed approach with subjective assessment. The proposed method is compared with conventional FBP and image domain IR algorithm (IRIS) in a low dose scan. In this case, we used the same raw data for image reconstructions. This study was conducted in compliance with the Health Insurance Portability and Accountability Act (HIPAA) and used a scan protocol approved by the Massachusetts General Hospital Institutional Review Board (IRB). We obtained written informed consent as per Federal U.S. guidelines. All procedures in this study were performed in accordance with the approved protocol.

A patient was scanned on a dual source 64-slice MDCT (1st generation DSCT Definition, Siemens Medical Solutions) using routine abdominal CT protocols. The scan parameters were $120kV$, $177mA$, and 0.5 second gantry rotation. The reconstruct-

Table 2. SNR comparison of the three reconstruction methods for the half-dose dataset in Figure 10.

	FBP	IRIS	TV with high fidelity term
m	173.43	169.78	169.60
σ	43.66	20.99	13.17
SNR (dB)	27.59	41.81	51.11

Table 3. CNR comparison of the three reconstruction methods for the half-dose dataset in Figure 10.

	FBP	IRIS	TV with high fidelity term
$S_A - S_B$	192.24	192.40	198.52
σ	35.78	18.55	6.88
CNR	5.37	10.37	28.84

ed images show low dose image quality by reconstructing images with only half the data (i.e., detector A).

For this case, images with the volume $512 \times 512 \times 100$ were reconstructed. For FBP, the sharp kernel on the scanner was utilized. For Iterative Reconstruction in Image Space (IRIS) [57,58], the corresponding sharp kernel was chosen. IRIS is developed on a novel mathematical algorithm through iterative formation. The image domain iteration is initiated after it reconstructs a master volume, which is reconstructed based on how the scan projections provide image detail information, while reducing noise and enhancing object contrast step by step. IRIS utilizes well-established convolution kernels so that it is very fast compared to raw data domain iterative reconstruction.

In this experiment, we compare three different reconstruction approaches: the conventional FBP method, image domain iterative IRIS, and raw data domain IRT with the proposed methods. We have used 10-iterations with $\alpha=2^5$ for IRT reconstruction with the proposed system modeling method.

To compare images, we defined a priori the regions of comparison. For SNR, the signal is defined over the region containing the hepatic artery, while the background standard deviation is chosen from patches (over 45 slices) of the liver without vasculature. We define CNR as:

$$CNR = \frac{|S_A - S_B|}{\sigma} \quad (7)$$

where S_A and S_B are mean signal intensities of signal producing structures of the liver (S_A) and the mean signal of the camper's fascia (S_B), respectively. To obtain CNR background statistics, the standard deviation of the camper's fascia over 45 slices was computed, and is denoted by σ by in Equation (7).

A comparison of reconstruction algorithms for the half-dose scan is shown in Figure 10. Although the added noise associated with this low-dose scan is apparent, no undesired texturing appears in this set of images either. The proposed method shows better visual impression compared to FBP and IRIS.

We also tabulate the SNR and CNR of the low-dose scans, in Table 2 and 3, respectively. The proposed method preserves the signal/contrast at much reduced noise for the low-dose acquisition. In this paper, we choose the regularization parameter based on clinician's feedback so it can be improved by processing more cases with broad feedback from multiple radiologists.

In this study, we showed the efficacy and impact of the proposed method in the real clinical scanner.

Discussions and Conclusions

Modern CT systems are highly complex, and different reconstruction algorithms go to various lengths to model such complexities. In this paper, we show that the accurate modeling of system components such as focal spot area, flying focal spot, and active detector area can make a significant difference in the quality of reconstructed images.

Our phantom and patient studies show that the proposed technique can improve image quality (low contrast, noise statistics, spatial resolution, and visual impression). We have introduced a modular system modeling framework for a sophisticated clinical CT scanner. Even within the same system, some functions can be turned off or manipulated for clinical purposes. The advanced functions of state-of-art CT scanners need to be modeled accordingly for high quality image reconstruction. These parameter changes are meticulously recorded in the header files of raw data. None of these functions can be ignored for accurate system modeling to develop high-fidelity characteristics of an iterative algorithm.

As shown in Figure 4, there are sub-modules of the system that cause a small mismatch in system modeling, but these can be propagated through iterations, making them very hard to correct or compensate for by post-processing or utilization of regularization terms. Many studies claim that they can produce high quality SNR images with simple phantoms (having a few high density structures with homogeneous background) in low dose imaging; however, it is very hard to contain the small low-contrast structure in the final results without advanced system modeling. Without satisfying the fidelity term of the energy functional in Equation (3), we cannot guarantee that the reconstructed image is "the only stable solution" of this ill-posed image reconstruction problem.

At 50% dose, both IRIS and the proposed TV with advanced system modeling were found to be diagnostically acceptable. Although the proposed TV provided objectively superior images in terms of SNR and CNR, this image quality was achieved through a significant amount of processing. As a technique that achieves fast computations while maintaining good image quality, a hybrid method (such as IRIS) may potentially be a promising approach.

Future work will also address a variety of dose reductions on cadavers, and we anticipate being able to reduce computation time for the proposed advanced system modeling by implementing it on parallel computing architectures.

Acknowledgments

The authors gratefully acknowledge Dr. Herbert Bruder, Dr. Karl Stierstofer, Christianne Leidecker, and Dr. Thomas G. Flohr (Siemens Healthcare) for providing system geometry and data structure information of CT sinogram.

Author Contributions

Conceived and designed the experiments: SD WCK TB HP. Performed the experiments: SS MK TB HP. Analyzed the data: SD WCK HP. Contributed reagents/materials/analysis tools: SD. Wrote the paper: SD ES HP.

References

1. Brenner DJ, Elliston CD, Hall EJ, Berdon WE (2001) Estimated risks of radiation-induced fatal cancer from pediatric CT. American Journal of Roentgenology 176: 289–296.
2. Brenner DJ, Hricak H (2010) Radiation Exposure From Medical Imaging. JAMA: The Journal of the American Medical Association 304: 208.
3. Kalra MK, Maher MM, Sahani DV, Blake MA, Hahn PF, et al. (2003) Low-Dose CT of the Abdomen: Evaluation of Image Improvement with Use of Noise Reduction Filters-Pilot Study1. Radiology 228: 251–256.
4. Pontana F, Duhamel A, Pagniez J, Flohr T, Faivre J-B, et al. (2011) Chest computed tomography using iterative reconstruction vs filtered back projection (Part 2): image quality of low-dose CT examinations in 80 patients. European radiology 21: 636–643.
5. Scheffel H, Alkadhi H, Leschka S, Plass A, Desbiolles L, et al. (2008) Low-dose CT coronary angiography in the step-and-shoot mode: diagnostic performance. Heart 94: 1132–1137.
6. Husmann L, Valenta I, Gaemperli O, Adda O, Treyer V, et al. (2007) Feasibility of low-dose coronary CT angiography: first experience with prospective ECG-gating. European heart journal.
7. Marin D, Nelson RC, Schindera ST, Richard S, Youngblood RS, et al. (2009) Low-Tube-Voltage, High-Tube-Current Multidetector Abdominal CT: Improved Image Quality and Decreased Radiation Dose with Adaptive Statistical Iterative Reconstruction Algorithm-Initial Clinical Experience 1. Radiology 254: 145–153.

8. Prakash P, Kalra MK, Kambadakone AK, Pien H, Hsieh J, et al. (2010) Reducing abdominal CT radiation dose with adaptive statistical iterative reconstruction technique. Investigative radiology 45: 202–210.
9. Fazel R, Krumholz HM, Wang Y, Ross JS, Chen J, et al. (2009) Exposure to low-dose ionizing radiation from medical imaging procedures. New England Journal of Medicine 361: 849–857.
10. Kan MW, Leung LH, Wong W, Lam N (2008) Radiation dose from cone beam computed tomography for image-guided radiation therapy. International Journal of Radiation Oncology* Biology* Physics 70: 272–279.
11. Kwan AL, Boone JM, Shah N (2005) Evaluation of x-ray scatter properties in a dedicated cone-beam breast CT scanner. Medical physics 32: 2967–2975.
12. Kalra MK, Maher MM, Toth TL, Hamberg LM, Blake MA, et al. (2004) Strategies for CT Radiation Dose Optimization 1. Radiology 230: 619–628.
13. Hsieh J (2009) Computed tomography: principles, design, artifacts, and recent advances. SPIE Bellingham, WA.
14. Hentschel D, Popescu S, Strauss K-E, Wolf H (1999) Adaptive dose modulation during CT scanning. Google Patents.
15. Kalra MK, Maher MM, D'Souza RV, Rizzo S, Halpern EF, et al. (2005) Detection of Urinary Tract Stones at Low-Radiation-Dose CT with Z-Axis Automatic Tube Current Modulation: Phantom and Clinical Studies 1. Radiology 235: 523–529.
16. McCollough CH, Bruesewitz MR, Kofler Jr JM (2006) CT Dose Reduction and Dose Management Tools: Overview of Available Options 1. Radiographics 26: 503–512.
17. Singh S, Kalra MK, Moore MA, Shailam R, Liu B, et al. (2009) Dose Reduction and Compliance with Pediatric CT Protocols Adapted to Patient Size, Clinical Indication, and Number of Prior Studies 1. Radiology 252: 200–208.
18. Li J, Udayasankar UK, Toth TL, Seamans J, Small WC, et al. (2007) Automatic patient centering for MDCT: effect on radiation dose. American Journal of Roentgenology 188: 547–552.
19. Shepp LA, Vardi Y (1982) Maximum likelihood reconstruction for emission tomography. Medical Imaging, IEEE Transactions on 1: 113–122.
20. Wang G, Snyder DL, O'Sullivan J, Vannier M (1996) Iterative deblurring for CT metal artifact reduction. Medical Imaging, IEEE Transactions on 15: 657–664.
21. Thibault J-B, Sauer KD, Bouman CA, Hsieh J (2007) A three-dimensional statistical approach to improved image quality for multislice helical CT. Medical physics 34: 4526.
22. Bittencourt MS, Schmidt B, Seltmann M, Muschiol G, Ropers D, et al. (2011) Iterative reconstruction in image space (IRIS) in cardiac computed tomography: initial experience. The international journal of cardiovascular imaging 27: 1081–1087.
23. Tang J, Nett BE, Chen G-H (2009) Performance comparison between total variation (TV)-based compressed sensing and statistical iterative reconstruction algorithms. Physics in medicine and biology 54: 5781.
24. Sidky EY, Pan X, Reiser IS, Nishikawa RM, Moore RH, et al. (2009) Enhanced imaging of microcalcifications in digital breast tomosynthesis through improved image-reconstruction algorithms. Medical physics 36: 4920.
25. Park JC, Song B, Kim JS, Park SH, Kim HK, et al. (2012) Fast compressed sensing-based CBCT reconstruction using Barzilai-Borwein formulation for application to on-line IGRT. Medical Physics 39: 1207.
26. Andersen A, Kak A (1984) Simultaneous algebraic reconstruction technique (SART): a superior implementation of the ART algorithm. Ultrasonic imaging 6: 81–94.
27. Levitan E, Herman GT (1987) A maximum a posteriori probability expectation maximization algorithm for image reconstruction in emission tomography. Medical Imaging, IEEE Transactions on 6: 185–192.
28. Fessler JA (1994) Penalized weighted least-squares image reconstruction for positron emission tomography. Medical Imaging, IEEE Transactions on 13: 290–300.
29. Browne JA, Boone JM, Holmes TJ (1995) Maximum-likelihood x-ray computed-tomography finite-beamwidth considerations. Applied optics 34: 5199–5209.
30. Fu L, Wang J, Rui X, Thibault J-B, De Man B (2013) Modeling and estimation of detector response and focal spot profile for high-resolution iterative CT reconstruction. Nuclear Science Symposium and Medical Imaging Conference (NSS/MIC), 2013 IEEE. IEEE. pp. 1–5.
31. Little K, La Riviere P (2012) An algorithm for modeling non-linear system effects in iterative CT reconstruction. Nuclear Science Symposium and Medical Imaging Conference (NSS/MIC), 2012 IEEE. IEEE. pp. 2174–2177.
32. Sauer K, Bouman C (1993) A local update strategy for iterative reconstruction from projections. Signal Processing, IEEE Transactions on 41: 534–548.
33. De Man B, Nuyts J, Dupont P, Marchal G, Suetens P (2001) An iterative maximum-likelihood polychromatic algorithm for CT. Medical Imaging, IEEE Transactions on 20: 999–1008.
34. Hudson HM, Larkin RS (1994) Accelerated image reconstruction using ordered subsets of projection data. Medical Imaging, IEEE Transactions on 13: 601–609.
35. Wang G, Snyder DL, O'Sullivan JA, Vannier M (1996) Iterative deblurring for CT metal artifact reduction. Medical Imaging, IEEE Transactions on 15: 657–664.
36. Ramani S, Fessler J (2010) A splitting-based iterative algorithm for accelerated statistical X-ray CT reconstruction. Medical Imaging, IEEE Transactions on: 1–1.
37. Do S, Cho S, Karl WC, Kalra MK, Brady TJ, et al. (2009) Accurate model-based high resolution cardiac image reconstruction in dual source CT. IEEE. pp. 330–333.
38. Hofmann C, Knaup M, Kachelrie M (2014) Effects of ray profile modeling on resolution recovery in clinical CT. Medical physics 41: 021907.
39. Alessio AM, Kinahan PE, Lewellen TK (2006) Modeling and incorporation of system response functions in 3-D whole body PET. Medical Imaging, IEEE Transactions on 25: 828–837.
40. Panin VY, Kehren F, Michel C, Casey M (2006) Fully 3-D PET reconstruction with system matrix derived from point source measurements. Medical Imaging, IEEE Transactions on 25: 907–921.
41. Tohme MS, Qi J (2009) Iterative image reconstruction for positron emission tomography based on a detector response function estimated from point source measurements. Physics in Medicine and Biology 54: 3709.
42. Beekman FJ, Slijpen ETP, de Jong HWAM, Viergever MA (1999) Estimation of the depth-dependent component of the point spread function of SPECT. Medical physics 26: 2311.
43. La Riviere PJ, Pan X (2004) Sampling and aliasing consequences of quarter-detector offset use in helical CT. Medical Imaging, IEEE Transactions on 23: 738–749.
44. Kachelrie M, Knaup M, Penel C, Kalender WA (2006) Flying focal spot (FFS) in cone-beam CT. Nuclear Science, IEEE Transactions on 53: 1238–1247.
45. Qi J, Huesman RH (2005) Effect of errors in the system matrix on maximum a posteriori image reconstruction. Physics in Medicine and Biology 50: 3297.
46. Vogel CR, Oman ME (1996) Iterative methods for total variation denoising. SIAM Journal on Scientific Computing 17: 227–238.
47. Sidky EY, Pan X (2008) Image reconstruction in circular cone-beam computed tomography by constrained, total-variation minimization. Physics in Medicine and Biology 53: 4777.
48. Chan TF, Mulet P (1999) On the convergence of the lagged diffusivity fixed point method in total variation image restoration. SIAM Journal on Numerical Analysis: 354–367.
49. Do S, Karl WC, Liang Z, Kalra M, Brady TJ, et al. (2011) A decomposition-based CT reconstruction formulation for reducing blooming artifacts. Physics in Medicine and Biology 56: 7109.
50. Hsieh J (2003) Computed tomography: principles, design, artifacts, and recent advances. Society of Photo Optical.
51. Siddon RL (1985) Fast calculation of the exact radiological path for a three-dimensional CT array. Medical Physics 12: 252.
52. Siddon RL (1985) Fast calculation of the exact radiological path for a three?dimensional CT array. Medical physics 12: 252–255.
53. Sunnegardh J, Danielsson PE (2007) A new anti-aliased projection operator for iterative CT reconstruction. pp. 124–127.
54. Jacobs F, Sundermann E, De Sutter B, Christiaens M, Lemahieu I (1998) A fast algorithm to calculate the exact radiological path through a pixel or voxel space. Journal of computing and information technology 6: 89–94.
55. Jang B, Do S, Pien H, Kaeli D (2009) Architecture-aware optimization targeting multithreaded stream computing. ACM. pp. 62–70.
56. Flohr T, Stierstorfer K, Ulzheimer S, Bruder H, Primak A, et al. (2005) Image reconstruction and image quality evaluation for a 64-slice CT scanner with z-flying focal spot. Medical physics 32: 2536.
57. Tipnis S, Ramachandra A, Huda W, Hardie A, Schoepf J, et al. Iterative reconstruction in image space (IRIS) and lesion detection in abdominal CT. pp. 76222K.
58. Bittencourt MS, Schmidt B, Seltmann M, Muschiol G, Ropers D, et al. (2010) Iterative reconstruction in image space (IRIS) in cardiac computed tomography: initial experience. The International Journal of Cardiovascular Imaging (formerly Cardiac Imaging): 1–7.

22

Feasibility Study of Dual Energy Radiographic Imaging for Target Localization in Radiotherapy for Lung Tumors

Jie Huo[1], Xianfeng Zhu[1], Yang Dong[2], Zhiyong Yuan[2], Ping Wang[2]*, Xuemin Wang[1], Gang Wang[1], Xin-Hua Hu[3], Yuanming Feng[1,2,4]*

1 Department of Biomedical Engineering, Tianjin University, Tianjin, China, **2** Department of Radiation Oncology, Tianjin Cancer Hospital, Tianjin, China, **3** Department of Physics, East Carolina University, Greenville, North Carolina, United States of America, **4** Department of Radiation Oncology, East Carolina University, Greenville, North Carolina, United States of America

Abstract

Purpose: Dual-energy (DE) radiographic imaging improves tissue discrimination by separating soft from hard tissues in the acquired images. This study was to establish a mathematic model of DE imaging based on intrinsic properties of tissues and quantitatively evaluate the feasibility of applying the DE imaging technique to tumor localization in radiotherapy.

Methods: We investigated the dependence of DE image quality on the radiological equivalent path length (EPL) of tissues with two phantoms using a stereoscopic x-ray imaging unit. 10 lung cancer patients who underwent radiotherapy each with gold markers implanted in the tumor were enrolled in the study approved by the hospital's Ethics Committee. The displacements of the centroids of the delineated gross tumor volumes (GTVs) in the digitally reconstructed radiograph (DRR) and in the bone-canceled DE image were compared with the averaged displacements of the centroids of gold markers to evaluate the feasibility of using DE imaging for tumor localization.

Results: The results of the phantom study indicated that the contrast-to-noise ratio (CNR) was linearly dependent on the difference of EPL and a mathematical model was established. The objects and backgrounds corresponding to ΔEPL less than 0.08 are visually indistinguishable in the bone-canceled DE image. The analysis of patient data showed that the tumor contrast in the bone-canceled images was improved significantly as compared with that in the original radiographic images and the accuracy of tumor localization using the DE imaging technique was comparable with that of using fiducial makers.

Conclusion: It is feasible to apply the technique for tumor localization in radiotherapy.

Editor: Masaru Katoh, National Cancer Center, Japan

Funding: The authors have no support or funding to report.

Competing Interests: The authors have declared that no competing interests exist.

* Email: fengyu@ecu.edu (YF); wangping@tjmuch.com (PW)

Introduction

As a method for tissue discrimination, dual energy (DE) imaging has been shown to be of good performance in thoracic [1], cardiac [2] and mammographic [3] imaging applications. In DE imaging the acquired images are combined to effectively separate an imaged object into distinct component images of specific tissue types or tissue-selection for generating high contrast images of targeted structures, which can be applied to improve tumor detection for diagnostic interpretation.

Planar kilovoltage (kV) imaging plays an important role in image guidance in radiation therapy (RT) systems, such as CyberKnife (Accuray, Inc., Sunnyvale, CA), ExacTrac (Brainlab AG, Feldkirchen, Germany) and others. It operates by acquiring two radiographs of the patient's anatomy in the treatment room at two different beam angles in real-time and comparing them with pre-generated digitally reconstructed radiographs (DRRs) from the computed tomography (CT) image data used in the RT planning. This procedure is designed to monitor the position variation of the patient's anatomy in the CT coordinate frame [4]. The projection of three dimensional (3D) structures into a two dimensional (2D) image can result in obscuration of the structure of interest such as a lung nodule by overlying structures such as the ribs, which has been identified as a major limiting factor in the detection of lung nodules in radiographs [5].

As DE imaging could provide tissue-selecting images by eliminating the overlying structures, it could bring potential benefits of improved tumor localization if DE imaging can be applied using the kV image guidance unit. Additionally, tumor localization without implanted metallic or radio frequency fiducials may eliminate a number of problems such as pneumothorax and hemorrhage [6]. Previous studies have explored the optimization of DE image acquisition parameters including kVp combinations [7], differential beam filtration and dose allocation [8] based on different image quality metrics such as contrast-to-noise ratio (CNR) [9], signal-to-noise ratio (SNR) [4], signal difference to noise ratio (SDNR) [10] and detectability index [11]. However, much more remains to be investigated quantitatively on the attenuation of x-ray as a function of the properties of the intervening tissues (such as atomic composition, mass density and thickness) in additional to the photon energy [12]. Enhanced discrimination of targeted structures such as tumor tissues through optimized DE imaging can only be achieved through a clear understanding of the effects of intrinsic tissue properties.

The purpose of this report was to quantify the effects of intrinsic tissue properties on tissue discrimination in DE images and to investigate the feasibility of applying the technique in radiotherapy image guidance systems such as the CyberKnife. We first derived the mathematical model for generating bone-canceled images. Then we conducted experimental studies with two phantoms to quantitatively analyze the influence of intrinsic tissue properties (represented by EPL) on the CNR of the image. Finally we applied the DE imaging technique to 10 lung cancer patients to evaluate the accuracy for tumor localization by comparing the results with that using the existing method of implanted fiducial markers.

Materials and Methods

1. Modeling of bone-canceled image

DE imaging exploits differences in the photoelectric and Compton cross sections of different type of tissues in the object as x-ray photon energy varies [13]. Since the photoelectric absorption is dependent sensitively on atomic number, bony structures with high calcium concentration present different image contrast in the high energy (HE) radiograph from that in the low energy (LE) radiograph. Therefore, tissue-selecting image can be obtained by combining the two radiographs of different energies. A common algorithm for DE image reconstruction, derived from the Beer–Lambert law, is to apply a weighted log-subtraction scheme [1]. If we assume that an object consists of bone, lung tissue and other soft tissues, the transmitted intensities of x-ray beams at two different energies of HE and LE can be written as

$$I^L = I_0^L \exp[-(\mu_{Bone}^L t_{Bone} + \mu_{Soft-tissue}^L t_{Soft-tissue} + \mu_{Lung}^L t_{Lung})] \quad (1a)$$

$$I^H = I_0^H \exp[-(\mu_{Bone}^H t_{Bone} + \mu_{Soft-tissue}^H t_{Soft-tissue} + \mu_{Lung}^H t_{Lung})] \quad (1b)$$

where L and H denote LE and HE, respectively, I_0 and I are the intensities of incident and transmitted x-ray beams, μ_{Bone}, $\mu_{Soft-tissue}$, and μ_{Lung} are the linear attenuation coefficients of bone, soft-tissue, and lung tissue respectively, and t_{Bone}, $t_{Soft-tissue}$, and t_{Lung} are the thicknesses of bone, soft-tissue, and lung tissue respectively. Because of the linear relationship with the transmitted intensities, the grey-level values of pixels in a HE or LE image can be expressed by Eq. (1) except a proportional constant.

A "bone-canceled" DE image can be calculated from a pair of HE and LE images as the following,

$$P_{Bone-canceled}^{DE} = \ln(I^H) - w_s \ln(I^L) \quad (2)$$

where $w_s = \mu_{Bone}^H / \mu_{Bone}^L$ is the ratio of the bone attenuation coefficients to the HE beam and to the LE beam used as a weighting coefficient. In practice, because of the difference of imaging systems (such as difference in beam filtration and spectrum of energy, etc.), the calculated value of w_s is not necessarily the ideal value for a specific DE imaging study. In this study, we set up w_s from 0.05 to 1 with a step size of 0.05 in the calculation of bone-canceled DE images and chose the optimized value to best eliminate the bony structures in the DE images. Substituting the I^L and I^H given by Eq. (1a) and (1b) into Eq. (2), one can derive the bone-canceled image as

$$P_{Bone-canceled}^{DE} = \ln(I_0^H) - w_s \ln(I_0^L) - t_{Lung}(\mu_{Lung}^H - w_s \mu_{Lung}^L) - t_{soft-tissue}(\mu_{Soft-tissue}^H - w_s \mu_{Soft-tissue}^L) \quad (3)$$

For the concerned energy range of diagnostic imaging, the x-ray interaction with tissues is dominated by photoelectric absorption and Compton scattering. Attenuation coefficient can therefore be decomposed into two components as given by the following approximate form [14],

$$\mu(E) \approx \rho_e (C_p Z^{3.8} / E^{3.2} + f_{KN}(E)) \quad (4)$$

where $\rho_e C_p Z^{3.8}/E^{3.2}$ provides the photoelectric absorption coefficient with a fitting parameter of $C_p = 9.8 \times 10^{-24}$, photon energy E in keV [14] and Z as the effective atomic number while the Klein-Nishina function $f_{KN}(E)$ yields the electronic cross section of Compton scattering which depends only on E with ρ_e as the electron density. Combining Eq. (3) with Eq. (4) leads to Eq. (5).

$$P_{Bone-canceled}^{DE} = \ln(I_0^H) - w_s \ln(I_0^L) - (t_{Soft-tissue}\rho_{eSoft-tissue} + t_{Lung}\rho_{eLung})\{[f_{KN}(E^H) - w_s f_{KN}(E^L)] + [1/(E^H)^{3.2} - w_s/(E^L)^{3.2}] C_p (Z_{Water})^{3.8}\} \quad (5)$$

Here, we used Z_{Water} to replace $Z_{Soft-tissue}$ and Z_{Lung} due to the following fact. Given the definition of effective atomic number as $Z = (\sum w_i Z_i^{3.5})^{1/3.5}$, with w_i as the weight fraction of the element i of atomic number Z_i [15], the effective atomic number of soft-tissue and lung tissue can be found as 7.5666 and 7.5881, respectively, which are close to Z_{Water} at 7.6843 [16]. To correlate the grey-level values of pixels in the bone-canceled image with the characteristics of the tissues that the x-ray photons transport through, a parameter of radiological equivalent path length (EPL) is used which is usually defined as the summed products of the thickness Δd_i of a bone-excluding tissue component i and the ratio of electron density of the tissue component to that of water ρ_{ei} as given by Eq. (6).

$$\mathrm{EPL} = \sum_i \Delta d_i \rho_{ei} \quad (6)$$

Hence, Eq. (5) can be simplified with EPL,

$$P_{Bone-canceled}^{DE} = \ln(I_0^H) - w_s \ln(I_0^L) - \rho_{eWater} \cdot EPL\{[f_{KN}(E^H) - w_s f_{KN}(E^L)] + [1/(E^H)^{3.2} - w_s/(E^L)^{3.2}] C_p (Z_{Water})^{3.8}\} \quad (7)$$

where EPL accounts for the accumulated equivalent path length that x-ray photons pass through except the tissue to be canceled, i.e., bone.

The model expressed in Eq. (7) correlates the grey-level values of pixels in the bone-canceled image with the characteristics of bone-excluding tissues in terms of the EPL and the photon energies clearly. Therefore, the dependence of the image quality on the tissue properties expressed by EPL and image acquisition parameters can be quantitatively analyzed.

2. Evaluation of image quality

The visibility of targeted structures in a radiograph is largely dependent upon the absolute signal difference and the noise in the image, which can be related to the parameter CNR as defined below,

$$CNR = (\overline{P_{object}} - \overline{P_{background}})/[0.5(\sigma_{object} + \sigma_{background})] \quad (8)$$

where $\overline{P_{object}}$ is the averaged grey-level values of pixels in an object region, and $\overline{P_{background}}$ is the averaged grey-level values of pixels in an adjacent background region. σ_{object} is the standard deviation (SD) of grey-level values in an object region, and $\sigma_{background}$ is the SD of grey-level values in an adjacent background region, which are calculated as the root-mean-square of the grey-level variance for all pixels in the regions respectively. CNR was used in this study for the quantitative evaluation of bone-canceled image quality.

3. Phantom study

We employed two phantoms to investigate the influence of the EPL on the DE image quality. HE and LE radiographs of the phantoms were acquired with the kV radiographic imaging unit of a CyberKnife system (G3, Version 7.1.1). The x-ray detector of the unit has a 20×20 cm^2 field of view (FOV) with a 392 μm pixel size. The geometry of the imaging unit is shown in Figure 1.

Two elliptic cylinder phantoms, a chest phantom (Model 002LFC, CIRS, Norfolk, VA) and an Xsight Lung Tracking (XLT) phantom (Model 18023, CIRS), were used to assess the impacts of the tissue EPL on the quality of bone-canceled image. The first phantom has dimensions of $30 \times 20 \times 30$ cm^3 and simulates the structure of human chest consisting of three tissue equivalent components mimicking soft tissue (water), lung, and bone of which the relative electron densities are 1.002, 0.207, and 1.506, respectively. The second one has an elliptic cylinder configuration with dimensions of $30 \times 20 \times 18$ cm^3 and tissue-equivalent inserts mimicking cortical bone, lung, soft tissue, and a tumor, of which the relative electron densities are 1.782, 0.207, 1.002, and 1.028, respectively.

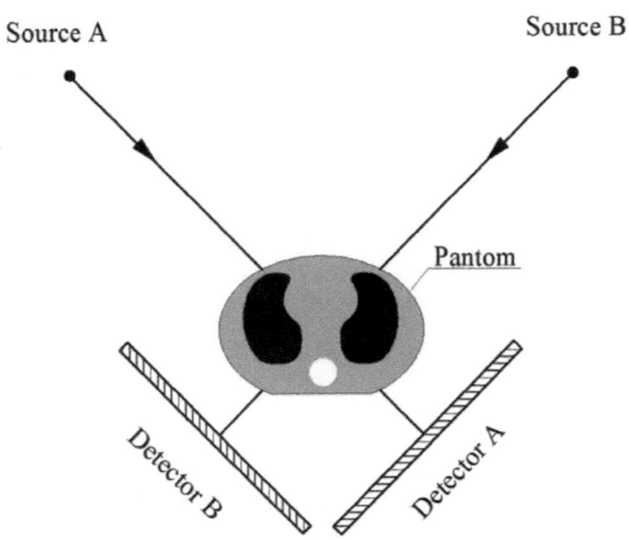

Figure 1. Geometric schematic of the radiographic imaging unit. The imaging system uses 2 diagnostic X-ray sources (Source A and Source B) mounted on the ceiling and paired with 2 flat panel detectors (Detector A and Detector B) with the same source-to-detector distance (SDD) of 3 m to acquire real-time digital radiographic images of the patient. The patient is imaged at 45 degree LAO (left anterior oblique) and RAO (right anterior oblique) angles to facilitate target localization in the 3D space.

According to the published data [8], optimal DE image quality can be achieved with the beam energy combination of 120 kVp and 60 kVp for HE and LE images respectively. With this combination, the milliampere seconds (mAs) were set at 7.5 and 90 for the HE and LE images respectively in our phantom study for obtaining optimal image quality and avoiding overheating of the x-ray tubes during the image acquisition. The bone-canceled images of the chest phantom were obtained by combining the HE and LE images according to Eq. (2). In order to quantify the quality of bone-canceled images with CNRs, twelve ROIs of 12 pixels × 12 pixels in each bone-canceled image were identified with six as the object regions and six as the background regions. Each ROI was divided into 9 sub-areas for the calculation of mean value and SD of CNR. Then the CNRs were calculated using Eq. (8) to quantitatively analyze the impact of EPL. The EPL difference between an object region and a background region normalized by the averaged EPL level of the two regions (ΔEPL) was derived and the correlation between the CNR and ΔEPL was established and tested by evaluating the agreement of the calculated relationship between ΔEPL and CNR among the two different phantoms.

The EPL of each ROI is the averaged value of the region and was calculated according to the method described in the next section.

4. Calculation of EPL

EPL calculation was performed in the volumes of objects represented by their 3D CT image data sets. We used the ray tracing algorithm [17] to track the exact radiological path by propagating the incident x-ray photons through an object's 3D voxels. Following steps were used in the calculation of EPL. First, the 3D volume of a calibration phantom with known electron densities (Model 062, CIRS, Norfolk, VA) was reconstructed from the CT image data acquired with a Brilliance Big Bore CT simulator (Philips, Cleveland, OH) at 120 kVp and 400 mAs. This allowed us to build a look-up table to correlate the electron density of the object with the CT numbers in the 3D image sets acquired by the same scanner. The next step was to identify all voxels on the trajectories of x-ray photons propagating through a study phantom, the XLT or chest phantom, from source to the corresponding pixels of a flat panel detector placed behind the phantom. Once the voxels were identified we could retrieve the electron density values of these voxels from the look-up table based on their CT numbers and distinguish the bony structures at the same time. Finally, the values of EPL on the photon trajectories were summed by integrating along the path excluding bones since they were performed on the bone-canceled images.

5. Feasibility study with patient data

Image data from 10 patients with lung cancers who underwent SBRT with the CyberKnife system were used with the approval of the Ethics Committee of Tianjin Cancer Hospital (#2013-10) and the patients' written consents. Before including a patient in the study, tumor movement range due to respiratory motion was evaluated with fluoroscopic imaging first to minimize the effect of motion artifacts. Patients with tumor movement ranges of less than

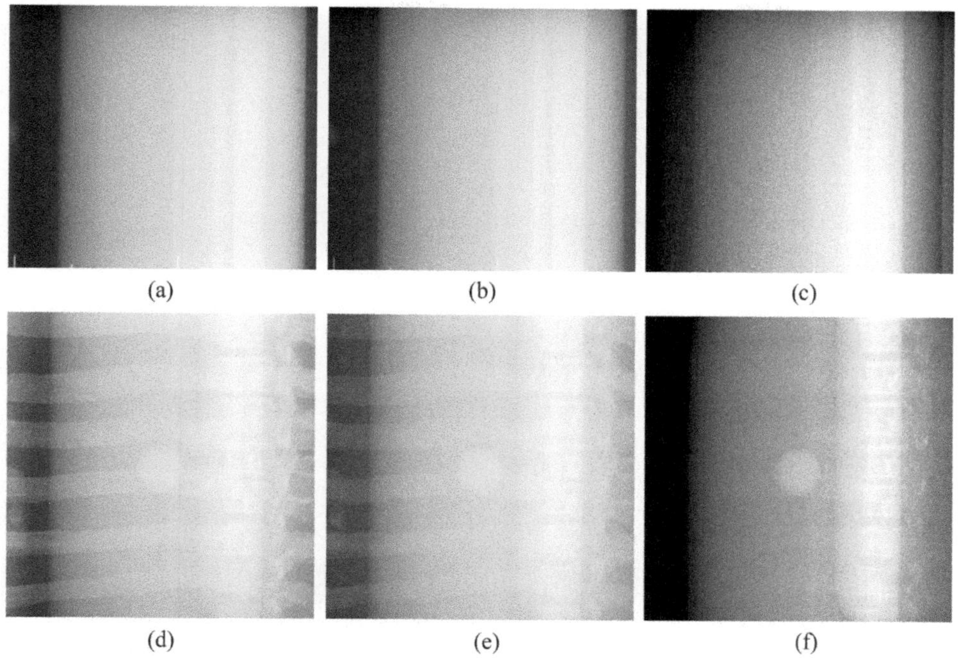

Figure 2. Radiographic images of chest phantom. (a), (b), and (c) are the images of chest phantom at 60 kVp, 120 kVp, and the bone-canceled image by combining (a) and (b), respectively. (d), (e), and (f) are the images of XLT phantom at 60 kVp, 120 kVp, and the bone-canceled image by combining (d) and (e), respectively.

12 mm in a respiration cycle were selected and then trained for holding their body still and exercising shallower breathing before the image acquisition. Radiographic images of HE and LE were obtained sequentially during the radiation delivery at the same phases of respiration which was guaranteed by the synchrony respiratory tracking system. We also chose to only include patients who had nodule size $\geq$ 10 mm in diameter as the identification of small nodules is still problematic for DE imaging [18]. Image data from 10 patients were selected. Each patient had at least three gold fiducial markers implanted before their CT simulation for treatment planning. And the maximum displacement of the tumors was checked with the markers to be $\leq$ 0.23 mm between the HE and LE images at the same phases of respiration.

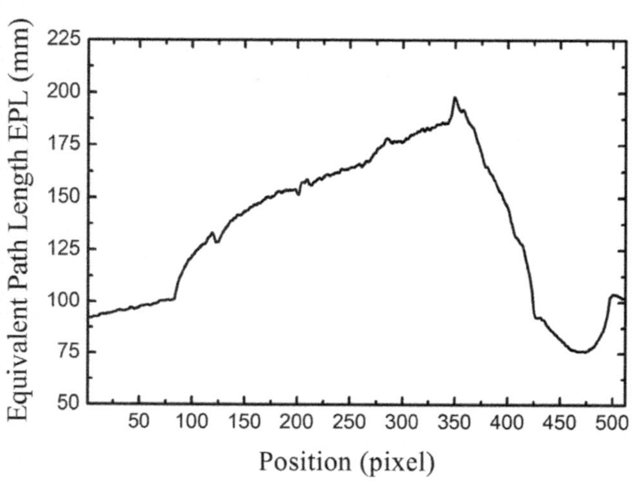

Figure 3. Averaged EPL per pixel column in the bone-canceled image of chest phantom.

The DRRs generated with the simulation CT image data for the image guidance of the treatment were used for comparison in the study, which carried the projected gross tumor volume (GTV) contours delineated in the CT images by an experienced radiation oncologist. HE and LE images (120 kVp, 100 mA, 75 ms and 60 kVp, 250 mA, 150 ms) were acquired with the image guidance unit before the start of treatment. Then bone-canceled images were obtained using the above discussed method and the GTVs were delineated in the bone-canceled images using an algorithm for automatically detecting pulmonary nodules in chest x-ray images [19]. The averaged displacement of the gold marker centroids between in the DRR and in the bone-canceled image was used as the reference for the GTV position variance analysis for each patient. The difference between the variation of the centroid of the delineated GTV in the DRR and in the bone-canceled image and the averaged variation of gold marker centroids in the two image sets was used to quantify the accuracy and evaluate the feasibility of the proposed DE imaging method for GTV localization. To quantitatively evaluate the improvement of tumor contrast, CNRs of the tumors in the radiographs at LE and HE, and in the bone-canceled DE images were calculated respectively using the same method as described in Section 2.3.

Statistical analysis was performed with GraphPad Prism 6 (GraphPad Software, Inc., La Jolla, CA). A 2-sided Student's t-test was used to compare the displacement between fiducial centroids and the GTV centroids, and evaluate the improvement of CNR of tumors with the DE imaging technique. A p-value of less than or equal to 0.05 was regarded as statistically significant.

Results

1. Influence of ΔEPL on CNR

Figures 2(a) and 2(b) show the planar x-ray images of the chest phantom at 60 kVp and 120 kVp, respectively, and Figure 2 (c) is the bone-canceled image calculated from these two images.

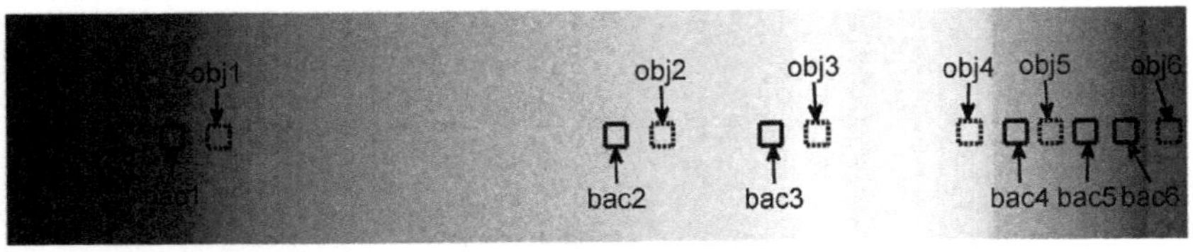

Figure 4. ROIs used in CNR-ΔEPL analysis of the bone-canceled image of chest phantom.

Figure 3 is the averaged EPL corresponding to every column in the image (512 columns) which was calculated according to the method described above. By comparing Figure 2(c) and Figure 3, it can be observed that the EPL is proportional to the grey-level value of the corresponding pixel, which corroborates with the model expressed in Eq. (7). Measurement of CNR in Figure 2(c) and data fitting using the linear-least-squares method showed that a linear relationship exists between CNR and ΔEPL. The result was evaluated with the parameter of coefficient of determination R^2, which indicates how well measured data fit a statistical model and ranges from 0 to 1 with 1 indicating a perfect fit. The evaluation yielded a very high R^2 value (0.99), which means that the CNR in bone-canceled image as a function of ΔEPL can be expressed by Eq. (9). Figure 4 plots the CNR against ΔEPL, the dots represent measured data and the solid line is the modeled result.

$$\mathrm{CNR} = 22.35 \times \Delta\mathrm{EPL} + \delta \tag{9}$$

Because of noise, CNR can fluctuate in DE image for tissue trajectories with same EPL which is represented by δ in Eq. (9). Figure 2 (d) and (e) show the planar x-ray images of the XLT phantom acquired at 60 kVp and 120 kVp, respectively, and Figure 2(f) is the bone-canceled image. The CNR dependence on ΔEPL as expressed in Eq. (9) was also verified with the XLT phantom with the slope given by 23.29 and the difference was 4.2% between the two phantoms. Therefore, for the image guidance unit, the correlation of CNR with ΔEPL can be written as

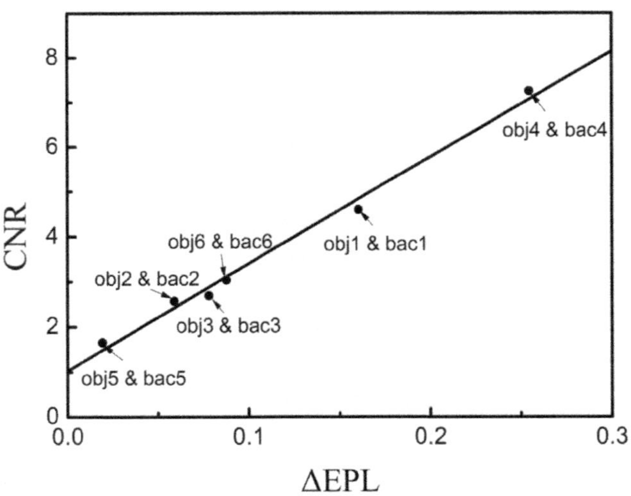

Figure 5. CNR versus ΔEPL in the bone-canceled image of chest phantom.

$$\mathrm{CNR} = k \times \Delta\mathrm{EPL} + \delta \tag{10}$$

where k is a system parameter with value around 22.8 and equal to the averaged value of the slope for the two phantoms.

Figure 4 presents the bone-canceled image with ROIs of the chest phantom selected for the CNR calculation, and the corresponding CNR values are indicated in Figure 5. The squares in dash line are the object ROIs (marked as obj) while the ones in solid line are the background ROIs (marked as bac). By visual inspection, one can find that the visual differences between the ROI pairs of obj2 and bac2, obj3 and bac3, obj5 and bac5 cannot be observed; the visual differences between the ROI pairs of obj1 and bac1, obj4 and bac4, obj6 and bac6 can be observed. And the smallest observable difference in the image is between the pair of obj6 and bac6, of which the CNR is 2.57 ± 0.34 (Mean ± SD). According to Figure 5, when CNR = 2.91 (2.57+0.34), ΔEPL is 0.08, therefore, when ΔEPL is greater than 0.08, the difference between the object and the background in the bone-canceled image can be discriminated. In comparison, objects and backgrounds corresponding to ΔEPL less than 0.08 are visually indistinguishable.

2. Study with patient data

Figure 6 shows the DRRs, radiographic images and bone-canceled images of one of the patients. Calculation of CNR for the tumors showed that the mean value and SD of CNR of the 10 tumors was 5.22 ± 2.96 in LE images, 7.43 ± 3.33 in HE images and 8.29 ± 3.56 in DE images, respectively. The p-value was 0.16 for the CNR in HE images versus in LE images, 0.01 for the CNR in DE images versus in LE images, and 0.03 for the CNR in DE images versus in HE images, respectively. This indicates that tumor contrast in the bone-canceled images is improved significantly as compared with those in the original planar radiographic images. The GTVs in the DRRs were projected from the planning RT data which were delineated and confirmed by an experienced radiation oncologist. And the contours in the radiographs were delineated with the automatic tumor detection algorithm as discussed above. Using the displacement of GTV centroid to represent the variation of tumor location, we compared the displacements of the fiducial centroids and the GTV centroids. The results are shown in Table 1. With a 2-sided Student's t-test, we found the p-value was 0.53 indicating that the variation measured by the two methods does not exhibit significant difference.

Discussion

Dual-energy imaging technique holds promise to provide valuable information for improving target or tumor localization. However, its implementation as a practical clinical tool requires a clear understanding of the underlying mechanism for optimizing the image acquisition process and quality assurance. Specifically

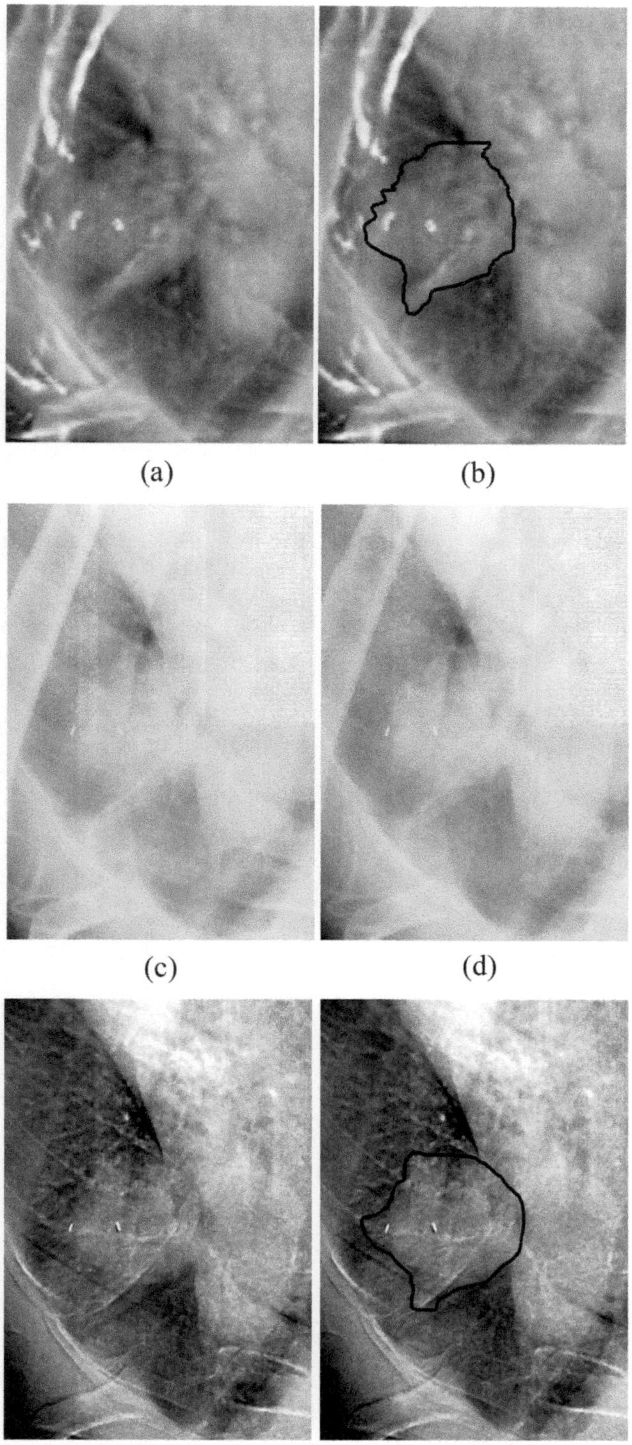

(a) (b) (c) (d) (e) (f)

Figure 6. DRRs and radiographs of a patient. (a) DRR of a patient, (b) DRR with the projected GTV contour, (c) radiograph at LE, (d) radiograph at HE, (e) bone-canceled image by pairing two original radiographs, and (f) bone-canceled image with the GTV contour automatically segmented.

one needs to quantitatively characterize the intrinsic tissue properties to accurately assess the discrimination of targets. For this purpose, we have analyzed the DE imaging process and derived an expression for the image contrast CNR in terms of EPL which allows quantification of the target localization in a DE image.

Table 1. Displacements of GTV centroids and fiducial markers.

Patient	D[a] of GTV centroids (mm)	D[a] of fiducials (mm)
1	4.22	4.22
2	6.36	4.36
3	5.63	3.05
4	6.67	6.06
5	9.37	7.82
6	6.09	6.63
7	1.11	0.40
8	15.03	11.94
9	3.11	3.15
10	2.81	2.50
Mean[b]	6.04	5.10
SD[c]	3.93	3.26

[a]D: Displacement.
[b]Mean: mean value.
[c]SD: standard deviation.

Previously published studies focused mainly on the effect of phantom size on the quality of image. For example, Kappadath et al. employed a phantom consisting of different aluminum strips to simulate calcifications and breast-tissue-equivalent materials to evaluate the CNR in tissue-canceled DE images under the conditions of different strip thicknesses or glandular ratios [9]. The results showed that the CNR increases with increasing aluminum strip thickness and decreases with increasing glandular ratio in DE image, which is consistent with our results. However, the strip thickness used in that study differs from the realistic clinical situations. In contrast we utilized the anthropomorphic phantoms and the EPL to study the influence of intrinsic tissue properties with of improved clinical relevance. Although the qualitative relationship between EPL and CNR agrees with previous studies, the values of CNR obtained in our study differ because of the large variation in the imaging systems. As the image quality is influenced by detector performance such as the modulation transfer function (MTF), the noise-power spectrum (NPS), and the noise-equivalent quanta (NEQ), the image quality of different imaging system and CNR can vary widely. Therefore, it is necessary to calibrate the CNR-ΔEPL curve according to the specifications of each imaging system.

Finally, we would like to point out that the feasibility study with data of 10 patients has indicated that the tumor in the bone-canceled image as shown in Figure 6 can be easily seen with higher contrast than those in the planar radiographs. We expect that the DE imaging technique has the potential as a powerful tool for tumor localization. There are other advanced image processing methods and imaging techniques, such as rib suppression method [20] or MRI, which could provide similar image quality or superior soft tissue discrimination. But the feasibility for tumor localization in radiotherapy treatment with these advanced methods yet to be quantitatively evaluated.

Conclusion

CNR is linearly dependant on ΔEPL in bone-canceled DE images and the relationship can be shown with a mathematical model as given by Eq. (10). The contrast for tumors in the bone-canceled images is improved significantly as compared with the one in the planar radiographic images and the accuracy of tumor localization using the DE imaging technique has been demonstrated to be comparable with that of using fiducial makers. Therefore, it is feasible to apply the technique for tumor localization in radiotherapy. Comprehensive clinical study with more patient data to model DE image quality with intrinsic tissue properties for tumor localization is ongoing and the results will be presented after completion of the study.

Author Contributions

Conceived and designed the experiments: JH YF PW. Performed the experiments: YD ZY PW. Analyzed the data: JH YF XW XZ GW. Wrote the paper: JH XH YF. Final approval of the version to be published: YF.

References

1. Sabol JM, Avinash GB, Nicolas F, Claus BEH, Zhao J, et al. (2001) The development and characterization of a dual-energy subtraction imaging system for chest radiography based on CsI: Tl amorphous silicon flat-panel technology. Proc. SPIE 2001: 399–408.
2. Ducote JL, Xu T, Molloi S. (2007) Dual-energy cardiac imaging: an image quality and dose comparison for a flat-panel detector and x-ray image intensifier. Phys. Med Biol 52(1):183–96.
3. Arvanitis CD, Speller R. (2009) Quantitative contrast-enhanced mammography for contrast medium kinetics studies. Phys Med Biol 54(20):6041–64.
4. Murphy MJ, Adler JR, Bodduluri M, Dooley J, Forster K, et al. (2000) Image-guided radiosurgery for the spine and pancreas. Comput Aided Surg 5(4):278–88.
5. Samei E, Flynn MJ, Eyler WR. (1999) Detection of subtle lung nodules: relative influence of quantum and anatomic noise on chest radiographs. Radiology 213(3):727–34.
6. Collins BT, Erickson K, Reichner CA, Collins SP, Gagnon GJ, et al. (2007) Radical stereotactic radiosurgery with real-time tumor motion tracking in the treatment of small peripheral lung tumors. Radiat Oncol 2(39): 2(39), 717X–2.
7. Williams DB, Siewerdsen JH, Tward DJ, Paul NS, Dhanantwari AC, et al. (2007) Optimal kVp selection for dual-energy imaging of the chest: Evaluation by task-specific observer preference tests. Med Phys 34(10):3619–25.
8. Shkumat NA, Siewerdsen JH, Dhanantwari AC, Williams DB, Richard S, et al. (2007) Optimization of image acquisition techniques for dual-energy imaging of the chest. Med Phys 34(10):3904–15.
9. Kappadath SC, Shaw CC. (2004) Quantitative evaluation of dual-energy digital mammography for calcification imaging. Phys Med Biol 49(12):2563–76.
10. Carton AK, Ullberg C, Lindman K, Acciavatti R, Francke T, et al. (2010) Optimization of a dual-energy contrast-enhanced technique for a photon-counting digital breast tomosynthesis system: I. A theoretical model. Med Phys 37(11):5896–5907.
11. Richard S, Siewerdsen JH. (2006) Optimization of dual-energy imaging systems using generalized NEQ and imaging task. Med Phys 34(1):127–39.
12. Yeh BM, Shepherd JA, Wang ZJ, Teh HS, Hartman R, et al. (2009) Dual-Energy and Low-kVp CT in the Abdomen. AJR 193(1):47–54.
13. Richard S, Siewerdsen JH, Jaffray DA, Moseley DJ, Bakhtiar B. (2005) Generalized DQE analysis of radiographic and dual-energy imaging using flat-panel detectors. Med Phys 32(5):1397–413.
14. Lehmann LA, Alvarez RE, Macovski A, Brody WR, Pelc NJ, et al. (1981) Generalized image combinations in dual KVP digital radiography. Med Phys 8(5):659–67.
15. Bazatova M, Carrier JF, Beautieu L, Verhaegen F. (2008) Tissue segmentation in Monte Carlo treatment planning: A simulation study using dual-energy CT images. Radiother Oncol 86(1):93–98.
16. International Commission on Radiation Units and Measurements. (1989) Tissue substitutes in radiation dosimetry and measurement. ICRU Report 44.
17. Siddon RL. (1985) Fast calculation of exact radiological path for a three-dimensional CT array. Med Phys 12(2):252–55.
18. Szucs-Farkas Z, Patak MA, Yuksel-Hatz S, Ruder T, Vock P. (2008) Single-exposure dual-energy subtraction chest radiography: Detection of pulmonary nodules and masses in clinical practice. Eur Radiol 18(1):24–31.
19. Schilham AMR, van Ginneken B, Loog M. (2006) Computer-aided diagnosis system for detection of lung nodules in chest radiographs with an evaluation on a public database. Med Image Anal 10(2):247–58.
20. Szucs-Farkas Z, Schick A, Cullmann JL, Ebnerl L, Megyeri B et al (2013) Comparison of Dual-Energy Subtraction and Electronic Bone Suppression Combined With Computer-Aided Detection on Chest Radiographs: Effect on Human Observers' Performance in Nodule Detection. AJR 200(5):1006–13.

Erythrocyte Stiffness during Morphological Remodeling Induced by Carbon Ion Radiation

Baoping Zhang[1,2,3], Bin Liu[3,4], Hong Zhang[4], Jizeng Wang[1,2,3]*

1 School of Civil Engineering and Mechanics, Lanzhou University, Lanzhou, 730000, PR China, 2 Key Laboratory of Mechanics on Disaster and Environment in Western China, The Ministry of Education of China, Lanzhou University, 730000, PR China, 3 Institute of Biomechanics and Medical Engineering, Lanzhou University, Lanzhou, 730000, PR China, 4 Department of Heavy Ion Radiation Medicine, Institute of Modern Physics, Chinese Academy of Sciences, Lanzhou 730000, PR China

Abstract

The adverse effect induced by carbon ion radiation (CIR) is still an unavoidable hazard to the treatment object. Thus, evaluation of its adverse effects on the body is a critical problem with respect to radiation therapy. We aimed to investigate the change between the configuration and mechanical properties of erythrocytes induced by radiation and found differences in both the configuration and the mechanical properties with involving in morphological remodeling process. Syrian hamsters were subjected to whole-body irradiation with carbon ion beams (1, 2, 4, and 6 Gy) or X-rays (2, 4, 6, and 12 Gy) for 3, 14 and 28 days. Erythrocytes in peripheral blood and bone marrow were collected for cytomorphological analysis. The mechanical properties of the erythrocytes were determined using atomic force microscopy, and the expression of the cytoskeletal protein spectrin-α1 was analyzed via western blotting. The results showed that dynamic changes were evident in erythrocytes exposed to different doses of carbon ion beams compared with X-rays and the control (0 Gy). The magnitude of impairment of the cell number and cellular morphology manifested the subtle variation according to the irradiation dose. In particular, the differences in the size, shape and mechanical properties of the erythrocytes were well exhibited. Furthermore, immunoblot data showed that the expression of the cytoskeletal protein spectrin-α1 was changed after irradiation, and there was a common pattern among its substantive characteristics in the irradiated group. Based on these findings, the present study concluded that CIR could induce a change in mechanical properties during morphological remodeling of erythrocytes. According to the unique characteristics of the biomechanical categories, we deduce that changes in cytomorphology and mechanical properties can be measured to evaluate the adverse effects generated by tumor radiotherapy. Additionally, for the first time, the current study provides a new strategy for enhancing the assessment of the curative effects and safety of clinical radiotherapy, as well as reducing adverse effects.

Editor: Juan Carlos del Alamo, University of California San Diego, United States of America

Funding: This work was supported by grants from the National Natural Science Foundation of China (grants No. 11032006, No. 11072094, and No. 11121202), the PhD Program Foundation of the Ministry of Education of China (grant No. 20100211110022), and New Century Excellent Talents in University (program No. NCET-10-0445). The funders had no role in study design, data collection and analysis, decision to publish, or preparation of the manuscript.

Competing Interests: The authors have declared that no competing interests exist.

* Email: jizengwangibme@gmail.com

Introduction

Ionizing radiation and radiotherapy commonly encounter problems not only due to the action of the treated tumor but also due to the adverse effects of irradiation on non-target cells or tissues [1]. Over the past decades, due to their high targeting ability and distinct curative effects, radioactive rays and ion beams have been intensively researched. Thus, special charged ion beam-carbon ion beams (CIBs) have great potential for the development of radiation therapy. Because CIBs have a special energy beam path, the so-called Bragg peak characteristic of its occurrence provides a higher relative biological effectiveness (RBE) than low linear energy transfer (LET) radiation (X-rays, γ-rays and electron beams) [2,3]. Thus, heavy ion beams ($^{12}C^{6+}$ ions) can precisely target the nidus and avoid energy loss, leading to improved targeting with greater curative effect and better local control at the tumor site than is possible with conventional X-rays or similar treatments [4,5]. However, although the beams have many advantages in their application, the adverse effects of treatment caused by the rays themselves remain an inevitable problem. Improving the maximum targeting of radiation therapy and reducing its adverse effects on normal cells remain major research focuses for tumor radiotherapy. Previous studies mainly emphasized the direct effects of cellular lethality caused by the irradiation of human organs or tissues [6] or investigated these aspects within the context of chromosomal rearrangement and mutation in the genetic material arising from energy deposition [7–9]. Additionally, whether the therapeutic success that is possible with X-ray treatment can also be achieved with heavy ion radiation is a major question.

The organs of the blood and hematopoietic systems are vulnerable to radiation [10–14]. Indeed, many studies have shown that radiation can cause a decrease in the visible components of blood [15], cell morphology changes, alterations to the electrolyte state in peripheral blood (PB), mild hyperplasia in the bone marrow (BM) [16], serious inhibition or even destruction of the bone marrow [17,18], a reduction in the production of erythrocytes [19], changes in the aggregation state of platelets [20], and induction of the transformation of normal stem cells into tumor stem cells [20–22]. Thus, a hemogram of the blood system is often used initially as an approximate guide to assess the adverse effects caused by radiotherapy to the human body. Indeed, CIR may cause changes of in the hemogram and myelogram. Likewise, biological function and morphology must be in conformity with each other to determine the occurrence of disease. However, several investigations have indicated that radiation induces a series of complex and dynamic changes in cell shape as well as membrane damage and that a close relationship exists among the membrane skeleton components [23] and the function and antioxidant effects of electrolytes [9], [24]–such as changes in cell membrane permeability and alterations of the membrane and cytoskeleton–which can cause changes in the membrane, including organizational and metabolic changes [25], eventually leading to cell dysfunction.

Some considerable insights have already been obtained concerning the physiological or pathological processes of cell movement, invasion and migration through cell biomechanics research. Presently, cell mechanics are favored for understanding the problem. Additionally, not only is the cell membrane considered a very important factor in the response to damage; the cytoskeleton also plays a key role, being the most direct embodiment of cell morphology changes. For instance, the role of cytoskeletal morphological remodeling in tumor development is a crucial problem. Thus far, very few studies have assessed the biomechanical principles underlying the cytoskeletal morphological remodeling induced by radiation to evaluate the safety of ion radiotherapy in the human body through using morphological remodeling mechanics at the cellular level to understand how heavy ion radiation affects organs and tissues of the body from the perspective of biomechanics. This study investigates the mechanical properties of the membrane surface, cytoskeletal morphological remodeling and cytoskeletal protein levels to clarify the morphological remodeling process of the cytoskeleton. Normal erythrocytes have good mechanical properties that depend on an equilibrium state between two parameters–morphological motion and deformations–in particular, the geometric shape and biophysical characteristics of the spherical surface area, the viscosity of the cytoplasm, and the elasticity of the membrane. Alteration of any of these factors can lead to the differences in the cell membrane and the cytoskeletal structure. Previous studies have shown that some erythrocyte-related diseases are associated with the following three significant characteristics: the typical biconcave disc shape, the phospholipid bilayer membrane and the cytoskeleton meshwork. If these shape-changing agents cause area differences between the change in membrane morphology and mechanical properties of the cell, the process of the disease is altered [26]. Therefore, the size and shape, the phospholipid bilayer membrane and the cytoskeletal network govern the deformation and damage of erythrocytes and are widely considered to represent changes in biological behavior or function [27–29]. Typical illnesses related to erythrocyte dysfunction include malaria [30–34], sickle cell anemia [35,36], hemolytic anemia [37,38], cancer [39], spherocytosis and elliptocytosis [30], [40], and diabetes mellitus [41]. Thus, it has been vital to study the pathophysiology of these diseases [27], [42,43].

Biological-type atomic force microscopy (BT-AFM) can allow the direct visualization of cell morphology changes in erythrocytes at the micro-nano level using an inverted microscope and measurement of the mechanical properties of biological specimens [44,45]. However, measurement of the dynamic properties of cells as a characteristic feature can provide important information regarding their physical state [46,47]. Current literature has suggested that altering the physical properties of the cytoplasm and membrane-cytoskeleton in erythrocytes can result in morphologically distinct signals [46], [48]. Thus, the remarkable changes in erythrocyte morphology result from a coupled dynamic response of the phospholipid bilayer membrane and an elastic spectrin molecular meshwork on the cytoplasmic face [27], [31], [42], [49–51]. Generally, erythrocyte damage depends on the phospholipid bilayer membrane of an adult red cell (mainly including membrane proteins or enzymatic erythrocyte defects), which is supported on its inner surface by a complex arrangement of spectrin-spectrin molecular interactions of cytoskeletal proteins (membrane skeleton). A major component of cytoskeletal proteins is the neofunctionalized protein spectrin, called an erythrocyte "ghost", that was first reported to be isolated from human erythrocytes in 1968 by Marchesi and Steers [52,53]. Studies have demonstrated that some examples of unhealthy cell morphology changes produce adverse outcomes, and these changes were focused on the interactions between the cell membrane and the cytoskeleton [50], [54,55]. Additionally, previous theoretical research has contributed to a reliance on numerical modeling for the analysis of the membrane shape and surface free energy [48], [56–60], partly revealing the time-dependent relationship between the shape changes and deformability of erythrocytes [61], as well as displaying the elastic response of erythrocytes to small and large deformations [62–65]. Therefore, through quantitative measurement of the inherent behavior of erythrocytes, such as the elasticity of the cell membrane (cell stiffness), cell membrane contributions to the local or nonlocal bending deformation in the process of damage, changes in tension in the membrane-skeleton system, and the membrane surface area and size of erythrocytes [66], the degree of erythrocyte damage can be further assessed.

Herein, this paper will provide further insight into the adverse effects in erythrocytes related to radiation by examining the changes in microstructure and mechanical properties that have been used to analyze the functional relationship of erythrocytes before and after irradiation. We investigated whether subtle changes in the morphology and mechanical properties of cells can be used to assess the effects of radiation and to better depict the correlations among signal molecules involved in the configuration of the cytoskeleton, cell morphology changes, and the dynamic mechanical properties of cells in the process of damage. Based on these attempts, we focused on a new method of explaining the deformation or damage via the mechanical mechanism of erythrocyte morphological remodeling in different irradiated groups. Thus, according to the established parameters and these insights, we hypothesized the quantitation of the degree of erythrocyte damage to better explain cytoskeleton signaling dominated by biochemical molecules involved in the erythrocyte cytoskeleton morphological remodeling process, the biomechanical mechanism underlying erythrocyte induction by irradiation, and the relationship between the erythrocyte shape and injury rate to provide a theoretical base. In the present article, cell stiffness was chosen to meticulously estimate biological and adverse effects in erythrocytes during irradiation. Finally, this new perspective should be exploited to develop biomechanics to better assess the onset or progression of damage caused by ionizing radiation and to identify novel potential biomechanical targets or characteristics for therapeutic interventions.

Materials and Methods

Animals

SPF-class female Syrian golden hamsters (6–8 weeks old and weighing 80–100 g) provided by the Lanzhou Institute of Biological Products (Lanzhou, China) were used in the current study. All of the animals were maintained under standardized conditions (temperature, 22±2°C; humidity, 40±10%; light/dark cycle, 12 h:12 h) and given standard food and water ad libitum. The animal experimental protocols were approved by the Animal Experiment Medicine Center of Lanzhou University. A total of 156 hamsters were randomly divided into three groups: a carbon ion irradiation group (1 Gy, 2 Gy, 4 Gy, or 6 Gy; six hamsters per group), an X-ray irradiation group (2 Gy, 4 Gy, 6 Gy, or 12 Gy; six hamsters per group), and a control non-irradiated group (0 Gy; twelve hamsters per group).

Irradiation procedure

Each hamster was positioned in a chamber attached to the irradiation equipment at the Heavy Ion Research Facility in Lanzhou (HIRFL, Institute of Modern Physics, Chinese Academy of Sciences, Lanzhou, China). The whole body of the hamster was irradiated with $^{12}C^{6+}$ ion beams at an energy of 270 MeV/u and LET of 10 keV/m, with a dose rate of 0.3 Gy/min. When $^{12}C^{6+}$ ion beams at 200 MeV/u and 31.3 keV/m of the beam entered the chamber, the $^{12}C^{6+}$ ion dose of 0.5 Gy corresponded to a fluence of 3.0×10^7 particles/cm^2. The carbon ions were equipped with a passive beam delivery system. The data were controlled automatically by a microcomputer during irradiation. Particle fluences were determined from an air-ionization chamber signal according to the calibration of the detector (PTW-UNIDOS; PTW-Freiburg Co., Wiesbaden, Germany). Similarly, animals exposed to X-rays were given whole-body radiation using an X-ray therapy machine (Elekta BMEI Medical Equipment Co. Ltd, Beijing, China) at a source-to-surface distance (SSD) of 100 cm and a dose rate of 2 Gy/min [67].

Preparation of erythrocytes in peripheral blood and bone marrow

The experiments complied with the laboratory animal disposal regulations of the Animal Ethics Committee at Lanzhou University. Animals were sacrificed at different time points to collect peripheral blood (PB) and bone marrow (BM) following treatment with different doses of radiation. Briefly, fresh peripheral blood and bone marrow were retrieved from the hamsters. First, the animals were anesthetized with 0.3% pentobarbital sodium at the injection concentration range of 30–35 mg/kg body weight. After adequate anesthetization, dissection was performed, the abdominal vein was exposed, and then the blood from the abdominal vein was retrieved using an anti-coagulated tube containing EDTA. After the plasma and buffy coat were removed, the erythrocytes were washed three times in an iso-osmotic HEPES-Ringer's buffer [68] (centrifugation at $1000\times g$ for 10 min at room temperature (RT)). Following the final wash, the erythrocytes were resuspended in HEPES-Ringer's buffer (100 mM NaCl, 10 mM HEPES, 4 mM KCl, 1 mM $CaCl_2$, 0.7 mM NaH_2PO_4, 0.6 mM $MgSO_4$, and 5 mM glucose) with 1 mg/mL of bovine serum albumin (BSA). The final dilution of the erythrocyte pellet ranged from 1:10,000 to 1:50,000, which was sufficient to separate individual erythrocytes by several cell diameters on a microscope slide. Erythrocyte ghosts were prepared from these samples by hemolysis using a standard procedure [69] and phosphate-buffered saline (PBS, 151.2 mmol/L NaCl, 5.6 mmol/L KCl, 5.48 mmol/L Na_2HPO_4, 0.32 mmol/L NaH_2PO_4, pH 7.4, osmotic pressure 300 mosmol/kg). First, one drop of the suspension was placed on a glass substrate treated with poly-L-lysine (P4832; Sigma) and was then incubated for 1 hour at 37°C. Next, one drop of 0.5% glutaraldehyde was added for 1.5 min to fix the erythrocyte membrane to the substrate. Finally, the pretreated cells were washed with phosphate buffer solution to remove the unbound cells and glutaraldehyde. The samples were immediately subjected to AFM.

The whole femurs of hamsters were dissected, and then the bone was cut from the knee to the hip buttock to better expose the bone marrow (BM). With a pointed tip, the area around the bone marrow was mixed evenly. The bone marrow was removed (approximately 0.5 mm^3) with the tips of a pair of tweezers, and its color and status were then recorded to prior loading into 1.5–2.0 mL of serum in vitro. The bone marrow-serum mixture was mixed by aspiration with a glass dropper tip approximately 20 times until the mixture was evenly dispersed, carefully avoiding the production of bubbles. Finally, using a trace sample gun, 50 μl of the bone marrow fluid (depending on the amount of bone marrow retrieved) was removed to be applied to a centrifugal smear machine small funnel at 600–800 r/min using a 10-min medium speed centrifuge. The pre-coated glass slide with the cells was removed, and the follow-up test was completed.

Cytological analysis of the proportion of irradiated erythrocytes in the bone marrow

BM smear samples were prepared on different of substrates using three glass slides: one slide was used for Swiss-Giemsa staining, another was used to determine the number of nucleated cells in the BM, and the third was counted at low magnification. The BM cytological report contained four grades of activity: hyperactive, active, reduced and significantly reduced. Additionally, the erythroid cells in the BM smear were classified into four clinical types–pronormoblasts, basophilic erythroblasts, polychromatophilic erythroblasts and normoblasts–and then the proportion of the total number of nucleated cells was determined under oil. According to cell counting principles, the samples were divided into three types–low, medium and high cell count. Additionally, each slide was observed no fewer than 30 times, and each observation involved the selection of several fields for statistical processing parameters.

Atomic force microscopy analysis of the changes in morphology and mechanical properties in erythrocytes induced by CIR or X-rays

A NanoWizard III AFM (JPK Instruments, Germany) mounted on an inverted optical microscope (Axiovert 200; Carl Zeiss Microimaging) was used for cell imaging and force spectroscopy. Silicon nitride cantilevers (PNP-DB; NanoWorld) with a nominal spring constant of 0.06 N/m (f_o: 17 kHz) were used in all of the experiments. For each cantilever, the spring constant was determined using the thermal noise constant calibration method. To ensure reproducibility in force application, the cantilever sensitivity and spring constant were calibrated before each experiment using JPK Instruments software 4.2.61. The optical microscope was used to select the desired cell and position the AFM tip. All of the AFM images and measurements were obtained in contact mode in air.

AFM imaging and measurement

Erythrocyte imaging was performed on glass slides at RT. The AFM had a maximum scanning range from 50×50 μm bar (Fast × Slow) to 5×5 μm bar (Fast × Slow) and a vertical range (Z-direction) of 15 μm. Pretreated cells were imaged using a pixel resolution of 512 pixels at a line rate of 0.10–0.30 Hz. The imaging parameters were carefully monitored to achieve good contrast with scanning forces as determined from force distance curves in the experiment. Elastic modulus (cell stiffness) determination is detailed in Section 2.5.2 below. Regarding radiation dose changes, a series of 50–100 curves of elastic modulus measurements in the erythrocytes was performed for each specimen in which the probe was placed over the sample surface and then pushed against the sample. The force acting between the tip and the sample caused a deflection of the cantilever that was recorded as a function of the relative sample position as a force curve. **Figure 1** shows two curves, one obtained from a soft erythrocyte and the other from a hard material. After subtraction of these two curves, the force-versus-indentation curve was obtained. In this experiment, the glass coverslip was taken as a zero-reference hard surface and was used for calibration, and the calibration curve was recorded each time together with a newly prepared erythrocyte sample. Ultimately, all of the AFM data were acquired and analyzed using two proprietary codes–a topographical image analysis code and a code for force curve analysis–using JPK instruments data processing software version 4.2.61.

Elastic modulus determination

Using AFM for nanoindentation is a useful tool to determine elastic properties such as the elastic modulus of biological samples [61], [70–73]. Cantilevers serve as soft nanoindenters that allow local testing of small and inhomogeneous samples such as cells or tissues. To calculate the parameter of interest, various models are used, but most of them are based on the Hertz model, modified to match the experimental conditions concerning the indenter's shape or the thickness of the sample [74–76]. The cell elastic modulus was calculated by applying the modified Hertz model contact theory to the force curves [35], [75], [77,78]. Thus, it is assumed that the surface is continuous, frictionless and incompressible (similar to rubber) at small deformations [79], and also consider the indentation is considered to be negligible compared with the sample thickness, to reflect the real situation of the cells and to ensure that the indentation depth is optimized. The Hertz model is valid for small indentations (5–10% of the height of the cell, approximately, 200–500 nm) where the substrate does not influence the calculations [45], [78], [80]. There may be additional limitations in the indentation depth if the tip shape model is an approximation.

In the present study, tiny force probes were employed during the entire experimental process, and the probes were modified by attaching 6-μm diameter polystyrene microspheres (Base Line Chromtech Research Centre, Tianjin, China) onto the cantilever with epoxy resin glue (Epoxy F-05 Clear; Alteco, Japan). Additionally, the cell deformation nonlinearity was reduced due to a more homogeneous contact between the cells and probe. Elastic modulus measurements were derived from the force-distance profiles (extended curves) acquired at different locations on the cells, and JPK instruments software was used for this purpose. Microprobes were positioned on the cell membrane under optical control, in accordance with the method described by Ketene [81], and force curves were acquired at a sampling rate of 5 kHz and a constant approach velocity of ~1.0 μm/s. The movement is sufficiently slow that the viscous contributions are small, and force measurements are dominated by elastic behavior [82,83]. A maximum force of 3.5±1.0 nN was implemented for all of the force curves to maintain a basis for comparison among the cells. In light of these claims, the parabolic model is often used if the indenter is a sphere because it is relatively easy to fit and yields a reasonable approximation for small indentations. Because the tip that comes in contact with the cell sample is spherical in shape, the model [84] predicts the relationship between the applied force and the indentation depth of the AFM cantilever into the soft sample by the following equation:

$$F = \frac{4E^*}{3}\sqrt{R}.\delta^{\frac{3}{2}} \tag{1}$$

where F is the applied force, R is the radius of the sphere, δ is the indentation, and $E^*$is the relative Young's modulus term:

$$\frac{1}{E^*} = \frac{(1\text{-}v_{tip}^2)}{E_{tip}} + \frac{(1\text{-}v_{cell}^2)}{E_{cell}} \tag{2}$$

Here, v is Poisson's ratio, and E_{tip} and E_{cell} represent the Young's

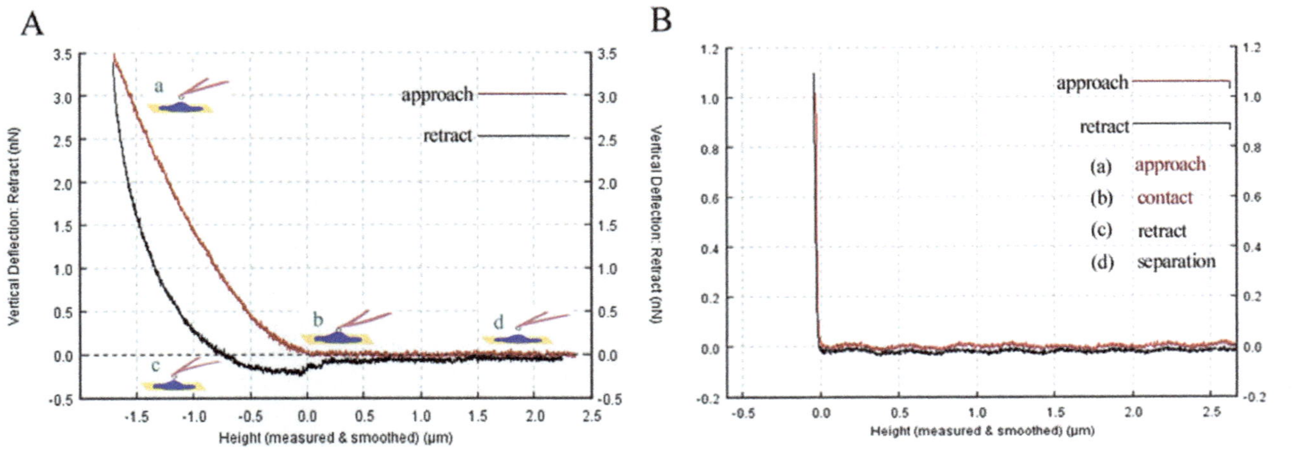

Figure 1. Force distance curve taken on the erythrocyte, Extend (or approach) (dark red) and retract (dark) curve clearly show hysteresis owing to the viscous and plastic behavior of the erythrocyte. (**A**) Cantilever deflection dependence on the tip sample distance (Z coordinate), and determination of the force-versus-indentation curves for control erythrocytes. (**B**) The straight line corresponds to curves measured on hard, non-deformable surface (glass coverslip) as the calibration curves. Lowercase letters show the marching trajectory of the probe in the whole process, and it consists of four steps, approach, contact, retract and separation (in **A**).

modulus of the tip and the cell, respectively. If the assumption of an infinitely hard needlepoint tip is employed, then $E_{tip} >> E_{cell}$. Thus, equation (2) could be simplified to the following:

$$\frac{1}{E^*} = \frac{(1-v_{cell}^2)}{E_{cell}} \quad (3)$$

where v depends on the material. For soft biological samples (i.e., cells, soft tissue, lipid bilayers and vesicles) [35], Poisson's ratio was assumed to be 0.5 in accordance with the incompressibility assumption usually employed for cells. Finally, the Hertz model equation assumes the following format:

$$F = \left[\frac{4\sqrt{R}}{3(1-v_{cell}^2)} E_{cell}\right] . \delta^{\frac{3}{2}} \quad (4)$$

However, regarding equation (4), it is difficult to determine the exact point at which the tip and the cell membrane come into contact, resulting in an inability to judge the most appropriate force curve to which the Hertz model is fitted. As a result, the following equation can be applied:

$$F^{2/3} = \left[\frac{4\sqrt{R}}{3(1-v_{cell}^2)} E_{cell}\right]^{2/3} . \delta \quad (5)$$

Additionally, when the dependence of the deformation on the force becomes linear, we use the indentation (δ) described as the difference in the relative changes of the piezo scanner displacement (z) and cantilever deflection (d). We obtain the following equation by replacing δ:

$$\delta = (z - z_0) - (d - d_0) \quad (6)$$

where z_0 and d_0 are both the x and y coordinates of initial contact between the tip and the cell sample to identify the initial contact point. To attain the use of visual means to approximate the contact point for the fit region range, we adopt a semi-automated, mathematical approximation for the contact point. To better calculate the Young's modulus, we substitute equation (6) into equation (5) to produce the formula below:

$$F^{2/3} = \left[\frac{4\sqrt{R}}{3(1-v_{cell}^2)} E_{cell}\right]^{2/3} (z - d) - \left[\frac{4\sqrt{R}}{3(1-v_{cell}^2)} E_{cell}\right]^{2/3} (z_0 - d_0) \quad (7)$$

Thus, this equation can be analyzed as a line in the ($F^{2/3}$, z–d) plane, from which the Young's modulus (E) can be directly calculated from the linear slope and contact point (z_0-d_0) through the intercept of Eq. (7) [82], [85–87]. In addition, the Hertz model assumes linearity, so it can be further analyzed according to the following formula:

$$y = kx + b \quad (8)$$

The slope information of the indentation curve (k) was used to calculate the Young's modulus (E):

$$\left[\frac{4\sqrt{R}}{3(1-v_{cell}^2)} E_{cell}\right]^{2/3} = slope_{indentation} = k \quad (9)$$

Solving for E_{cell}, we obtain the following:

$$E_{cell} = k^{3/2} \left[\frac{3(1-v_{cell}^2)}{4\sqrt{R}}\right] \quad (10)$$

Equation (7) should give a good linear fit line for the indentation data. The Young's modulus of the cell is considered a constant within the range of force applied to it. Presently, the contact point can be approximately represented by the b term in the following equation:

$$b = -\left[\frac{4\sqrt{R}}{3(1-v_{cell}^2)} E_{cell}\right]^{2/3} (z_0 - d_0) \quad (11)$$

However, z_0 and d_0 are both the x and y coordinates of the initial point of contact. d_0 refers to the deflection offset that is experienced during force curve acquisition and can be determined conveniently by simply observing the raw deflection *vs.* piezo position data. We solve for z_0 as follows:

$$z_0 = -\frac{b}{k} + d_0 \quad (12)$$

Ultimately, we will acquire a more accurate fitting region (z_0, d_0) for the Hertz model. All of the data analysis and curve fitting of the Hertz model to the collected force-indentation data were performed using JPK IP software, which offered automatic fitting for all of the indenter shapes. Finally, the elastic modulus (E) calculations were performed using the JPK IP software.

Extraction and purification of scaffolding protein in irradiated erythrocytes, and western blot analysis of the expression of spectrin-α1

First, the erythrocytes were purified within 48 hours from hamster whole blood and were then isolated by centrifugation at 600×*g* for 20 min at 4°C. After removing the plasma and buffy coat by careful aspiration, the erythrocyte pellet was resuspended in cold isotonic buffer (145 mM NaCl, 5 mM KCl, 5 mM HEPES, pH 7.4) and then centrifuged again at 2,000×*g* for 10 min at 4°C. Thereafter, the erythrocyte suspension was washed with isotonic buffer four times to completely remove the plasma and buffy layers. Next, to remove white blood cells from the erythrocyte suspensions, the samples were passed through white blood cell filters (Leukotrap RC; Pall Corporation, East Hills, NY) twice. In each step of the purification process, the upper layer was removed. The erythrocytes were finally resuspended in cold isotonic buffer at pH 7.4, made up to a hematocrit of approximately 50%, and stored at 4°C until further analysis.

Erythrocyte samples were purified as described above and were incubated for 10 min at 4°C in buffer containing 1% Triton X-100, 100 mg/mL PMSF, and 1 mM EDTA. The cell lysates were then centrifuged at 30,000×*g* at 4°C. The obtained supernatants and pellets, as well as the control (intact cell suspension in PBS), were treated with sample buffer (125 mmol/L Tris-HCl, pH 6.8, 2% sodium dodecyl sulfate (SDS), 10% β-mercaptoethanol, 10% glycerol, and 0.01% bromophenol blue) and heated at 100°C for 8 min. Standard immunoblot procedures were used for all of the samples using the indicated antibody combinations. The protein samples were subjected to 6% SDS-PAGE gel electrophoresis followed by electrotransfer onto PVDF membranes in 0.2 M glycine-NaOH transfer buffer with 0.01% SDS. Filters were blocked for 2 h at RT with blocking buffer (10% FSC, 0.1% Tween-20, and PBS) and subsequently incubated for 2 h at RT in blocking buffer containing monoclonal spectrin-α1 primary antibody (sc-15371; Santa Cruz Biotechnology) at a dilution of 1:1,000. Membranes were washed and incubated for 2 h at RT in blocking buffer containing 1:10,000 affinity-purified goat anti-rabbit IgG (H&L) antibody (7074; Cell Signaling Technology) secondary antibody and then were extensively washed. Next, the antibody conjugate was decanted and washed for 30 min with agitation in wash buffer (TBS with 0.1% Tween-20), changing the wash buffer every 5 min. Protein visualization was performed using ECL reagents (Super Signal West Pico Chemiluminescent Substrate; 34077; Pierce) followed by photography. Normal untreated cells with extraction buffer were used as controls. Western blot analysis was performed using a color scanner by densitometry (HP Scan jet Enterprise 7000n) and analyzed using the Image J software (NIH).

Statistical analysis

Except where noted, data are reported as the mean ± standard error, and statistical comparisons were performed using one-way ANOVA followed by the Tukey-Kramer HSD test for pair-wise comparisons. p values less than 0.05 were considered significant. All statistical analyses were performed using SPSS 11.5 (Statistical Product and Service Solutions) (Stanford University, USA).

Results

3.1 Radiation-induced morphological changes of erythrocytes in hamster peripheral blood via optical microscope observation

Morphological changes were observed in normal and irradiated erythrocytes by optical microscopy. Non-irradiated erythrocytes in peripheral blood were typically biconcave discs, resembling round cakes that were thinner at the center and thicker at the edges. However, after irradiation with CIR for 3 days, these cells appeared to have undergone shrinkage and were irregular, and the edges of some cells exhibited abnormal spines or ruffles. As shown in **Figure 2**, these changes were associated with decreased erythrocyte levels, and the number of abnormally shaped cells increased gradually. Moreover, quantitative analysis was performed on the inherent physicochemical parameters of the erythrocytes, such as the size, shape, effective area of the membrane, and average volume of the cells after irradiation by CIR and X-rays. The results showed that these morphological changes were closely correlated with ionizing irradiation, and a dose-time effect relationship was observed in the irradiated group of erythrocytes with respect to the different radiation doses (**Table 1**).

3.2 Influence of the proportion of erythroid cells in bone marrow exposed to radiation

Changes in the BM erythrocytes after irradiation were analyzed using a tangible cell-counting method. The purpose of our observations was to compare the characteristics among the different cell population types in the total number of BM cells and to understand the distribution characteristics of erythroid cells in BM caused by irradiation. The results revealed a mild myeloproliferative effect with small doses of radiation. Additionally, given the priority of the early development of erythroid cells, the pronormoblasts and basophilic erythroblasts seemed to demonstrate a tendency to increase with increasing absorbed doses of CIR; however, this change in the X-ray radiation group was not obvious. When the radiation dose increased, an obvious inhibitory effect was shown on BM. However, the proportions of polychromatophilic erythroblasts and normoblasts decreased significantly following both types of irradiation. In addition, the data indicated the presence of the myeloid maturation stage in a significantly higher proportion of granulocytes. Furthermore, the annular core, class changes and lack of particles were easily observed via the additive pleochroism of the erythrocytes (**Figure 3** and **Figure 4**).

3.3 Alterations of erythrocyte morphology and mechanical properties triggered by radiation evaluated using atomic force microscopy

3.3.1 AFM topographic imaging. AFM experiments were performed on erythrocytes that were spin-coated onto glass slides, representing the surface effects of the measurement period. Image acquisition was performed in contact mode, and the mechanical properties of the erythrocytes were measured using the force spectrum of the AFM. The AFM probe not only senses the differences in the surface and local mechanical properties in the cell, it also leads to differential surface deformation and contributes to image contrast. During AFM raster scanning, the AFM tip presses against the soft cell membrane into the cytosol until the membrane is resisted by the underlying stiffer structures, resulting in the sub-membrane structures appearing elevated and being detected in deflection images. Thus, through the analysis of AFM topographic images, including height-measured images, deflection images and 3D images, the imaging results can connect the membranous structure and function to reveal the variations in the microstructure of erythrocytes exposed to radiation. Unaffected erythrocytes are typically smooth, biconcave discs; when the cells were irradiated, a series of changes, ranging from minute to major, was captured throughout the whole process using BT-AFM, as detailed below (**Figure 5**).

3.3.2 AFM measurement of the elastic modulus (cell stiffness) of irradiated erythrocytes. The elastic modulus is often used to describe the mechanical properties of cells and other biological samples. The modified Hertz model fit well to the experimental data obtained by AFM measurement, and the calculated value of the elastic modulus was obtained using JPK Instruments data processing software. Stiffness measurements for the erythrocytes treated with different radiation doses were recorded relative to the reference hard material at 3, 14 and 28 days. The results are shown as histograms in **Figure 6** (including, carbon ion beams and X-rays), with the bin size reflecting the confidence interval of the measurements. The average values of the elastic modulus were obtained by fitting the Gaussian distribution to the histograms. Justification for using a normal distribution function for the analysis of the experimental data was provided by performing the Shapiro–Wilk normality test. This procedure indicated that all of the distributions from **Figure 6** were normal at the level of $\alpha = 0.05$. Furthermore, the equality of variance was successfully verified using Levene's test, and the statistical evaluation of the differences among the distributions was performed using analysis of variance (ANOVA). The ANOVA results showed that the means were different at the

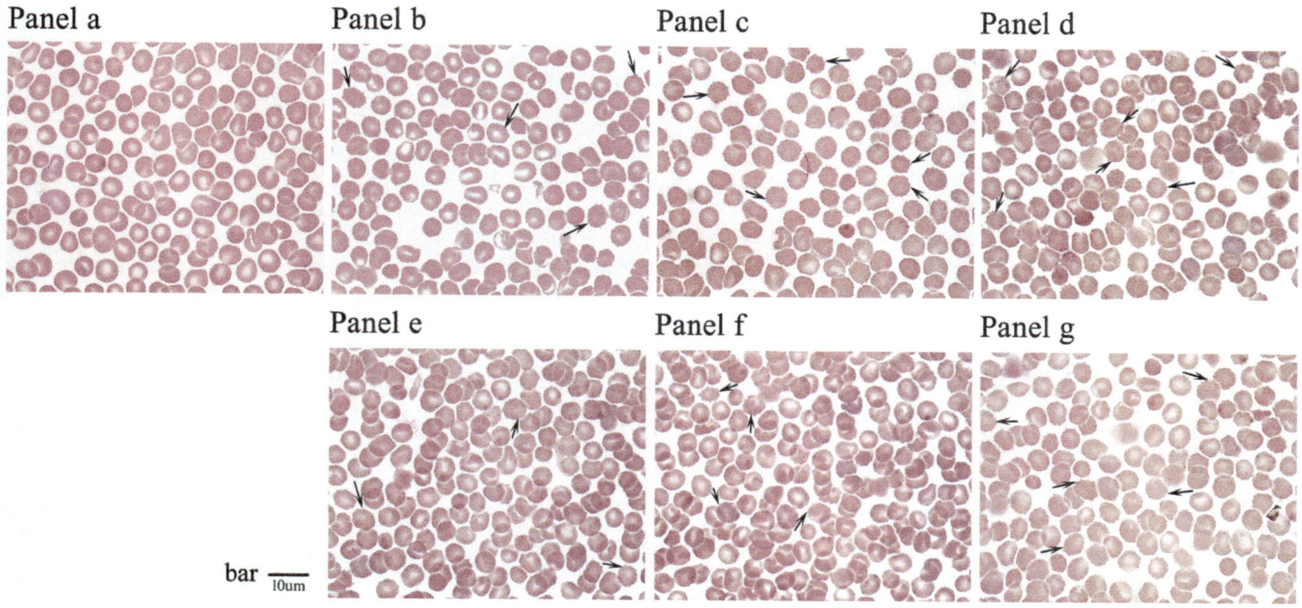

Figure 2. Photographs of analysis the changes of gross morphology of erythrocytes in blood smear at 3d after whole-body exposure to $^{12}C^{6+}$ ions or X-rays (by 100×oil immersion observation). Panel **a**: Non-irradiated control group erythrocytes (0 Gy); Panel **b–d**: erythrocytes of carbon ions radiation groups (Radiation dose: 2 Gy, 4 Gy and 6 Gy); and Panel **e–g**: erythrocytes of X-rays radiation groups (Radiation dose: 4 Gy, 6 Gy and 12 Gy). Black arrows indicate the morphological changes of erythrocytes. The scale bar is 10 μm.

level of $\alpha = 0.01$. The time dependence of the average elastic modulus is shown in **Figure 7**. The error bars in this figure represent half-widths of the normal distributions from **Figure 7**. It could be concluded that the elastic modulus of the phospholipid bilayer membrane in erythrocytes decreases slightly over time with exposure to large doses of radiation. Additionally, an interesting phenomenon is evident in the figure: with the increasing radiation doses, the elastic modulus also decreased. In the experiment, the changes in the elastic modulus were due to different radiation doses with CIR or X-rays, triggering injury to the membrane-cytoskeleton system.

Figure 8 shows scatter plots of the elastic modulus values of the irradiated and non-irradiated groups over 3, 14, and 28 days calculated from the average of the approach force curves, and the results are shown as box-plots in which the scattered dots represent the effective sample point number. The data indicate that there were similar trends in variations of the elastic modulus according to the different doses of radiation in the erythrocyte samples, possibly indicating that the elastic modulus was proportional to the radiation dose.

3.4 Spectrin-α1 specifically participates in the morphological remodeling of irradiated erythrocytes

After exposure to CIR, the expression of spectrin-α1 protein significantly decreased in erythrocytes. With increasing radiation doses, spectrin-α1 protein expression was reduced. From 3 to 28 days after exposure to CIR, spectrin-α1 expression steadily decreased with increasing radiation doses. However, for X-rays, when small doses (<4 Gy) of radiation were utilized, spectrin-α1 expression was slightly augmented for a short time (approximately 14 days); with larger doses of radiation, spectrin-α1 expression appeared to be inhibited. As shown in **Figure 9**, the changes in erythrocyte morphology at the micro-nano scale level illustrate the integrity of the cell membrane and the stability of the cytoskeleton, which are dependent on protein conformation.

3.5 Comparison of the variation between the average of the elastic modulus and the mean density levels of spectrin-α1 caused by radiation

As indicated in **Table 2**, noticeable differences were observed for all of the data before and after irradiation. The mean density values of spectrin-α1 protein expression were significantly lower in the irradiated samples than in the non-irradiated samples (*$p<0.05$*), and the difference in the elastic modulus of both groups is clearly shown in **Table 2**. In particular, after exposure to CIR for 3 days, with increasing radiation dose from 2 Gy to 6 Gy, the mean density values of spectrin-α1 protein expression ranged from 0.99±0.16 to 0.75±0.15, which was significantly different from those of the control non-irradiated group (*$p<0.05$*). However, at 14 days, the radiation-exposed cells showed mean density values of spectrin-α1 protein expression between 1.03±0.19 to and 0.71±0.17 with increasing radiation dose. At 28 days, the mean density values of spectrin-α1 protein expression ranged from 1.39±0.12 to 0.57±0.13. Furthermore, the mean elasticity modulus values of the irradiated group were reduced with increasing radiation dose from 10.62±1.57 kPa to 5.08±0.59 kPa after irradiation for 3 days; at 14 and 28 days, the average value of the Young's modulus ranged from 9.42±0.66 kPa to 4.98±0.76 kPa and from 8.22±1.33 kPa to 4.72±0.74 kPa, respectively. For X-ray radiation, results similar to those obtained with CIR were observed (**Table 2**). Thus, in summary, the results indicate that when the micromorphology and microstructure of an erythrocyte change from a typically smooth, biconcave disc to a cell surface with corrugated, irregular, and rolling regional topography, changes in the elastic modulus and morphology occur in parallel with the irradiation process. Additionally, the fact is the elastic modulus values always increase when young cells become old cells in process, the form of change coexist in the process of erythrocyte changes by CIR induced, but the radiation induce the cell apoptosis that is a programmed cell death process along with the evolution of time, the activation of

Table 1. Measurement of the changes of erythrocytes shape by induced of $^{12}C^{6+}$ ions and X-rays radiation in *Mesocricetus auratus*.

Group	Cells No.	Length(μm)	Width(μm)	Perimeter(μm)	Thickness(μm)	ROI area(μm²)	Volume(μm³)
Control 0Gy	1500	7.25±0.13	6.12±0.10	584.14±36.78	2.0	20517.44±3651.02	41.03±7.30
$^{12}C^{6+}$ions 2Gy	410	6.85±0.15▲	5.96±0.20	563.95±57.72▲	2.0	19019.15±3120.58	38.04±6.24▲
4Gy	376	6.72±0.16▲	5.85±0.11▲	547.98±47.86▲	2.0	18178.41±2933.45	36.36±5.87▲
6Gy	373	5.96±0.24▲	5.55±0.15▲	529.38±40.77▲	2.0	17317.20±2419.97	34.63±4.84▲
X-rays 4Gy	652	7.0±0.11▲▲	5.8±0.16▲▲	570.7±57.43▲▲	2.0	19496.54±2975.36	38.99±5.95▲▲
6Gy	325	6.8±0.15▲▲	5.6±0.12▲▲	535.6±37.50▲▲	2.0	18659.76±2260.22	37.32±4.52▲▲
12Gy	554	6.1±0.18▲▲	5.4±0.10▲▲	519.0±45.65▲▲	2.0	17734.23±2747.42	35.47±5.49▲▲

Note, Measurement of the morphological differences of erythrocytes had indicated the obvious impact of $^{12}C^{6+}$ ions or X-rays radiation with Image J software. And these general varies mainly includes the physical and chemical parameters of the erythrocyte, such as length, width, perimeter, thickness, ROI area and volume (of average value). Because of the average thickness of erythrocytes in mammals is around in the range of 1.0–2.5 μm, and using an optical microscope in the experiment, so as to calculate the volume, we taken the average thickness value of 2.0 μm to obtain the relative size of erythrocytes. And in the list of **Tab.**, ▲ Black triangle symbols significant statistical significance compared with the control group in carbon ion radiation ($p<0.05$), but ▲▲ double triangle line represent the differences results by inducing X-rays ($p<0.05$). (In detail, for length, Control *vs* C ions-2Gy, p = 0.000, $p<0.05$; Control *vs* C ions-4Gy, p = 0.000, $p<0.05$; Control *vs* C ions-6Gy, p = 0.000, $p<0.05$; Control *vs* X rays-4Gy, p = 0.000, $p<0.05$; Control *vs* X rays-6Gy, p = 0.000, $p<0.05$; Control *vs* X rays-12Gy, p = 0.000, $p<0.05$; for width, Control *vs* C ions-2Gy, p = 0.479, $p>0.05$; Control *vs* C ions-4Gy, p = 0.000, $p<0.05$; Control *vs* C ions-6Gy, p = 0.000, $p<0.05$; Control *vs* X rays-4Gy, p = 0.000, $p<0.05$; Control *vs* X rays-6Gy, p = 0.000, $p<0.05$; Control *vs* X rays-12Gy, p = 0.000, $p<0.05$; for perimeter, Control *vs* C ions-2Gy, p = 0.002, $p<0.05$; Control *vs* C ions-4Gy, p = 0.000, $p<0.05$; Control *vs* C ions-6Gy, p = 0.000, $p<0.05$; Control *vs* X rays-4Gy, p = 0.027, $p<0.05$; Control *vs* X rays-6Gy, p = 0.000, $p<0.05$; Control *vs* X rays-12Gy, p = 0.000, $p<0.05$; for volume, Control *vs* C ions-2Gy, p = 0.000, $p<0.05$; Control *vs* C ions-4Gy, p = 0.000, $p<0.05$; Control *vs* C ions-6Gy, p = 0.000, $p<0.05$; Control *vs* X rays-4Gy, p = 0.000, $p<0.05$; Control *vs* X rays-6Gy, p = 0.000, $p<0.05$; Control *vs* X rays-12Gy, p = 0.000, $p<0.05$.).

signaling molecules, then the series of cascading effects of transduction pathway [88,89]. Specific mechanisms with age may be different from the mechanism of apoptosis, maybe there are some commonness, and also differences. Clearly, age-related changes have showed a transitions from physiological to pathological state, and the change of age relative to the apoptosis process is negligible. Therefore, the elastic modulus may function as a "biomarker" in the process and can be used to assess the harmful effects to erythrocytes or other cell types/tissues triggered by irradiation. The assessment of a single cell or group of cells may be sufficient to connect the biomechanical properties of cells and the protein molecular signaling cascade.

3.6 Spatial correlation of the expression of cytoskeletal protein spectrin-α1 and the elastic modulus in irradiated erythrocytes

After the experimental groups were exposed to CIR or X-rays, the spatial relationships between spectrin-α1 protein expression and the elastic modulus in erythrocytes were examined. We correlated the value measured for the elastic modulus of the erythrocyte membrane using BT-AFM with the expression of the cytoskeletal protein spectrin-α1. Qualitatively, the elastic modulus appeared to be positively correlated with the relative expression of spectrin-α1 (i.e., a high modulus was observed in regions with higher protein expression in the context of irradiation) and was also correlated with radiation dose (low modulus in regions with lower protein level in the context of irradiation). Additionally, there was a special dose-response relationship between the elastic modulus and the radiation dose: when the irradiation dose increased, the elastic modulus increased as well (**Figure 10**). Based on these findings, Pearson's correlation coefficient (r) was calculated between the elastic modulus and the relative level of cytoskeletal protein spectrin-α1. In control erythrocyte samples, there appeared to be no correlation among high-modulus regions, low-modulus regions and spectrin-α1 protein expression. After treatment with radiation, the average modulus was reduced, and the area of the cell membrane appeared to be more correlated with the modulus. Reflecting these findings, after exposure to CIR for 3 days, Pearson's correlation coefficient (r) between the modulus and spectrin-α1 protein expression was relatively strong and significant ($r_{3c} = 0.678$, $p<0.01$) compared with the other time points. At 14 days of irradiation with CIR, Pearson's correlation coefficient showed a positive correlation ($r_{14c} = 0.639$, $p<0.01$); at 28 days of irradiation by CIR, the correlation coefficient was also positive ($r_{28c} = 0.438$, $p<0.01$). For X-rays, there were radiation effects similar to those of CIR among the different groups: at 3, 14 and 28 days, the correlation coefficients were ($r_{3x} = 0.390$, $p<0.05$), ($r_{14x} = 0.301$, $p<0.01$) and ($r_{28x} = 0.353$, $p<0.01$), respectively.

Discussion

The inherent mechanical characteristics of cells are an important manifestation of their physical state under external perturbation

The mechanical properties of individual cells have been regarded as unique indicators that can constantly reflect the changes in their states caused by cellular events and pathological conditions. Simply put, alterations in biological activity or transformation of cell states can also trigger changes in the mechanical properties of cells. In particular, alterations in cell stiffness or the elastic modulus have been used as biological markers for cellular phenotypic events and diseases [90]. The

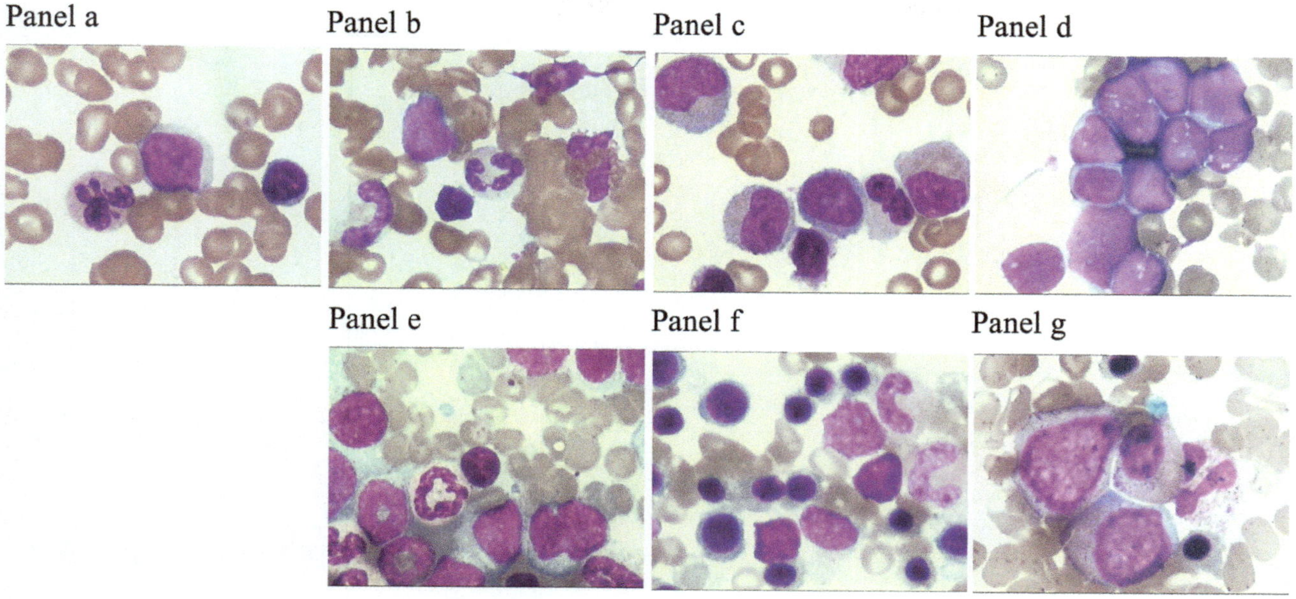

Figure 3. The distribution characteristics of erythrocytes in BM at 3d after exposed by different doses of $^{12}C^{6+}$ ions or X-rays. Cytology analysis the distribution of erythrocytes in BM. In detailed, Panel **a**: Non-irradiated control group erythrocytes (0Gy); Panel **b–d**: erythrocytes of carbon ions radiation groups (Radiation dose: 2Gy, 4Gy and 6Gy); panel **e–g**: erythrocytes of X-rays radiation groups (Radiation dose: 4Gy, 6Gy and 12Gy). And BM aspirate smear from irradiated golden hamster showing abnormal erythroblasts indicative of a cell-division defect, or dysplasia. The cytology image was observed with 100×oil immersion, in the picture, pink represents the erythrocytes.

mechanical properties of cells are largely attributable to the cytoskeleton components and the cytoskeletal architecture, which maintain the basic form of cells. Thus, for the abovementioned changes in a cell's life cycle, visualizing the changes in the mechanical properties of cells exposed to some type of stimulus and the association of these changes with the biomechanics of

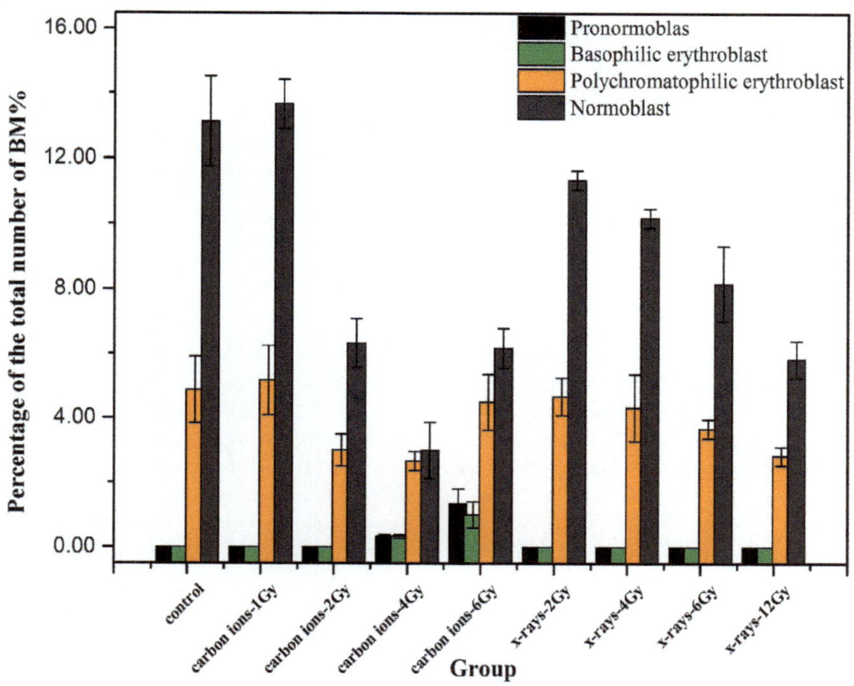

Figure 4. The number of erythroid cells in BM accounted for the relative percentage of the total of BM cells after exposed carbon ion beams or X-rays. From the column chart showed that the pronormoblast and basophilic erythroblast seemed upward tendency with the increasing of absorbed dose in carbon ions radiation, but the change in X-rays radiation groups seemed to be not obvious, as for the polychromatophilic erythroblast and normoblast, the percentage of cells number had decreased significantly in two types of irradiation, and the differences between groups had significant statistical significance ($p<0.05$).

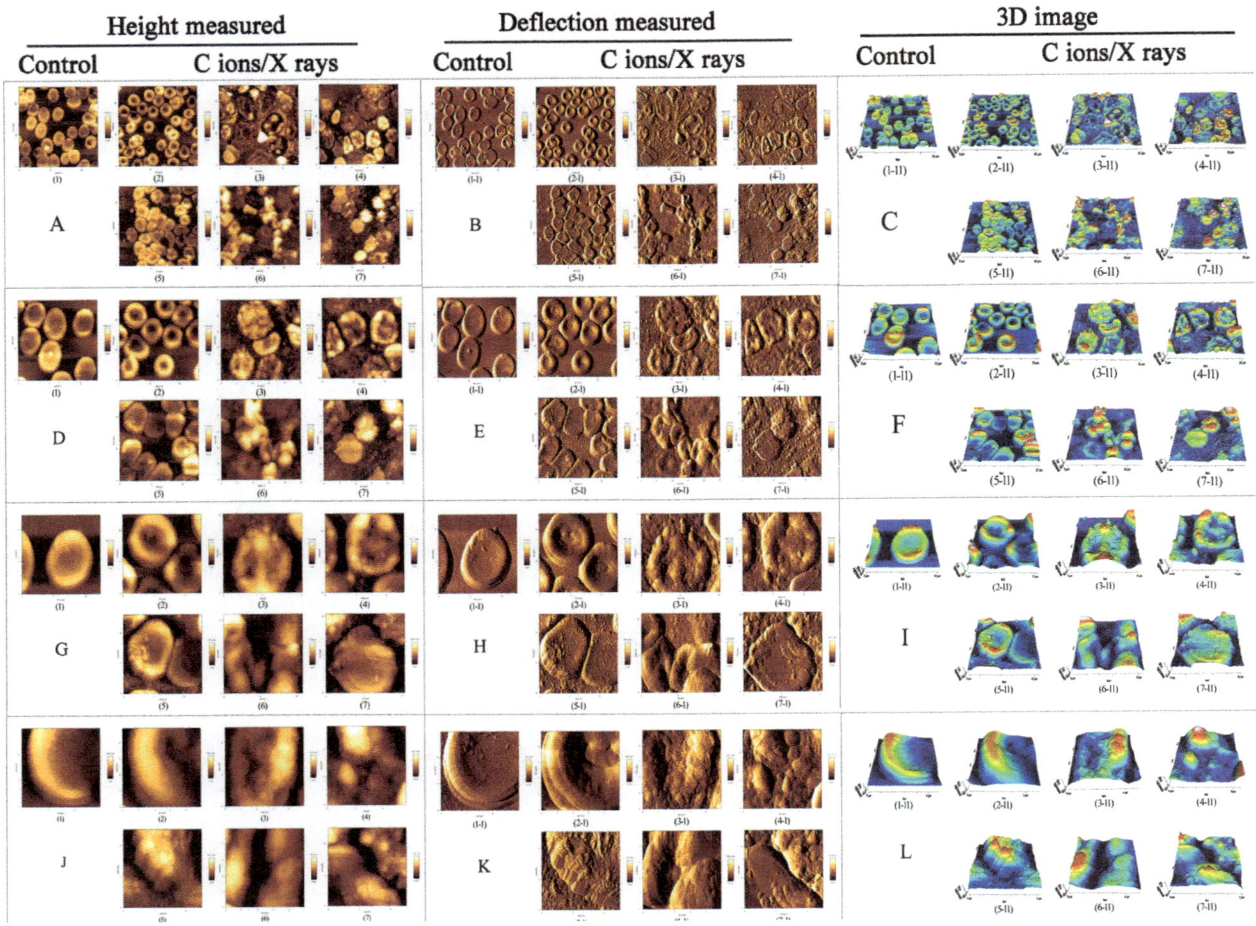

Figure 5. Effects of radiation on micromorphology in erythrocytes membrane. (**A–L**) Surface imaging of erythrocytes induced by carbon ion beams and X-rays radiation using biological type atomic force microscopy; and the graph **A**, **B** and **C** showed respectively for the Height measured image, Deflection image and 3D image at scan scale of 50 μm (Fast)×50 μm bar (Slow), [for **A**:(1) Control; (2) C ions 2Gy; (3) C ions 4Gy; (4) C ions 6Gy; (5) X-rays 4Gy; (6) X-rays 6Gy; (7) X-rays 12Gy; for **B**: (1–1) Control; (2–1) C ions 2Gy; (3–1) C ions 4Gy; (4–1) C ions 6Gy; (5–1) X-rays 4Gy; (6–1) X-rays 6Gy; (7–1) X-rays 12Gy; for **C**: (1–11) Control; (2–11) C ions 2Gy; (3–11) C ions 4Gy; (4–11) C ions 6Gy; (5–11) X-rays 4Gy; (6–11) X-rays 6Gy; (7–11) X-rays 12Gy]. But the graph **D–F** showed respectively for the Height measured image, Deflection image and 3D image at scan scale of 25 μm (Fast) ×25 μm bar (Slow); the graph **G–I** showed respectively for the Height measured image, Deflection image and 3D image at scan scale of 12.5 μm (Fast) ×12.5 μm bar (Slow); the graph **J–L** showed respectively for the Height measured image, Deflection image and 3D image at scan scale of 5 μm (Fast) × 5 μm bar (Slow). In addition, for a smaller scan scale was the same grouping as 50 μm (Fast) × 50 μm bar (Slow) bar. Here, the schematic showed different doses and type radiation for the influence of micromorphology of erythrocytes, and this fine change was captured by AFM.

cellular events have very important significance. Previously, the spectrin skeleton of erythrocytes was studied as a model tethered membrane [91], and many results have suggested that spectrin is a vital scaffold protein involved in signaling pathway organization, influencing changes in cytoskeletal structure and controlling membrane function.

Radiation induces changes in erythrocyte stiffness during morphological remodeling

In the present study, the mechanical properties of erythrocytes were assessed by combining the use of biological-type AFM, cytological analysis of samples of peripheral blood and optical microscopy of bone marrow after irradiation by CIR or X-rays. The experimental results suggested that there was a clear relationship between changes in cell morphology and variations in mechanical properties; this relationship was mainly manifested in the following respects. First, in terms of morphology, a normal erythrocyte is a biconcave disc resembling a round cake, has a uniform size, has no nucleus, appears as a bilaterally indented sphere of approximately 4–8 μm in diameter (in mammals; in humans, 6–9 μm), has a thickness of approximately 1.0–2.5 μm, and has a relatively uniform, flat, and smooth membrane surface that is structured and maintains some continuity. However, after 3 days of irradiation with CIR, these cells underwent shrinkage and became irregular, and some exhibited abnormal spines or ruffles on the edges; additionally, the membrane area exhibited discontinuities and an undulating surface (**Figure 1**). Furthermore, the cytological smear method was used and analyzed with the NIH Image J software to reveal changes in the cell form in peripheral blood samples and in the proportions of different cell types in the marrow. The inherent parameters, such as the length, width, perimeter, thickness, ROI area and volume were quantitatively analyzed. Measurement of the results showed that the average value of the length was reduced from approximately 7.25±0.13 μm to 5.96±0.24 μm, the average value of the width was reduced from approximately 6.12±0.10 μm to

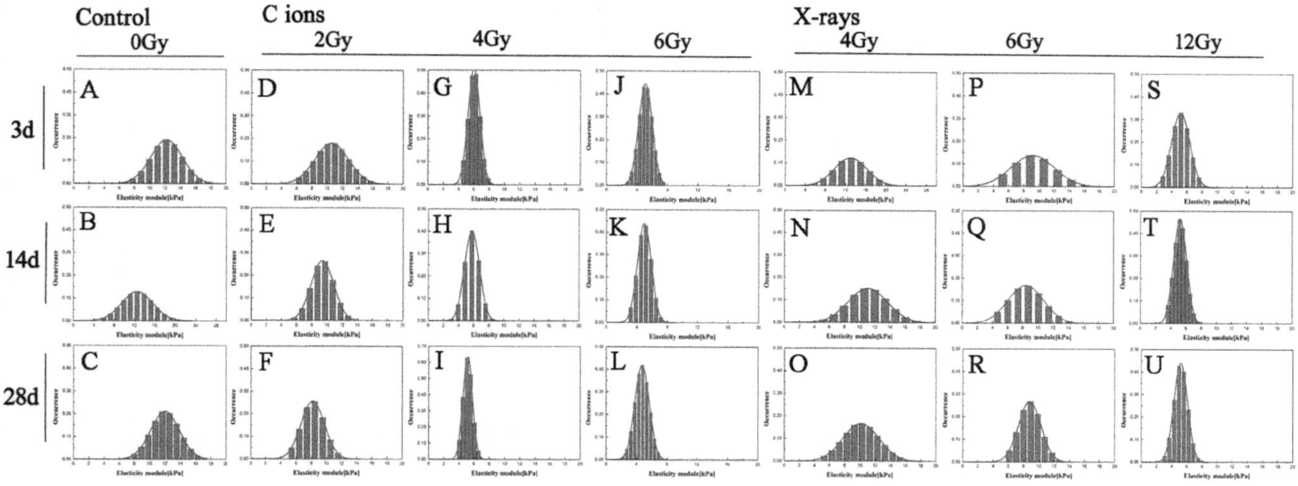

Figure 6. Histograms of erythrocytes elasticity modulus distributions induced by C ions or X-rays exposed for 3, 14 and 28 days. The bar graph (**A**), (**B**) and (**C**) represented control erythrocytes (0 Gy), 3d, 14d and 28d, respectively; the bar graph (**D**), (**E**) and (**F**) represented carbon ions 2 Gy, 3d, 14d and 28d, respectively; the bar graph (**G**), (**H**) and (**I**) represented carbon ions 4 Gy, 3d, 14d and 28d, respectively; the bar graph (**J**), (**K**) and (**L**) represented carbon ions 6 Gy, 3d, 14d and 28d, respectively. But the bar graph (**M**), (**N**) and (**O**) showed X-rays 4 Gy, 3d, 14d and 28d, respectively; the bar graph (**P**), (**Q**) and (**R**) showed X-rays 6 Gy, 3d, 14d and 28d; the bar graph (**S**), (**T**) and (**U**) showed X-rays 12 Gy, 3d, 14d and 28d, respectively.

5.40±0.10 μm, the average value of the perimeter was reduced from approximately 584.14±36.78 μm to 519.0±45.65 μm, the ROI area was reduced from approximately 20517.44±3651.02 μm^2 to 17317.20±2419.97 μm^2, and the average volume was reduced from approximately 41.03±7.30 μm^3 to 34.63±4.84 μm^3. Additionally, the average thickness of erythrocytes in mammals is in the range of approximately 1.0–2.5 μm. Using an optical microscope, an average thickness value of 2.0 μm was found and used to calculate the relative volume of the erythrocytes. Additionally, using the tangible cell counting method to analyze the proportion of erythroid cells in BM, there was a mild myeloproliferative effect of small doses of radiation. Furthermore, given the priority of the early development of erythroid cells, the pronormoblasts and basophilic erythroblasts seemed to demonstrate a tendency to increase with increasing absorbed CIR doses; however, this change was not obvious in the X-ray radiation group. Taken together, these results indicated that when the radiation dose increased, there was an obvious inhibitory effect on BM; thus, the proportions of polychromatophilic erythroblasts and normoblasts decreased significantly with both types of irradiation (**Figure 2** and **Figure 3**).

Most importantly, BT-AFM was employed in this study as a powerful and versatile tool to study the mechanical properties at the micro-nano scale for the analysis of fine surface structure changes on erythrocytes, emphasizing the role of the cell membrane and the integrity of the membrane in cell mechanical stability following radiation exposure. This study investigated the microstructural and mechanical properties of erythrocytes and quantified the deformation and damage to the membrane skeleton. In particular, as shown in **Figure 5**, AFM topographic images reveal the fine variations induced by radiation, and the images were obtained of shrunken, irregular, ruffled-edge shapes and progressively discontinuous membrane structures. Next, a conclusion can be drawn based on the relative elastic modulus or stiffness, which depends on the precise measurement of the mechanical properties of the cell membrane. The mean elastic modulus of erythrocytes irradiated with increasing CIR doses was decreased to between 10.62±1.57 (kPa) and 5.08±0.59 (kPa) at 3 days after irradiation; at 14 and 28 days, the average values of the elastic modulus ranged from 9.42±0.66 (kPa) to 4.98±0.76 (kPa) and 8.22±1.33 (kPa) to 4.72±0.74 (kPa), respectively. For X-ray radiation, similar results were observed to those obtained with CIR. Thus, fundamental alterations in erythrocyte stiffness were triggered by the different radiation types, at different times and with different doses. Furthermore, the combination, the distribution, and the changes in stiffness were also different, as shown in **Figures 6, 7** and **8**. This strategy allowed us to perform nanobiological analysis of the erythrocytes after irradiation, further improving our knowledge of the aspects and dynamics of the mechanical properties of erythrocytes.

Spectrin-α1, a neofunctionalized cytoskeletal protein of erythrocytes, is involved in mediating changes in erythrocyte stiffness during the morphological remodeling process induced by radiation

The membrane skeleton, a dense proteinaceous network, is thought to be responsible for the remarkable morphological changes and mechanical properties of erythrocytes [92], allowing them to withstand and respond to different mechanical stresses and tension caused by external perturbations experienced throughout their 120-day lifespan [93]. The basic shape of an erythrocyte can be visualized by observing the spectrin-containing sub-membranous cytoskeleton because this structure preserves the outline of the cell. The spectrin molecules form pentagonal or hexagonal arrangements, which are composed of tetramers of spectrin subunits associating with short actin filaments at either end of the tetramer. These short actin filaments act as junctional complexes, allowing the formation of a hexagonal mesh and scaffolding. This assembly configuration not only plays an important role in the maintenance of plasma membrane shape, integrity, and cytoskeletal structure, influence influencing deformability or resulting in damage [90], [94,95] and finally determining biological behavior and functional aspects [96–99]; it can also produce a rapid response and break the tetramers [100]. A dysfunctional underlying membrane skeleton results in the erythrocyte membrane being partially devoid of a spectrin-actin

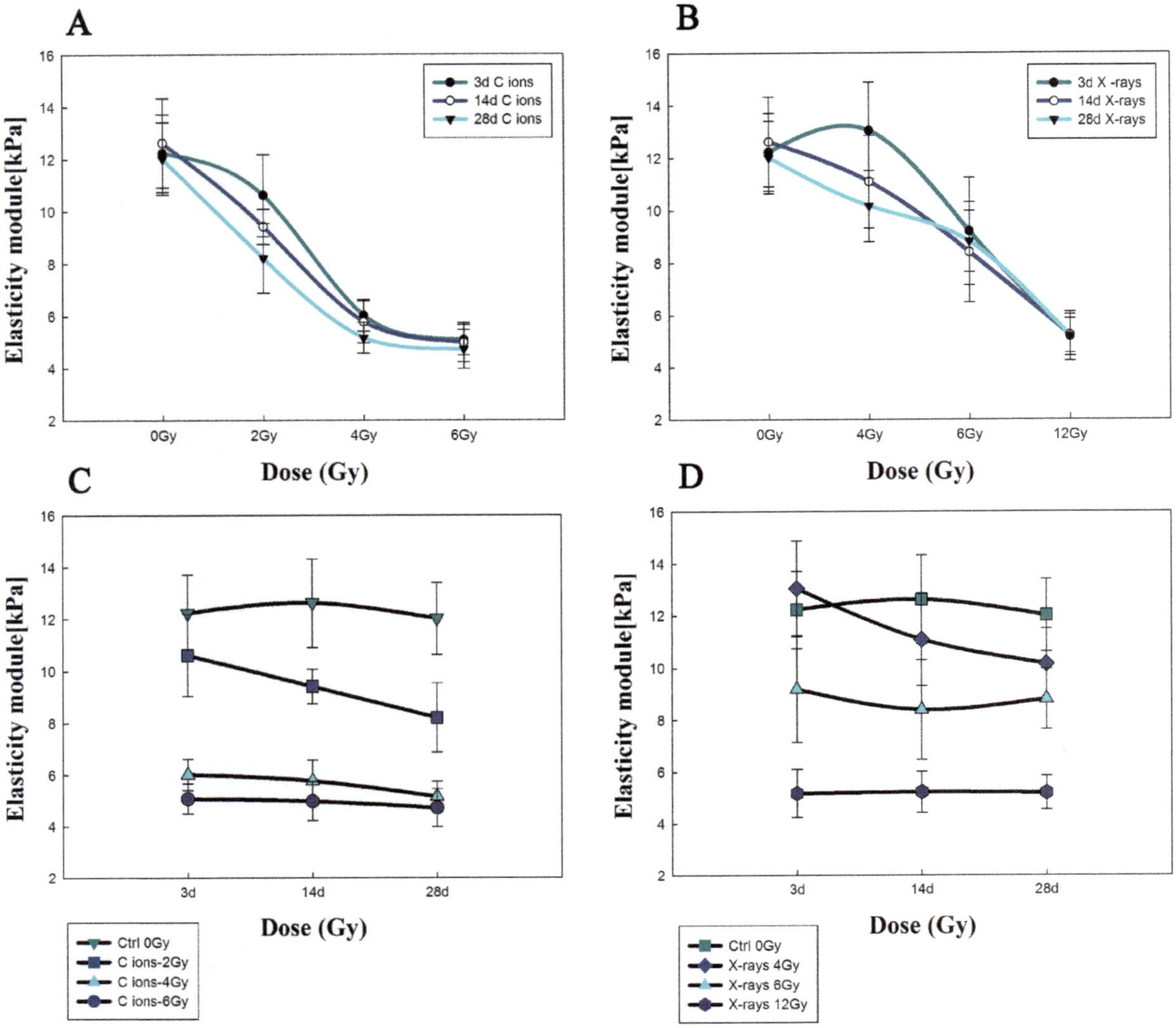

Figure 7. The change of elasticity modules of erythrocytes induced by C ions or X-rays radiation. And the groups displayed as a function of the dependent manner on dosage (**A** and **B**) and time (**C** and **D**). Error bars represent half-widths of the normal distributions fitted to the respective histograms.

network, no longer existing as a ghost, and causing disruption of the unique arrangement of spectrin, F-actin, protein 4.1 and ankyrin, with direct and indirect connections to the membrane bilayer with its immersed integral proteins [101] (**Figure 11**). Consequently, the distribution of membrane tension is regulated by signaling molecules through the activated complex signaling transduction pathway to mediate the biochemical reaction between target proteins or molecules [102–104] and triggering exquisite changes in cell shape or membrane damage [105]. Similarly, it was reported that the skeleton began to fragment and became a small, approximately 50-nm inverted vesicle [52], producing changes in cell shape and stability regarding the filamentous network. Consequently, the importance of this structure is highlighted by the above discussion noting that spectrin is a structural platform for the stabilization and activation of membrane channels, receptors and transporters in mammals; however, it is also closely related to cell physiology and pathology [106,107].

Many studies have shown that the measurement of mechanical properties in biological samples can explain the biomechanical mechanism of organism units in various physiological and pathological states. Recent evidence suggests that shear can induce the unfolding of spectrin within erythrocytes [108], forcing changes in protein structure by the unfolding of specific regions, and that the spectrin repeat unit can be subjected to reversible unfolding and refolding using 20-pN forces [109]. Regarding the erythrocyte cytoskeleton, spectrin comprises a tetrameric or higher oligomeric protein arranged as antiparallel filamentous heterodimers of α and β subunits [52], [110], which is easy to open or fold; moreover, spectrin is organized in a scaffold located at the intracellular side of the plasma membrane in eukaryotic cells, and is linked to several integral membrane proteins through a helical repeating unit. Additionally, spectrin and a few other proteins assemble into a building block and share a common structural fold with all of the spectrin repeat units [52]. Ultimately, the crystal structure of the assembled protein shows that it maintains an uninterrupted helical structure [111], creating a steady state for the cytoskeleton meshwork and maintaining the native cell shape. In the present study, the expression of the cytoskeletal protein spectrin-α1 was analyzed using a quantitative immunoblot technique after irradiation, and the results showed that CIR or X-rays can cause the expression of spectrin-α1 to decrease

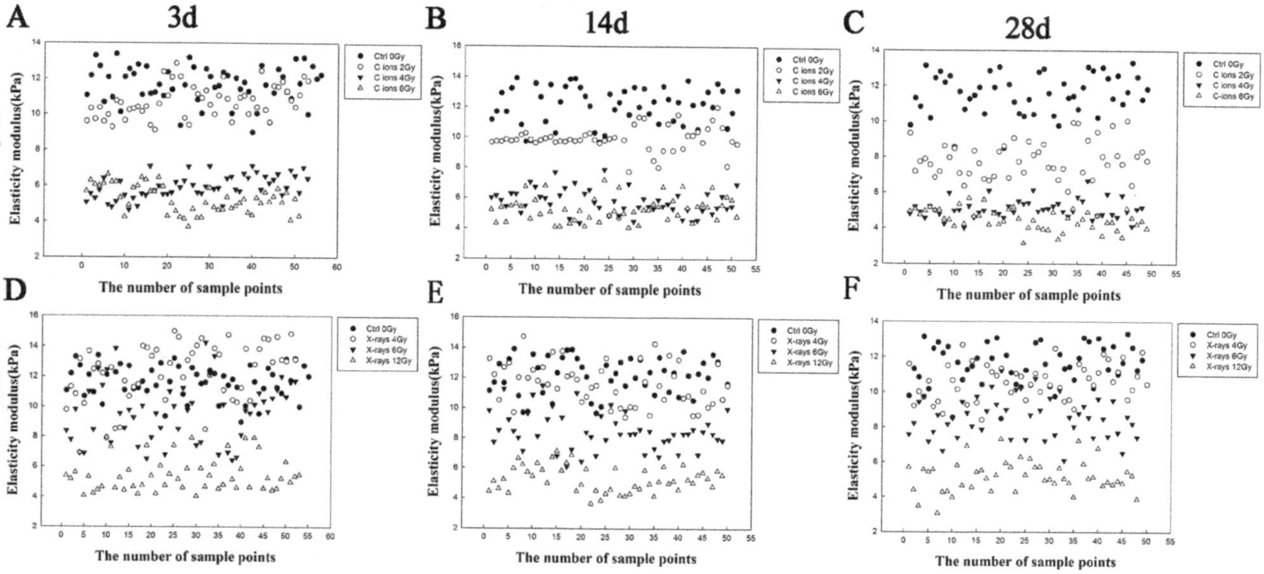

Figure 8. Variations of elasticity modulus for different doses of radiation in erythrocyte samples–control erythrocytes, and after suffering from the irradiation dose, the distribution effect of elasticity modulus was showed by scatters dots (A–F).

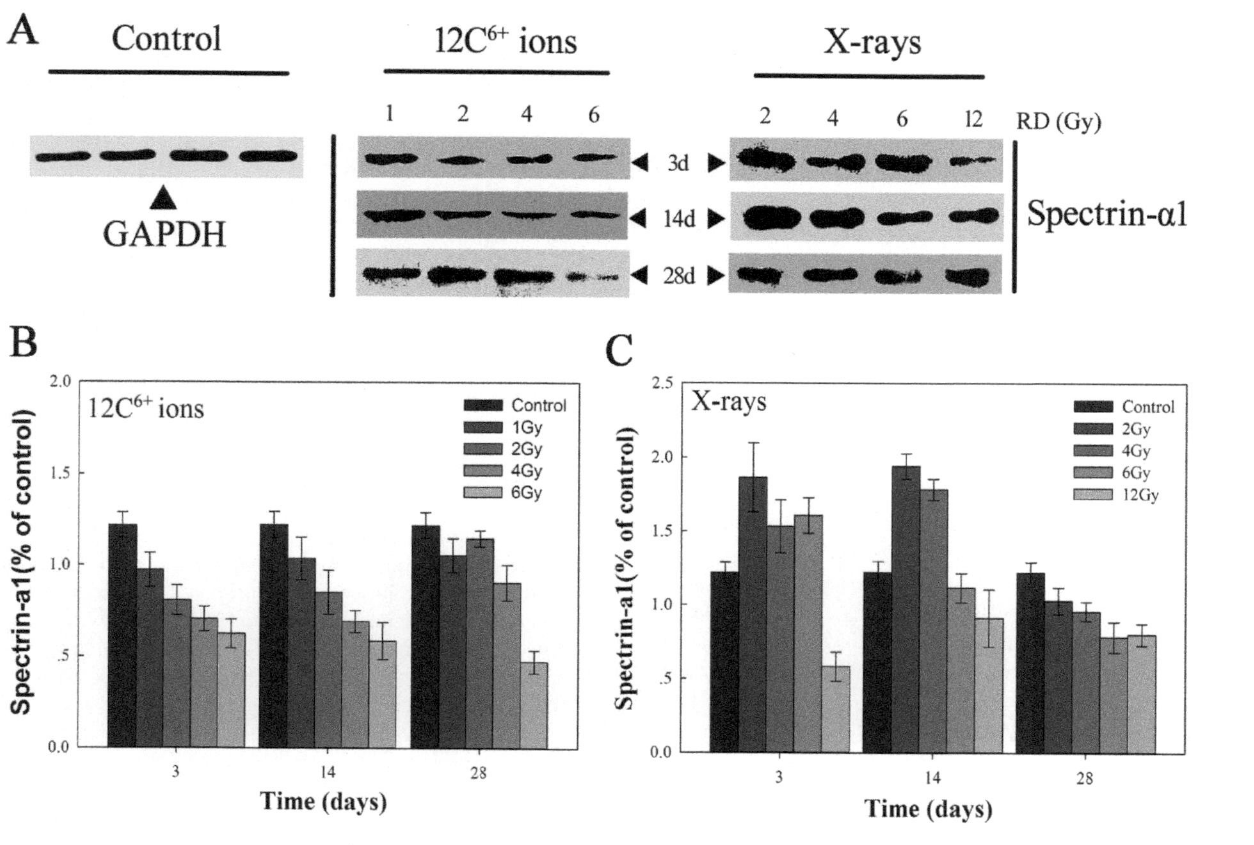

Figure 9. Spectrin-α1 is specifically targeted to drive erythrocyte skeleton impairment by C ions or X-rays radiation induction. Western blotting analyzed of the change of erythrocytes skeleton proteins spectrin-α1 expression after treated with radiation (**A**). (**B**) After C ions exposed at 3, 14 and 28d, the change of skeleton protein expression in different radiation groups. (**C**) After X-rays exposed at 3, 14 and 28d, and skeleton protein expression was also monitored by WB in different radiation groups. Error bars represent standard deviation from more triplicate valid data.

Table 2. Average values of Young's modulus and mean density values of spectrin-α1 expression for the change of RBCs distributions according to different radiation groups.

Group	Spectrin-α1 protein expression (mean density)			Young's modulus (kPa)		
	3d	14d	28d	3d	14d	28d
Control	1.21±0.07	1.22±0.62	1.22±0.64	12.23±1.48	12.62±1.71	12.02±1.38
C ions 2Gy	0.99±0.16$^{\blacktriangledown}$	1.03±0.19$^{\blacktriangledown}$	1.39±0.12$^{\blacktriangledown\#\#}$	10.62±1.57	9.42±0.66	8.22±1.33
4Gy	0.88±0.14$^{\blacktriangledown}$	0.82±0.13$^{\blacktriangledown}$	1.10±0.18$^{\blacktriangledown\#\#}$	6.02±0.60$^{\Delta\#}$	5.77±0.80$^{\Delta\#}$	5.17±0.60$^{\Delta\#}$
6Gy	0.75±0.15$^{\blacktriangledown}$	0.71±0.17$^{\blacktriangledown}$	0.57±0.13$^{\blacktriangledown\#\#}$	5.08±0.59$^{\Delta\#}$	4.98±0.76$^{\Delta\#}$	4.72±0.74$^{\Delta\#}$
X-rays 4Gy	1.86±0.26$^{\blacktriangledown}$	2.17±0.14	1.16±0.14$^{\#\#}$	13.05±1.84	11.09±1.77	10.16±1.35
6Gy	1.95±0.20$^{\blacktriangledown}$	1.36±0.17	0.95±0.17$^{\blacktriangledown\#\#}$	9.20±2.05$^{\Delta}$	8.40±1.91$^{\Delta}$	8.82±1.17$^{\Delta}$
12Gy	0.67±0.16$^{\blacktriangledown}$	1.11±0.27$^{\blacktriangledown}$	0.97±0.14$^{\blacktriangledown}$	5.18±0.94$^{\Delta\#}$	5.23±0.80$^{\Delta\#}$	5.21±0.66$^{\Delta\#}$

Errors are a standard deviation of the mean (SEM).

Note, $^{\Delta}$ White triangles represents the statistical significance compared with the control group, $^{\#}$the pound sign shows the plot as time goes on and the difference mean Young's modulus(E) between each dose group (*mean ± SEM*). (for 3d, Control *vs* C ions-2Gy, p = 0.114, *p>0.05*; Control *vs* C ions-4Gy, p = 0.000, *p<0.01*; Control *vs* C ions-6Gy, p = 0.000, *p<0.01*; Control *vs* X rays-4Gy, p = 0.200, *p>0.05*; Control *vs* X rays-6Gy, p = 0.000, *p<0.01*; Control *vs* X rays-12Gy, p = 0.000, *p<0.01*; for 14d, Control *vs* C ions-2Gy, p = 0.000, *p<0.01*; Control *vs* C ions-4Gy, p = 0.000, *p<0.01*; Control *vs* C ions-6Gy, p = 0.000, *p<0.01*; Control *vs* X rays-4Gy, p = 0.243, *p>0.05*; Control *vs* X -rays-6Gy, p = 0.000, *p<0.01*; Control *vs* X rays-12Gy, p = 0.000, *p<0.01*;for 28d, Control *vs* C ions-2Gy, p = 0.095, *p>0.05*; Control *vs* C ions-4Gy, p = 0.000, *p< 0.01*; Control *vs* C ions-6Gy, p = 0.000, *p<0.01*; Control *vs* X -rays-4Gy, p = 0.871, *p>0.05*; Control *vs* X rays-6Gy, p = 0.000, *p<0.01*; Control *vs* X rays-12Gy, p = 0.000, *p< 0.01*). But $^{\blacktriangledown}$ blank triangles standards for the differences of spectrin-α1 protein average level (sp) and mean Young's modulus (E) in different time points (*mean ± SEM*). The distinction was analyzed and we obtained an obvious statistical significance. $^{\#\#}$Double pound sign shows the plot as time goes on and the difference of protein between each dose group. (for 3d, Control *vs* C ions-2Gy, p = 0.000, *p<0.01*; Control *vs* C ions-4Gy, p = 0.000, *p<0.01*; Control *vs* C ions-6Gy, p = 0.000, *p<0.01*; Control *vs* X rays-4Gy, p = 0.013, *p<0.05*; Control *vs* X rays-6Gy, p = 0.000, *p<0.01*; Control *vs* X rays-12Gy, p = 0.000, *p<0.01*; for 14d, Control *vs* C ions-2Gy, p = 0.000, *p<0.01*; Control *vs* C -ions-4Gy, p = 0.000, *p<0.01*; Control *vs* C ions-6Gy, p = 0.000, *p<0.01*; Control *vs* X rays-4Gy, p = 0.000, *p<0.01*; Control *vs* X rays-6Gy, p = 0.020, *p<0.05*; Control *vs* X rays-12Gy, p = 0.023, *p<0.05*; for 28d, Control *vs* C -ions-2Gy, p = 0.010, *p<0.05*; Control *vs* C ions-4Gy, p = 0.046, *p<0.05*; Control *vs* C ions-6Gy, p = 0.000, *p< 0.01*; Control *vs* X rays-4Gy, p = 0.341, *p>0.05*; Control *vs* X rays-6Gy, p = 0.000, *p<0.01*; Control *vs* X rays-12Gy, p = 0.002, *p<0.01*).

significantly in irradiated erythrocytes. This effect relied on different radiation doses, and the data obtained showed a relationship between the expression of cytoskeletal protein spectrin-α1 and changes in cell stiffness in the irradiated group, as well as a negative correlation regarding changes in erythrocyte stiffness during the morphological remodeling process. Additionally, regarding the AFM experimental data, examination of these changes in mechanical properties by the response to force is one of the most straightforward visual indices to evaluate the membrane damage mechanism caused by radiation, assess the overall performance of protein conformation and the protein grid in the erythrocyte membrane skeleton, and increase the understanding of the radiation-induced morphological remodeling-cytoskeletal remodeling process.

Erythrocyte stiffness during morphological remodeling can be used as a biomarker to estimate the adverse effects induced by ionizing radiation

Based on the established parameters, the present study evaluated the roles of cell morphology and cell stiffness during the erythrocyte morphological remodeling process to determine the adverse effects on erythrocytes following exposure to radiation. The influence of the combination of cell signaling with the interactions of membrane phospholipids in vertical force interactions, horizontal interactions, and lateral network interactions of the spectrin structure were emphasized in the current study. Thus, it is necessary to clarify two basic problems of the mechanics induced by the effects of radiation. The first problem is the relationship between the stability of the membrane-associated cytoskeleton and changes in the mechanical properties (e.g., the stiffness or elastic modulus and the viscosity) of the erythrocytes. Another problem is that the shear stress or tension created by the effects of deformation or damage after radiation might influence how the radiation alters the cell behavior in various mechano-signaling processes, such as changes in cell shape, cell migration, cell movement and cell apoptosis. Thus, to solve these two problems, a link must be created between the biochemical molecules (proteins) and the response to force (cell stiffness) to improve our understanding of why mechanically induced changes in the protein structure within erythrocytes are likely to be important not only to cell deformability or damage but also to various mechano-signaling processes [35], [112].

When the erythrocytes were subjected to radiation, the cells first responded to the radiation at the cellular level. Next, the effect was further expanded via a signaling cascade starting at the level of proteins and molecules. Similarly to a scaffold protein, spectrin functions as a supporting protein of the erythrocyte membrane skeleton. Spectrin can organize and mediate signaling molecules into particular domains of specific signaling pathways that depend not only on the targeting affinity of proteins of the signaling pathway but also on the circumstances under which the expression of these signaling pathway components were increased and position these components in response to the radiation that activated the signal transduction pathway. Next, using this procedure, membrane proteins (comprising membrane channels, receptors and adhesion molecules) on the erythrocyte surface were activated to recruit target proteins to a specified location, organize them by affinity, and bind them into large biological macromolecular complexes. However, for spectrin proteins, posttranslational protein modifications of phosphorylation and dephosphorylation are involved in positioning and recruiting target proteins [52], resulting in a disturbance of the dynamic balance of the formation and depolymerization of scaffolding proteins [113]. This disturbance leads to the openings in the structure, rotation, and fracture, causing cytoskeleton rearrangement and collapse of the membrane skeleton due to radiation effects, in addition to directly affecting and modulating the mechanical stability of the erythro-

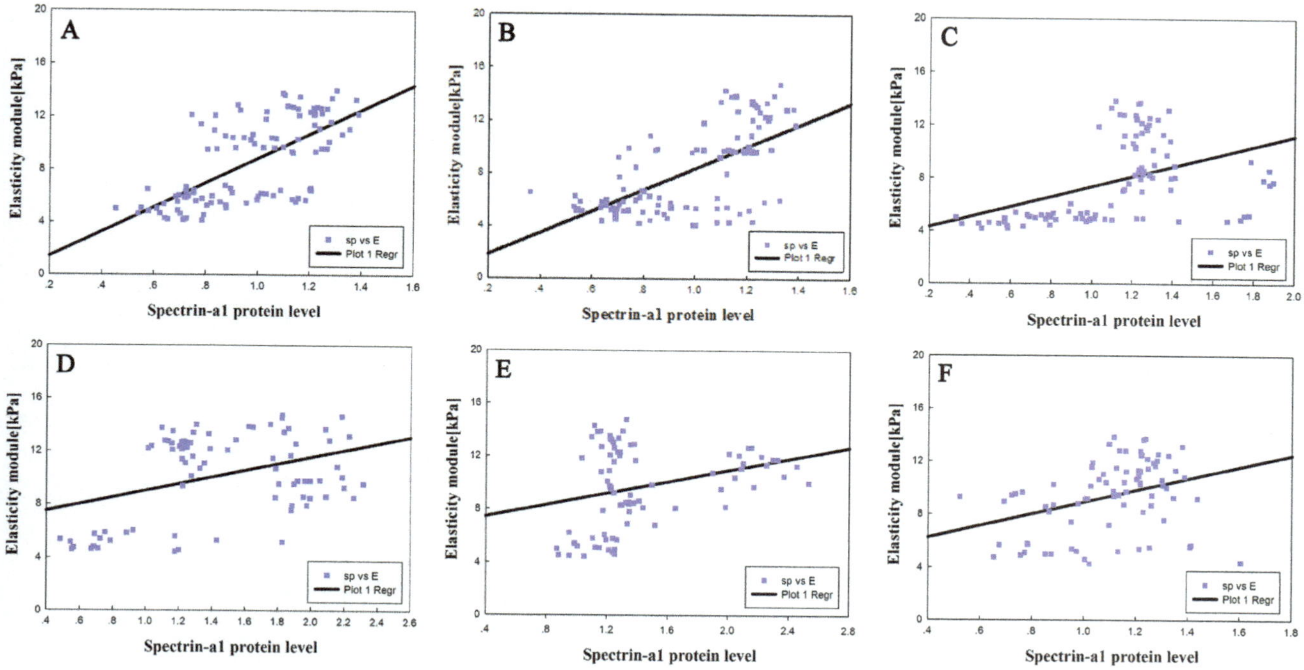

Figure 10. Spatial correlation of nanoscale modulus and spectrin-α1 protein expression with different doses of C ions or X-rays irradiated. With the increasing of radiation dosage, the relative protein expression of spectrin-α1 (sp) seemed more spatially correlated to elastic modulus (E) than low dose radiation (**A–F**). Comparison of correlation of the modulus in the same areas with Pearson's testing. In control erythrocyte samples, there appeared to be non-correlation among the Young's modulus in high-modulus regions, or low-modulus regions and the expression of spectrin-α1 protein. After treated with the radiation, the average elastic modulus was reduced and areas of cell membrane appeared to be more correlated with the modulus. Through the Pearson's correlation coefficient between modulus and spectrin-α1protein level by western blotting detection. Reflective of these findings, after exposure by carbon ion beams at 3 days, Pearson's correlation coefficient (r) between modulus and spectrin-α1 protein expression were relatively strong but significant ($r_{3c}=0.678$, $p<0.01$) compared with others time points; At 14 days irradiated by carbon ions, Pearson's correlation coefficient between them showed positive correlation ($r_{14c}=0.639$, $p<0.01$); at 28 days irradiated by carbon ions, the correlation coefficient was ($r_{28c}=0.438$, $p<0.01$). For X-rays, there were similar radiation effects with carbon ion beams in different groups, respectively, at 3, 14 and 28 days, the correlation coefficient were ($r_{3x}=0.390$, $p<0.05$), ($r_{14x}=0.301$, $p<0.01$) and ($r_{28x}=0.353$, $p<0.01$).

cyte plasma membrane. The direct effects manifest as uneven changes in the regional distribution of tension forces on the cell membrane surface; thus, the deformation or damage to the erythrocyte morphological remodeling process can be assessed.

However, for morphology-cytoskeleton remodeling, tension or stress forces are always involved in this complex coupling process. The cascade effects in the pathway are caused by biological composite macromolecules that can produce changes in the cytoskeleton-associated proteins in the spatial conformation of the erythrocyte–e.g., spectrin. There is a rigorous procedure to facilitate the interaction and fine-tune the activity and crosstalk among the proteins within the entire assembly. This targeted protein expression shows increased biological activity, which influences the activity of downstream proteins under their control, until the dynamic balance of the molecules is again coordinated. Thus, different molecular assemblies in different regions operate on the functions or implement local "microdomains" of the cell. However, the complexity of this response relies on several components of the membrane skeleton, and the stiffness of spectrin upon phosphorylation may permit the formation of many junctions to allow fast, reversible rearrangement of the spectrin network upon large deformations, thus indirectly modulating the mechanical stability of the membrane [114]. Certainly, the membrane stability depends largely on resultant forces in three directions to transfer the spatial effects of deformation or damage to the scaffolding proteins. If the protein chains are to be studied as a geometric unit, some of the mechanical behavior must be evaluated under the stress-induced load bearing of the protein structural unit (**Figure 11**). Additionally, the surface density of the filaments decreases from the center to the edge of the membrane-skeleton, and the overall thickness of the membrane-skeleton also increases from the edge of the cells (54 nm) to the center (110 nm) [115], suggesting a distribution imbalance between the surface density and the membrane-skeleton thickness, leading to tension of the membrane surface. The stress of the cytoskeleton protein chain as a unit inside the cell is unevenly distributed in partial regions or across the entire cell span. The direction of force is along the three axes; thus, the spectrin tetramers can dissociate transiently into dimers, and some of the repeating units of the spectrin chains can unfold. The dissociation of the spectrin tetramers leads to relatively unimpeded translational diffusion of transmembrane proteins and may be expected to allow them to form irregular clusters [116]. Therefore, in horizontal-plane interactions, including spectrin dimers, tetramers, hexamers and octamers, and even higher oligomeric proteins, the tension generates the interactions between the protein chains. In vertical-force interactions, the direction of the force mainly originates from two complexes, which produce shear force by the junctional complex and the AE1-ankyrin complex. The force of the lateral network interactions is more complex and presents numerous binding sites and binding proteins for a broad diversity of partners. There are mainly F-actin binding sites, actin-binding sites, and tropomyosin-, tropomodulin-, adducin-, and dematin-binding proteins participating in local regions of the network to dynamically change the mechanical properties, thus facilitating reversible deformations that the erythrocyte undergoes in different external environments

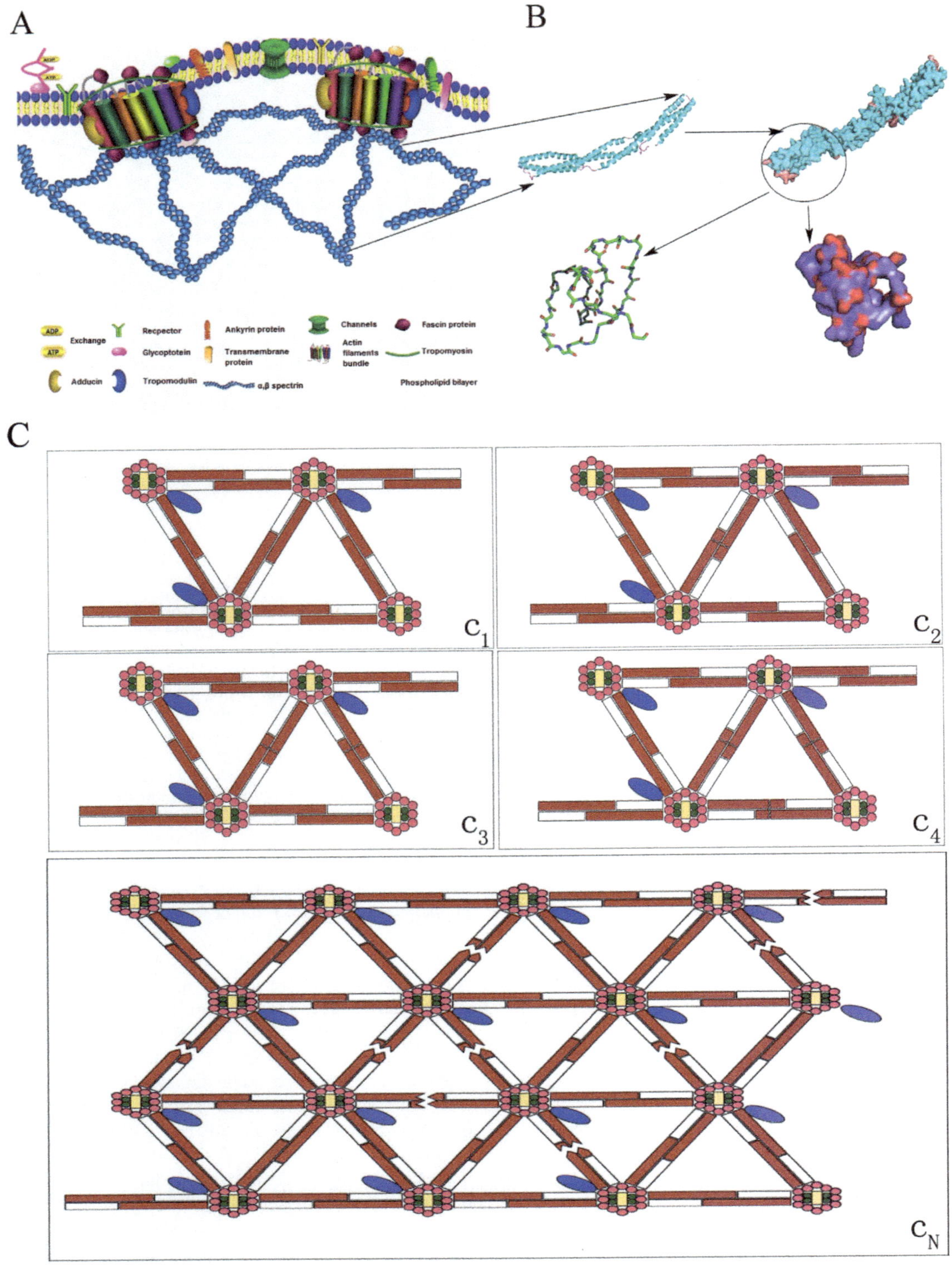

Figure 11. This picture shown the assembly structure of the scaffold protein spectrin and its spatial configuration, and were proposed a deformation hypothesis of our model. (**A**) The figure was a schematic diagram of spectrin and other cytoskeletal molecules. (**B**) Stereoview ribbon diagram of the overall structure of spectrin protein in all the repeats around the kink region. The first and second repeat (α, β subunit) were shown in light blue, and the linker region between repeats in purple, Residues were numbered according to the SWISS-PROT NP_003117.2 entry, and the residues from 1 to 2149 aa of Homo sapiens. Lastly, the software of the PyMOL Molecular Graphics Systerm was used to simulate the molecular structure, including a complete of the molecular structure and partial structure were displayed. (**C**) A series of random deformation process will be shown. The figure was α-spectrin in dark red band, and β-spectrin with a white band, the shape of saw tooth was rupture boundary. C_1 represented for completely without any deformation, then, C_2, C_3 and C_4 respectively shown that from a set of skeleton to three groups of skeleton were broken. But the case of C_N manifested randomly the fracture of cytoskeletal protein. Thus, this phenomenon could reflect the uninterrupted and dynamic of changes from small deformation to large deformation during the radiation, and more details were explained in the article.

[117,118] (as shown in **Figure 11**). The topographic and mechanical mapping of single components at the cytoplasmic face reveal that, surprisingly, the erythrocyte membrane mechanics are regulated by spectrin phosphorylation related to the metabolic state and the assembly of structural elements in the membrane [111]. Of course, to a certain extent, the local distortion or ratio of damage in cells is mainly determined by the radiation dose. Thus, the spectrins can fully dominate the deformation or damage of the cytoskeletal meshwork in the morphological remodeling process [119]. Considering the current knowledge that spectrin proteins can trigger a biological effect sufficient to change the local or overall cell morphology, as well as the mechanical and structural properties that are changed, few data are available on the interactions of spectrin with several participants in a particular pathway, organizing it into a chain of signaling events. However, according to the present study, the spectrins could be considered docking proteins in the morphological remodeling process induced by radiation.

Conclusion

In summary, our results suggest that CIR could influence the amount of components and reorganize the spectrin-α1 protein of the membrane-skeleton system, as well as affect the distribution of the regional tension or stress (force), resulting in changes in the surface topographical microstructure and mechanical properties (cell stiffness) in the erythrocyte morphological remodeling process. Additionally, we show how spectrin-α1 protein could be used as a biomarker to detect erythrocyte membrane deformation or damage and how this protein promotes the study of the biomechanical properties of signaling domains extending from the cell surface to deeper parts within the erythrocytes. These findings may bridge the gap between numerous interdependent behaviors of biological molecules and their mechanical properties to reveal the effects of deformation or damage or to assess the adverse effects on erythrocytes induced by radiation, thereby providing an inherent force-biochemical coupling analytical approach. The use of heavy ion radiation ($^{12}C^{6+}$ ions) has been proven to possess unique biological advantages in radiation therapy. Incidentally, we also suggest using heavy ion beam radiation pretreatment for the storage of erythrocytes, an application that has not yet been reported in the literature.

Author Contributions

Conceived and designed the experiments: BPZ JZW. Performed the experiments: BPZ BL. Analyzed the data: BPZ JZW. Contributed reagents/materials/analysis tools: BPZ BL. Contributed to the writing of the manuscript: BPZ. Obtained permission for use of Heavy ion radiation: HZ. Reviewed the manuscript: HZ.

References

1. Umegaki K, Sugisawa A, Shin SJ, Yamada K, Sano M (2001) Different onsets of oxidative damage to DNA and lipids in bone marrow and liver in rats given total body irradiation. Free Radic Biol Med 31: 1066–1074. PubMed: 11677039.
2. Matsunaga A, Ueda Y, Yamada S, Harada Y, Shimada H, et al. (2010) Carbon-ion beam treatment induces systemic antitumor immunity against murine squamous cell carcinoma. Cancer 116: 3740–3748. PubMed: 20564091.
3. Suzuki Y, Nakano T, Ohno T, Oka K (2008) Comparison of the radiobiological effect of carbon ion beam therapy and conventional radiation therapy on cervical cancer. J Radiat Res 49: 473–479. PubMed: 18622131.
4. Ghosh S, Narang H, Sarma A, Krishna M (2011) DNA damage response signaling in lung adenocarcinoma A549 cells following gamma and carbon beam irradiation. Mutat Res/Fundamental and Molecular Mechanisms of Mutagenesis 716: 10–19. PubMed: 21839752.
5. Afrin R, Nakaji M, Sekiguchi H, Lee D, Kishimoto K, et al. (2012) Forced extension of delipidated red blood cell cytoskeleton with little indication of spectrin unfolding. Cytoskeleton (Hoboken) 69: 101–112. PubMed: 22213694.
6. Nomura T, Hongyo T, Nakajima H, Li LY, Syaifudin M, et al. (2008) Differential radiation sensitivity to morphological, functional and molecular changes of human thyroid tissues and bone marrow cells maintained in SCID mice. Mutat Res/Genetic Toxicology and Environmental Mutagenesis 657: 68–76. PubMed: 18778792.
7. Coates PJ, Lorimore SA, Wright EG (2004) Damaging and protective cell signalling in the untargeted effects of ionizing radiation. Mutat Res/ Fundamental and Molecular Mechanisms of Mutagenesis 568: 5–20. PubMed: 15530535.
8. Gavara N, Chadwick RS (2012) Determination of the elastic moduli of thin samples and adherent cells using conical atomic force microscope tips. Nat Nanotechnol. 7: 733–736. PubMed: 23023646.
9. Wang Y, Liu L, Pazhanisamy SK, Li H, Meng A, et al. (2010) Total body irradiation causes residual bone marrow injury by induction of persistent oxidative stress in murine hematopoietic stem cells. Free Radic Biol Med 48: 348–356. PubMed: 19925862.
10. Bao Y, Chen H, Hu Y, Bai Y, Zhou M, et al. (2012) Combination effects of chronic cadmium exposure and gamma-irradiation on the genotoxicity and cytotoxicity of peripheral blood lymphocytes and bone marrow cells in rats. Mutat Res/Genetic Toxicology and Environmental Mutagenesis 743: 67–74. PubMed: 22245108.
11. Mukherjee D, Coates PJ, Rastogi S, Lorimore SA, Wright EG (2013) Radiation-induced bone marrow apoptosis, inflammatory bystander-type signaling and tissue cytotoxicity. Int J Radiat Biol 89: 139–146. PubMed: 23078404.
12. Li Q, Sun H, Xiao F, Wang X, Yang Y, et al. (2014) Protection against radiation-induced hematopoietic damage in bone marrow by hepatocyte growth factor gene transfer. Int J Radiat Biol 90: 36–44. PubMed: 24059647.
13. Liesveld JL, Rubin P, Constine LS (2014) Hematopoietic System. ALERT• Adverse Late Effects of Cancer Treatment: Springer. pp. 623–655.
14. Wang C, Nakamura S, Oshima M, Mochizuki-Kashio M, Nakajima-Takagi Y, et al. (2013) Compromised hematopoiesis and increased DNA damage following non-lethal ionizing radiation of a human hematopoietic system reconstituted in immunodeficient mice. Int J Radiat Biol 89: 132–137. PubMed: 23020858.
15. Hu S, Cucinotta FA (2011) Characterization of the radiation-damaged precursor cells in bone marrow based on modeling of the peripheral blood granulocytes response. Health Phys 101: 67–78. PubMed: 21617393.
16. Li W, Wang G, Cui J, Xue L, Cai L (2004) Low-dose radiation (LDR) induces hematopoietic hormesis: LDR-induced mobilization of hematopoietic progenitor cells into peripheral blood circulation. Exp Hematol 32: 1088–1096. PubMed: 15539087.
17. Grande T, Bueren JA (2006) The mobilization of hematopoietic progenitors to peripheral blood is predictive of the hematopoietic syndrome after total or partial body irradiation of mice. Int J Radiat Oncol Biol Phys 64: 612–618. PubMed: 16414374.
18. Moroni M, Coolbaugh TV, Lombardini E, Mitchell JM, Moccia KD, et al. (2011) Hematopoietic radiation syndrome in the Gottingen minipig. Radiat Res 176: 89–101. PubMed: 21520996.
19. Peslak SA, Wenger J, Bemis JC, Kingsley PD, Frame JM, et al. (2011) Sublethal radiation injury uncovers a functional transition during erythroid maturation. Exp Hematol 39: 434–445. PubMed: 21291953.
20. Moroni M, Elliott TB, Deutz NE, Olsen CH, Owens R, et al. (2014) Accelerated Hematopoietic Syndrome after Radiation Doses Bridging Hematopoietic (H-ARS) and Gastrointestinal (GI-ARS) Acute Radiation Syndrome: Early Hematological Changes and Systemic Inflammatory Response Syndrome in Minipig. Int J Radiat Biol: 90: 363–372. PubMed: 24524283.
21. Manda K, Kavanagh JN, Buttler D, Prise KM, Hildebrandt G (2014) Low dose effects of ionizing radiation on normal tissue stem cells. Mutat Res Rev Mutat Res pii: S1383–5742(14)00017-9. PubMed: 24566131.
22. Kulkarni S, P Ghosh S, Hauer-Jensen M, Sree Kumar K (2010) Hematological targets of radiation damage. Curr Drug Targets 11: 1375–1385. PubMed: 20583980.
23. Lara PC, López-Peñalver JJ, Farias VdA, Ruiz-Ruiz MC, Oliver FJ, et al. (2013) Direct and bystander radiation effects: A biophysical model and clinical perspectives. Cancer Lett pii: S0304–3835(13)00659-9. PubMed: 24045041.
24. Garaj-Vrhovac V, Gajski G, Pažanin S, Šarolić A, Domijan A-M, et al. (2011) Assessment of cytogenetic damage and oxidative stress in personnel occupationally exposed to the pulsed microwave radiation of marine radar equipment. Int J Hyg Environ Health 214: 59–65. PubMed: 20833106.
25. Park HJ, Griffin RJ, Hui S, Levitt SH, Song CW (2012) Radiation-induced vascular damage in tumors: implications of vascular damage in ablative hypofractionated radiotherapy (SBRT and SRS). Radiat Res 177: 311–327. PubMed: 22229487.
26. Weng H, Guo X, Papoin J, Wang J, Coppel R, et al. (2014) Interaction of Plasmodium falciparum knob-associated histidine-rich protein (KAHRP) with

erythrocyte ankyrin R is required for its attachment to the erythrocyte membrane. Biochim Biophys Acta 1838: 185–192. PubMed: 24090929.
27. Park Y, Best CA, Badizadegan K, Dasari RR, Feld MS, et al. (2010) Measurement of red blood cell mechanics during morphological changes. Proc Natl Acad Sci U S A 107: 6731–6736. PubMed: 20351261.
28. Zou S, Chisholm R, Tauskela JS, Mealing GA, Johnston LJ, et al. (2013) Force Spectroscopy Measurements Show That Cortical Neurons Exposed to Excitotoxic Agonists Stiffen before Showing Evidence of Bleb Damage. PLoS One 8: e73499. PubMed: 24023686.
29. de Oliveira M, Vera C, Valdez P, Sharma Y, Skelton R, et al. (2010) Nanomechanics of multiple units in the erythrocyte membrane skeletal network. Ann Biomed Eng 38: 2956–2967. PubMed: 20490687.
30. Lim CT, Li A (2011) Mechanopathology of red blood cell diseases-Why mechanics matters. Theoretical and Applied Mechanics Letters 1: 014000-014000-014006.
31. Rojas-Aguirre Y, Hernández-Luis F, Mendoza-Martínez C, Sotomayor CP, Aguilar LF, et al. (2012) Effects of an antimalarial quinazoline derivative on human erythrocytes and on cell membrane molecular models. Biochim Biophys Acta 1818: 738–746. PubMed: 22155684.
32. Samanta S, Dutta D, Ghoshal A, Mukhopadhyay S, Saha B, et al. (2011) Glycosylation of Erythrocyte Spectrin and Its Modification in Visceral Leishmaniasis. PLoS One 6: e28169. PubMed: 22164239.
33. Shi H, Liu Z, Li A, Yin J, Chong AG, et al. (2013) Life Cycle-Dependent Cytoskeletal Modifications in Plasmodium falciparum Infected Erythrocytes. PLoS One 8: e61170. PubMed: 23585879.
34. An X, Mohandas N (2010) Red cell membrane and malaria. Transfus Clin Biol 17: 197–199. PubMed: 20674435.
35. Mohandas N, Evans E (1994) Mechanical properties of the red cell membrane in relation to molecular structure and genetic defects. Annu Rev Biophys Biomol Struct 23: 787–818. PubMed: 7919799.
36. Maciaszek JL, Lykotrafitis G (2011) Sickle cell trait human erythrocytes are significantly stiffer than normal. J Biomech 44: 657–661. PubMed: 21111421.
37. Delaunay J (2007) The molecular basis of hereditary red cell membrane disorders. Blood Rev 21: 1–20. PubMed: 16730867.
38. Debaugnies F, Cotton F, Boutique C, Gulbis B (2011) Erythrocyte membrane protein analysis by sodium dodecyl sulphate-capillary gel electrophoresis in the diagnosis of hereditary spherocytosis. Clin Chem Lab Med 49: 485–492. PubMed: 21231903.
39. Katira P, Zaman MH, Bonnecaze RT (2012) How changes in cell mechanical properties induce cancerous behavior. Phys Rev Lett 108: 028103. PubMed: 22324713.
40. Li J, Lykotrafitis G, Dao M, Suresh S (2007) Cytoskeletal dynamics of human erythrocyte. Proc Natl Acad Sci U S A 104: 4937–4942. PubMed: 17360346.
41. Lekka M, Fornal M, Pyka-Fościak G, Lebed K, Wizner B, et al. (2005) Erythrocyte stiffness probed using atomic force microscope. Biorheology 42: 307–317. PubMed: 16227658.
42. Bao G, Suresh S (2003) Cell and molecular mechanics of biological materials. Nat Mater 2: 715–725. PubMed: 14593396.
43. Suresh S, Spatz J, Mills J, Micoulet A, Dao M, et al. (2005) Connections between single-cell biomechanics and human disease states: gastrointestinal cancer and malaria. Acta Biomater 1: 15–30. PubMed: 16701777.
44. Stewart MP, Toyoda Y, Hyman AA, Müller DJ (2012) Tracking mechanics and volume of globular cells with atomic force microscopy using a constant-height clamp. Nat Protoc 7: 143–154. PubMed: 22222789.
45. Zuk A, Targosz-Korecka M, Szymonski M (2011) Effect of selected drugs used in asthma treatment on morphology and elastic properties of red blood cells. Int J Nanomedicine 6: 249–257. PubMed: 21499423.
46. Szarama KB, Gavara N, Petralia RS, Kelley MW, Chadwick RS (2012) Cytoskeletal changes in actin and microtubules underlie the developing surface mechanical properties of sensory and supporting cells in the mouse cochlea. Development 139: 2187–2197. PubMed: 22573615.
47. Li M, Liu L, Xi N, Wang Y, Dong Z, et al. (2012) Atomic force microscopy imaging and mechanical properties measurement of red blood cells and aggressive cancer cells. Sci China Life Sci 55: 968–973. PubMed: 23160828.
48. Heinrich V, Ritchie K, Mohandas N, Evans E (2001) Elastic thickness compressibilty of the red cell membrane. Biophys J 81: 1452–1463. PubMed: 11509359.
49. Park Y, Best CA, Auth T, Gov NS, Safran SA, et al. (2010) Metabolic remodeling of the human red blood cell membrane. Proc Natl Acad Sci U S A 107: 1289–1294. PubMed: 20080583.
50. Peng Z, Li X, Pivkin IV, Dao M, Karniadakis GE, et al. (2013) Lipid bilayer and cytoskeletal interactions in a red blood cell. Proc Natl Acad Sci U S A 110: 13356–13361. PubMed: 23898181.
51. Svetina S, Kuzman D, Waugh RE, Ziherl P, Žekš B (2004) The cooperative role of membrane skeleton and bilayer in the mechanical behaviour of red blood cells. Bioelectrochemistry 62: 107–113. PubMed: 15039011.
52. Machnicka B, Czogalla A, Hryniewicz-Jankowska A, Bogusławska DM, Grochowalska R, et al. (2013) Spectrins: A structural platform for stabilization and activation of membrane channels, receptors and transporters. Biochim Biophys Acta 1838: 620–634. PubMed: 23673272.
53. Marchesi VT, Steers E, Jr. (1968) Selective solubilization of a protein component of the red cell membrane. Science 159: 203–204. PubMed: 5634911.
54. Švelc T, Svetina S (2012) Stress-free state of the red blood cell membrane and the deformation of its skeleton. Cell Mol Biol Lett 17: 217–227. PubMed: 22302416.
55. Foretz M, Hébrard S, Guihard S, Leclerc J, Do Cruzeiro M, et al. (2011) The AMPKγ1 subunit plays an essential role in erythrocyte membrane elasticity, and its genetic inactivation induces splenomegaly and anemia. FASEB J 25: 337–347. PubMed: 20881209.
56. Kim Y, Kim M, Shin JH, Kim J (2011) Characterization of cellular elastic modulus using structure based double layer model. Med Biol Eng Comput 49: 453–462. PubMed: 21221828.
57. Strey H, Peterson M, Sackmann E (1995) Measurement of erythrocyte membrane elasticity by flicker eigenmode decomposition. Biophys J 69: 478–488. PubMed: 8527662.
58. Cardamone L, Laio A, Torre V, Shahapure R, DeSimone A (2011) Cytoskeletal actin networks in motile cells are critically self-organized systems synchronized by mechanical interactions. Proc Natl Acad Sci U S A 108: 13978–13983. PubMed: 21825142.
59. Fedosov DA, Caswell B, Karniadakis GE (2010) Systematic coarse-graining of spectrin-level red blood cell models. Comput Methods Appl Mech Eng 199: 1937–1948. PubMed: 24353352.
60. Zhu Q, Vera C, Asaro RJ, Sche P, Sung LA (2007) A hybrid model for erythrocyte membrane: a single unit of protein network coupled with lipid bilayer. Biophys J 93: 386–400. PubMed: 17449663.
61. Kozlova EK, Chernysh AM, Moroz VV, Kuzovlev AN (2012) Analysis of nanostructure of red blood cells membranes by space Fourier transform of AFM images. Micron 44: 218–427. PubMed: 22854216.
62. Li X, Peng Z, Lei H, Dao M, Karniadakis GE (2014) Probing red blood cell mechanics, rheology and dynamics with a two-component multi-scale model. Philos Trans A Math Phys Eng Sci 372: 20130389. PubMed: 24982252.
63. Callan-Jones A, Albarran Arriagada OE, Massiera G, Lorman V, Abkarian M (2012) Red Blood Cell Membrane Dynamics during Malaria Parasite Egress. Biophys J 103: 2475–2483. PubMed: 23260049.
64. Boey SK, Boal DH, Discher DE (1998) Simulations of the Erythrocyte Cytoskeleton at Large Deformation. I. Microscopic Models. Biophys J 75: 1573–1583. PubMed: 9726958.
65. Discher DE, Boal DH, Boey SK (1998) Simulations of the Erythrocyte Cytoskeleton at Large Deformation. II. Micropipette Aspiration. Biophys J 75: 1584–1597. PubMed: 9726959.
66. De Nunzio C, Aronson W, Freedland SJ, Giovannucci E, Parsons JK (2012) The correlation between metabolic syndrome and prostatic diseases. Eur Urol 61: 560–570. PubMed: 22119157.
67. Ma X, Zhang H, Wang Z, Min X, Liu Y, et al. (2011) Chromosomal aberrations in the bone marrow cells of mice induced by accelerated (12) C (6+) ions. Mutat Res/Fundamental and Molecular Mechanisms of Mutagenesis 716: 20–26. PubMed: 21843535.
68. Sheetz MP, Casaly J (1980) 2, 3-Diphosphoglycerate and ATP dissociate erythrocyte membrane skeletons. J Biol Chem 255: 9955–9960. PubMed: 7430109.
69. Lin S, Snyder C (1977) High affinity cytochalasin B binding to red cell membrane proteins which are unrelated to sugar transport. J Biol Chem 252: 5464–5471. PubMed: 407226.
70. Kunda P, Pelling AE, Liu T, Baum B (2008) Moesin controls cortical rigidity, cell rounding, and spindle morphogenesis during mitosis. Curr Biol 18: 91–101. PubMed: 18207738.
71. Ludwig T, Kirmse R, Poole K, Schwarz US (2008) Probing cellular microenvironments and tissue remodeling by atomic force microscopy. Pflugers Arch 456: 29–49. PubMed: 18058123.
72. Takeuchi M, Miyamoto H, Sako Y, Komizu H, Kusumi A (1998) Structure of the erythrocyte membrane skeleton as observed by atomic force microscopy. Biophys J 74: 2171–2183. PubMed: 9591644.
73. Swihart A, Mikrut J, Ketterson J, Macdonald R (2001) Atomic force microscopy of the erythrocyte membrane skeleton. J Microsc 204: 212–225. PubMed: 11903798.
74. Alonso JL, Goldmann WH (2003) Feeling the forces: atomic force microscopy in cell biology. Life Sci 72: 2553–2560. PubMed: 12672501.
75. Sneddon IN (1965) The relation between load and penetration in the axisymmetric Boussinesq problem for a punch of arbitrary profile. Int J Engi Sci 3: 47–57. doi.org/10.1016/0020-7225(65)90019-4.
76. Rico F, Roca-Cusachs P, Gavara N, Farré R, Rotger M, et al. (2005) Probing mechanical properties of living cells by atomic force microscopy with blunted pyramidal cantilever tips. Phys Rev E Stat Nonlin Soft Matter Phys 72: 021914. PubMed: 16196611.
77. Johnson K, Kendall K, Roberts A (1971) Surface energy and the contact of elastic solids. Proc Roya Soci Lond 324: 301–313. doi.jstor.org/stable/78058.
78. Dimitriadis EK, Horkay F, Maresca J, Kachar B, Chadwick RS (2002) Determination of elastic moduli of thin layers of soft material using the atomic force microscope. Biophys J 82: 2798–2810. PubMed: 11964265.
79. Carl P, Schillers H (2008) Elasticity measurement of living cells with an atomic force microscope: data acquisition and processing. Pflugers Arch 457: 551–559. PubMed: 18481081.
80. Li Q, Lee G, Ong C, Lim C (2008) AFM indentation study of breast cancer cells. Biochem Biophys Res Commun 374: 609–613. PubMed: 18656442.

81. Ketene AN (2011) The AFM Study of Ovarian Cell Structural Mechanics in the Progression of Cancer: Virginia Polytechnic Institute and State University. doi.scholar.lib.vt.edu/theses/available/etd-05182011-152552.
82. Ketene AN, Schmelz EM, Roberts PC, Agah M (2012) The effects of cancer progression on the viscoelasticity of ovarian cell cytoskeleton structures. Nanomedicine 8: 93–102. PubMed: 21704191.
83. Lu Y-B, Franze K, Seifert G, Steinhäuser C, Kirchhoff F, et al. (2006) Viscoelastic properties of individual glial cells and neurons in the CNS. Proc Natl Acad Sci U S A 103: 17759–17764. PubMed: 17093050.
84. Strobl JS, Nikkhah M, Agah M (2010) Actions of the anti-cancer drug suberoylanilide hydroxamic acid (SAHA) on human breast cancer cytoarchitecture in silicon microstructures. Biomaterials 31: 7043–7050. PubMed: 20579727.
85. Darling EM, Topel M, Zauscher S, Vail TP, Guilak F (2008) Viscoelastic properties of human mesenchymally-derived stem cells and primary osteoblasts, chondrocytes, and adipocytes. J Biomech 41: 454–464. PubMed: 17825308.
86. Guo S, Akhremitchev BB (2006) Packing density and structural heterogeneity of insulin amyloid fibrils measured by AFM nanoindentation. Biomacromolecules 7: 1630–1636. PubMed: 16677048.
87. Nikkhah M, Strobl JS, De Vita R, Agah M (2010) The cytoskeletal organization of breast carcinoma and fibroblast cells inside three dimensional (3-D) isotropic silicon microstructures. Biomaterials 31: 4552–4561. PubMed: 20207413.
88. Ghorai A, Bhattacharyya NP, Sarma A, Ghosh U (2014) Radiosensitivity and Induction of Apoptosis by High LET Carbon Ion Beam and Low LET Gamma Radiation: A Comparative Study. Scientifica (Cairo) 2014: 438030. PubMed: 25018892.
89. Xu H, Gao L, Che T, Du W, Li Q, et al. (2012) The effects of $^{12}C^{6+}$ irradiation on cell cycle, apoptosis, and expression of caspase-3 in the human lung cancer cell line h1299. Cancer Biother Radiopharm 27: 113–118. PubMed: 22242595.
90. Haghparast SMA, Kihara T, Shimizu Y, Yuba S, Miyake J (2013) Actin-based biomechanical features of suspended normal and cancer cells. J Biosci Bioeng 116: 380–385. PubMed: 23567154.
91. Schmidt CF, Svoboda K, Lei N, Petsche IB, Berman LE, et al. (1993) Existence of a flat phase in red cell membrane skeletons. Science 259: 952–955. PubMed: 8438153.
92. Machnicka B, Grochowalska R, Bogusławska D, Sikorski A, Lecomte M (2012) Spectrin-based skeleton as an actor in cell signaling. Cell Mol Life Sci 69: 191–201. PubMed: 21877118.
93. Franke R, Scharnweber T, Fuhrmann R, Mrowietz C, Jung F (2013) Effect of radiographic contrast media (Iodixanol, Iopromide) on the spectrin/actin-network of the membranous cytoskeleton of erythrocytes. Clin Hemorheol Microcirc 54: 273–285. PubMed: 23666115.
94. Sonmez M, Ince HY, Yalcin O, Ajdžanović V, Spasojević I, et al. (2013) The effect of alcohols on red blood cell mechanical properties and membrane fluidity depends on their molecular size. PloS One 8: e76579. PubMed: 24086751.
95. Kuriakose S, Dimitrakopoulos P (2013) Deformation of an elastic capsule in a rectangular microfluidic channel. Soft Matter. 9: 4284–4296. PubMed: 23585769.
96. Hansen J, Skalak R, Chien S, Hoger A (1996) An elastic network model based on the structure of the red blood cell membrane skeleton. Biophys J 70: 146–166. PubMed: 8770194.
97. Kabaso D, Shlomovitz R, Auth T, Lew VL, Gov NS (2010) Curling and local shape changes of red blood cell membranes driven by cytoskeletal reorganization. Biophys J 99: 808–816. PubMed: 20682258.
98. Afrin R, Nakaji M, Sekiguchi H, Lee D, Kishimoto K, et al. (2012) Forced extension of delipidated red blood cell cytoskeleton with little indication of spectrin unfolding. Cytoskeleton 69: 101–112. PubMed: 22213694.
99. Liu F, Burgess J, Mizukami H, Ostafin A (2003) Sample preparation and imaging of erythrocyte cytoskeleton with the atomic force microscopy. Cell Biochem Biophys 38: 251–270. PubMed: 12794267.
100. Salomao M, An X, Guo X, Gratzer WB, Mohandas N, et al. (2006) Mammalian αI-spectrin is a neofunctionalized polypeptide adapted to small highly deformable erythrocytes. Proc Natl Acad Sci U S A 103: 643–648. PubMed: 16407147.
101. Chan MM, Wooden JM, Tsang M, Gilligan DM, Hirenallur-S DK, et al. (2013) Hematopoietic Protein-1 Regulates the Actin Membrane Skeleton and Membrane Stability in Murine Erythrocytes. PloS One 8: e54902. PubMed: 23424621.
102. Nambiar R, McConnell RE, Tyska MJ (2009) Control of cell membrane tension by myosin-I. Proc Natl Acad Sci U S A 106: 11972–11977. PubMed: 19574460.
103. Muravyov AV, Tikhomirova IA (2013) Role molecular signaling pathways in changes of red blood cell deformability. Clin Hemorheol Microcirc 53: 45–59. PubMed: 22951624.
104. Corre I, Niaudet C, Paris F (2010) Plasma membrane signaling induced by ionizing radiation. Mutat Res 704: 61–67. PubMed: 20117234.
105. Daniels G (2007) Functions of red cell surface proteins. Vox Sang 93: 331–340. PubMed: 18070278.
106. Buys AV, Van Rooy M-J, Soma P, Van Papendorp D, Lipinski B, et al. (2013) Changes in red blood cell membrane structure in type 2 diabetes: a scanning electron and atomic force microscopy study. Cardiovasc Diabetol 12: 25. PubMed: 23356738.
107. Dubreuil RR (2006) Functional links between membrane transport and the spectrin cytoskeleton. J Membr Biol 211: 151–161. PubMed: 17091212.
108. Johnson CP, Tang H-Y, Carag C, Speicher DW, Discher DE (2007) Forced unfolding of proteins within cells. Science 317: 663–666. PubMed: 17673662.
109. Discher DE, Carl P (2001) New insights into red cell network structure, elasticity, and spectrin unfolding-a current review. Cell Mol Biol Lett 6: 593–606. PubMed: 11598637.
110. Broderick M, Winder S (2005) Spectrin, alpha-actinin, and dystrophin. Adv Protein Chem 70: 203–246. PubMed: 15837517.
111. Kusunoki H, MacDonald RI, Mondragón A (2004) Structural insights into the stability and flexibility of unusual erythroid spectrin repeats. Structure 12: 645–656. PubMed: 15062087.
112. Pan CQ, Sudol M, Sheetz M, Low BC (2012) Modularity and functional plasticity of scaffold proteins as p(l)acemakers in cell signaling. Cell Signal 24: 2143–2165. PubMed: 22743133.
113. Zhu Q, Asaro RJ (2008) Spectrin folding versus unfolding reactions and RBC membrane stiffness. Biophys J 94: 2529–2545. PubMed: 18065469.
114. Picas L, Rico Fl, Deforet M, Scheuring S (2013) Structural and Mechanical Heterogeneity of the Erythrocyte Membrane Reveals Hallmarks of Membrane Stability. ACS Nano 7: 1054–1063. PubMed: 23347043.
115. Nans A, Mohandas N, Stokes DL (2011) Native ultrastructure of the red cell cytoskeleton by cryo-electron tomography. Biophys J 101: 2341–2350. PubMed: 22098732.
116. Blanc L, Salomao M, Guo X, An X, Gratzer W, et al. (2010) Control of erythrocyte membrane-skeletal cohesion by the spectrin-membrane linkage. Biochemistry 49: 4516–4523. PubMed: 20433199.
117. Koshino I, Mohandas N, Takakuwa Y (2012) Identification of a novel role for dematin in regulating red cell membrane function by modulating spectrin-actin interaction. J Biol Chem 287: 35244–35250. PubMed: 22927433.
118. Baines A (2010) Evolution of the spectrin-based membrane skeleton. Transfus Clin Biol 17: 95–103. PubMed: 20688550.
119. Zhang R, Brown FL (2008) Cytoskeleton mediated effective elastic properties of model red blood cell membranes. J Chem Phys 129: 065101. PubMed: 18715105.

Associated Factors of Atrophic Gastritis Diagnosed by Double-Contrast Upper Gastrointestinal Barium X-Ray Radiography: A Cross-Sectional Study Analyzing 6,901 Healthy Subjects in Japan

Nobutake Yamamichi[1]*, Chigaya Hirano[2], Takeshi Shimamoto[1,2], Chihiro Minatsuki[1], Yu Takahashi[1], Chiemi Nakayama[1], Rie Matsuda[1], Mitsuhiro Fujishiro[1], Maki Konno-Shimizu[1], Jun Kato[3], Shinya Kodashima[1], Satoshi Ono[1], Keiko Niimi[1], Satoshi Mochizuki[1], Yosuke Tsuji[1], Yoshiki Sakaguchi[1], Itsuko Asada-Hirayama[1], Chihiro Takeuchi[1], Seiichi Yakabi[1], Hikaru Kakimoto[1], Ryoichi Wada[2], Toru Mitsushima[2], Masao Ichinose[3], Kazuhiko Koike[1]

1 Department of Gastroenterology, Graduate School of Medicine, The University of Tokyo, Tokyo, Japan, **2** Department of Gastroenterology, Kameda Medical Center Makuhari, Chiba, Japan, **3** Second Department of Internal Medicine, Wakayama Medical University, Wakayama, Japan

Abstract

Background: Double-contrast upper gastrointestinal barium X-ray radiography (UGI-XR) is one of the most widely conducted gastric cancer screening methods. It has been executed to find gastric cancer, but has not been usually executed to detect premalignant atrophic mucosa of stomach. To understand the meaning of UGI-XR-based atrophic gastritis, we analyzed its association with several causative factors including *Helicobacter pylori* (HP) infection.

Methods: We evaluated 6,901 healthy adults in Japan. UGI-XR-based atrophic gastritis was diagnosed based on the irregular shape of areae gastricae and its expansion in the stomach.

Results: Of the 6,433 subjects with no history of HP eradication and free from gastric acid suppressants, 1,936 were diagnosed as UGI-XR-based atrophic gastritis (mild: 234, moderate: 822, severe: 880). These were univariately associated with serum HP IgG and serum pepsinogen I/II ratio with statistical significance. The multiple logistic analysis calculating standardized coefficients (β) and odds ratio (OR) demonstrated that serum HP IgG (β = 1.499, OR = 4.48), current smoking (β = 0.526, OR = 1.69), age (β = 0.401, OR = 1.49), low serum pepsinogen I/II ratio (β = 0.339, OR = 1.40), and male gender (β = 0.306, OR = 1.36) showed significant positive association with UGI-XR-based atrophic gastritis whereas drinking and body mass index did not. Among the age/sex/smoking/drinking-matched 227 pairs derived from chronically HP-infected and successfully HP-eradicated subjects, UGI-XR-based atrophic gastritis was detected in 99.1% of the former but in only 59.5% of the latter subjects ($p<0.0001$). Contrastively, UGI-XR-based atrophic gastritis was detected in 13 of 14 HP-positive proton pump inhibitor users (92.9%) and 33 of 34 HP-positive histamine H_2-receptor antagonist users (97.1%), which are not significantly different from gastric acid suppressant-free subjects.

Conclusions: The presence of UGI-XR-based atrophic gastritis is positively associated with *Helicobacter pylori* infection, current smoking, age, decreased serum pepsinogen I/II ratio, and male gender. Eradication of *Helicobacter pylori* seems to superficially improve UGI-XR-based atrophic gastritis whereas intake of gastric acid suppressants does not.

Editor: Mitsunobu R. Kano, Okayama University, Japan

Funding: This work was supported in part by a research grant from Takeda Science Foundation, in part by a research grant from the Daiwa Security Health Foundation, and also in part by Grant-in-Aid for Scientific Research (C) from the Japan Society for the Promotion of Science. All the funders had no role in study design, data collection and analysis, decision to publish, or preparation of manuscript.

Competing Interests: The authors have declared that no competing interests exist.

* Email: nyamamic-tky@umin.ac.jp

Introduction

The incidence and mortality of gastric cancer has gradually fallen in the recent several decades, but it is still the second leading cause of cancer death worldwide [1,2]. Many gastric cancer screening methods have been developed and executed especially in East Asia, where a high incidence of gastric cancer is observed [3]. Among them, the double-contrast upper gastrointestinal barium X-ray radiography (UGI-XR) is one of the most widely used screening methods for gastric cancer. It has been conducted in

Japan since 1960's as the nationwide mass screening for stomach cancer [3,4,5]. Many previous studies suggested that regularly-scheduled UGI-XR may lead to a reduced risk of mortality from gastric cancer [4,6,7,8]. Therefore, UGI-XR is at present the only one method of gastric cancer screening officially authenticated in Japan [9], though other screening methods with endoscopy or serum pepsinogens are gradually spreading [10,11].

Nowadays, an issue to be solved for UGI-XR-based gastric cancer screening is coming about. UGI-XR has been mainly performed to find gastric cancer and other lesions such as erosion, ulcer, polyp, and so on. But regrettably, atrophic gastritis detected by UGI-XR has not been usually assessed. One of the reasons for that is probably the time when UGI-XR-based gastric cancer screening began: around 1960's in Japan, the prevalence of *Helicobacter pylori* (*H. pylori*)-induced gastritis was extremely high [3,5]. In the past several decades, however, the infection rate of *H. pylori* has been decreased worldwide [12,13,14,15]: consequently, clinical significance of evaluating UGI-XR-based atrophic gastritis become relatively higher today. Another more important reason is inadequate validation of the meaning of "atrophic gastritis" diagnosed by UGI-XR. At present, it is well established that chronic *H. pylori* infection mostly causes pathological gastritis with mucosal atrophy and precancerous intestinal metaplasia [16,17,18,19,20]. However, there is no clear evidence that "UGI-XR-based" atrophic gastritis coincides with *H. pylori*-induced "pathological" gastritis or "endoscopy-based" atrophic gastritis.

Based on these backgrounds, the purpose of this study is evaluating associations of "UGI-XR-based" atrophic gastritis with several causative factors including chronic *H. pylori* infection. Through the large-scale analysis of healthy adults in Japan, we have challenged the unsolved but important problem: the meaning of "atrophic gastritis" diagnosed by UGI-XR. We further expect that our results will improve the efficacy of gastric cancer screening via establishing precise evaluation of premalignant UGI-XR-based atrophic gastritis. Prediction of future cancer risk based on UGI-XR-based atrophic gastritis should increase the value of gastric cancer screening with barium X-ray.

Materials and Methods

Study Subjects

The study population was 20,773 subjects who received medical checkup at Kameda Medical Center Makuhari (Chiba-shi, Chiba, Japan) in 2010 and agreed with participating in our study. In cases where health checkup was performed twice in 2010, the former data was used. Criteria for exclusion were insufficient data for analysis or history of gastrectomy. This study was approved by the ethics committee of the University of Tokyo, and written informed consents were obtained from all the study participants according to the Declaration of Helsinki.

Double-contrast Upper Gastrointestinal Barium X-ray Radiography (UGI-XR)

Five minutes after intramuscular injection of spasmolytic agent (10 mg of scopolamine butylbromide), the subject drank 150 ml of barium (220 w/v %) in one gulp. X-ray images were then taken as follows; 1) double-contrast right anterior oblique view of the upper and lower esophagus in the near-supine standing position, 2) single-contrast frontal view of the stomach in the supine standing position, 3) double-contrast frontal image of the stomach in the supine position, 4) double-contrast right anterior oblique view of the stomach in the near-supine position, 5) double-contrast left anterior oblique view of the stomach in the near-supine position, 6) double-contrast right lateral view of the stomach in the horizontal position, 7) single-contrast frontal view of the stomach in the prone position, 8) double-contrast frontal view of the stomach in the prone position with the head down, 9) double-contrast frontal view of the stomach in the prone standing position, 10) double-contrast left anterior oblique view of the stomach in the prone position with the head down, 11) double-contrast left lateral view of the stomach in the horizontal position, 12) double-contrast left anterior oblique view of the stomach in the near-supine half-standing position (Schatzki's position), 13) double-contrast left anterior oblique view of the stomach in the near-supine position ("Barium divided" image), and 14) double-contrast right anterior oblique view of the stomach in the near-supine half-standing position.

Definition of Atrophic Gastritis Based on the Double-contrast Barium X-ray Radiography (UGI-XR-based atrophic gastritis)

The characteristics of gastritis in the double-contrast barium X-ray images have been described by a few reports [21,22]. By referring to them, in our previous report [23], we diagnosed gastritis based on the enlarged areae gastricae and/or hypertrophic gastritis with thickened folds on the greater curvature. It is also well known that atrophic gastritis usually extends from the antrum to body and fornix [19]. Taken these into consideration, we classified the double-contrast barium X-ray images of stomach into four types, on the basis of the irregular shapes of areae gastricae and their expansion as follows;

(A: normal) No atrophic change can be observed in stomach. The areae gastricae cannot be detected or can be recognized as small, round, and regular shapes in all the mucosal surface of stomach (Figure 1a).

(B: mild) The mucosal atrophy is mostly limited to gastric antrum. The enlarged areae gastricae with slight angularity and irregularity are observed in the restricted mucosal surface of stomach (Figure 1b).

(C: moderate) The mucosal atrophy extends from gastric antrum to body (corpus) and/or fornix. The obviously enlarged areae gastricae with considerable angularity and irregularity are observed in most or all mucosal surface of stomach (Figure 1c).

(D: severe) The severe atrophic change entirely covers the mucosal surface of stomach. The small or even absent areae gastricae diffusely extend in stomach, accompanied with irregularly rugged mucosal surface (Figure 1D).

Disgnosis of Atrophic Gastritis by Endoscopy

Atrophic patterns of gastric mucosa by endoscopy were classified into seven classes according to the Kimura-Takemoto classification [24,25]: no atrophic change (C0), three closed type atrophy patterns (C1, C2, C3), and three open type atrophy patterns (O1, O2, O3).

Evaluation of Serum anti-*Helicobacter pylori* IgG, Serum Pepsinogens (PGs), Alcohol Intake, and Smoking

Serum anti-*H. pylori* IgG, pepsinogen I, and pepsinogen II were measured using commercial kits (E-plate "EIKEN" Helicobacter pylori antibody and E-Plate "EIKEN" Pepsinogen I and II, Eiken Chemical Co LTD., Tokyo, Japan) as we had previously reported [26,27,28]. According to the manufacture's instruction, titer of *H. pylori* IgG $\geq$10 U/ml was considered as *H. pylori*-positive. Recently, it has been suggested that titer of *H. pylori* IgG $<$ 10 U/ml should be reconsidered from the standpoint of mucosal

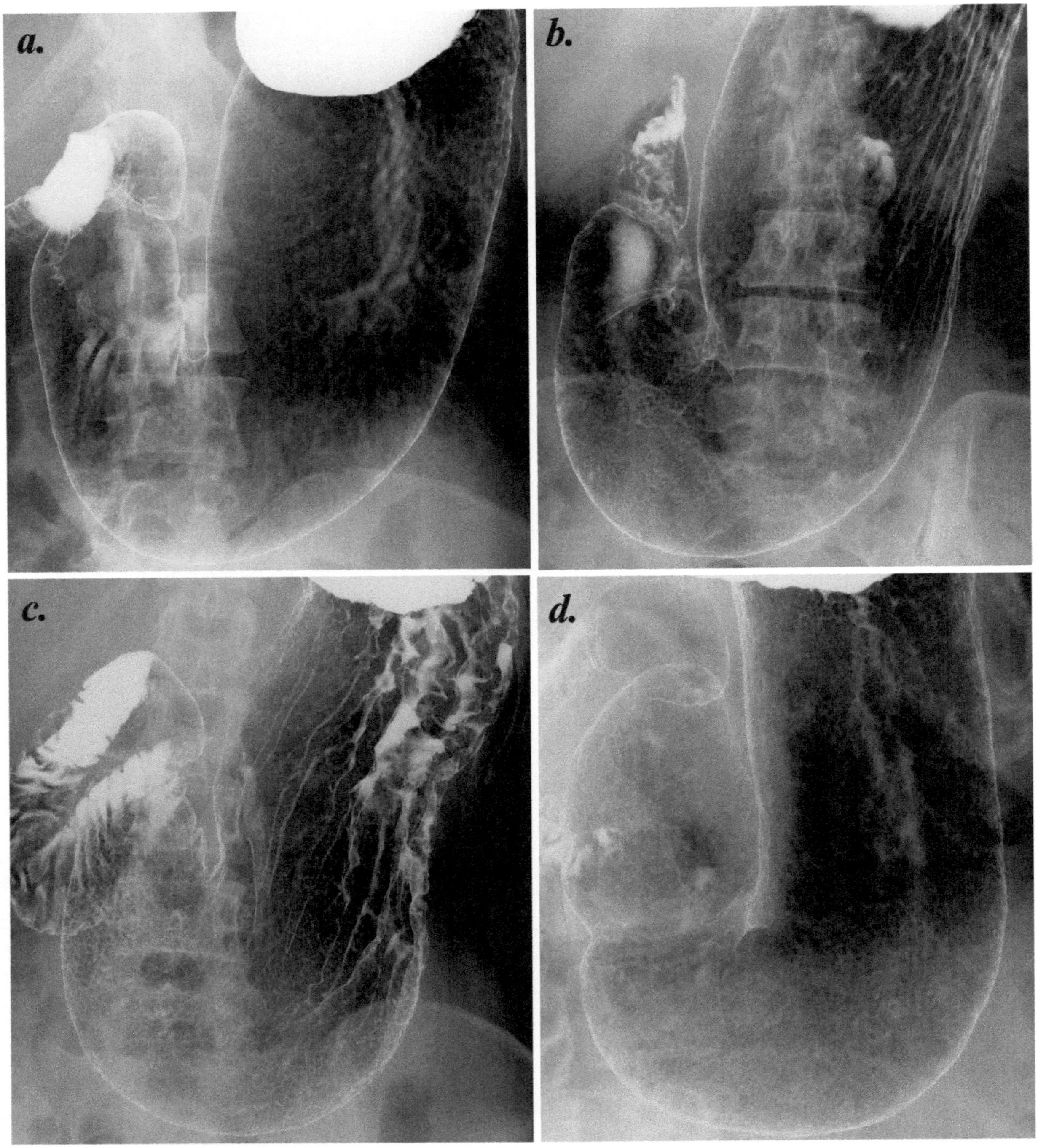

Figure 1. Typical four images of stomach by double-contrast upper gastrointestinal barium X-ray radiography (UGI-XR). (a) Normal stomach with no atrophic change of gastric mucosa. (b) Mild gastritis in which atrophic change mostly exists in gastric antrum and angle, accompanied with slightly enlarged irregular areae gastricae. (c) Moderate gastritis in which atrophic change extends from gastric antrum to body and/or fornix, accompanied with obviously enlarged irregular areae gastricae. (d) Severe gastritis in which atrophic change covers the entire stomach, accompanied with obscured small or even absent areae gastricae.

atrophic change or gastric cancer risk [29,30]. Therefore, we further divided "*H. pylori*-negative" subjects into "≥3 and < 10 U/ml (gray-zone titer of *H. pylori* IgG)" and "<3 U/ml (absolutely negative for *H. pylori* IgG)". In accordance with previous reports [28,31,32], ratios of serum pepsinogen I and II (pepsinogen I [ng/ml]/pepsinogen II [ng/ml]) were classified into ">3", ">2 and ≤3", and "≤2".

For alcohol intake, the study subjects were scored according to the 5-grade scale (never, seldom, sometimes, often, and always), and further categorized into "rarely drinking" group (never or seldom) and "usually drinking" group (sometimes, often, or always). For smoking, the subjects were classified into three groups: "current smoker" group, "past habitual smoker" group, and "lifelong nonsmoker" group.

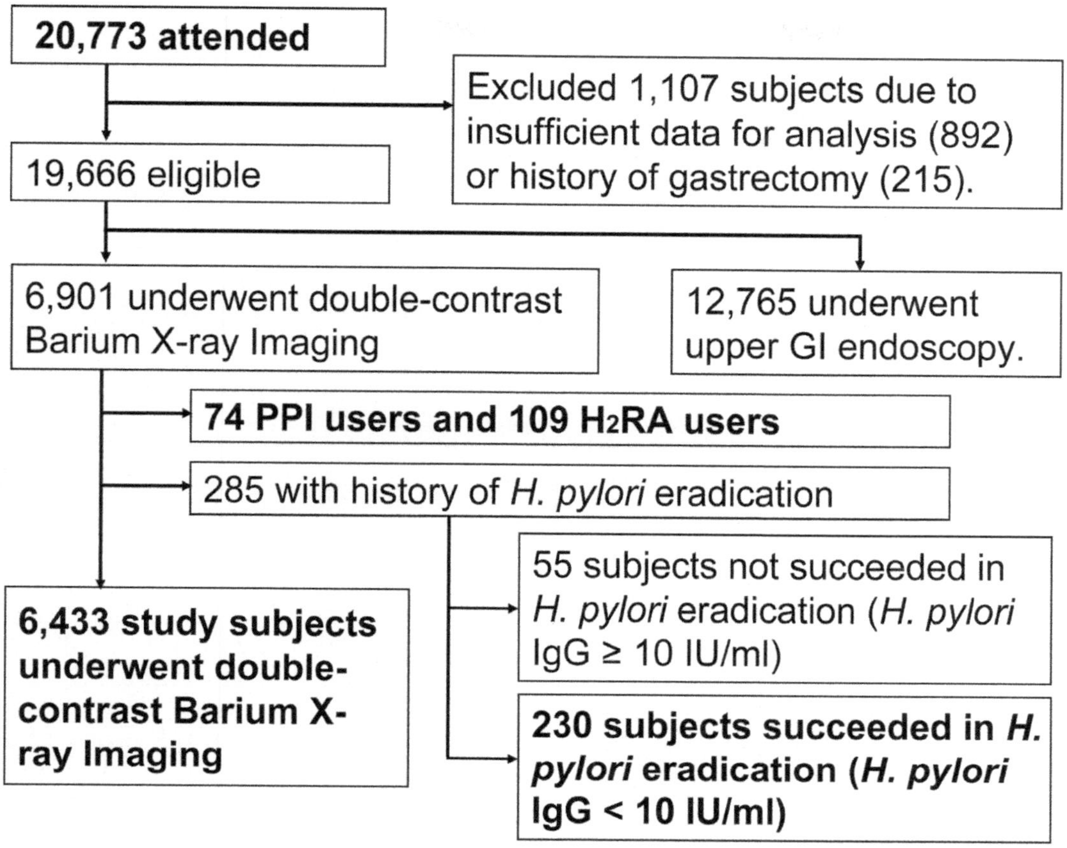

Figure 2. Study flowchart of the present study.

Endoscopy-based atrophic gastritis (Kimura-Takemoto classification of mucosal atrophic change in stomach)		UGI-XR-based atrophic gastritis: − Normal	+: Mild	+: Moderate	+: Severe	Total
−	C0	84	1	3	0	88
+	C1	6	0	1	1	8
+	C2	4	2	5	4	15
+	C3	1	0	3	1	5
+	O1	0	0	9	7	16
+	O2	0	0	3	11	14
+	O3	0	0	0	4	4
	Total	95	3	24	28	150

(Polychoric correlation coefficient: r=0.9330)

Figure 3. Relationship between the four grades of UGI-XR-based atrophic gastritis and the extent of endoscopy-based atrophic gastritis classified into seven categories according to the Kimura-Takemoto classification (C0 with no atrophic change and C1-O3 with various degrees of endoscopy-based atrophic change of gastric mucosa).

a.

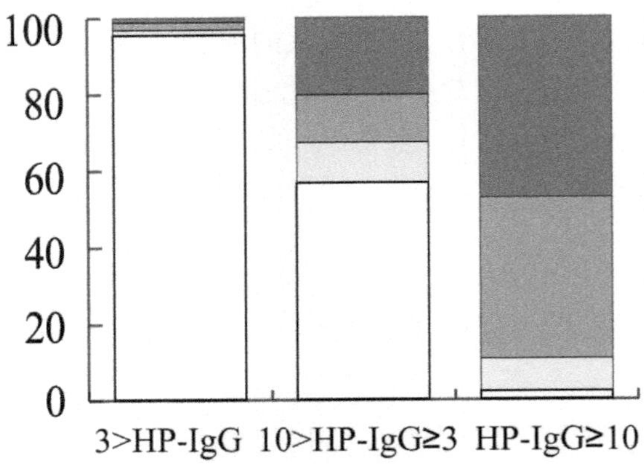

UGI-XR-based Gastritis	A	B	C	D	Total
3 > HP-IgG	4337 (95.5%)	66 (1.5%)	90 (2.0%)	48 (1.1%)	4541
10 > HP-IgG ≥ 3	124 (56.9%)	23 (10.6%)	27 (12.4%)	44 (20.2%)	218
HP-IgG ≥ 10	36 (2.2%)	145 (8.7%)	705 (42.1%)	788 (47.1%)	1674
Total	4497 (69.9%)	234 (3.6%)	822 (12.8%)	880 (13.7%)	6433

(p value<0.0001 by Cochran-Mantel-Haenszel trend test)

b.

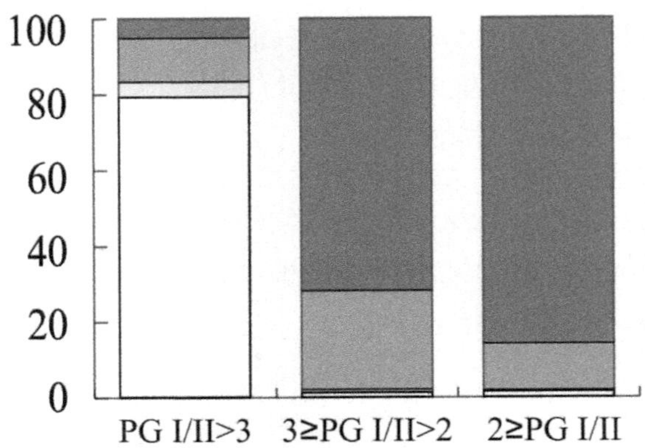

UGI-XR-based Gastritis	A	B	C	D	Total
PG I/II > 3	4486 (79.2%)	229 (4.0%)	656 (11.6%)	293 (5.2%)	5664
3 ≥ PG I/II > 2	7 (1.4%)	4 (0.8%)	135 (26.2%)	369 (71.7%)	515
2 ≥ PG I/II	4 (1.6%)	1 (0.4%)	31 (12.2%)	218 (85.8%)	254
Total	4497 (69.9%)	234 (3.6%)	822 (12.8%)	880 (13.7%)	6433

(p value<0.0001 by Cochran-Mantel-Haenszel trend test)

Figure 4. Distribution of our proposed four types of atrophic gastritis by double-contrast upper gastrointestinal barium X-ray radiography (A: normal, B: mild, C: moderate, D: severe) with titer of serum *Helicobacter pylori* IgG (a) or serum pepsinogen I/II ratio (b).

Statistical Analyses

We used JMP 10 software or SAS 9.1.3 (SAS Institute Inc. Cray, NC, USA) for statistical analyses and matching process. In the univariate analysis, associations between the presence of UGI-XR-based atrophic gastritis and seven variables were compared using the χ^2 test and Cochran-Mantel-Haenszel trend test. In the multivariate analysis, standardized coefficient and odds ratio of each variable were calculated using multiple logistic regression analysis. In the both analyses, p values <0.05 were considered as statistically significant.

To estimate the association between UGI-XR-based atrophic gastritis (normal, mild, moderate, and severe) and endoscopy-based atrophic gastritis (C0, C1, C2, C3, O1, O2, and O3 according to Kimura-Takemoto classification) [24,25], the polychoric correlation coefficient was calculated.

To evaluate the effect of *H. pylori* eradication on UGI-XR-based atrophic gastritis, the matching was performed to control age (±2 years), sex, smoking (current, past habitual, or lifelong non-smoking), and drinking ("rarely" or "usually") between the successfully *H. pylori*-eradicated subjects (negative for serum *H. pylori* IgG with history of eradication therapy) and the chronically *H. pylori*-infected subjects (positive for serum *H. pylori* IgG with no history of eradication therapy). Using the matched pairs of subjects, we applied Cochran-Mantel-Haenszel trend test, in which p value <0.05 was considered as statistically significant.

To evaluate the influence of gastric acid suppressants (proton pump inhibitors (PPI) and histamine H_2-receptor antagonist (H_2RA)) upon UGI-XR-based atrophic gastritis, we used Fisher's exact test in which p value <0.05 was considered as statistically significant.

Results and Discussion

Characteristics of the Study Subjects

Of the 20,773 subjects who participated in the study (Figure 2), we excluded 1,107 subjects with insufficient data or history of gastrectomy, and also excluded 12,765 subjects who underwent upper gastrointestinal (GI) endoscopy. Of the residual 6,901 subjects, we further excluded 74 PPI users, 109 H_2RA users, and 285 subjects who had underwent eradication therapy for *H. pylori*. The eligible 6,433 subjects comprised of 3,405 men and 3,028 women (a mean age of 47.4±8.8 years; range 20–83 years) were mainly analyzed in our present study (Figure 2).

Among the 6,433 main subjects for this study, only 1,674 (26.0%) were positive for *H. pylori*, which is consistent with the rapid decrease in prevalence of *H. pylori* infection in Japan [12,33]. Actually, for the data of healthy adults in our institutes located at Chiba prefecture in Japan, the seropositivity of *H. pylori* infection has markedly reduced from 47.0% (2,695 of 5,732

Table 1. Characteristics of the study subjects from the standpoint of atrophic gastritis diagnosed by double-contrast upper gastrointestinal barium X-ray radiography (UGI-XR-based atrophic gastritis).

Factor	Total 6,433 study subjects	1,936 subjects with UGI-XR-based atrophic gastritis	234 subjects with mild UGI-XR-based atrophic gastritis	822 subjects with moderate UGI-XR-based atrophic gastritis	880 subjects with severe UGI-XR-based atrophic gastritis	Residual 4,497 subjects without UGI-XR-based atrophic gastritis (normal)	*p* value
Age	47.7±8.8 y.o.	51.1±8.9 y.o.	48.4±8.4 y.o.	49.8±8.8 y.o.	53.0±8.7 y.o.	45.8±8.3 y.o.	<.0001*
<30	53 (0.8%)	5 (0.3%)	0 (0.0%)	3 (0.4%)	2 (0.2%)	48 (1.1%)	
≥30 and <40	1,274 (19.8%)	212 (11.0%)	40 (17.1%)	107 (13.0%)	65 (7.4%)	1,062 (23.6%)	
≥40 and <50	2,579 (40.1%)	600 (31.0%)	94 (40.2%)	286 (34.8%)	220 (25.0%)	1,979 (44.0%)	
≥50 and <60	1,909 (29.7%)	774 (40.0%)	76 (32.5%)	304 (37.0%)	394 (44.8%)	1,135 (25.2%)	
≥60 and <70	558 (8.7%)	308 (15.9%)	22 (9.4%)	111 (13.5%)	175 (19.9%)	250 (5.6%)	
≥70	60 (0.9%)	37 (1.9%)	2 (0.9%)	11 (1.3%)	24 (2.3%)	23 (0.5%)	
Sex							<.0001*
female	3,028 (47.1%)	828 (42.8%)	77 (32.9%)	366 (44.5%)	385 (43.8%)	2,200 (48.9%)	
male	3,405 (52.9%)	1,108 (57.2%)	157 (67.1%)	456 (55.5%)	495 (56.3%)	2,297 (51.1%)	
BMI	22.8±3.4	23.0±3.3	23.3±3.4	22.9±3.3	22.8±3.4	22.8±3.4	0.0079*
<18.5	451 (7.0%)	120 (6.2%)	17 (7.3%)	42 (5.1%)	61 (6.9%)	331 (7.4%)	
≥18.5 and <25	4,508 (70.1%)	1,337 (69.1%)	147 (62.8%)	587 (71.4%)	603 (68.5%)	3,171 (70.5%)	
≥25	1,474 (22.9%)	479 (24.7%)	70 (29.9%)	193 (23.5%)	216 (24.5%)	995 (22.1%)	
H. pylori IgG							<.0001*
<3	4,541 (70.6%)	204 (10.5%)	66 (28.2%)	90 (10.9%)	48 (5.5%)	4,337 (96.4%)	
<10 and ≥3	218 (3.4%)	94 (4.9%)	23 (9.8%)	27 (3.3%)	44 (5.0%)	124 (2.8%)	
≥10	1,674 (26.0%)	1,638 (84.6%)	145 (62.0%)	705 (85.8%)	788 (89.5%)	36 (0.8%)	
PG I/II ratio							<.0001*
>3	5,664 (88.0%)	1,178 (60.9%)	229 (97.9%)	656 (79.8%)	293 (33.3%)	4,486 (99.8%)	
≤3 and >2	515 (8.0%)	508 (26.2%)	4 (1.7%)	135 (16.4%)	369 (41.9%)	7 (0.2%)	
≤2	254 (3.9%)	250 (12.9%)	1 (0.4%)	31 (3.8%)	218 (24.8%)	4 (0.1%)	
Smoking							<.0001*
non smoker	3,511 (54.6%)	950 (49.1%)	92 (39.3%)	422 (51.3%)	436 (49.5%)	2,561 (57.0%)	
former smoker	1,622 (25.2%)	548 (28.3%)	73 (31.2%)	197 (24.0%)	278 (31.6%)	1,074 (23.9%)	
current smoker	1,300 (20.2%)	438 (22.6%)	69 (29.5%)	203 (24.7%)	166 (18.9%)	862 (19.2%)	
Alcohol							0.8881
rarely drinking	2,567 (39.9%)	770 (39.8%)	75 (32.1%)	319 (38.8%)	376 (42.7%)	1,797 (40.0%)	
usually drinking	3,866 (60.1%)	1,166 (60.2%)	159 (67.9%)	503 (61.2%)	504 (57.3%)	2,700 (60.0%)	

BMI, body mass index; *H. pylori*, *Helicobacter pylori*; PG, pepsinogen. The levels of significance (*p* value) for analyzing associations between UGI-XR-based atrophic gastritis and the seven causative factors were set at <0.05 (*), which were calculated by χ^2 test or Cochran-Mantel-Haenszel trend test.

Table 2. Multivariate analysis of the 6,433 study subjects evaluating associations of the seven background factors with UGI-XR-based atrophic gastritis (atrophic gastritis diagnosed by double-contrast upper gastrointestinal barium X-ray radiography).

Factor	Standardized coefficients	Odds ratio (95% C.I.)	*p* value
Age	0.401	1.49 (1.31–1.70)	<.0001*
Sex			
female	reference	reference	reference
male	0.306	1.36 (1.16–1.59)	0.0002*
BMI	−0.100	0.90 (0.80–1.03)	0.124
H. pylori IgG			
<3	reference	reference	reference
<10 and ≥3	0.479	1.61 (1.52–1.72)	<.0001*
≥10	1.499	4.48 (4.12–4.91)	<.0001*
PG I/II ratio			
>3	reference	reference	reference
≤3 and >2	0.270	1.31 (1.18–1.48)	<.0001*
≤2	0.339	1.40 (1.26–1.59)	<.0001*
Smoking			
non smoker	reference	reference	reference
former smoker	0.137	1.15 (0.98–1.33)	0.0773
current smoker	0.526	1.69 (1.49–1.93)	<.0001*
Alcohol			
rarely drinking	reference	reference	reference
usually drinking	0.051	1.05 (0.92–1.20)	0.449

BMI, body mass index; *H. pylori*, *Helicobacter pylori*; PG, pepsinogen. The level of significance in each factor was set at $p<0.05$ (*).

subjects in 1996–1997 [34]) to 26.0% (1,674 of 6,433 subjects in the present study) in only 14 short years.

The 285 subjects after *H. pylori* eradication therapy comprised of 230 subjects with serum *H. pylori* IgG <10 U/ml (certainly succeeded in *H. pylori* eradication) and 55 subjects with serum *H. pylori* IgG ≥10 U/ml (probably not succeeded in *H. pylori* eradication or on the way of negative conversion of serum *H. pylori* IgG). Aside from the main 6,433 study subjects, we additionally analyzed the above-mentioned 74 PPI users, 109 H_2RA users, and 230 "successfully *H. pylori*-eradicated" subjects (Figure 2).

Validation of our defined "UGI-XR-based" Atrophic Gastritis by comparing "Endoscopy-based" Atrophic Gastritis

In our previous work [23], 29 (97%) of 30 subjects positive for serum anti-*H. pylori* IgG were diagnosed as gastritis by UGI-XR, which convinced us the sufficient detection of *H. pylori*-induced chronic gastritis by barium X-ray. In the present study, we classified the UGI-XR-based atrophic gastritis into four types as above-mentioned (Figure 1). To validate this classification, the extent of endoscopy-based atrophic gastritis were simultaneously evaluated among the 150 subjects randomly selected (Figure 3).

Table 3. Comparison between the matched pairs of 227 subjects with chronic infection of *H. pylori* and after successful eradication of *H. pylori*, focusing on the presence of UGI-XR-based atrophic gastritis (atrophic gastritis diagnosed by double-contrast upper gastrointestinal barium X-ray radiography).

	Presence of UGI-XR-based atrophic gastritis (mild, moderate, severe)	Absence of UGI-XR-based atrophic gastritis (normal)	Total
The 227 matched subjects after successful eradication of *H. pylori*	135 (59.5%)	92 (40.5%)	227 (100%)
The 227 matched subjects with chronic *H. pylori* infection	225 (99.1%)	2 (0.9%)	227 (100%)

($p<0.0001$ by Cochran-Mantel-Haenszel test).

Table 4. Comparison between the *H. pylori*-positive gastric acid suppressant (PPI or H_2RA) users and *H. pylori*-positive gastric acid suppressant-free subjects, focusing on the presence of UGI-XR-based gastritis (gastritis diagnosed by double-contrast upper gastrointestinal barium X-ray radiography).

	Presence of UGI-XR-based atrophic gastritis (mild, moderate, severe)	Absence of UGI-XR-based atrophic gastritis (normal)	Total	*p* value
H. pylori-positive and gastric acid suppressant-free subjects among the 6,433 main study subjects	1,638 (97.8%)	36 (2.1%)	1,674 (100%)	reference
H. pylori-positive subjects among the 74 PPI users	13 (92.9%)	1 (7.1%)	14 (100%)	0.2677
H. pylori-positive subjects among the 109 H_2RA users	33 (97.1%)	1 (2.9%)	34 (100%)	0.5286

For the PPI and H_2RA users each, the level of significance was set at $p<0.05$ (*) by Fisher's exact test.

On the basis of endoscopy-based atrophic gastritis, sensitivity and specificity of UGI-XR-based atrophic gastritis were 82.3% (51/62) and 95.5% (84/88) respectively. In addition, the four-grade categories of UGI-XR-based atrophic gastritis showed significant association with seven-grade classes of endoscopy-based atrophic gastritis (polychoric correlation coefficient: $r = 0.9330$). Actually, all the subjects (34/34) with severe endoscopy-based atrophic gastritis (namely, open type (O1–O3) atrophy according to Kimura-Takemoto classification [24,25]) were diagnosed as UGI-XR-based atrophic gastritis (Figure 3). Based on these results, we concluded that UGI-XR-based diagnosis used in this study can certainly reflect the atrophic mucosa of stomach.

The Four-grade Types of UGI-XR-based Atrophic Gastritis are Significantly Associated with the Titer of Serum *H. pylori* IgG and the Ratio of Serum Pepsinogen I and II

Based on the UGI-XR-based mucosal atrophy of stomach, the total 6,433 subjects with no history of *H. pylori* eradication and free from gastric acid suppressants were classified into four classes (Figure 4): 234 subjects with mild gastritis, 822 subjects with moderate gastritis, 880 subjects with severe gastritis, and residual 4,497 subjects without atrophic gastritis (normal).

We first evaluated associations of the four-grade UGI-XR-based atrophic gastritis with two serum markers: the titer of *H. pylori* IgG and the ratio of pepsinogen I and II reflecting the mucosal atrophy of stomach [32,35]. As shown in Figure 4a, UGI-XR-based atrophic gastritis significantly extends in proportion to rise in serum *H. pylori* IgG titer ($p<0.0001$). And as also shown in Figure 4b, the grade of UGI-XR-based atrophic gastritis meaningfully advances accompanied with decline in pepsinogen I/II ratio ($p<0.0001$). Though the effects of other causative factors should not be groundlessly underestimated, these results suggest that the four-grade categorization of UGI-XR-based atrophic gastritis strongly reflects chronic *H. pylori* infection and consequent mucosal atrophy of stomach.

Associated Background Factors of UGI-XR-based Atrophic Gastritis

The detailed characteristics of the 6,433 study subjects focusing on UGI-XR-based atrophic gastritis and the seven putative background factors are shown in Table 1. The results of univariate analyses concerning the seven factors are also denoted. It is clear that old age, male gender, a high titer of serum *H. pylori* IgG, low ratio of serum pepsinogen I/II, and a habit of smoking show strongly positive association with the presence of UGI-XR-based atrophic gastritis.

We next executed multivariate analyses with these seven causative factors (Table 2). As was expected, a high titer of serum *H. pylori* IgG is the strongest associated factor for UGI-XR-based atrophic gastritis. Current smoking, old age, low ratio of serum pepsinogen I/II, and male gender also show significant association. In contrast, drinking as well as BMI (body mass index) has no meaningful association with UGI-XR-based atrophic gastritis: this unexpected but clear difference between drinking and smoking should be noted when considering the establishment of atrophic gastritis.

Eradication of *Helicobacter pylori* Seems to Superficially Improve UGI-XR-based Atrophic Gastritis

We next tried to evaluate the effect of *H. pylori* eradication upon UGI-XR-based atrophic gastritis. For this purpose, the matching was performed to control age (within±2 years), sex, smoking, and drinking between the 230 subjects succeeded in *H. pylori* eradication (negative for serum *H. pylori* IgG with history of eradication therapy) and the 1,674 subjects with chronic *H. pylori* infection (positive for serum *H. pylori* IgG with no history of eradication therapy).

Between the 227 matched pairs of subjects, prevalences of UGI-XR-based atrophic gastritis were markedly different with statistical significance (Table 3): it was detected in only 59.5% of the *H. pylori*-eradicated subjects but was detected in 99.1% of the chronically *H. pylori*-infected subjects ($p<0.0001$). These suggest that eradication of *H. pylori* diminishes the typical images of UGI-XR-based atrophic gastritis. In other words, chronic infection of *H. pylori* in the past cannot be efficiently detected by UGI-XR, after eradication therapy has been completed.

It has been reported that eradication of *H. pylori* can improve gastritis both pathologically [20,36,37] and endoscopically [38]. The result of our present study suggests that eradication of *H. pylori* can also relieve UGI-XR-based atrophic gastritis, which is defined by the irregular shapes of areae gastricae and their expansion in the stomach. However, this is not always a preferable result, since the superficial improvement of chronic gastritis does not considerably reduce the risk of gastric tumorigenesis [39,40,41,42]. It can be otherwise considered that UGI-XR cannot adequately distinguish the lifelong *H. pylori*-negative stomach (having a very low risk of gastric cancer [17,30,43]) from the *H. pylori*-eradicated stomach keeping a considerable risk for gastric canceration [40]. We are apprehensive that the difficulty in detecting *H. pylori*-eradicated stomach will be a formidable problem for UGI-XR-based gastric cancer screening.

Intakes of PPI and H_2RA Mostly do not Affect UGI-XR-based Atrophic Gastritis

We further evaluated the influence of gastric acid suppressants upon UGI-XR-based atrophic gastritis. Among the gastric acid suppressant users positive for serum *H. pylori* IgG (Table 4), UGI-XR-based atrophic gastritis was detected in 13 of 14 PPI users (92.9%) and 33 of 34 H_2RA users (97.1%). Though the statistical evaluation cannot be accurately calculated due to the small number of subjects, there seems to be no obvious differences compared to the *H. pylori*-positive 1,674 subjects free from gastric acid suppressants. To say the least, our results indicate that intakes of PPI and H_2RA mostly do not deteriorate the diagnostic quality of UGI-XR-based atrophic gastritis.

Conclusions

The presence of atrophic gastritis diagnosed by double-contrast upper gastrointestinal barium X-ray radiography (UGI-XR-based atrophic gastritis) is positively associated with *Helicobacter pylori* infection, current smoking, old age, decreased pepsinogen I/II ratio, and male gender. Eradication of *Helicobacter pylori* seems to superficially improve UGI-XR-based gastritis whereas intake of proton pump inhibitors or histamine H_2-receptor antagonist does not.

Acknowledgments

We are grateful to Mr. Minoru Okada, Mr. Masanori Fujiwara, and Mr. Masami Muraoka (Kameda Medical Center Makuhari, Chiba-shi, Chiba, Japan) for assistance with establishment and maintenance of the study database.

Author Contributions

Conceived and designed the experiments: NY CH TS TM MI. Performed the experiments: NY CH CM Y. Takahashi CN RM MKS. Analyzed the data: NY TS SK SO KN SM Y. Tsuji YS IAH CT SY HK RW. Contributed reagents/materials/analysis tools: NY CH TM. Contributed to the writing of the manuscript: NY CH TS MF JK MI KK.

References

1. Crew KD, Neugut AI (2006) Epidemiology of gastric cancer. World J Gastroenterol 12: 354–362.
2. Yamamichi N, Inada K, Ichinose M, Yamamichi-Nishina M, Mizutani T, et al. (2007) Frequent loss of Brm expression in gastric cancer correlates with histologic features and differentiation state. Cancer Res 67: 10727–10735.
3. Leung WK, Wu MS, Kakugawa Y, Kim JJ, Yeoh KG, et al. (2008) Screening for gastric cancer in Asia: current evidence and practice. Lancet Oncol 9: 279–287.
4. Lee KJ, Inoue M, Otani T, Iwasaki M, Sasazuki S, et al. (2006) Gastric cancer screening and subsequent risk of gastric cancer: a large-scale population-based cohort study, with a 13-year follow-up in Japan. Int J Cancer 118: 2315–2321.
5. Tsubono Y, Hisamichi S (2000) Screening for gastric cancer in Japan. Gastric Cancer 3: 9–18.
6. Oshima A, Hirata N, Ubukata T, Umeda K, Fujimoto I (1986) Evaluation of a mass screening program for stomach cancer with a case-control study design. Int J Cancer 38: 829–833.
7. Hisamichi S, Sugawara N (1984) Mass screening for gastric cancer by X-ray examination. Jpn J Clin Oncol 14: 211–223.
8. Mizoue T, Yoshimura T, Tokui N, Hoshiyama Y, Yatsuya H, et al. (2003) Prospective study of screening for stomach cancer in Japan. Int J Cancer 106: 103–107.
9. Hamashima C, Shibuya D, Yamazaki H, Inoue K, Fukao A, et al. (2008) The Japanese guidelines for gastric cancer screening. Jpn J Clin Oncol 38: 259–267.
10. Hosokawa O, Miyanaga T, Kaizaki Y, Hattori M, Dohden K, et al. (2008) Decreased death from gastric cancer by endoscopic screening: association with a population-based cancer registry. Scand J Gastroenterol 43: 1112–1115.
11. Miki K, Morita M, Sasajima M, Hoshina R, Kanda E, et al. (2003) Usefulness of gastric cancer screening using the serum pepsinogen test method. Am J Gastroenterol 98: 735–739.
12. Nakajima S, Nishiyama Y, Yamaoka M, Yasuoka T, Cho E (2010) Changes in the prevalence of Helicobacter pylori infection and gastrointestinal diseases in the past 17 years. J Gastroenterol Hepatol 25 Suppl 1: S99–S110.
13. Lee SY, Park HS, Yu SK, Sung IK, Jin CJ, et al. (2007) Decreasing prevalence of Helicobacter pylori infection: a 9-year observational study. Hepatogastroenterology 54: 630–633.
14. Brown LM (2000) Helicobacter pylori: epidemiology and routes of transmission. Epidemiol Rev 22: 283–297.
15. Bures J, Kopacova M, Koupil I, Seifert B, Skodova Fendrichova M, et al. (2012) Significant decrease in prevalence of Helicobacter pylori in the Czech Republic. World J Gastroenterol 18: 4412–4418.
16. Dixon MF, Genta RM, Yardley JH, Correa P (1996) Classification and grading of gastritis. The updated Sydney System. International Workshop on the Histopathology of Gastritis, Houston 1994. Am J Surg Pathol 20: 1161–1181.
17. Uemura N, Okamoto S, Yamamoto S, Matsumura N, Yamaguchi S, et al. (2001) Helicobacter pylori infection and the development of gastric cancer. N Engl J Med 345: 784–789.
18. Polk DB, Peek RM Jr (2010) Helicobacter pylori: gastric cancer and beyond. Nat Rev Cancer 10: 403–414.
19. Satoh K, Kimura K, Taniguchi Y, Yoshida Y, Kihira K, et al. (1996) Distribution of inflammation and atrophy in the stomach of Helicobacter pylori-positive and -negative patients with chronic gastritis. Am J Gastroenterol 91: 963–969.
20. Ohkusa T, Fujiki K, Takashimizu I, Kumagai J, Tanizawa T, et al. (2001) Improvement in atrophic gastritis and intestinal metaplasia in patients in whom Helicobacter pylori was eradicated. Ann Intern Med 134: 380–386.
21. Dheer S, Levine MS, Redfern RO, Metz DC, Rubesin SE, et al. (2002) Radiographically diagnosed antral gastritis: findings in patients with and without Helicobacter pylori infection. Br J Radiol 75: 805–811.
22. Rubesin SE, Levine MS, Laufer I (2008) Double-contrast upper gastrointestinal radiography: a pattern approach for diseases of the stomach. Radiology 246: 33–48.
23. Yamamichi N, Shimamoto T, Minatsuki C, Yoshida Y, Fujishiro M, et al. (2011) Postprandial fullness correlates with rapid inflow of gastric content into duodenum but not with chronic gastritis. BMC Gastroenterol 11: 140.
24. Kimura K (1972) Chronological transition of the fundic-pyloric border determined by stepwise biopsy of the lesser and greater curvatures of the stomach. Gastroenterology 63: 584–592.
25. Kimura K, Takemoto T (1969) An Endoscopic Recognition of the Atrophic Border and its Significance in Chronic Gastritis. Endoscopy 3: 87–97.
26. Takahashi Y, Yamamichi N, Shimamoto T, Mochizuki S, Fujishiro M, et al. (2013) Helicobacter pylori infection is positively associated with gallstones: a large-scale cross-sectional study in Japan. J Gastroenterol.
27. Minatsuki C, Yamamichi N, Shimamoto T, Kakimoto H, Takahashi Y, et al. (2013) Background factors of reflux esophagitis and non-erosive reflux disease: a cross-sectional study of 10,837 subjects in Japan. PLoS One 8: e69891.
28. Shimamoto T, Yamamichi N, Kodashima S, Takahashi Y, Fujishiro M, et al. (2013) No association of coffee consumption with gastric ulcer, duodenal ulcer, reflux esophagitis, and non-erosive reflux disease: a cross-sectional study of 8,013 healthy subjects in Japan. PLoS One 8: e65996.
29. Tatemichi M, Sasazuki S, Inoue M, Tsugane S (2009) Clinical significance of IgG antibody titer against Helicobacter pylori. Helicobacter 14: 231–236.
30. Ohata H, Kitauchi S, Yoshimura N, Mugitani K, Iwane M, et al. (2004) Progression of chronic atrophic gastritis associated with Helicobacter pylori infection increases risk of gastric cancer. Int J Cancer 109: 138–143.
31. Oishi Y, Kiyohara Y, Kubo M, Tanaka K, Tanizaki Y, et al. (2006) The serum pepsinogen test as a predictor of gastric cancer: the Hisayama study. Am J Epidemiol 163: 629–637.
32. Watabe H, Mitsushima T, Yamaji Y, Okamoto M, Wada R, et al. (2005) Predicting the development of gastric cancer from combining Helicobacter pylori antibodies and serum pepsinogen status: a prospective endoscopic cohort study. Gut 54: 764–768.
33. Shiota S, Murakami K, Fujioka T, Yamaoka Y (2010) Population-based strategies for Helicobacter pylori-associated disease management: a Japanese perspective. Expert Rev Gastroenterol Hepatol 4: 149–156.
34. Yamaji Y, Mitsushima T, Ikuma H, Okamoto M, Yoshida H, et al. (2001) Inverse background of Helicobacter pylori antibody and pepsinogen in reflux oesophagitis compared with gastric cancer: analysis of 5732 Japanese subjects. Gut 49: 335–340.
35. Miki K (2006) Gastric cancer screening using the serum pepsinogen test method. Gastric Cancer 9: 245–253.

36. Sung JJ, Lin SR, Ching JY, Zhou LY, To KF, et al. (2000) Atrophy and intestinal metaplasia one year after cure of H. pylori infection: a prospective, randomized study. Gastroenterology 119: 7–14.
37. Ito M, Haruma K, Kamada T, Mihara M, Kim S, et al. (2002) Helicobacter pylori eradication therapy improves atrophic gastritis and intestinal metaplasia: a 5-year prospective study of patients with atrophic gastritis. Aliment Pharmacol Ther 16: 1449–1456.
38. Kato M, Terao S, Adachi K, Nakajima S, Ando T, et al. (2013) Changes in endoscopic findings of gastritis after cure of H. pylori infection: multicenter prospective trial. Dig Endosc 25: 264–273.
39. Correa P, Fontham ET, Bravo JC, Bravo LE, Ruiz B, et al. (2000) Chemoprevention of gastric dysplasia: randomized trial of antioxidant supplements and anti-helicobacter pylori therapy. J Natl Cancer Inst 92: 1881–1888.
40. Fuccio L, Zagari RM, Eusebi LH, Laterza L, Cennamo V, et al. (2009) Meta-analysis: can Helicobacter pylori eradication treatment reduce the risk for gastric cancer? Ann Intern Med 151: 121–128.
41. Wong BC, Lam SK, Wong WM, Chen JS, Zheng TT, et al. (2004) Helicobacter pylori eradication to prevent gastric cancer in a high-risk region of China: a randomized controlled trial. JAMA 291: 187–194.
42. Leung WK, Lin SR, Ching JY, To KF, Ng EK, et al. (2004) Factors predicting progression of gastric intestinal metaplasia: results of a randomised trial on Helicobacter pylori eradication. Gut 53: 1244–1249.
43. Correa P, Houghton J (2007) Carcinogenesis of Helicobacter pylori. Gastroenterology 133: 659–672.

Role of Gist and PHOG Features in Computer-Aided Diagnosis of Tuberculosis without Segmentation

Arun Chauhan[1], Devesh Chauhan[2], Chittaranjan Rout[1]*

1 Department of Biotechnology and Bioinformatics, Jaypee University of Information Technology, Solan, Himachal Pradesh, India, 2 Department of Radiology, National Institute of TB and Respiratory Diseases, New Delhi, India

Abstract

Purpose: Effective diagnosis of tuberculosis (TB) relies on accurate interpretation of radiological patterns found in a chest radiograph (CXR). Lack of skilled radiologists and other resources, especially in developing countries, hinders its efficient diagnosis. Computer-aided diagnosis (CAD) methods provide second opinion to the radiologists for their findings and thereby assist in better diagnosis of cancer and other diseases including TB. However, existing CAD methods for TB are based on the extraction of textural features from manually or semi-automatically segmented CXRs. These methods are prone to errors and cannot be implemented in X-ray machines for automated classification.

Methods: Gabor, Gist, histogram of oriented gradients (HOG), and pyramid histogram of oriented gradients (PHOG) features extracted from the whole image can be implemented into existing X-ray machines to discriminate between TB and non-TB CXRs in an automated manner. Localized features were extracted for the above methods using various parameters, such as frequency range, blocks and region of interest. The performance of these features was evaluated against textural features. Two digital CXR image datasets (8-bit DA and 14-bit DB) were used for evaluating the performance of these features.

Results: Gist (accuracy 94.2% for DA, 86.0% for DB) and PHOG (accuracy 92.3% for DA, 92.0% for DB) features provided better results for both the datasets. These features were implemented to develop a MATLAB toolbox, TB-Xpredict, which is freely available for academic use at http://sourceforge.net/projects/tbxpredict/. This toolbox provides both automated training and prediction modules and does not require expertise in image processing for operation.

Conclusion: Since the features used in TB-Xpredict do not require segmentation, the toolbox can easily be implemented in X-ray machines. This toolbox can effectively be used for the mass screening of TB in high-burden areas with improved efficiency.

Editor: Hans A. Kestler, University of Ulm, Germany

Funding: The authors have no support or funding to report.

Competing Interests: The authors have declared that no competing interests exist.

* Email: chittaranjan.rout@juit.ac.in

Introduction

X-rays were discovered by Wilhelm Röntgen, a German physicist in 1895 and have revolutionized the field of diagnostics. Chest radiographs (CXRs) are ubiquitous in clinical diagnostics and make up about one-third of all radiological examinations. Chest radiographs are inexpensive and least invasive primary diagnostic tool for tuberculosis (TB). They are used in routine medical checkups and immigrant medical examinations even in well-equipped hospitals where blood and skin tests are available [1]. The CXRs are also used for mass screening of TB in human immunodeficiency virus (HIV) endemic areas.

Tuberculosis is one of the leading infectious diseases with high mortality rate in developing and under-developed countries. Approximately 1.1 and 0.35 million of deaths were caused worldwide by the disease in non-HIV and HIV people respectively from about 8.8 million incidents reported in 2011 [2]. The disease is diagnosed on the basis of patient's symptoms, CXR and smear microscopy tests. Since the accuracy of smear microscopy test has been less than 50%, diagnosis relies primarily on the interpretation of radiological patterns found in a CXR. Early detection of TB often leads to success of anti-TB therapy, and also helps in gaining control over the transmission of infection as well as development of drug resistant TB. However, lack of resources and skilled radiologists particularly in rural areas of developing countries impedes its effective diagnosis. Therefore, computer-aided diagnosis (CAD) tools assume a lot of significance as they not only reduce diagnostic errors but also increase the efficiency of mass screening in poor-resource settings.

The CAD may be referred to a diagnosis made by a radiologist taking into account the results obtained through computer analysis. Success of the CAD methods in better diagnosis of breast cancer, colon cancer, lungs cancer, prostate cancer, coronary artery disease, congenital heart defects, etc., has suggested that TB may be detected more effectively by incorporating CAD methods [3–6]. The CAD techniques have been helpful in providing second opinion to the radiologists for their findings as well as assisting them in making their final decision regarding diagnosis with increased accuracy. Interpretation of CXRs is dependent on the expertise and skills of the radiologist, which is subject to human error. Even many district level hospitals in developing countries do not have skilled radiologists and incorrect diagnosis of TB takes place due to erroneous interpretation of CXR patterns. A well-trained CAD method can assume the role of a second CXR reader to some extent and may assist the radiologist in some facets of disease detection and decision making. Although these techniques may by no means be able to achieve the level of cognitive ability and knowledge of a radiologist, nonetheless, a trained classifier can perform the prediction consistently without the intra-observer and inter-observer variability. A recent study has also shown that the performance of CXR readers in diagnosing TB improved with the support of CAD [7].

Basic methodology employed in most of the earlier reported CAD studies was segmentation and extraction of grey-level co-occurrence matrix (GLCM) textural features [8]. Ginneken *et al.* used the GLCM textural features on two datasets for classification of CXRs as TB or non-TB, but the performance of both varied significantly [9]. For one dataset, specificity of 90% was obtained while only 50% was achieved for the other. Detection of clavicle, and abnormalities in texture and shape in the CXRs were combined to develop a TB classification model by Hogeweg *et al* [10]. The area under the receiver operating characteristic curve (AUC) for the method was 0.86 [9]. Semi-automated segmentation based classification model using textural features provided a prediction accuracy of 92.9% with sensitivity of 0.91 [1].

Current CAD methods employed for classification of CXR images are either object or region based [11–13]. These methods require segmentation and are prone to magnifying and carrying over low-level errors. The performance of GLCM features was inconsistent across various datasets [9], and these features lose significance when lungs have different shapes or CXRs have complex appearances due to overlapping of anatomical structures [1]. Commonly used manual or semi-automatic segmentation methods not only require high expertise but also make the classification model data and machine dependent. Although automated segmentation methods have potential to be used for development of CAD techniques, but studies have shown that automated segmentation of TB CXRs failed in many cases leading to incorrect classification [1]. Textural features are based on the implicit hypothesis that there exist some specific texture signatures which are dissimilar between non-TB and TB CXRs (Figure 1). The effectiveness of these textural signatures greatly depends on their ability to correlate with the disease. Since context of the features obtained with respect to the whole image are expected to be more useful than local textural features, therefore, contextual scene based Gist features were used in this study for the prediction of TB from CXR. This method captures biologically plausible features into a signatory low-dimensional vector [14]. These features identify salient locations within the image which differ significantly from their neighbours and also accumulate image statistics over the entire scene. Gabor [15], histogram of oriented gradients (HOG) [16], and pyramid histogram of oriented gradients (PHOG) [17] features were also used in this study. PHOG features were computed as they contain local as well as global spatial information. The advantage with these methods is that they can be incorporated to X-ray machines for fully automated detection of TB. Localisation of features was done through optimising and fine-tuning various parameters, like region of interest (ROI), blocks and frequency range.

Materials and Methods

The methodology is based on pixel-based classification which is illustrated in Figure 2. The proposed methodology was implemented in MATLAB 2010a.

Ethics statement

This study was approved by the institution, National Institute of TB and Respiratory Diseases, and the requirement to obtain informed consent was waived. The data was obtained and analysed anonymously.

Dataset

Two CXR digital image datasets were obtained from two different X-ray machines available at the National Institute of Tuberculosis and Respiratory Diseases, New Delhi. These CXRs were taken in standard practice conditions followed by clinicians. In developing countries like India, the posterior-anterior (PA) CXRs are mostly taken and lateral CXRs are taken rarely. Therefore, only PA CXRs were used in the creation of the datasets. The CXRs were randomly collected over a period of one year with varied lung presentations. Dataset A (DA) was taken from Diagnox-4050 X-ray machine manufactured by Meditronics with CXRs digitised by AGFA CR35-X. Dataset B (DB) was obtained from PRORAD URS with Canon CXDI detectors. The tube voltage was set to 50 kV and 55 kV for DA and DB respectively. E-7252X and E-7254X X-ray tubes manufactured by Toshiba, Japan were used by Diagnox-4050 and PRORAD URS respectively. Although AGFA CR35-X acquires 12-bit grayscale CXRs, but 8-bit CXRs (DA) were obtained due to imaging system used by the radiologists. 14-bit CXR digital images (DB) were obtained by using PRORAD URS. For both the datasets DA and DB, the acquired images were resized to 1024×1024 resolutions to obtain images with identical dimensions. No change in classification accuracy was noticed with respect to original sized images. CXRs from each dataset were randomly divided into training and test sets. DA comprised of training set (52 non-TB and 52 TB CXRs) and the independent test set (26 non-TB and 26 TB CXRs). Similarly, DB comprised of training set (50 non-TB and 50 TB CXRs) and the independent test set (25 non-TB and 25 TB CXRs). Selection of all non-TB and TB cases was based on the consensus of independent review of each CXR by two highly experienced chest radiologists from National Institute of Tuberculosis and Respiratory Diseases, New Delhi, India and Indira Gandhi Medical College, Shimla, India. The selection of abnormal CXRs, varying from subtle to severe TB findings, was based on radiological findings through the consensus of the radiologists. Datasets are available freely at http://sourceforge.net/projects/tbxpredict/files/data/.

Segmentation

Segmentation is the process of dividing an image into a set of distinctive areas or regions that differ significantly qualitatively or quantitatively. It is a critical intermediate step in high level object-recognition tasks. Since existing methods required segmentation of CXRs, manual and automatic segmentation of CXRs for the dataset DA was done merely to evaluate the performance of our method (features extracted from whole image) against features extracted from manual and automatic segmentation. Manual segmentation of CXRs was done with the help of ImageJ software [18]. To evaluate the effectiveness of classification using features extracted from automated segmentation methods, Chan-Vese method [19] was used for the segmentation of CXRs from the dataset DA (Figure 3). The Chan-Vese algorithm is a type of

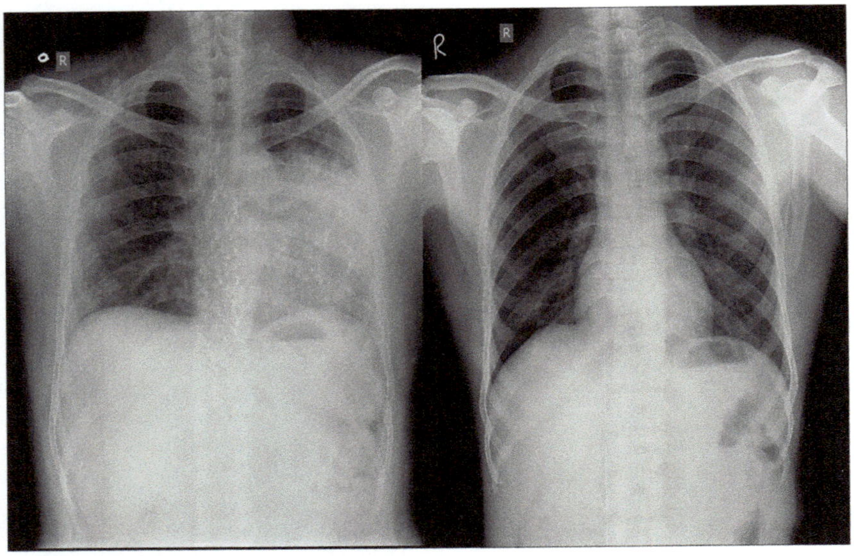

Figure 1. CXRs. Left: TB patient Right: Normal person.

geometric active contour model which begins with a contour in the image plane defining an initial segmentation, and then this contour evolves with respect to evolution equation. The contour is evolved using level set method in such a manner that it terminates on the foreground boundaries. The level set function minimizes the Mumford-Shah functional, which is a type of "fitting energy" functional.

Initial contour was developed using Euler-number [20] based segmentation with an auto-tuned threshold value as shown in Figure 4. The optimal threshold value for this segmentation is obtained on the basis of minimum and maximum values of the correlated image Euler numbers. Chan-Vese active contours segmentation was then used and the number of iterations for segmentation was fixed to 4000. The terminating criterion for segmentation does not depend on the gradient of the image.

Preprocessing

Preprocessing involves denoising of the image. Wavelet-based denoising is a well-known method in the field of digital image processing. Mean, Gaussian, anisotropic diffusion, Fourier transformation and the SURE orthonormal wavelet filters [21] were

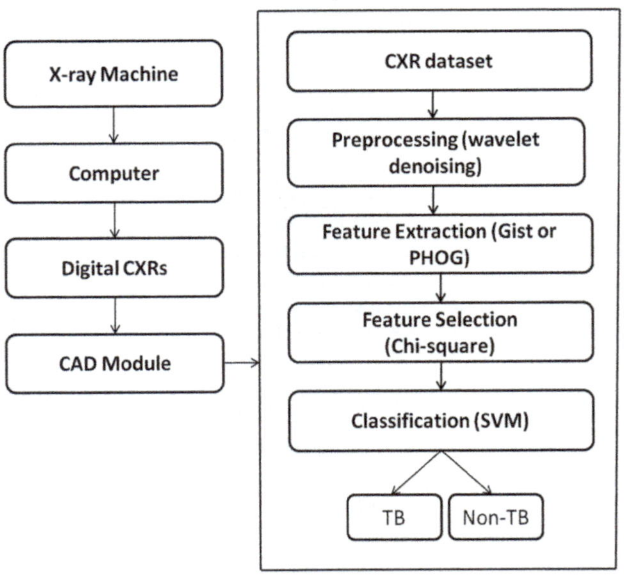

Figure 2. Schematic representation of CAD implementation for TB. CAD module is applied to the digital CXRs obtained from the computer attached to the the X-ray machine. The CAD module preprocesses (denoises) the image using SURE wavelet denoising, extract features (Gist and PHOG), selects relevant features using chi-square based feature selection method and finally classifies the CXR into TB and non-TB.

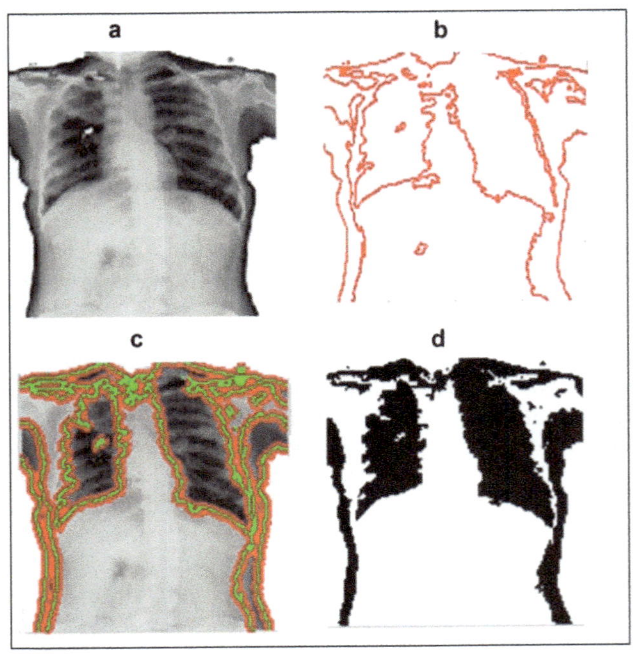

Figure 3. Chan-Vese active contour segmentation of a CXR. a. Original CXR image b. Initial contour c. Iterations for foreground segmentation, and d. Segmented image.

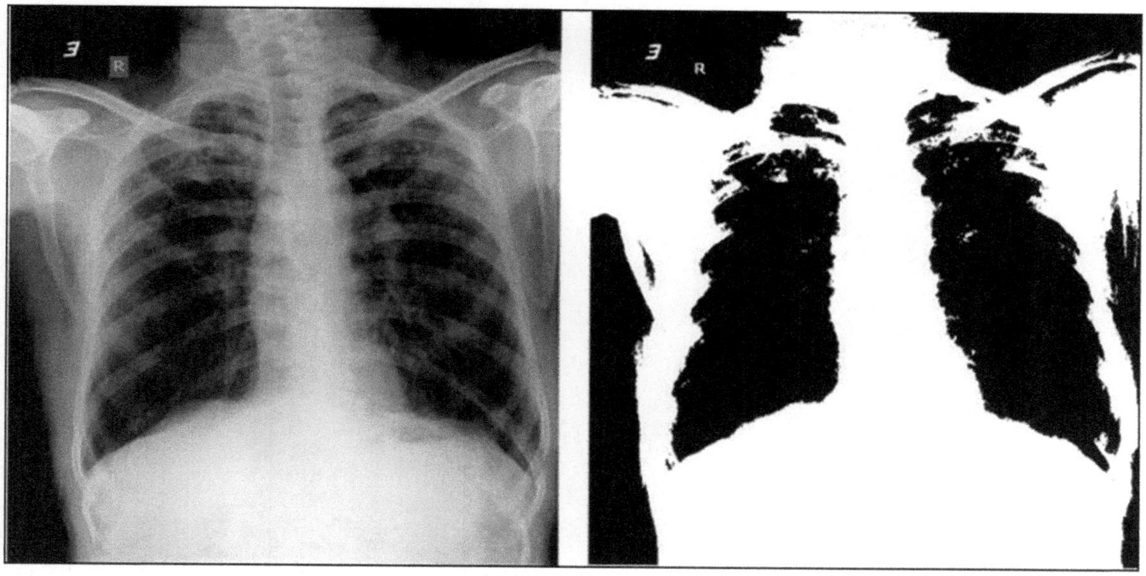

Figure 4. X-ray image before and after Euler-based segmentation. The Euler-based segmented image provides initial contour for Chan-Vese segmentation.

evaluated in this study for denoising of the images. Finally, orthonormal wavelet denoising of the image was used for this study as it provided best denoising effect with respect to visual inspection. The denoising process is parameterized as the sum of elementary non-linear processes with unknown weights. The estimate of mean square error (MSE) between denoised and clean image is minimized using Stein's unbiased risk estimate (SURE), a statistically unbiased estimate that depends only on the noisy image. The existence of this as a priori estimate avoids the requirement of statistical model for wavelet coefficients.

Feature extraction

Textural (GLCM and Gabor) as well as other features, like Gist, HOG and PHOG were extracted from the digital CXRs. Details of the feature extraction methods used in this study are given below:

GLCM textural features

Textural features are calculated based on the statistical distribution of combinations of pixel intensities at specific positions relative to each other. Based on the number of pixels in each combination, statistics are categorized into first-, second- and higher-order statistics. The GLCM method extracts second-order statistics textural features. GLCM is a matrix with rows and columns equal to the number of grey levels. The matrix element G(i,j | dx,dy) is the relative frequency with which two pixels occur within a given neighbourhood, where i and j are pixel intensities separated by distance (dx,dy). Various textural features were extracted from this matrix (for details refer to Table S1). A two pixel offset (2,0 and 0,2) was used in this study.

Gabor features

Gabor filters have been found to be very effective in texture representation and discrimination [15,22,23]. These filters with different frequencies and orientations are used for extracting textural features from an image. A 2-D Gabor function g(x,y) and its Fourier transform G(u,v) are calculated using Eq. (1) and Eq. (2) respectively:

$$g(x,y)=\left(\frac{1}{2\pi\sigma_x\sigma_y}\right)\exp\left[-\frac{1}{2}\left(\frac{x^2}{\sigma_x{}^2}+\frac{y^2}{\sigma_y{}^2}\right)+2\pi jWx\right] \quad \text{Eq.(1)}$$

Where, j $=\sqrt{-1}$, and W is the frequency of the Gabor function

$$G(u,v)=\exp\left\{-\frac{1}{2}\left[\frac{(u-W^2)}{\sigma_u{}^2}+\frac{v^2}{\sigma_v{}^2}\right]\right\} \quad \text{Eq.(2)}$$

Where $\sigma_u=\frac{1}{2}\pi\sigma_x,\sigma_v=\frac{1}{2}\pi\sigma_y$

Impulse responses of Gabor filters are rotated and scaled versions of the above function. The Gabor filters can be considered as edge detectors with adjustable orientations and scales. A self similar filter dictionary is obtained by the association of rotation parameter θ and scale factor α with the Gabor function g(x,y). Scales and orientations of the Gabor wavelets are represented by M and N respectively.

$$g_{mn}(x,y)=\alpha(x',y'),0\leq m\leq M-1,0\leq n\leq N-1 \quad \text{Eq.(3)}$$

$$x'=\alpha^{-m}(xcos\theta+ysin\theta),y'=\alpha^{-m}(xsin\theta+ycos\theta),$$

where $\theta=n\pi/K$ and K is the total number of orientations.

Gabor wavelet transform for a given image I(x,y) is defined as in Eq. (4):

$$G_{mn}(x,y)=\int I(x_1,y_1)g^*_{mn}(x-x_1,y-y_1)dx_1dy_1 \quad \text{Eq.(4)}$$

Where, * represents complex conjugate.

Spatial homogeneity of local textural regions is assumed. μ_{mn} and σ_{mn} are the mean and standard deviation of the magnitude of Gabor wavelet transform coefficients respectively, and are used to represent regions for classification and retrieval of images.

$$\mu_{mn} = \iint |G_{mn}(xy)|dxdy,$$

and

$$\sigma_{mn} = \sqrt{\iint (|G_{mn}(x,y)| - \mu_{mn})^2 dxdy} \qquad \text{Eq.}(5)$$

Gabor features are created using μ_{mn} and σ_{mn} as feature components. Number of scales and orientations was set to six and ten respectively for creating feature vectors in this study. Frequency range was set between 0.01 and 0.4.

Gist features

These are global image features and they assist in characterizing various important statistics of a scene. These features are computed by convoluting the filter with an image at different scales and orientations. Thus, high and low frequency repetitive gradient directions of an image can be measured. The scores for filter convolution at each orientation and scale are used as Gist features for an image. These features are currently being used for scene classification [14,24–26]. The first step of Gist feature extraction is filtering of input image into a number of low level visual feature channels, like intensity, colour, orientation, motion and flicker at multiple spatial scales. Center-surround operations within each sub-channel i are performed between filter output maps, $O_i(s)$, at different scales s. This yields feature maps $M_i(c, s)$, given a "center" scale c and "surround" scale s. Across scale difference (Θ) between two feature maps is computed by interpolation to the center scale and pointwise absolute difference.

For color and intensity channels, feature maps are computed usingEq. (6):

$$M_i(c,s) = |O_i(c)\Theta O_i(s)| = |O_i(c) - interp_{s-c}(O_i(s))| \qquad \text{Eq.}(6)$$

Feature maps are used to detect conspicuous regions in each channel and are merged linearly to yield a saliency map. Information from the orientation channel is incorporated by employing Gabor filters to the grayscale image (Eq. (7)) at four spatial center scales (c = 0, 1, 2, 3) and at four different angles ($\theta_i = 0^\circ, 45^\circ, 90^\circ, 135^\circ$).

For orientation channels, feature maps are computed using Eq. (7):

$$M_i(c) = Gabor(\theta_i, c) \qquad \text{Eq.}(7)$$

After the computation of low-level center-surround features, each sub-channel extracts a gist vector from its corresponding feature map. Averaging operations are applied in a 4×4 grid of subregions over the map. Sixteen raw gist features ($G_i^{k,l}(c, s)$) are computed per feature map using Eq. (8):

$$G_i^{k,l}(c,s) = \frac{1}{16WH} \sum_{u=\frac{kW}{4}}^{\frac{(k+1)W}{4}-1} \sum_{v=\frac{lH}{4}}^{\frac{(l+1)H}{4}-1} [M_i(c,s)](u,v) \qquad \text{Eq.}(8)$$

where W and H are width and height of the image respectively.

k and l are the indices in horizontal and vertical directions respectively.

12 orientations per scale and 8 blocks were used for this study.

HOG features

This method was first introduced by Dalal and Trigg [16]. HOG breaks up a CXR image into small cells, computes the HOGs for each cell, normalizes HOGs using block pattern, and provides a descriptor for each cell [27]. These features are generally used for object detection in an image. The basic idea behind HOG features is that shape and appearance of local objects within an image can be described by the intensity gradients distribution. This method involves counting the occurrence of gradient orientation and thereby maintains photometric transformations and geometric invariance. The descriptor generation is comprised of four main steps: gradient computation, orientation binning, descriptor blocks generation, and block normalization. In gradient computation, the filtering of intensity or color data of the image is done with 1-D centred discrete derivative masks ($D_x = [-1,0,1]$ and $D_y = [-1,0,1]^T$) in horizontal and/or vertical directions. For a given image I, x and y derivatives are obtained using a convolution operation $I_x = I * D_x$ and $I_y = I * D_y$. Magnitude and orientation of the gradient is computed by the following equations Eq. (9) and Eq. (10) respectively:

$$[G] = I_x^2 + I_y^2 \qquad \text{Eq.}(9)$$

$$\theta = \arctan\frac{I_y}{I_x} \qquad \text{Eq.}(10)$$

Orientation binning involves the creation of a cell histogram. Weighted vote is cast by each pixel within a cell based on the gradient computation values. The histogram channels are uniformly spread over 0 to 360 or 0 to 180 degrees depending on signed or unsigned gradient respectively. The cells are then grouped together into spatially connected blocks to account for changes in contrast and illumination. These blocks usually overlap, and two main geometries R-HOG (rectangular) and C-HOG (circular) blocks exist. The blocks are normalised using one of the following normalization factors:

L1-norm: $f = v/(\|v\|_1 + e))$

L1-sqrt: $f = \sqrt{v/(\|v\|_1 + e)}$

L2-norm: $f = v/\sqrt{\|v\|_2^2 + e^2}$

L2-hys: L2-norm equation with maximum value of v limited to 0.2 followed by renormalization.

In this study, block size and number of bins were set to 6×6 and 9 respectively. R-HOG was used as it provided better classification accuracy as compared to C-HOG.

PHOG features

These are spatial shape descriptors which describe an image by its spatial layout and local shape [17]. These descriptors are comprised of HOGs over each sub-region of an image at each pyramid resolution level. Local shapes in an image are captured by the distribution over edge orientations within a region while the spatial layout is captured by tiling an image into regions at multiple resolutions.

Initially, the HOG for entire image is computed. The bin size for HOG is fixed to N bins. The CXR is divided into a sequence of increasingly finer spatial grids by repetitively doubling the number of divisions along each axis. The number of points in each grid cell is stored. Since the number of points in a cell at one level is equal to the sum of points contained in the four cells it is divided into at the next level, this is a pyramid representation. HOG is computed for each of these levels. The bin count for the histogram representing a level is the cell count at that level of resolution. This process is repeated until a depth L. During pyramid formation, 2^L cells are present along each dimension for the grid at level L. PHOG features obtained for an image is a weighted combination of the above HOG features. The summation of calculated PHOG values is then normalized to unity to ascertain that texture rich images are not weighted more strongly than others. In this study, the number of bins on histogram and number of pyramid levels at 360 degrees were set to 8 and 3 respectively.

Feature selection

Feature selection was performed using chi-square based method. Although several other feature selection methods such as correlation based feature selection, info gain and kernel principal component analysis were evaluated, but the performance of chi-square based feature selection method using WEKA software [28] was found to be the best with respect to classification results. This method uses chi-square statistics to discretize features repeatedly until some inconsistency is found in the data. Feature ranking was also done by this method and the best features were used for classification of a CXR as TB or non-TB.

Classification

Support vector machines (SVMs) [29], a machine learning algorithm, is commonly used for classification and regression. The objective of SVM is to find the hyperplane which maximizes distance between data points from two classes. Training data points closest to the hyperplane are called support vectors (Figure 5). The hyperplane can be defined as:

$$f(x) = \beta_0 + \beta^T x$$

where β, β_0 and x are the weight vector, bias and support vectors respectively.

The SVM is a non-probabilistic binary linear classifier, but it can also perform a non-linear classification using the kernel trick by mapping the data points into high-dimensional feature spaces. Some common kernel methods are polynomial homogeneous, polynomial inhomogeneous, Gaussian radial basis function and hyperbolic tangent. Gaussian radial basis function was used in the study. LIBSVM [30], a supervised machine learning software, was used for labelling (classification) of a given CXR as TB or non-TB.

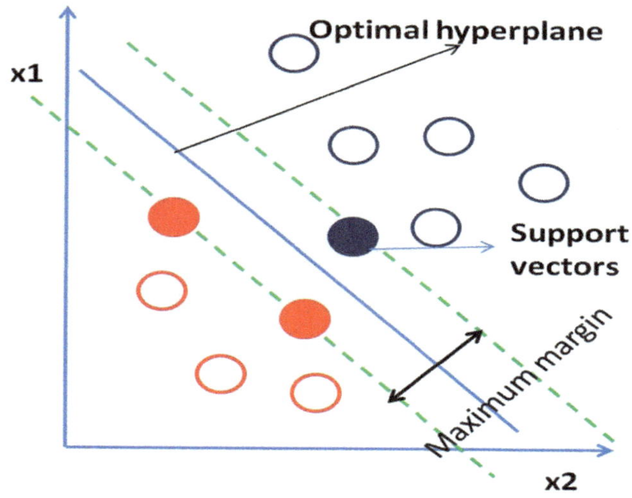

Figure 5. Hyperplane (blue line) representation in SVM. Red and blue circles represent data points from two different classes. Solid filled circles denote support vectors.

Results and Discussion

Current CAD methods use local GLCM textural features extracted from segmented CXRs for the classification of CXRs. Segmentation is an important step for the optimal extraction of features. Implementation of CAD method into X-ray machines for the automatic prediction requires features to be extracted from automatically segmented or whole CXR images. The ground truth that we were striving to reproduce by this CAD method for the two datasets was the judgement or decision of radiologists who read the CXRs.

Performance of features extracted from automatically segmented CXRs

The performance of the GLCM textural features was quite low for the CXR dataset DA (Table 1). Prediction accuracy of only 65.4% was obtained for GLCM textural features extracted from automatically segmented CXRs, while 80.8% was obtained for manually segmented CXRs from dataset DA. The poor performance of the features extracted from automatic segmented CXRs may be attributed to severe intensity distortions [1], variability in lungs shape, and complex appearances of CXRs due to overlapping of anatomical structures.

Performance of features extracted from whole-CXR and manually segmented CXRs

Since low prediction accuracy was obtained using GLCM method, therefore, features extracted from the whole image, like Gabor, Gist, HOG, and PHOG were evaluated for their ability to discriminate between the TB and non-TB CXRs. The parameters were fine-tuned, so that the features relevant to TB discrimination were extracted. The Gabor, Gist, HOG, and PHOG features extracted from the whole CXR provided a prediction accuracy of 86.5%, 94.2%, 86.5%, and 92.3% respectively for dataset DA, and 92.0%, 86.0%, 86.0%, and 90% respectively for dataset DB (Table 1 and 2). The Gist features provided the maximum sensitivity of 0.961 for the dataset DA. This outcome is significant because sensitivity is considered as major criterion when measuring the effectiveness of a classification model for the detection of diseases. Although Gabor features provided comparable predic-

Table 1. Performance of classification of CXRs dataset, DA using various feature extraction methods.

Feature*	Accuracy	Sensitivity	Specificity	Precision	F-score	GMean	AUC	CI#	SE#
Gabor[1]	0.865	0.808	0.923	0.913	0.857	0.864	0.888	0.769–0.958	0.0482
Gab[2]	0.865	0.885	0.846	0.852	0.868	0.865	0.919	0.809–0.976	0.0392
Gab[3]	0.712	0.654	0.769	0.739	0.694	0.709	0.771	0.633–0.876	0.0668
Gist[1]	0.942	0.961	0.923	0.925	0.943	0.942	0.957	0.861–0.994	0.0301
Gist[2]	0.885	0.846	0.923	0.917	0.880	0.884	0.905	0.792–0.969	0.0444
Gist[3]	0.827	0.808	0.846	0.840	0.824	0.827	0.868	0.746–0.946	0.0497
HOG[1]	0.865	0.846	0.885	0.880	0.863	0.865	0.904	0.790–0.968	0.0456
HOG[2]	0.846	0.769	0.923	0.909	0.833	0.843	0.880	0.760–0.954	0.0483
HOG[3]	0.865	0.846	0.885	0.880	0.863	0.865	0.907	0.793–0.970	0.0440
PHOG[1]	0.923	0.885	0.962	0.958	0.920	0.922	0.956	0.859–0.993	0.0294
PHOG[2]	0.827	0.769	0.885	0.870	0.816	0.825	0.859	0.735–0.940	0.0520
PHOG[3]	0.808	0.846	0.769	0.786	0.815	0.807	0.828	0.698–0.919	0.0577
GLCM[2]	0.808	0.769	0.846	0.833	0.800	0.807	0.859	0.735–0.940	0.0510
GLCM[3]	0.654	0.769	0.538	0.625	0.690	0.644	0.623	0.478–0.753	0.0803

*Features extracted from: [1] indicates whole CXR, [2] indicates manually segmented CXR and [3] indicates automatic segmented CXR.
#CI refers to confidence interval at 95% at P-value <0.0001 whereas SE refers to standard error for AUC.

Table 2. Performance of classification of CXRs dataset, DB using various feature extraction methods.

Feature*	Accuracy	Sensitivity	Specificity	Precision	F-score	GMean	AUC	CI#	SE#
Gab[1]	0.920	0.920	0.920	0.920	0.920	0.920	0.936	0.829–0.986	0.0377
Gist[1]	0.860	0.880	0.840	0.846	0.863	0.860	0.893	0.773–0.962	0.0520
HOG[1]	0.860	0.800	0.920	0.909	0.851	0.858	0.909	0.793–0.972	0.0434
PHOG[1]	0.900	0.920	0.880	0.885	0.902	0.900	0.918	0.806–0.977	0.0404

*Features extracted from: [1] indicates whole CXR, [2] indicates manually segmented CXR and [3] indicates automatic segmented CXR.
#CI refers to confidence interval at 95% at P-value <0.0001 whereas SE refers to standard error for AUC.

tion accuracy to PHOG for dataset DB, but the latter provided significantly better 5-fold cross-validation accuracy of 86.6% in comparison to the former's 81.5%. Also, Gabor feature extraction is a computationally intensive process than PHOG method. For 5-fold cross-validation, the dataset were divided into five equal parts. One part was used for testing while the other four parts were used for the training of SVM. The procedure was repeated five times. The performance of features extracted from manually segmented images was comparable or lower than to those extracted from whole CXR image (Table 1). This may be attributed to the better spatial and contextual information provided by the whole CXR in comparison to the segmented one. Comparable performance between the whole and manually lung segmented CXRs indicated that these features (Gist, Gabor, HOG, and PHOG) were able to capture discriminative features without the need for segmentation of lungs (Table 1). Comparison of performance for various features is provided in the form bar graph in Figure 6.

Validation

The performance of various feature extraction methods used in this study is provided in Table 1 and 2. To validate the proposed methodology, five-fold cross validation and ROC curve analysis were done. PHOG features provided five-fold cross-validation accuracies of 83.2% and 86.6% for the datasets DA and DB respectively while 84.4% and 86.6% were obtained for the same datasets using Gist features.

The AUC is a plot between true positive and false positive rates and it determines how well a model can distinguish between the TB and non-TB CXRs [31,32]. Figure 7 and 8 show high value of AUC for both Gist and PHOG features indicating a good discrimination between the TB and non-TB CXRs [33]. Every point on the ROC curve represents a specificity and sensitivity pair corresponding to a certain decision threshold. Higher is the overall accuracy of classification; closer is the ROC curve to the upper left corner. When a classifier cannot discriminate between the two classes or groups, the AUC would be equal to 0.5. When there is a perfect discrimination, the AUC would be equal to 1. The 95% confidence interval (CI) is the interval in which the true AUC lies with 95% confidence. P-value is the probability that the observed AUC is found when actually the true AUC is 0.5. If P is smaller than 0.05, it can be concluded that the AUC is significantly different from 0.5 and the classifier has the ability to discriminate between the two classes. High AUC values were obtained (Table 1 and 2) at 95% confidence interval for our methods at P-level (AUC = 0.5) smaller than 0.0001. Standard error (SE) of AUC was also calculated using the method of Delong *et al.* [34] and SE values were found to be quite low (Table 1 and 2). As inferred from the results of this study, the Gist and PHOG features were quite robust and provided better results without segmentation.

TB-Xpredict

Gist and PHOG features were implemented to develop TB-Xpredict, a MATLAB toolbox available at http://sourceforge.net/projects/tbxpredict/. It has a user-friendly graphical user interface (GUI), which provides both training and prediction modules (Figure 9 and 10). The former enables the user to develop a model trained on his/her own CXRs (TB and non-TB CXRs) while the latter can be used for the classification of digital CXR(s). The user can independently upload CXRs into the prediction module to classify them using already trained model provided with the software. Training and prediction modules of the toolbox are available for Gist and PHOG features separately with the use of Gist as default. The toolbox automatically identifies the bit size and file format (dicom or jpeg) of the CXR images.

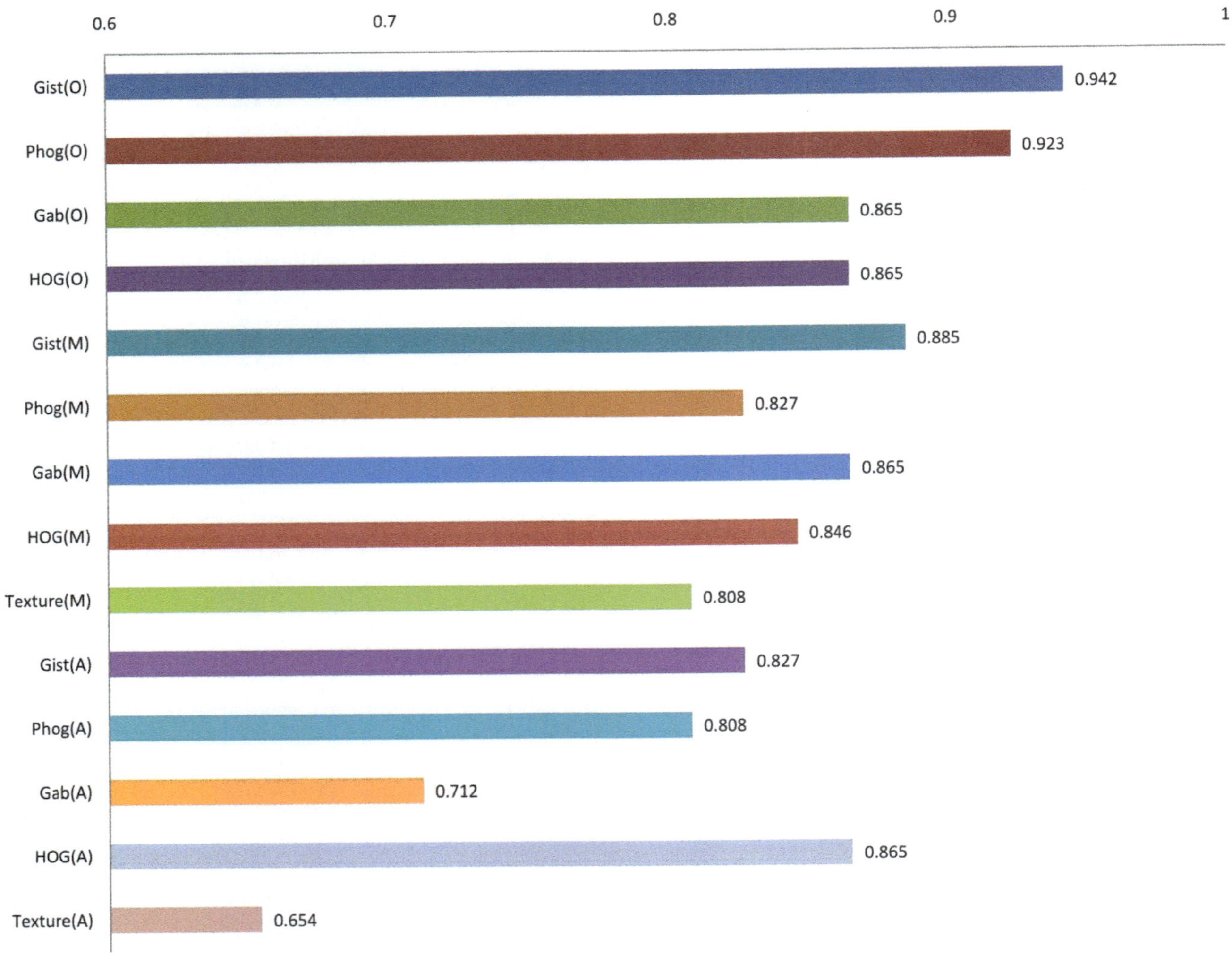

Figure 6. Comparison of performance for various features from whole, manually segmented, and automatically segmented CXRs.

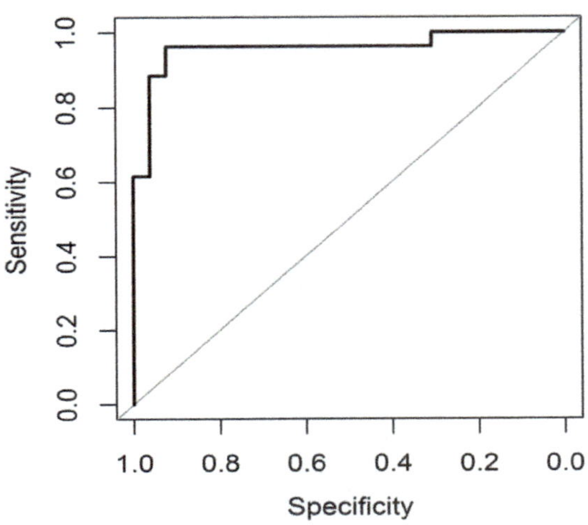

Figure 7. ROC plot for classification between TB and non-TB CXRs (DA) using Gist features.

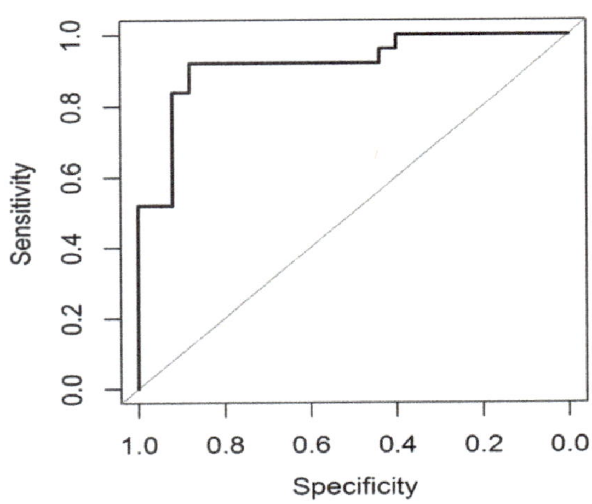

Figure 8. ROC plot for classification between TB and non-TB CXRs (DA) using PHOG features.

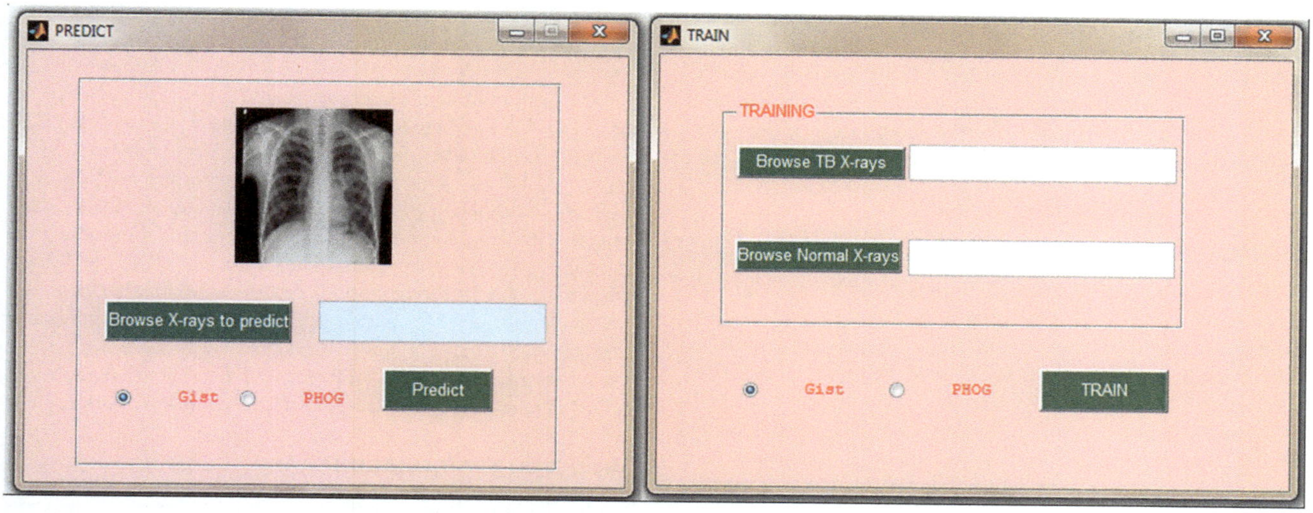

Figure 9. GUI of Prediction and Training Modules in Matlab toolbox, TB-Xpredict.

Since TB-Xpredict does not require prior segmentation of digital CXR images, this toolbox can easily be incorporated into existing X-ray machines for the automated classification of CXR as TB or non-TB. X-ray machines with such modules can effectively be used for the mass screening of TB in high-burden areas. GUI of TB-Xpredict enables user to train and classify CXRs without the need of expertise in image processing. User only needs to upload positive and negative CXRs separately, and the module trains the model in an automatic manner. The newly developed model can be used for the prediction of CXRs using

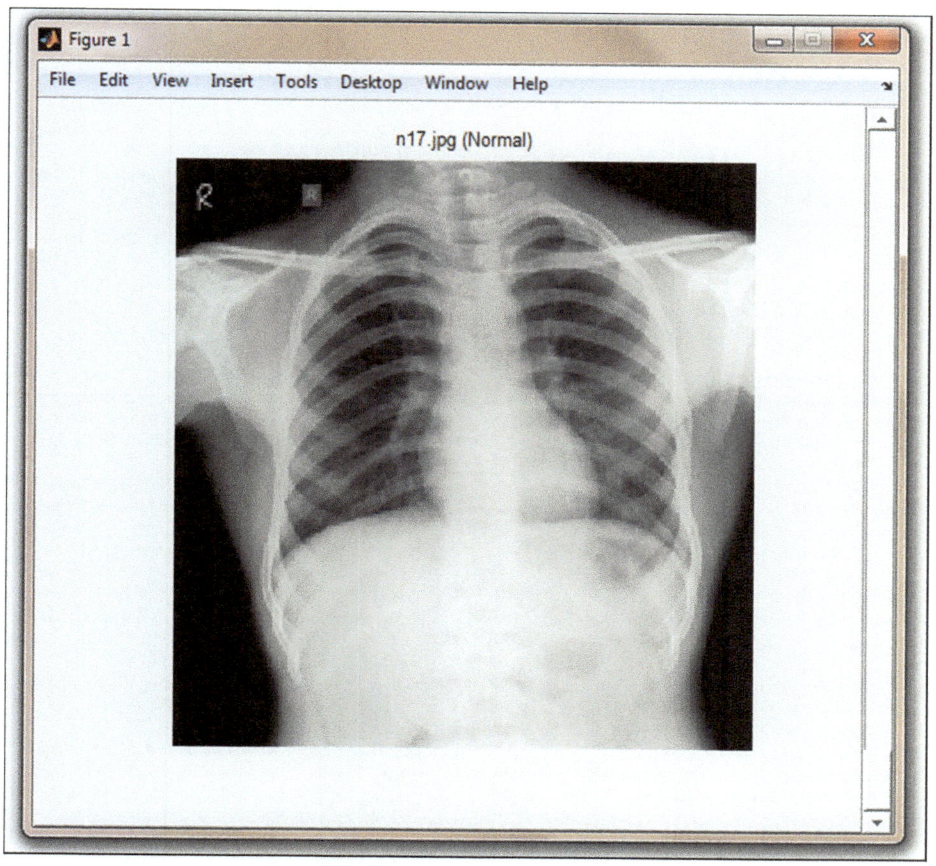

Figure 10. GUI of sample output provided by Matlab toolbox, TB-Xpredict.

prediction module. Since illumination and other parameters do not differ significantly in test data with respect to training model, automated prediction methods which use CXRs from the same X-ray machine for training as well as classification generally may lead to better prediction accuracy. Furthermore, such model may become more efficient as the number and diversity of training data increases over time.

Conclusions

CAD techniques provide second opinion to the clinicians for their findings, so its implementation is expected to improve their performance in the diagnosis of TB. Features extracted by methods such as Gabor, Gist, HOG, and PHOG enabled SVM to efficiently discriminate between the TB and non-TB whole CXR images. Validations of results using five-fold cross-validation and independent datasets have shown that the performance of these features is significantly higher than that of textural features (Table 1 and 2). CAD techniques proposed earlier were mainly based on the segmentation of CXRs followed by the extraction of GLCM textural features. The major limitation with these methods is that they cannot be incorporated into existing X-ray machines for automated detection of TB due to their dependency on manual or semi-automated segmentation. Although GLCM textural features extracted from the automatically segmented CXRs can be used for automated detection, however, the performance of this method is exceedingly poor (Table 1). Since the features (Gabor, Gist, HOG, and PHOG) extracted from the whole CXR do not require ROI identification using segmentation, these features can easily be implemented to existing digital X-ray machines for the automated TB detection. As Gist and PHOG features provided the best discrimination between the non-TB and TB for both 8-bit and 14-bit CXRs, these features were used to develop a MATLAB toolbox, TB-Xpredict, which can effortlessly train as well as predict CXRs as TB or non-TB. TB-Xpredict has a very simple GUI for automated training and classification of CXRs, and requires only basic knowledge of computer to operate. It also gives users the option to choose between Gist and PHOG for feature extraction. One of the limitations of the toolbox is that since TB has similar radiological patterns to cancer and some interstitial lung diseases (ILDs), it may wrongly classify CXRs with these diseases as TB CXRs. This toolbox will assist in better diagnosis as well as efficient mass screening of TB in high burden areas.

Supporting Information

Table S1 Various grey-level co-occurrence matrix (GLCM) textural features used for the classification.

Author Contributions

Conceived and designed the experiments: AC DC CR. Performed the experiments: AC. Analyzed the data: AC DC CR. Contributed reagents/materials/analysis tools: AC DC CR. Wrote the paper: AC CR. Designed and implemented the Matlab Toolbox: AC CR. Compilation of data sets: AC DC CR.

References

1. Tan C, Lim CM, Acharya UR, Tan JH, Abraham KT (2012) Computer-Assisted Diagnosis of Tuberculosis: A First Order Statistical Approach to Chest Radiograph. J Med Syst 36: 2751–2759. doi:10.1007/s10916-011-9751-9.
2. Global TB Control Report 2012 (2012) World Health Organization, Geneva.
3. Doi K (2007) Computer-aided diagnosis in medical imaging: historical review, current status and future potential. Comput Med Imaging Graph 31: 198–211.
4. Noble M, Bruening W, Uhl S, Schoelles K (2009) Computer-aided detection mammography for breast cancer screening: systematic review and meta-analysis. Arch Gynecol Obstet 279: 881–890. doi:10.1007/s00404-008-0841-y.
5. Gur D, Sumkin JH, Rockette HE, Ganott M, Hakim C, et al. (2004) Changes in breast cancer detection and mammography recall rates after the introduction of a computer-aided detection system. J Natl Cancer Inst 96: 185–190. doi:10.1093/jnci/djh067.
6. Dean JC, Ilvento CC (2006) Improved cancer detection using computer-aided detection with diagnostic and screening mammography: prospective study of 104 cancers. AJR Am J Roentgenol 187: 20–28. doi:10.2214/AJR.05.0111.
7. Ginneken BV, Hogeweg L, Maduskar P, Peters-Bax L, Dawson R, et al. (2012) Performance of inexperienced and experienced observers in detection of active tuberculosis on digital chest radiographs with and without the use of computer-aided diagnosis. Annual Meeting of the Radiological Society of North America.
8. Haralick RM, Shanmugam K, Dinstein I (1973) Textural Features for Image Classification. IEEE Trans Syst Man Cybern 3: 610–621. doi:10.1109/TSMC.1973.4309314.
9. Ginneken BV, Katsuragawa S, ter Haar Romeny BM, Doi K, Viergever MA (2002) Automatic detection of abnormalities in chest radiographs using local texture analysis. IEEE Trans Med Imaging 21: 139–149. doi:10.1109/42.993132.
10. Hogeweg L, Mol C, de Jong PA, Dawson R, Ayles H, et al. (2010) Fusion of local and global detection systems to detect tuberculosis in chest radiographs. Med Image Comput Comput Assist Interv 13: 650–657. doi:10.1007/978-3-642-15711-0_81.
11. Arzhaeva Y, Hogeweg L, de Jong PA, Viergever MA, van Ginneken B (2009) Global and local multi-valued dissimilarity-based classification: application to computer-aided detection of tuberculosis. Med Image Comput Comput Assist Interv 12: 724–731. doi:10.1007/978-3-642-04271-3_88.
12. Ginneken BV, Tax DMJ, Arzhaeva Y (2009) Dissimilarity-based classification in the absence of local ground truth: Application to the diagnostic interpretation of chest radiographs. Pattern Recognit 42: 1768–1776. doi:10.1016/j.patcog.2009.01.016.
13. Shen RSR, Cheng I, Basu A (2010) A Hybrid Knowledge-Guided Detection Technique for Screening of Infectious Pulmonary Tuberculosis From Chest Radiographs. IEEE Trans Biomed Eng 57. doi:10.1109/TBME.2010.2057509.
14. Oliva A, Hospital W, Ave L (2001) Modeling the Shape of the Scene: A Holistic Representation of the Spatial Envelope. Int J Comput Vis 42: 145–175.
15. Manjunath BS, Ma WY (1996) Texture features for browsing and retrieval of image data. IEEE Trans Pattern Anal Mach Intell 18: 837–842. doi:10.1109/34.531803.
16. Dalal N, Triggs B (2005) Histograms of oriented gradients for human detection. 2005 IEEE Comput Soc Conf Comput Vis Pattern Recognit 1. doi:10.1109/CVPR.2005.177.
17. Bosch A, Zisserman A, Munoz X (2007) Representing shape with a spatial pyramid kernel. Image Process 5: 401–408.
18. Abràmoff MD, Magalhães PJ, Ram SJ (2004) Image processing with ImageJ. Biophotonics international, 11: 36–43.
19. Chan TF, Sandberg BY, Vese LA (2000) Active Contours without Edges for Vector-Valued Images. J Vis Commun Image Represent 11: 130–141.
20. Wong LP, Ewe HT (2005) A study of lung cancer detection using chest x-ray images. Proc. 3rd APT Telemedicine Workshop, Kuala Lumpur 3: 210–214
21. Luisier F, Blu T, Unser M (2007) A new SURE approach to image denoising: interscale orthonormal wavelet thresholding. IEEE Trans Image Process 16: 593–606.
22. Grigorescu SE, Petkov N, Kruizinga P (2002) Comparison of texture features based on Gabor filters. IEEE Trans Image Process 11: 1160–1167. doi:10.1109/ICIAP.1999.797585.
23. Yang Y, Newsam S (2008) Comparing SIFT descriptors and gabor texture features for classification of remote sensed imagery. 2008 15th IEEE Int Conf Image Process. doi:10.1109/ICIP.2008.4712139.
24. Siagian C, Itti L (2007) Rapid biologically-inspired scene classification using features shared with visual attention. IEEE Trans Pattern Anal Mach Intell 29: 300–312. doi:10.1109/TPAMI.2007.40.
25. Oliva A, Torralba A (2006) Building the gist of a scene: the role of global image features in recognition. Prog Brain Res 155: 23–36. doi:10.1016/S0079-6123(06)55002-2.
26. Itti L, Siagian C (2010) Comparison of gist models in rapid scene categorization tasks. J Vis 8: 734–734. doi:10.1167/8.6.734.
27. Ludwig O, Delgado D, Goncalves V, Nunes U (2009) Trainable classifier-fusion schemes: An application to pedestrian detection. 2009 12th Int IEEE Conf Intell Transp Syst. doi:10.1109/ITSC.2009.5309700.

28. Hall M, Frank E, Holmes G, Pfahringer B, Reutemann P, et al. (2009) The WEKA Data Mining Software: An Update. ACM SIGKDD Explor Newsl 11: 10–18. Available: http://dl.acm.org/citation.cfm?id=1656278.
29. Cortes C, Vapnik V (1995) Support-vector networks. Machine learning 20: 273–297.
30. Chang C-C, Lin C-J (2011) LIBSVM: a library for support vector machines. ACM Trans Intell Syst Technol 2: 1–39.
31. Zweig MH, Campbell G (1993) Receiver-operating characteristic (ROC) plots: a fundamental evaluation tool in clinical medicine. Clin Chem 39: 561–577.
32. Metz C (1978) Basic principles of ROC analysis. Semin Nucl Med 8: 283–298. Available: papers2://publication/uuid/7A60F045-4E92-43C3-9586-6994FE10B463.
33. Robin X, Turck N, Hainard A, Tiberti N, Lisacek F, et al. (2011) pROC: an open-source package for R and S+ to analyze and compare ROC curves. BMC Bioinformatics 12: 77. doi:10.1186/1471-2105-12-77.
34. DeLong ER, DeLong DM, Clarke-Pearson DL (1988) Comparing the areas under two or more correlated receiver operating characteristic curves: a nonparametric approach. Biometrics 44: 837–845. doi:10.2307/2531595.

Permissions

All chapters in this book were first published in PLOS ONE, by The Public Library of Science; hereby published with permission under the Creative Commons Attribution License or equivalent. Every chapter published in this book has been scrutinized by our experts. Their significance has been extensively debated. The topics covered herein carry significant findings which will fuel the growth of the discipline. They may even be implemented as practical applications or may be referred to as a beginning point for another development.

The contributors of this book come from diverse backgrounds, making this book a truly international effort. This book will bring forth new frontiers with its revolutionizing research information and detailed analysis of the nascent developments around the world.

We would like to thank all the contributing authors for lending their expertise to make the book truly unique. They have played a crucial role in the development of this book. Without their invaluable contributions this book wouldn't have been possible. They have made vital efforts to compile up to date information on the varied aspects of this subject to make this book a valuable addition to the collection of many professionals and students.

This book was conceptualized with the vision of imparting up-to-date information and advanced data in this field. To ensure the same, a matchless editorial board was set up. Every individual on the board went through rigorous rounds of assessment to prove their worth. After which they invested a large part of their time researching and compiling the most relevant data for our readers.

The editorial board has been involved in producing this book since its inception. They have spent rigorous hours researching and exploring the diverse topics which have resulted in the successful publishing of this book. They have passed on their knowledge of decades through this book. To expedite this challenging task, the publisher supported the team at every step. A small team of assistant editors was also appointed to further simplify the editing procedure and attain best results for the readers.

Apart from the editorial board, the designing team has also invested a significant amount of their time in understanding the subject and creating the most relevant covers. They scrutinized every image to scout for the most suitable representation of the subject and create an appropriate cover for the book.

The publishing team has been an ardent support to the editorial, designing and production team. Their endless efforts to recruit the best for this project, has resulted in the accomplishment of this book. They are a veteran in the field of academics and their pool of knowledge is as vast as their experience in printing. Their expertise and guidance has proved useful at every step. Their uncompromising quality standards have made this book an exceptional effort. Their encouragement from time to time has been an inspiration for everyone.

The publisher and the editorial board hope that this book will prove to be a valuable piece of knowledge for researchers, students, practitioners and scholars across the globe.

List of Contributors

Jeongeun Ryu, Sungsook Ahn, Seung-Gon Kim and Sang Joon Lee
Department of Mechanical Engineering, Pohang University of Science and Technology (POSTECH), Pohang, Gyeongbuk, Republic of Korea
Center for Biofluid and Biomimic Research, Pohang University of Science and Technology (POSTECH), Pohang, Gyeongbuk, Republic of Korea

TaeJoo Kim
Neutron Science Division, Korea Atomic Energy Research Institute (KAERI), Daejeon, Republic of Korea

Marrigje F. Meijer, Alexander L. Boerboom, Martin Stevens and Sjoerd K. Bulstra
Department of Orthopaedics, University of Groningen, University Medical Center Groningen, Gronigen, The Netherlands

Inge H. F. Reininga
Department of Trauma Surgery, University of Groningen, University Medical Center Groningen, Groningen, The Netherlands

Shinichi Shimizu and Hiroki Shirato
Department of Radiation Oncology, Hokkaido University Graduate School of Medicine, Sapporo, Hokkaido, Japan

Naoki Miyamoto
Department of Medical Physics, Hokkaido University Graduate School of Medicine, Sapporo, Hokkaido, Japan

Taeko Matsuura
Section of Medical Physics, Hokkaido University Hospital Proton Beam Therapy Center, Sapporo, Hokkaido, Japan

Yusuke Fujii and Masumi Umezawa
Hitachi, Ltd., Hitachi Research Laboratory, Omika, Ibaraki, Japan

Kikuo Umegaki
Division of Quantum Science and Engineering, Hokkaido University Graduate School of Engineering, Sapporo, Hokkaido, Japan

Kazuo Hiramoto
Hitachi, Ltd., Research & Development Group, Omika, Ibaraki, Japan

Yuan Zhang, Zhengxue Quan, Zenghui Zhao, Xiaoji Luo, Ke Tang, Jie Li, Xu Zhou andDianming Jiang
Department of Orthopedic Surgery, The First Affiliated Hospital of Chongqing Medical University, Chongqing, China

Ming Chen and Ming Ling
Department of Orthopedics, Shaanxi Provincial Peoples Hospital, Xi'an, Shaanxi, China

Qun Huang, Wei Xu, Chang She, Zong-Gang Xie, Yong-Tao Mao and Qi-Rong Dong
Department of Orthopedics, Second Affiliated Hospital of Soochow University, Suzhou, Jiangsu, China

Keith K. W. Chan
School of Public Health and Primary Care, Faculty of Medicine, The Chinese University of Hong Kong, Hong Kong

Regina W. S. Sit
Jockey Club School of Public Health and Primary Care, Faculty of Medicine, The Chinese University of Hong Kong, Hong Kong

Ricky W. K. Wu and Allen H. Y. Ngai
The Hong Kong Institute of Musculoskeletal Medicine, Hong Kong

Timothy D. Butters, Simon J. Castro and Henggui Zhang
School of Physics and Astronomy, The University of Manchester, Manchester, Greater Manchester, United Kingdom

Tristan Lowe and Philip J. Withers
School of Materials Science, The University of Manchester, Manchester, Greater Manchester, United Kingdom

Yanmin Zhang and Ming Lei
Institute of Cardiovascular Sciences, Faculty of Medical and Human Sciences, The University of Manchester, Manchester, Greater Manchester, United Kingdom

Department of Pharmacology, University of Oxford, Oxford, Oxfordshire, United Kingdom

Qingsong Yang, Wenxiang Cong and Ge Wang
Biomedical Imaging Center, Center for Biotechnology and Interdisciplinary Studies, Department of Biomedical Engineering, Rensselaer Polytechnic Institute, Troy, New York, United States of America

Fenglin Liu
Key Lab of Optoelectronic Technology and System, Engineering Research Center of Industrial Computed Tomography Nondestructive Testing, Ministry of Education, Chongqing University, Chongqing, China
Biomedical Imaging Center, Center for Biotechnology and Interdisciplinary Studies, Department of Biomedical Engineering, Rensselaer Polytechnic Institute, Troy, New York, United States of America

Bram van Ginneken and Rick H. H. M. Philipsen
Diagnostic Image Analysis Group, Radboud University Medical Center, Nijmegen, The Netherlands

Francis Mhimbira, Jerry J. Hella and Fred Lwilla
Ifakara Health Institute, Bagamoyo, United Republic of Tanzania

Jan van den Hombergh
PharmAccess International, Dar es Salaam, United Republic of Tanzania

Dirk Wagner
Center for Infectious Diseases and Travel Medicine, University Hospital Freiburg, Freiburg, Germany

Amanda Ross
Swiss Tropical and Public Health Institute, Basel, Switzerland
University of Basel, Basel, Switzerland

Marianne Breuninger
Swiss Tropical and Public Health Institute, Basel, Switzerland
Ifakara Health Institute, Bagamoyo, United Republic of Tanzania
Center for Infectious Diseases and Travel Medicine, University Hospital Freiburg, Freiburg, Germany

Levan Jugheli and Klaus Reither
Swiss Tropical and Public Health Institute, Basel, Switzerland
Ifakara Health Institute, Bagamoyo, United Republic of Tanzania
University of Basel, Basel, Switzerland

Ekrem Misimi, Svein Martinsen, John Reidar Mathiassen and Ulf Erikson
SINTEF Fisheries and Aquaculture, Trondheim, Norway

Audrey Baudet
Centre d'Investigation Clinique INSERM 1432, Plateforme d'Investigation Technologique, Dijon University Hospital, Dijon, France

Philippe d'Athis
Medical Information department, Dijon University Hospital, Dijon, France

Claire Morisset and Davy Laroche
Centre d'Investigation Clinique INSERM 1432, Plateforme d'Investigation Technologique, Dijon University Hospital, Dijon, France
INSERM U1093, Dijon, France

Jean-Francis Maillefert and Paul Ornetti
INSERM U1093, Dijon, France
University of Burgundy, Dijon, France
Department of rheumatology, Dijon University Hospital, Dijon, France

Jean-Marie Casillas
Centre d'Investigation Clinique INSERM 1432, Plateforme d'Investigation Technologique, Dijon University Hospital, Dijon, France
INSERM U1093, Dijon, France
University of Burgundy, Dijon, France
Department of physical medicine, Dijon University Hospital, Dijon, France

João Valente-dos-Santos, Manuel J. Coelho-e-Silva and Aristides M. Machado-Rodrigues
Faculty of Sport Sciences and Physical Education, University of Coimbra, Coimbra, Portugal

Édio L. Petroski
Research Centre for Kinanthropometry and Human Performance, Federal University of Santa Catarina, Florianópolis, Santa Catarina, Brazil

Cláudia S. Minderico, Analiza M. Silva, Fátima Baptista and Luís B. Sardinha
Exercise and Health Laboratory, CIPER, Faculdade de Motricidade Humana, Universidade de Lisboa, Cruz-Quebrada, Portugal

Marije T. Elferink-Gemser
Center for Human Movement Sciences, University Medical Center Groningen, University of Groningen, Groningen, The Netherlands
Institute for Studies in Sports and Exercise, HAN University of Applied Sciences, Nijmegen, The Netherlands

Robert M. Malina
Department of Kinesiology and Health Education, University of Texas at Austin, Austin, Texas, United States of America
Department of Kinesiology, Tarleton State University, Stephenville, Texas, United States of America

Weiqing Liu, Shiwen Zhang, Dan Zhao, Huawei Zou, Ningyuan Sun, Xing Liang and Quan Yuan
State Key Laboratory of Oral Diseases, West China Hospital of Stomatology, Sichuan University, Chengdu, China

Michel Dard
Department of Periodontology and Implant Dentistry, New York University College of Dentistry, New York, United States of America

Beate Lanske
Department of Oral Medicine, Infection, and Immunity, Harvard School of Dental medicine, Boston, Massachusetts, United States of America

Marcus J. Kitchen
School of Physics, Monash Institute of Medical Research, Clayton, Victoria, Australia

Melissa L. Siew, Megan J. Wallace and Stuart B. Hooper
The Ritchie Centre, Monash Institute of Medical Research, Clayton, Victoria, Australia

Andreas Fouras
Department of Mechanical and Aerospace Engineering, Monash University, Clayton, Victoria, Australia

Naoto Yagi and Kentaro Uesugi
SPring-8/Japan Synchrotron Radiation Research Institute, Sayo, Hyogo, Japan

Arjan B. te Pas
Department of Pediatrics, Leiden University Medical Centre, Leiden, Netherlands

Robert A. Lewis
Department of Medical Imaging and Radiation Science, Monash University, Clayton, Victoria, Australia
Biomedical Engineering, University of Saskatchewan, Saskatoon, Canada

Yasunori Enomoto, Eri Hagiwara, Shigeru Komatsu, Ryuichi Nishihira, Tomohisa Baba, Hideya Kitamura, Akimasa Sekine, Atsuhito Nakazawa and Takashi Ogura
Department of Respiratory Medicine, Kanagawa Cardiovascular and Respiratory Center, Yokohama, Japan

Kai Scherer, Lorenz Birnbacher, Michael Chabior and Franz Pfeiffer
Lehrstuhl für Biomedizinische Physik, Physik-Department & Institut für Medizintechnik, Technische Universität München, Garching, Germany

Julia Herzen
Centre for Materials and Coastal Research, Helmholtz-Zentrum Geesthacht, Geesthacht, Germany

Doris Mayr
Department of Pathology, Ludwig Maximilian University, Munich, Germany

Susanne Grandl, Karin Hellerhoff, Fabian Bamberg and Anikó Sztrókay-Gaul
Department of Clinical Radiology, Ludwig Maximilian University, Munich, Germany

Steven Schalekamp, Bram van Ginneken, Miranda M. Snoeren and Nico Karssemeijer
Dept. Of Radiology, Radboud University Medical Center, Nijmegen, The Netherlands

Inge A. H. van den Berk and Laura J. Schijf
Dept. Of Radiology, Academic Medical Center, Amsterdam, The Netherlands

Ieneke J. C. Hartmann
Dept. Of Radiology, Maasstad Hospital, Rotterdam, The Netherlands

Arlette E. Odink and Winnifred van Lankeren
Dept. Of Radiology, Erasmus Medical Center, Rotterdam, The Netherlands

Sjoert A. H. Pegge
Dept. Of Radiology, Meander Medical Center, Amersfoort, The Netherlands

Cornelia M. Schaefer-Prokop
Dept. Of Radiology, Radboud University Medical Center, Nijmegen, The Netherlands
Dept. Of Radiology, Meander Medical Center, Amersfoort, The Netherlands

Jun Li, Mingshu Wu, Linan Dong, Lu Zhang, Hongli Shi and Shuqian Luo
School of Biomedical Engineering, Capital Medical University, Beijing, China

Huihui Yuan
Department of Rheumatology and Immunology, Capital Medical University, Beijing, China

Wei Yu
Key Laboratory of Optoelectronic Technology and System of the Education Ministry of China, Chongqing University, Chongqing, China
Engineering Research Center of Industrial Computed Tomography Nondestructive Testing of the Education Ministry of China, Chongqing University, Chongqing, China

Li Zeng
Key Laboratory of Optoelectronic Technology and System of the Education Ministry of China, Chongqing University, Chongqing, China
College of Mathematics and Statistics, Chongqing University, Chongqing, China

Astrid Velroyen, Irene Zanette, Jolanda Schwarz and Franz Pfeiffer
Chair of Biomedical Physics, Department of Physics (E17), Munich, Bavaria, Germany

Alexander Rack
European Synchrotron Radiation Facility, Grenoble, France

Christiane Tympner
Institute of Pathology, Ludwig-Maximilians-University Munich, Munich, Germany

Tanja Herrler
Department of General, Trauma, Hand, and Plastic Surgery, Ludwig-Maximilians-University Hospital Munich, Munich, Germany

Margarita Braunagel and Maximilian Reiser
Institute for Clinical Radiology, University Hospitals Munich, Munich, Germany

Martin Bech
Chair of Biomedical Physics, Department of Physics (E17), Munich, Bavaria, Germany
Medical Radiation Physics, Lund University, Lund, Sweden

Claudia Staab-Weijnitz
Institute for Clinical Radiology, University Hospitals Munich, Munich, Germany
Comprehensive Pneumology Center, University Hospital, Ludwig-Maximilians-University and Helmholtz Zentrum Munich, Munich, Germany

Fabian Bamberg and Mike Notohamiprodjo
Institute for Clinical Radiology, University Hospitals Munich, Munich, Germany
Department of Radiology, University Hospital Tuebingen, Tuebingen, Germany

Synho Do, Sarabjeet Singh, Mannudeep Kalra, Tom Brady, Ellie Shin and Homer Pien
Department of Radiology, Massachusetts General Hospital and Harvard Medical School, Boston, Massachusetts, United States of America

William Clem Karl
Department of Electrical and Computer Engineering, Boston University, Boston, Massachusetts, United States of America

Jie Huo, Xianfeng Zhu, Xuemin Wang and Gang Wang
Department of Biomedical Engineering, Tianjin University, Tianjin, China

Yang Dong, Zhiyong Yuan and Ping Wang
Department of Radiation Oncology, Tianjin Cancer Hospital, Tianjin, China

Xin-Hua Hu
Department of Physics, East Carolina University, Greenville, North Carolina, United States of America

Yuanming Feng
Department of Biomedical Engineering, Tianjin University, Tianjin, China
Department of Radiation Oncology, Tianjin Cancer Hospital, Tianjin, China

Department of Radiation Oncology, East Carolina University, Greenville, North Carolina, United States of America

Hong Zhang
Department of Heavy Ion Radiation Medicine, Institute of Modern Physics, Chinese Academy of Sciences, Lanzhou 730000, PR China

Bin Liu
Institute of Biomechanics and Medical Engineering, Lanzhou University, Lanzhou, 730000, PR China
Department of Heavy Ion Radiation Medicine, Institute of Modern Physics, Chinese Academy of Sciences, Lanzhou 730000, PR China

Baoping Zhang and Jizeng Wang
School of Civil Engineering and Mechanics, Lanzhou University, Lanzhou, 730000, PR China
Key Laboratory of Mechanics on Disaster and Environment in Western China, The Ministry of Education of China, Lanzhou University, 730000, PR China
Institute of Biomechanics and Medical Engineering, Lanzhou University, Lanzhou, 730000, PR China

Nobutake Yamamichi, Chihiro Minatsuki, Yu Takahashi, Chiemi Nakayama, Rie Matsuda, Mitsuhiro Fujishiro, Maki Konno-Shimizu, Shinya Kodashima, Satoshi Ono, Keiko Niimi, Satoshi Mochizuki, Yosuke Tsuji, Yoshiki Sakaguchi, Itsuko Asada-Hirayama, Chihiro Takeuchi, Seiichi Yakabi, Hikaru Kakimoto and Kazuhiko Koike
Department of Gastroenterology, Graduate School of Medicine, The University of Tokyo, Tokyo, Japan

Chigaya Hirano, Ryoichi Wada and Toru Mitsushima
Department of Gastroenterology, Kameda Medical Center Makuhari, Chiba, Japan

Jun Kato and Masao Ichinose
Second Department of Internal Medicine, Wakayama Medical University, Wakayama, Japan

Takeshi Shimamoto
Department of Gastroenterology, Graduate School of Medicine, The University of Tokyo, Tokyo, Japan
Department of Gastroenterology, Kameda Medical Center Makuhari, Chiba, Japan

Arun Chauhan and Chittaranjan Rout
Department of Biotechnology and Bioinformatics, Jaypee University of Information Technology, Solan, Himachal Pradesh, India

Devesh Chauhan
Department of Radiology, National Institute of TB and Respiratory Diseases, New Delhi, India

Index